Surgery - Procedures, Complications, and Results

nova
Medicine & Health
New York

Surgery - Procedures, Complications, and Results

Ovarian Cancer: The "Gynaecological Challenge" from Diagnostic Work-Up to Cytoreduction and Chemotherapy. Volume 1
Christos Iavazzo, Alexandros Fotiou, MD and John Spiliotis, PhD (Editors)
2023. ISBN: 979-8-88697-633-5 (Hardcover)
2023. ISBN: 979-8-89113-034-0 (eBook)

Nosocomial Infection in Abdominal Surgery
Andrés García Marín, MD, PhD and Jaime Ruiz-Tovar, MD, PhD (Editors)
2022. ISBN: 978-1-68507-603-0 (Softcover)
2022. ISBN: 978-1-68507-666-5 (eBook)

Neurointerventional Surgery: Current Status and Future Prospects
Xianli Lv, MD and Zhongxue Wu, MD (Editors)
2022. ISBN: 978-1-68507-863-8 (Hardcover)
2022. ISBN: 979-8-88697-062-3 (eBook)

A Clinical Guide to Thyroidectomies
Anand Mishra (Editor)
2022. ISBN: 978-1-68507-814-0 (Hardcover)
2022. ISBN: 979-8-88697-033-3 (eBook)

Tracheostomy: Indications, Safety and Outcomes
Amit Agrawal, MD (Editor)
2021. ISBN: 978-1-68507-188-2 (Hardcover)
2021. ISBN: 978-1-68507-263-6 (eBook)

Enhanced Recovery after Surgery (ERAS) in Bariatric Surgery
Jaime Ruiz-Tovar, MD, PhD (Editor)
2021. ISBN: 978-1-53619-976-5 (Hardcover)
2021. ISBN: 978-1-68507-026-7 (eBook)

More information about this series can be found at https://novapublishers.com/product-category/series/surgery-procedures-complications-and-results/

Christos Iavazzo
Alexandros Fotiou
and John Spiliotis
Editors

Ovarian Cancer

The "Gynaecological Challenge" from Diagnostic Work-Up to Cytoreduction and Chemotherapy

Volume 1

nova
Medicine & Health
New York

DOI: https://doi.org/10.52305/XRTT7855

NOTICE TO THE READER

Library of Congress Cataloging-in-Publication Data

Names: Iavazzo, Christos, editor. | Fotiou, Alexandros, editor. | Spiliotis, John D., editor.
Title: Ovarian cancer : the "gynaecological challenge" from diagnostic work-up to cytoreduction and chemotherapy / Christos Iavazzo (editor), Metaxa Memorial Cancer Hospital, Piraeus, Greece, Alexandros Fotiou, MD (editor), Metaxa Memorial Cancer Hospital, Piraeus, Greece, John Spiliotis, PhD (editor), Department of Surgical Oncology and HIPEC, Athens Medical Centre, Athens, Greece; Department of Surgical Oncology and HIPEC, European Interbalkan Medical Centre, Thessaloniki, Greece.
Description: New York : Nova Science Publishers, [2023]- | Series: Surgery - procedures, complications, and results | Includes bibliographical references and index. |
Identifiers: LCCN 2023030101 (print) | LCCN 2023030102 (ebook) | ISBN 9798886976335 (volume 1 : hardcover) | ISBN 9798891130340 (volume 1 : adobe pdf)
Subjects: LCSH: Ovaries--Cancer. | Ovaries--Cancer--Diagnosis. | Ovaries--Cancer--Treatment.
Classification: LCC RC280.O8 O92765 2023 (print) | LCC RC280.O8 (ebook) | DDC 616.99/465--dc23/eng/20230720
LC record available at https://lccn.loc.gov/2023030101
LC ebook record available at https://lccn.loc.gov/2023030102

Published by Nova Science Publishers, Inc. † New York

Contents

Preface

We are proud to present our book entitled: "Ovarian Cancer: The "Gynaecological Challenge" from diagnostic work-up to cytoreduction and chemotherapy".

Ovarian cancer is one of the deadliest gynaecological cancers. In most cases, it is detected as an advanced tumor, since early diagnosis is challenging for most forms of the disease. Surgery and platinum-based compounds have been the mainstay of therapy for many years. The prognosis for ovarian cancer depends on the type of surgery and on the response to chemotherapy. Other regimens have little effect if the disease does not respond to platinum. However, several new therapies are emerging including bevacizumab and PARP-inhibitors, among others.

This book provides a detailed body of information important to an understanding of the clinical aspects and management of such a challenging disease. The authors strive to provide the physician with insights and illustrations as well as useful tips and tricks for the everyday clinical practice.

Several world-known experts in the field participated in this fruitful effort offering their knowledge and everyday experience, as well as valuable and original photos from their personal archives as well as the most recent and up-to-date guidelines in the field.

In this book, we evaluate all the challenging pathways from the moment of diagnosis to the surgical and medical therapies. The pathogenesis, the variation of the morphological types and the problems in differential diagnosis are also discussed.

Moreover, we provide an overview of recent attempts to improve the diagnosis and prognosis of ovarian cancer as well as a discussion of fertility sparing alternatives and minimal invasive (laparoscopic and robotic) approaches. All the new diagnostic and therapeutic strategies that lay out the foundation for these improvements are presented. Areas of future research are also discussed, supported by a wealth of up-to-date referenced material.

The book is written at a level appropriate for both medical students, physicians as well as gynaecological oncologists, pathologists, and medical oncologists.

We hope you find this book both educational and a trusted reference as you care for your patient achieving a long "shelf life" and becoming an everyday tool of diagnosis and management.

Dr. Christos Iavazzo, Metaxa Memorial Cancer Hospital, Greece
Dr. Alexandros Fotiou, Metaxa Memorial Cancer Hospital, Greece
Dr. John Spiliotis, Athens Medical Centre, Greece
(Editors)

Chapter 1

Ovarian Cancer Pathology and Surgery, Historical Pearls from the Pioneering Greeks and the General Term Gynecologic Cancer to Modern Histopathology and Ovarian Malignancy

G. Tsoucalas[1,*], MD, PhD
Christos Iavazzo[2], MD, PhD
and M. Karamanou[3], MD, PhD

[1]Anatomy Department, Democritus University of Thrace, Alexandroupoli, Greece
[2]Gynecologic Oncology Department, Metaxa Cancer Hospital of Piraeus, Piraeus, Greece
[3]History of Medicine and Medical Deontology, Medical School of University of Crete, Heraklion, Greece

Introduction

Ovarian cancer constitutes one of the most frequently encountered cancers among female patients worldwide. Some researchers say it is the 6th fatal malignancy. For someone to comprehend such a significant pathological entity, an in-depth knowledge of all its aspects is fundamental. Medical history provides an inquiry from the point of origin in the past, when a discovery was made, up to modern times, when knowledge is perfected or at least is evolved and matured. This chapter records and presents the history of ovarian cancer, progress in the field, a summary of drugs, tools and innovative ideas from the Hellenic philosophy in antiquity until today.

During antiquity, in the Hellenic peninsula and colonies, ancient Greek medico-philosophers and physicians tried to explain cancer in a logical way. But how to rationalize such a disease that presents itself with both fatality and vanity upon confrontation. In the 5th century BC, Hippocrates (460-377 BC) and his pupils provided a rational and systemic basis to medical science a rational and systemic basis, an influential legacy of the Hippocratic approach, introducing the theory of the four humors to explain all diseases in a pathophysiological manner. According to the humoral doctrine, disease was determined as a disturbance affecting the whole person through some imbalance in the four bodily fluids, or

* Corresponding Author's Email: gregorytsoucalas@yahoo.gr.

In: Ovarian Cancer
Editors: Christos Iavazzo, Alexandros Fotiou and John Spiliotis
ISBN: 979-8-88697-633-5

humors, of blood, phlegm, yellow bile, and black bile. Thus, health was defined as a balance between the body fluids (eukrasia) and external environment. If this balance was to be disturbed, the result was the disease itself (dyskrasia). Based mainly on humoral theory, ancient Greek physicians developed the black bile theory of cancer, stating that an excess of the black bile in the body could provoke malignancy. It was the Hippocratic Corpus in which the terms "karkinos" (cancer) and "karkinoma" were coined, referring to the shape of a crab. The terms "phumata," "theria," "elkoi," and "oidemata" all described the neoplastic nature of tumors. Tumors thus arose from a localised inflammation when flux caused an overconcentration of the black bile from the veins into the fleshy or parenchymal components of the body part, resulting in "karkinoma apertus," the superficial type and "karkinoma occlusus," the in-depth type of cancer. All those terms described a non-healing swelling or ulceration of a probable malignant origin. Hippocrates also introduced the term "scirrhus" to describe hard-in-substance tumorous lesions [1-3].

The Hellenic concept to clash with cancer was to operate superficial types like breast or manipulate into the cavities that is in the mouth, ear, nose, vagina and rectum. A palliative approach based mainly on herbal and mineral drugs was to follow to alleviate cancerous symptoms. Supportive measures had also been proposed to strengthen the immune system and provide a rich nourishment diet, as malignant cachexia which affected the whole body, was prevalent at the time. Postmortem examination of the human body was strictly prohibited due to social and religion reasons, instating the detailed topographic anatomy and the physiology of the internal organs somewhere in the terra incognita. Surgical intervention was limited to operations with minor (or less as possible) amputations to remove or cauterize the formations when tumors developed. A plethora of surgical tools had been manufactured by the ingenious Greek metalworkers and all were at the surgeon's disposal alongside with gauzes, compresses, bandages, and drugs (powders, liquids, ointments, creams etc). Namely, Dioptras, hedrodiastoleus, mochliskos, ostagra, kauterion, motos moloubus, catheters, metrechytes, agkistra, tricholabis, embryoulkos, staphylagra, osteotomes, scalpels, psalis, spathomele, cyathiscomele, had been in use for operations" [4-5] all placed harmonically inside the surgeon's medical bag, arranged in the most appropriate way, following a methodical layout, as physicians cannot keep everything in mind, as Hippocrates stated [6]. For extensive operations, Hippocrates introduced the famous Thessaly's endemic plant, mandrake, as a general anaesthetic (it contains scopolamine), combined with morus alba and hedera, known sedatives of the era. A strict protocol of antisepsis was to be followed, performed by multiple rinses of clean boiled rainwater, firewater, salt, hot sea water (hypertonic serum), copper, tar (contains carbolic acid), resin, perfumes (myrrha, boswellia, thymus, cinnamomum, salvia, pinus, cypressus sempervirens, artemisia absinthium, aloe), milk and fire (spirit?). For less invasive operations, in the case of minor or more superficial tumors, "only a careful superficial excision and cauterization should be performed, and the wounds should be dusted with Black Hellebore plant when rot, cleaned afterwards with copper flower (an oxide) and poured with honey" to finish the therapeutic approach [2]. Dyspnoea (mostly caused by the phlegm), could sometimes have been severe, and an acute death could have occurred during an operation, or due to the tumor's volume. In a more daring thought, to avoid such an incident, or to help the patient undertake the surgical interventions needed, Hippocrates introduced the endotracheal intubation, by using a thin pliable stannum (tin) tube through the larynx, "for the lung to attract pneuma" (pneuma ≈ air = the vital force of the soul) [2, 7]. All were there, a Greek perspective, surgical tools, palliative drugs, antiseptics and tube ventilation. The enemy was known, understood and fatal. Its types described. Breasts, nose, ear, rectum, skin, internal organs, urinary and gynecologically. Although a notorious entity, described by various Greek scholars, surprisingly, gynecological cancer takes up little space in the treatises of ancient Greek physicians. Nonetheless, the term "gynecologic" in most works included all types - cervical, ovarian, uterine, vaginal, vulvar and fallopian, as physiology, cell, tissues and pathology were blurred at the time. Meanwhile, the term uterine in the writings of most scholars also meant gynecological and it included malignancies of the area [8].

The Hippocratics, famous for their observation and record skills, recognized both general and local pathological symptoms of gynecological malignancy. The first included cessation of menstruation, bitter taste, anorexia, pain (mild to severe), a hemorrhagic predisposition, cachexia and emaciation. Then later, the appearance of vaginal bleeding, oedema, inflammation, and ulceration. Therapeutically, Hippocrates (460-377 AD) recommended a conservative approach, applying an intravaginal enema, made of pumpkin crumb and honeycomb mixed with water. The patient was also regularly receiving laxatives and bloodletting phlebotomies for the extraction of the bad humors (mainly black bile) to re-balance the homeostasis of the organism, while a daily body examination was to follow. Repeated daily fumigations of the vagina, with special heated device containing dried garlic, water and seal oil was in order. In the case when the uterus felt softer in palpation, fumigations with fennel roots were applied for five or six days. For a holistic and personalized approach, every female patient was monitored, and her diet was specific. In advanced cancer stages, Hippocrates suggested that the physician should proceed with a progressive opening of the "mouth" (orifice) of the uterus with numbered waxes, and when the expansion permitted, pessaries made from rods of pine covered with oil, were to be placed as deep as it could. Having an innovative type of thinking, the Hippocrates suggested a hollow lead pessary to be inserted in the cavity, in attempt to create an artificial vaginal opening and to prevent the formation of adhesions. Pain palliation, care in the ulcerated area, and antiseptic were used. Hippocrates wrongfully believed that gynecological cancer was a disease of the elderly, while on the other hand realized the importance of the vascular system for the circulation of "malignant matter" (black bile). Surgical intervention was to be avoided, preserved only in small part amputations of the tumorous mass and bleeding-prevention cauterizations during the process of the lead pessary insertion. This concept dominated medical thought and for the following centuries endured as a standard-setting example of medical practice [8-9].

Aristotle (384-322 BC), the famous Greek philosopher and scientist was among the few who added some stones in the wall of gynecological cancer history after Hippocrates. In his masterpiece the "History of Animals," described the first combined surgical removal of ovaries and uterus (hysterectomy) on animals. Although the reason for this operation was not a malignancy, Aristotle made a noteworthy observation, noting that the removal of the ovaries from the pigs had decreased their sexual appetite. Comparative anatomy and animals' dissections provided at least some knowledge to carry out a difficult for the era surgical operation, allowing us to suppose that ancient Greek physicians had probably tried to perform removal of the uterus in an attempt to cure gynecologic carcinomas. Adequate evidence to support this hypothesis may be found in the centuries that followed [10].

Eons later, the distinguished Roman encyclopaedist Celsus (25 BC-50 AD) in his work "De Medicina" devoted a whole chapter on uterine cancer. Celsus writings were forgotten for a while, being rediscovered during the Renaissance and highly appreciated by physicians for their medical content. He mentioned, "females are subject to a malignant disease of the womb...Sometimes this affection deprives the patient of all sensibility, in the same manner as if she falls in epilepsia. Yet with a difference, neither the eyes are turned nor does foam flow from the mouth...there is only a profound sleep." Celsus described the anterior groin swelling, the local oedema due to the vein compression, and probably he was the first to recognize nodal metastases. To confront it he had proposed bloodletting, cataplasms, frictions and a diet free of wine, following the example of Hippocrates. He had proposed "a cerate of rose oil, or fresh hog's lard and the whites of eggs may be mixed together and applied," while in the case when "the womb is in pain it ought to be fumigated with Sulphur." Still the possibility of surgical intervention was vague [11].

Soranus of Ephesus (98-138 AD), the magnificent Greek physician and gynaecologist who practiced in Rome, left us a palatial treatise on obstetrics and gynaecology. His great skills in surgical anatomy gave us a vivid delineation of the uterus, "the uterus presents sometimes without ulceration sometimes with ulceration. In this case we may experience pains, sharp pains in the kidney, in the vertebrae, in umbilicus. The evolution of the disease is malignant." He was the first who documented hysterectomy, strengthening the hypothesis that from the era of Aristotle such an operation was probably possible. Soranus believed that the "uterus should not be considered as an essential organ for life, not only because it is usually prolapsed but, in some cases, it can even be cut, without death to occur... if the entire uterus is bruised (blackened), we must cut it off entirely, not only because some previously mentioned writers noticed that resection is harmless, but also because it has ceased to be a vital organ. In the case of ulcer (cancerous) from continuous prolapse and the creation of adhesion to the labia..., more preferably and most secure is to spare the uterus something from the labia as the separation cannot be accurate...in the case of a more local bruise, uterus could be excised partially." Soranus, although a precursor in operative gynecology, was fortunate as already advanced surgical instruments, such as vaginal endoscopes (speculum-dioptras) and "kauteria" (cautery), antiseptic protocols and sedatives as well as herbal drugs were at his disposal. This was the era when surgical removal of the ovaries due to cancer originated [4, 12-13].

Galen (ca. 130-210 AD), the greatest medical authority of antiquity after Hippocrates. Although he was a great anatomist, establishing his dogma in anatomy for more than 15 centuries, he had surprisingly followed and supported the non-invasive approach of the Hippocratic school on uterine cancer. In his opinion a surgical ablation could lead to death. He had described scleroma of the uterus as a hard tumor which originated from phlegmon of the organ and which might be of long duration. Concerning the diagnosis of uterine cancer after a clinical examination, Galen wrote that "when the mouth of the womb is closed, and the neck is at the same time hard to the touch, this points to the uterus being diseased." He had also noted that the affected women were suffering from extreme pain reflecting towards mouth cavity and lower extremities [8, 14]. Aretaeus of Cappadocia (ca. 2nd-3rd century AD) in his book "On the causes and symptoms of acute and chronic diseases," in the chapter entitled "On uterine affections," notably mentioned the predisposition of uterus to malignancy "the womb of the female…is conductive to many bad diseases," recognizing the high prevalence of this type of cancer among the female population. He classified the disease into two types, the non-ulcerated and the ulcerated one, with the latter being worse in prognosis. He had masterfully recorded a vivid description, "the purulent discharge is large ...the lips of the ulcer are harsh and rough, there is certain offensive ichor, and the pain is severe. The ulcer corrodes the uterus and sometimes a loose fleshy substance protrudes which does not cicatrize for a long time but occasions death... the veins in the uterus become swollen with tension of the surrounding parts."

Ovaries were known since the era of classical Greece, yet, malignancies on the area through Hellenistic and Roman periods was veiled by the term "uterine" [15-16].

Late Eastern Roman Empire (Byzantium) notions on uterine cancer were drawn directly from ancient Greek and Greco-Roman medical authorities. Uterine cancer was an incurable disease, and "black bile" is the main reason. Byzantine physicians pointed out various concepts of palliative treatment, or at least most of them [17]. Oribasius (ca. 325-403 AD) of Pergamus, was among those scholars who did not make any original contribution in the field of medicine. However, his books and the Medical Collections (Iatrikai Synagogai) are of great importance, as they contain numerous extracts from earlier and contemporary medical writers, whose works could have perished forever. The work of Oribasius contains a few facts on uterine cancer. He had pointed out the painful nature of the disease and mentioned its origin from polyps and fibroids, identifying the tissue necrosis of uterine cancer. For him, gynecological cancer was incurable, while surgery could be fatal. Nonetheless, he had advocated early diagnosis and surgical excision of all endometrial tumors and opium pessaries to alleviate pain [18].

Aetius of Amida (ca. 502-575 AD) was the writer of a medical encyclopedia - the "Tetrabiblon" or "Libri Medicinales," in 16 books. The sixteenth book of Aetius work is considered the epitome of gynecological knowledge of the Greco-Roman world, while a chapter is devoted to uterine cancer. His description includes all types of cancers in the area, "when there is no ulceration, the tumor found round the os uteri is hard and resistant to the touch, uneven, prominent, feculent in color, red or livid; sharp pains are felt in the groins, belly, vulva, and loins, and these are increased by manual examination and by various medications. Should the cancer be an ulcerated one, in addition to pain, hardness, and swelling, we find ulcers spreading and irregular, and for the most part foul, prominent, and white in color; some, however, appear feculent, livid, red and bloody." Aetius was among those who believed malignancies of the female genital would be incurable, painful and occasionally with hemorrhage which could be worsened soon after a surgical intervention. He had suggested various drugs to alleviate both pain and hemorrhage, such as baths of fenugreek and mallow, and cataplasms of a similar kind. Paul of Aegina (ca. 625-690 AD), a century later, composed his medical encyclopedia in seven books, named "Medical Compendium." He was also in favor of conservative and palliative treatment, noting that it was preferable to the surgeon to avoid the removal of the uterine cancer as there was a risk that it would grow worse. This fact probably means that he had understood the high risk of cancer cells spreading through adjacent tissues and nearby blood vessels. He recommended surgery only in cases of uterine abscesses that do not respond to medication and may provoke a fast cachexia-sepsis of the female patient [19].

None of the great Byzantine surgeons mentioned ovaries as an individual entity during cancer confrontation. All but the supreme Cleopatra Metrodora (ca. 7th century AD), a unique example of a highly educated woman physician who lived most probably around the seventh century AD, or according to some, was a contemporary of Soranus of Ephesus. Among her great number of works, "On the Uterus, Abdomen and Kidneys" contains a chapter on uterine cancer. Cleopatra Metrodora also sustained that it was a fatal and painful disease. However, he had surprisingly declared that it is of the patient's interest to have the surgical removal of the tumor. Able to perform vaginal operations or combined hysterectomies, he had suggested that simultaneously the surgeon should surgically reconstruct the vagina and the labia and if needed to insert a tube-pesso in order for the vagina to preserve an opening. She was also fond of the application of a tuber porridge mixed with goose fat, or a mixture of cinnamon, cob and ginger in a form of intravaginal pessary to alleviate pain and delay ulceration [20].

Theophanes Nonnus (ca. 10th century AD), originally Theophanes Chrysobalantes, a famous Byzantine physician, composed a synopsis known simply as "Synopsis" or "Epitome." He had added nothing new, noting for the treatment of uterine cancer, that ointments and intravaginal pessaries based on mixtures of honey, wax, eggs, fat, bone marrow of several animals and birds, sheep wool, sea sponge and oxymeli (Greek: a mixture of aged sweet wines, honey=meli, raisins and fig extract) should be used to confront gynecological cancer [21]. Prominent Byzantine physicians emerged during the era of the Late Eastern Roman Empire in the lands of the Hellenic peninsula and the areas surrounding Aegean and Eastern Mediterranean seas. By compiling and refining the Hippocratic-Galenic scientific ideas they were mostly based on the knowledge acquired from their predecessors, adding only some of their own observations and clinical experience. Their work through translations and copying in monastic libraries survived the Middle Ages and contributed to the foundation of our current concepts of disease, while the Arabs soon recognized their significant role and adopted them all [17].

The contribution of Byzantine physicians to gynecological oncology was limited because of the restrictions imposed on their practice by the Church and social beliefs. The Arabs during the Late Eastern Roman Empire, through commercial and social channels, contacted scholars who were acquainted with medical knowledge of the past and soon perceived the weighty role of the ancient Greeks. Greco-Roman medicine was introduced to the Arabic world by Abu Bakr Mohammad Ibn Zakariya Razi, known in the west as Rhazes (865 to 925 AD), who translated the writings of Hippocrates and Galen. A strong supporter of the "Theory of the Four Humors," he was convinced not only that the purging of bad humors by venesection and purgatives might be curative, but also that bloodletting might be used as a preventive measure as blood itself, containing the causative material of cancer. For gynecological cancer, he noted hematuria, and supported that malignancies could not be cured by surgery and that sometimes surgery was inferior to treatment with medicinal substances, introducing the idea of chemotherapy. He is known to have often tested his chemicals in animals. Hot oil, mercurial ointments, arsenic, carbonate of lead, chicory, opium were used in cases when ulcers had been appearing in the vaginal area. Abu Marwan ibn Zuhr (1073-1162 AD), or Latinized Avenzoar was among those who practiced the dissection of animals and postmortem autopsy examinations of his patients for medical teaching according to Islamic laws. For him, anatomy was fundamental. Although he had described a case of uterine cancer (akila, gangrene), he did not perform a pelvic examination as he believed that it was a taboo, condemned by religion. Avenzoar proposed drugs and the woman died by massive bleeding. Ali Ibn al-Abbas al-Majusi (949-982 AD), Latinized as Haly Abbas Ahwazi, the author of "Complete Book of the Medical Art" prescribed black myrobalan, dodder, common polypody, French lavender, nafti salt and black hellebore that should all be pulverized, pasted and then formed into a pill, introducing a per os variant. After the Islamic Empire came to an end in 1258 when the Mongols occupied Baghdad, a plethora of Arabic and Greek writings were translated into Latin by monks in monasteries and were distributed in Christian Europe [22].

The fall of the Western Roman Empire with the Church having shed the veil of conservatism slowed down the scientific evolution. However, progressively the point of progress in medical achievements shifted towards the West mainly because the conviction of importance of human autopsy weakened over time. The first medical school of Salerno, the combined introduction of Arabic and ancient Greek medicine, the Hippocratic concept of medical ethics and the Galenic anatomic dogma, the first public dissections by Mondino de Luzzi (ca 1270-1326 AD), the first Anatomy laboratory under Jacques Dubois (1478-1555 AD) in Paris and the great new society of anatomist with Andreas Vesalius (1514-1564 AD) as the greatest, boosted knowledge and surgical skills. Joseph-Claude-Anthelme Récamier (1774-1852) was credited for the first successful vaginal hysterectomy for cancer. The time of ovaries to emerge to the spotlight of the operating table was closer than ever before [18].

German physician Johannes Schenck von Grafenberg (1530-1598 AD) was the first modern scholar to report an ovarian malignancy in 1595. Jan Baptist van De Lamzweerde (ca 17th century) reported ovarian cysts in 1686, while Justus Theodor Schorkopff (ca 17th century) at the same period gave us the first work entirely dedicated to ovarian cysts, "De hydrope ovarii muliebris" in 1685 [23]. Scottish anatomist and obstetrician William Hunter (1718-1783) was the first to propose the removal of the ovarian cyst but did not perform it. German surgeon Johann CA Theden (1714-1797 AD) in 1771, Samuel Hartman d 'Escher in 1807 and Ameri can physician and pioneer surgeon Ephraim McDowell (1771-1830 AD) in 1809 performed surgical removal of ovarian cysts and tumors. McDowell paved the way and Robert Lawson Tait (1845-1899 AD) who was a pioneer in pelvic and abdominal surgery became one of the most famous ovariotomists of the 19th century. French surgeon Jacques Mathieu Delpech (1777-1832 AD) was the first to introduce the hypothesis that malignant change in benign ovarian cysts may occur. Austrian gynecologist Ernst Wertheim (1864-1920 AD), a pioneer in the surgical treatment of cervical cancer in his treatise "The extended abdominal operation for carcinoma uteri," published in 1912, had proposed a hysterectomy with removal of the ovaries. American obstetrician and gynecologist Joe Vincent Meigs (1892-1963 AD) and American physician John W. Cass in 1937 documented the association of hydrothorax, ascites, and ovarian tumor commonly seen in association with ovarian fibromas (its presence also noted in ovarian cancer). Similar research was previously documented by gynecologists Otto Spiegelberg (1830-1881 AD) from Germany and Charles James Cullingworth (1841-1908 AD) from England [24].

Meigs of Boston is widely credited with the original description of the surgical approach to ovarian cancer in his 1934 landmark treatise "Tumors of the Female Pelvic Organs." Meigs focused his career on gynecologic cancer, including malignant tumors of the ovary, despite his early observation that "the outlook for patients with this disease is hopeless." In the third chapter of his book, he had described a consecutive series of 67 women diagnosed with "solid carcinomas" and "malignant papillary cystadenomas." As chemotherapy had not been yet developed, he stated that surgical removal was extremely important, while the effects of X-ray application treatment had mixed results. By 1961, Meigs had refined his surgical technique, advocating for hysterectomy and bilateral salpingooophorectomy in the cases when childbearing was not of importance for the female patient. Meigs did not appreciate the minimally invasive peritoneoscope in helping to determine the diagnosis and resectability of advanced ovarian cancer, as relatively low-resolution imaging in a surface-spreading disease with wide variation in the amount and location of intraperitoneal dissemination could be obvious only after a direct inspection. His opinion has led to the reintroduction of preoperative laparoscopy. Despite intraoperative limitations for the surgeon in being unable to manually palpate and explore the abdomen, current data support the efficacy of laparoscopic or robotic interval cytoreductive surgery. Indeed, in the decades which followed and despite the original justified reverse, the value of the peritoneoscope in advanced ovarian cancer had increased.

Meigs understood that ovaries were radio-resistant and for the years to come, he insisted on surgical removal. He had noted an operative mortality rate of 1.7%, an incidence of fistulae of 9%, and a 5-year survival rate for Stage I cervical carcinoma of 74%. Meigs gained his place in history with namely the "Meigs' radical hysterectomy," an extended Wertheim radical hysterectomy with pelvic lymphadenectomy [25].

Outstanding German gynaecologists Christian Gerhard Leopold (1846-1911) and Friedrich Ernst Ktukenberg (1871-1946) definite a relationship between gastric and breast cancer and ovarian malignancy [24]. Surprisingly, the ovary was found to be a striking exception to Virchow's dictum which held that organs which were frequently the point of origin for primary cancer to be seldom involved in a secondary malignancy and vice versa [26]. Robert Meyer in 1930 was the first to write a review on ovarian cancer. He had analyzed several series of reported cases and determined that carcinoma of the ovaries could present itself as a solid or cystic structure with the latter being more common. He also noted that almost 15% of all ovarian tumors were cancerous, while 50% of those were bilateral. The second important review was conducted by Stanley Way in 1951, when he studied cases from 1930 and 1940, and quoted an incidence of 20-28% of all reported malignant tumors in females. In 1983, DL Creasman and WT Clarke-Pearson estimated in their analyses that one out of every nine females in the USA would die from ovarian malignancy. Now the ovary was exactly at the center of a fatal disease, tumors of which were needed to be classified in order to be confronted in the best way possible [24].

German gynecologist Hermann Johannes Pfannenstiel (1862-1909) introduced a classification of ovarian tumors in 1898 which was the accepted global standard until the 1920s. Robert Meyer was the one who amended his classification in 1915 and went on to describe granulosa cell tumors, arrhenoblastoma and dysgerminoma. HC Taylor in 1929 under the terms of pathology defined three groups of ovarian cancer: i) those in which well-differentiated columnar epithelium was present; ii) tumors with glandular or papillary structure and actively malignant; and iii) tumors showing undifferentiated epithelial cells with marked nuclear changes and little or no glandular or papillary structure. In 1930, Robert Meyer proposed his classification based on primary cystic ovarian carcinomas, i) carcinoma arising in pseudomucinous cystadenoma; ii) carcinoma arising in serous cystadenoma; and iii) carcinoma arising in dermoid cysts. In the late 1970s, the World Health Organization classification of ovarian tumors became widely accepted, being present in various modified versions by many authors. In the late 1980s, the International Federation of Gynaecology and Obstetrics was used as the global classification, submitted in updates. The classification was there, the pathology was known but the treatment was under study [24].

Staging the disease was fundamental for the treatment. The staging of ovarian cancer was based on the findings during surgical exploration combined with histological grade and the type of tumor. For the proper treatment, an interdisciplinary team of expertise physicians had been proposed, including the gynecologist, pathologist, chemotherapist, and radiation expert. RW Rundles and WB Burton in 1952 were the first to report the use of alkylating agents in patients with advanced ovarian cancer and reported a favorable response in about 30% of the cases. The door of chemotherapy in modern medicine opened once more after the old Arabian concept [24]. It was in 1961 when the pioneer in medical oncology, Ezra M Greenspan (1919-2004 AD),introduced a combination of methotrexate with thiotepa [27], while in 1976 Eve Wiltshaw (1927-2008 AD) and T Kroner demonstrated the activity of cisplatin against epithelial ovarian cancer [28]. JP Smith and F Rudedge in 1975 and WT Creasman and his colleagues in 1979 suggested a triple therapy treatment. The first vincristine, actinomycin-D and cyclophosphamide, while the later methotrexate, actinomycin-D, and cyclophosphamide. Chemotherapy had been found to present various disagreeable side effects including depression of the hematological system, gastrointestinal upset, severe nephrotoxicity and alopecia and long-term development of myeloblastic leukaemia. Skepticism arose but chemotherapy became a main modality of treatment, usually combined with surgical removal of the ovary affected. FA Pemberton in 1940 was the first after Meigs to add an innovative surgical maneuver when he advised an omenectomy, whether or not gross metastases can be seen, for 2 reasons. Omentum is so often affected by metastatic cells and moreover, it may be a source of recurrence in a later period. In 1971, Harrith M. Hasson pioneered an open laparoscopy for direct visualization and dissection of the tissues, an option which remained the favorite entry method for laparoscopic surgeons in the next decades. In 1973, CM Bagley and his colleagues proposed laparoscopy in the initial staging. To surgery and chemotherapy, emerged a third treatment variant, radiotherapy. During the 1950s, external radiation of the pelvis and abdomen was used as a treatment after surgery. However, studies reported that radiation was effective only when the ovarian tumor was properly debulked. The first use of radioisotopes, a novel modality in the ovarian carcinoma's confrontation was reported by JH Muller in 1945 who used radioactive zinc as palliative therapy. A decade later, two great virologists, Scottish Alick Isaacs (1921-1967) and Swiss Jean Lindenmann (1924-2015) thought that immunotherapy could play a synergistic role with alkylating agent therapy and in 1957, introduced the use of Interferon [24].

In the 21st century, taxanes as chemotherapy agents entered ovarian oncology. Despite measured improvement in survival, little additional progress has been made with conventional cytotoxic agents. Intraperitoneal therapy in standard management was introduced with mixed results. In addition, several ways of administration improvement were under study, including patient eligibility, proper catheter management, and determination of the optimal infusate. A significant advantage in progression-free and overall survival with a combination of intravenous paclitaxel and intraperitoneal cisplatin and paclitaxel was introduced. A metronomic dose studied in ovarian cancer proved to have some effect in smaller volume tumors [29]. British surgeon Thomas Spencer Wells (1818-1897) proposed in 1873 the hypothesis that ovarian cancer developed from cells on the surface of the ovary. For more than a century, physicians assumed this concept as true. However, they almost never found early-stage cancers, or even precursor lesions, that were confined to the ovary. In 1999, Louis Dubeau proposed a credible alternative innovative hypothesis. He had pointed out that ovarian tumor cells shared characteristics with healthy cells from the fallopian tubes and endometrium. He concluded that ovarian cancer therefore may arise from those tissues. Nowadays, it is widely accepted that most, if not all the most common types of ovarian cancer (high-grade serous ovarian carcinoma), arise in one of the two fallopian tubes that transport eggs from the ovaries to the uterus. According to scientists, this creates an opportunity for ovarian cancer prevention with, for example, a prophylactic removal of the tubes which may alter future cancer especially in women with a predisposition.

Conclusion

Despite the progress of medical science, ovarian cancer remains a silent killer, holding many secrets which need to be unveiled [30].

References

[1] Retief FP, Cilliers L. Tumours and cancers in Graeco-Roman times. *S Afr Med J* 2001;91: 344-348.

[2] Hippocrates. De locis in homine & De mulierum affectibus i-iii & De natura muliebri & De fracturis & De articulis & De medico & De Visu De morbis i-iii (ed. É. Littré). *Oeuvres complètes d'Hippocrate* [Hippocrates of places in man & of women's affections i-iii & of woman's nature & of fractures & of joints & of physician & of sight of diseases i-iii (ed. É. Littré). *Complete Works of Hippocrates*]. Paris, Baillière; 1849-1853 (repr. Amsterdam: Hakkert, 1962).

[3] Weiss L. Early concepts of cancer. *Cancer Metastasis Rev* 2000;19: 205-217.

[4] Milne JS. *Surgical instruments in Greek and Roman times.* Oxford, USA: Clarendon Press; 1907.

[5] Tsoucalas G, Sgantzos M, Androutsos G. Hippocrates: Principles on Abdominal Surgery in Ancient Greece During the Fifth Century BC. *Surg Innov* 2016;23: 212-213.

[6] Tsoucalas G, Kousoulis, AA Tsoukalas I, Androutsos G. The earliest mention of a black bag. *Scand J Primary Health Care* 2011;29: 196-197.

[7] Actuarius J. Opera, *Methodi Medendi* (*Méthodes Thérapeutiques*) [*Methods of Healing* (*Therapeutic Methods*)], Lib. vi. Paris: Bernard Turrisan; 1556.

[8] Tsoucalas G, Karamanou M, Sgantzos M, Deligeoroglou E, Androutsos G. Uterine cancer in the writings of ancient Greek physicians. *J BUON* 2015;20(5): 1382-1385.

[9] Kouzis A. *Cancer among ancient Greek physicians.* Athens: Konstantinidis; 1902 [in Greek].

[10] Aristotle. *History of the Animals*. Cresswell R. (transl) London: Bell; 1883.

[11] Celsus. *On Medicine in eight books*. Greive J (transl) London: Chidley; 1837.

[12] Karamanou M, Tsoucalas G, Creatsas G, Androutsos G. The effect of Soranus of Ephesus (98-138) on the work of midwives. *Women Birth* 2013;26: 226-228.

[13] Soranus. *On women diseases*. Athens: Kaktos; 1996 [in Greek].

[14] Galen. Œuvres médicales choisis. Daremberg C (transl) Paris: Gallimard; 1994.

[15] Tsoucalas G, Karamanou M, Laïos K, Androutsos G. Aretaeus of Cappadocia and the first accurate description of uterine carcinoma. *J BUON* 2013;18: 805-807.

[16] Aretaeus of Cappadocia. *On the causes and signs of acute and chronic disease*. Reynolds TF (transl) London: Pichering; 1837.

[17] Karamanou M, Tsoucalas G, Laios K, Deligeoroglou E, Agapitos E, Androutsos G. Uterine cancer in the writings of Byzantine physicians. *J BUON* 2015;20(6): 1645-1648.

[18] Buck AH. *The growth of medicine*. New Haven: Yale University Press; 1917.

[19] Adams F. *The Seven Books of Paulus Aegineta*. London: Sydenham Society; 1844-1857.

[20] Tsoucalas G, Karamanou M, Androutsos G. Metrodora, an Innovative Gynecologist, Midwife, and Surgeon. *Surg Innov* 2013;20: 648-649.

[21] Sonderkamp JAM. Theophanes Nonnus: Medicine in the Circle of Constantine Porphyrogenitus. *Dumbarton Oaks Papers* 38. Symposium on Byzantine Medicine, 1984.

[22] Hajdu SI. Pathfinders in oncology from ancient times to the end of the Middle Ages. *Cancer* 2016;122(11): 1638-1646.

[23] Cianfrani T. *A Short History of Obstetrics and Gynecology*. Springfield Illinois: C. C. Thomas; 1960.

[24] O'Dowd MJ, Phillipp EE. *The history of obstetrics and gynaecology.* New York: Informa Healthcare; 2011.

[25] Schorge JO, Bregar AJ, Durfee J, Berkowitz RS. Meigs to modern times: The evolution of debulking surgery in advanced ovarian cancer. *Gynecol Oncol* 2018;149(3): 447-454.

[26] Novak E. *Gynecological and Obstetrical Pathology With Clinical and Endocrine Relations*, 2nd edn. Philadelphia, London: W. B. Saunders; 1947.

[27] Greenspan EM. Thiotepa and methotrexate chemotherapy of advanced ovarian carcinoma. *Mount Sinai J Med* 1968;35: 52-67.

[28] Wiltshaw E, Kroner T. Phase II study of cis-dichlorodiaminepla tinum (II) (NSC-119875) in advanced adenocarcinoma of the ovary. *Cancer Treatment Reports* 1976;60: 55-60.

[29] Coleman RL, Sood AK. Historical progress in the initial management of ovarian cancer: intraperitoneal chemotherapy. *Curr Oncol Rep* 2006;8(6): 455-464.

[30] DeWeerdt S. The origins of ovarian cancer. *Nature* 2021;600(7889): S42-S44.

Chapter 2

Ovarian Cancer Screening

Aleksandra Gentry-Maharaj*,[1,2] and Aarti Sharma[3]

[1]Medical Research Council Clinical Trials Unit at UCL, Institute of Clinical Trials and Methodology, University College London, London, UK
[2]Department of Women's Cancer, EGA Institute for Women's Health, University College London, London, UK
[3]Department of Obstetrics and Gynaecology, University Hospital of Wales, Cardiff, UK

Introduction

We live in a society of fast evolving medicine yet advances in treatment do not always translate into improved outcomes for the sufferers. Despite numerous efforts in improving surgical approaches and introduction of a number of novel chemotherapy/targeted therapy agents, ovarian cancer remains the most lethal gynaecological cancer with the mortality rates decreasing by around 21% since the 1970s [1]. The 10-year survival rates of 35% are the worst amongst all women's cancers [2]. As in other cancers, detecting the disease early has the most encouraging survival of over 90% if detected in Stage I, sharply declining to 13% in Stage IV [3]. The efforts have therefore focused on detecting the disease at an early stage with screening for ovarian cancer explored since the mid-1980s [4-9].

How best to screen for the disease has been and still remains a challenge. Due to a precursor lesion not being identified until recently, all efforts have focused on the detection of ovarian cancer at an early stage. In 2010, Kurman *et al.* proposed a unifying theory regarding the origin and pathogenesis of ovarian cancer suggesting that the disease arises in the fallopian tube or other pelvic structures prior to implanting itself on the ovary and presenting as ovarian cancer [10]. It was also suggested that there are two types of tumors, Type I tumors (low-grade serous, endometroid, clear cell, mucinous) which are thought to be indolent, slow growing cancers, and Type II, mainly high-grade serous cancers accounting for most of the ovarian cancer mortality [10]. The entire premise of screening for any cancer is to detect either a precursor lesion or the most aggressive cancers. Our knowledge of the precursor lesion, serous tubal intraepithelial carcinoma (STIC) [11], is very recent and despite these lesions harboring a p53 signature on the tissue level, a circulating or imaging marker for STICs is not yet available. All efforts to

* Corresponding Author's Email: a.gentry-maharaj@ucl.ac.uk.

In: Ovarian Cancer
Editors: Christos Iavazzo, Alexandros Fotiou and John Spiliotis
ISBN: 979-8-88697-633-5

date have therefore focused on the detection of early stage disease. The impetus is to detect mainly high-grade serous cancers, which account for most of ovarian cancer mortality. More recent data suggests poor outcomes in some of the other histotypes [12] which are less chemosensitive and will almost certainly recur. The focus should therefore be on detecting poorer prognostic subtypes at an earlier stage or earlier in their natural history.

The lifetime risk of ovarian cancer in the general population is ~2% [13]. This is low risk when compared to women who have a familial risk due to the inheritance of mutations in genes such as BRCA1/2, whose lifetime risk of ovarian cancer ranges from 15-40% [14]. The remit of this chapter is to focus on advances in screening for ovarian cancer in the general population.

Keywords: ovarian cancer, screening, CA125, risk of ovarian cancer algorithm (ROCA), ultrasound, biomarkers, PLCO, UKCTOCS

Screening for Ovarian Cancer in the General Population

In the early 1980s, a transabdominal ultrasound scan approach was trialed in the King's Study in the UK. This was a single arm ultrasound-only study of 5,479 asymptomatic women aged 18-78, screened annually for 3 years. This approach was able to detect ovarian cancer at an early stage in 5 patients (Stage IA: 4; Stage IB:1) [4].

In parallel, with the discovery of CA125 in 1981, screening strategies incorporating biomarker measurements commenced. The Stockholm study of 5,550 asymptomatic women aged >40 which was also a single arm study used the discovery of CA125 and the advancement in imaging with the introduction of transvaginal ultrasound (TVS), the latter able to provide a better view of the ovaries. Women were screened with CA125 (>35U/ml) and TVS with the study showing not only that such a contemporaneous approach can detect the disease early (primary ovarian cancer in 6 patients; Stage IA: 2, Stage IIB: 2, Stage IIIC: 2; with 20 ovarian cancers diagnosed after the end of screening) but it also demonstrated improved survival (100 months) in those detected during screening compared with 20 months for those diagnosed after screening ended [15].

A sequential approach was trialed next in the Barts pilot randomised controlled trial (RCT) of 21,935 postmenopausal women aged >45 who were screened annually with CA125 (>30U/ml) followed by TVS. The trial reported encouraging survival of 72.9 months in those in the screened group compared with 41.9 months for those in the control group who underwent no screening [5]. The trial introduced the multimodal approach where the screening strategy includes CA125 as a first line and TVS as a second line test.

From the mid-1980s to date, there was a large single arm transvaginal ultrasound scan (TVS) study in women over 50 years old or women over 25 years old who had a family history of ovarian cancer in Kentucky [6]. In their first report, on 25,327 asymptomatic women, the study demonstrated that the annual TVS screening detected 35 invasive ovarian cancers and 9 serous ovarian tumors with low malignant potential, suggesting that using such an approach may have detected low malignant potential tumors in a higher proportion than presented in the previous studies using CA125. The sensitivity for ovarian cancer was 85.0%, specificity 98.7%, PPV 14.01% and NPV 99.9%. The study showed that 82% of the cancers were detected at an early stage (I/II). This finding, however, has to be taken with caution due to the lead time of screening and the single arm nature of the study. At a mean follow-up of 5.8 years, the 5-year survival rates were higher (74.8%+/-6.6%) in the screened women compared with those treated at the same institution during the same period who were not study participants (53.7%+/-2.3%) [6].

Table 1. Summary of the performance of the different ovarian cancer screening strategies and their impact on mortality in PLCO and UKCTOCS

Study	PLCO [8, 9, 16, 17]	UKCTOCS [24, 27, 28, 31, 36]
Population size	78,215 randomised (68,557 eligible for ovarian cancer screening)	202,638 randomised (202,562 eligible for mortality analysis)
Design	Randomised control trial with 1 screening strategy versus control group	Randomised control trial with 2 screening strategies versus control group
Randomisation	1993-2003	2001-2005
Setting	10 centres in USA	13 centres in England, Wales and Northern Ireland
Age (eligibility)	55-74	50-74
Population	General population (~2% risk)	General population (~2% risk)
Tests/strategy used	Both CA125 (using a 35U/ml cut-off) and ultrasound for 4 years, followed by CA125 alone in years 5-6	CA125 using the Risk of Ovarian Cancer Algorithm (ROCA) as a first line and TVS as a second line test (MMS) and Ultrasound as first and second line test (USS)
Number of annual screens	6	7 to 11
Definition of ovarian cancer	Primary ovarian, tubal and peritoneal cancer	Primary ovarian and tubal cancer WHO 2003 (*Lancet 2016*) [31] and WHO 2014 definition (*Lancet 2021*) [36]
Sensitivity for detection of primary ovarian cancer	86% (65% for Type II cancers)	MMS: 89% Prevalence/86% Incidence; USS: 85% Prevalence/68% Incidence
Specificity	98.4%	MMS: 99.8%; USS: 99.7%
Number of operations per cancer detected	21.1	MMS: 4; USS: 11
Proportion of Early stage (I/II) disease detected by screening	22.2% (screen arm) vs 21.6% (control)	47.1% MMS; 50% USS (Prevalence, *Lancet Onc 2009*)
		36.1% (MMS) vs 23.9% Control p = 0.00013; 22.4% (USS) vs 23.9% Control p = 0.642 (Invasive ovarian/tubal cancer, Initial mortality analysis, *Lancet 2016*) [31]
		MMS: 47.2% (95%CI 19.7-81.1) higher incidence of stage I disease and a 24.5% (–41.8 to –2.0) lower incidence of stage IV disease (Final mortality analysis on long term follow up, *Lancet 2021*) [36]
Mortality (initial report)[8,31]	Ratio 1.18 (95%CI 0.91-1.54) *(Weighted log rank test)*	0-14 years: MMS: 15% mortality reduction (95% CI -3 to 30; p = 0.10); USS: Mortality reduction 11% (-7 to 27; p = 0·2) *Cox Proportional Hazards*
		0-7 years: MMS: Mortality reduction 8% (-20 to 31); USS: 2% (-27 to 26) *Royston-Parmar flexible parametric model*
		7-14 years: MMS: Mortality reduction 23% (1-46); USS: 21% (-2 to 42) *Royston-Parmar flexible parametric model*
		0-14 years: MMS: Mortality reduction of 22% (3-38, p=0·023), USS: 20% (0-35, p=0·049) (Weighted log rank test, post-hoc)
		Excluding prevalent cases (0-14 years): MMS: Mortality reduction 20% (-2 to 40); 8% (-27 to 43) in 0-7 years and 28% (-3 to 49) in years 7-14

Table 1. (Continued)

Study	PLCO [8, 9, 16, 17]	UKCTOCS [24, 27, 28, 31, 36]
Median follow up (years, IQR) for initial report	12.4 years (IQR 10.9-13)	11.1 years (IQR 10.0-12.0)
Mortality (long term follow up) [9, 36]	Ratio 1.06 (95% CI: 0.87-1.30, p = 0.16) *(Weighted log rank test)*	MMS vs control (p = 0.58 *Versatile test*); HR = 0·96 (0·83 to 1·10; p = 0.52) *Cox Proportional Hazards* USS vs control (p = 0.36 *Versatile test*); HR = 0·94 (0·82 to 1·08; p = 0.37) *Cox Proportional Hazards*
Median follow up for long term follow up	14.7 years (maximum follow-up 19.2 years)	16.3 years (IQR 15.1-17.3)
Final impact	Stage shift not noted. No reduction in mortality	Stage shift noted. No reduction in mortality

Between 1985-1999, the Japanese Shizuoka Cohort Study of Ovarian Cancer Screening, an RCT of 82,487 postmenopausal women, set in 212 hospitals in the Shizuoka prefecture utilised an annual CA125 (>35U/ml), physical examination and TVS approach. Although a higher proportion of Stage I ovarian cancer were detected in the screened (63%) group compared with the control group (38%), this was not statistically significant [7].

In the Prostate Lung Colorectal Ovarian (PLCO) cancer screening trial, set across 10 centres in the United States, 78,286 postmenopausal women aged 55-74 years were assigned to the ovarian cancer screening part of the trial. The screening strategy was based on CA125 using a fixed cut-off (35U/mL) and TVS for 4 years, followed by CA125 only for a further 2 years [8]. This screening trial was initially designed to assess screening for prostate, colorectal and lung malignancies. The ovarian cancer arm was the last to be added. For this reason, 4,852 women in the screened and 4,818 in the control arm had a previous oophorectomy. The ovarian arm therefore had a total of 68,557 women randomized to screening or no screening (control arm) in a 1:1 ratio [16]. The sensitivity for the detection of ovarian cancer was 86% which decreased to 65% for the detection of Type II cancers [17]. At a median follow up of 12.4 years (10.9 -13), the trial reported no reduction in ovarian cancer mortality (ratio 1.18 95% CI 0.91-1.54) (Table 1). Fifteen percent (163/1080) of patients who had 'false positive' surgery had major complications [8]. On an extended follow up of a median of 14.7 years (maximum follow-up 19.2 years), there was no reduction in ovarian cancer mortality (ratio 1.06, 95% CI: 0.87-1.30, p = 0.16) [9]. Following the initial mortality results and the long-term follow up mortality results from this trial in 2016, the American Cancer Society [18] and the US Preventive Services Task Force (USPSTF) [19] updated their guidance that ovarian cancer screening should not be offered in the general population as it is not effective in reducing mortality from the disease. This was followed by many countries issuing a similar guidance.

The largest and last trial to report, the United Kingdom Collaborative Trial of Ovarian Cancer Screening (UKCTOCS) was set up in 13 centres across England, Wales and Northern Ireland. The trial commenced in 2001. In total, 1,243,282 women aged 50-74 were invited and 202,638 postmenopausal women randomised to either (1) multimodal screening using annual CA125 interpreted using the Risk of Ovarian Cancer Algorithm (ROCA) (50,640) (MMS), (2) annual TVS (50,639) screening (USS) or (3) control group (101,359 women) in a 1:1:2 ratio [20]. All women were to receive 6 annual screens. However, midway through the trial, a healthy volunteer effect was observed with lower mortality from any cause [21]. At a mean of 5.55 years from randomisation, the observed all-cause mortality was 37% of that expected for the age matched UK population [21]. The screening therefore had to be extended to 7-11 annual screens with all women screened up to 31st Dec 2011. The primary outcome was ovarian and fallopian tube cancer mortality by 31st Dec 2014. The trial also assessed acceptability, compliance, physical and psychological morbidity as well as cost-effectiveness of screening.

Other than UKCTOCS, all studies and trials interpreted CA125 using a single cut-off. The MMS arm in UKCTOCS used a longitudinal algorithm to interpret CA125 [22]. The ROCA is a computerised algorithm based on the Bayes theorem which compares serial CA125 levels to patterns in cases and controls and presents the results as an estimated risk of ovarian cancer. The premise of this is that women who do not have ovarian cancer have a static CA125 profile over time. However, in those developing ovarian cancer, CA125 may initially be low but then rises. It is this change that the algorithm picks up and signals that the woman is at an 'elevated' risk of ovarian cancer. The major challenge of this approach is that in asymptomatic women, CA125 levels are likely to be below the 35U/ml cut-off and any rise above baseline may indicate increased risk. Therefore, small rises in CA125 (e.g., 8 to 16U/ml) may mean that the woman is at an increased risk. The quality control (QC) of the CA125 assay in UKCTOCS therefore had to be run very tightly daily as even a unit change would require many women to be called back for a repeat CA125. The design of the trial with processing of all blood samples in a central laboratory closely monitored by the same team for the duration of the trial ensured tight QC and consistency when a large number of samples had to be processed daily. It must be noted that although ROCA was built using serial CA125 data from previous studies before UKCTOCS, its performance had to be assessed prospectively before it could be implemented in UKCTOCS. A pilot feasibility RCT of 13,582 postmenopausal women >50 years was therefore set up in the mid-1990s which showed that for detection of primary invasive epithelial ovarian cancer, the ROCA-based multimodal approach to screening demonstrated a high specificity of 99.8% (95% CI, 99.7-99.9) and PPV 19% (95% CI, 4.1-45.6) [23].

The initial (prevalence) screen on UKCTOCS showed that TVS is acceptable with 48,230 of the 50,639 women randomised to the USS arm undergoing the first scan [24] despite a transvaginal approach to scanning in this older population of women. A survey of 800 women randomised to this arm showed that TVS caused very little discomfort and pain and was acceptable to the women [25]. The ultrasound arm was set up in a way that each centre was provided with the same ultrasound machine. The Quality Assurance (QA) set for the trial was further developed during the course of the trial [26]. As postmenopausal ovaries can be difficult to visualise, an accreditation process was set up within the trial under the oversight of the UKCTOCS Ultrasound Subcommittee, appointment of a national lead sonographer, assessment of the scanning on the trial including visits to all centres to physically assess the scanning of all sonographers and personnel who scanned on the trial, a fail-safe monitoring approach, archiving and ongoing review of the ultrasound images by an expert. This contributed to the improvement in visualisation rate of postmenopausal ovaries at each individual centre [26].

From the initial prevalence screen data, it became apparent that the MMS strategy had higher sensitivity (89.4%) compared with USS (84.9%) for ovarian cancer overall and when restricted to invasive disease (89.5% MMS vs 75% USS) [24]. Encouragingly, ~50% of cancers across both arms were detected at an early stage (I/II) [24]. During the incidence screening in the MMS arm, of the 296,911 screens, 3,329 (1.1%) women underwent clinical assessment and 640 (0.2%) underwent surgery [27]. Of these, 113 women were diagnosed with primary invasive ovarian cancer of whom 56 (50%) women had annual CA125 of under 35U/ml. Lower annual CA125 levels seemed to be associated with higher proportion of Stage I/II cancers. This indicates that previous studies/trials would not have had the opportunity to detect these cancers as they were using a single cut off for CA125 at 30 or 35U/ml. Encouragingly, even at the incidence screening (which more likely reflects the performance of a strategy in a screening programme scenario), the MMS strategy had a sensitivity for invasive ovarian cancer of 85.8%. Over 40% (41.4%) of ovarian/tubal cancers were detected at Stage I/II [27]. The majority (81.9%) of screen detected cancers in the MMS group were Type II. Moreover, there were only 4.8 operations per case detected [27].

In the USS group, the incidence screening showed a lower sensitivity for invasive ovarian cancer of 61.5%, with a similar proportion of Stage I/II (37.5%) cancers as in the MMS arm. However, there were more operations per case detected (11) mainly due to benign ovarian neoplasms being detected in the USS but not the MMS arm [28, 29]. The large set of ultrasound data captured in the trial enabled exploring the risk of ovarian cancer in women across the various radiological morphologies [29, 30]. A prospective cohort study undertaken within UKCTOCS to evaluate the malignant potential of radiologically detected inclusion cysts did not show an increased risk of ovarian or other hormone dependent cancers such as breast or endometrial cancers [29]. Another prospective cohort study within the trial in the ultrasound group was undertaken to assess the absolute risk of epithelial ovarian cancers/borderline tumors/Type I and Type II tumors who had an ultrasound detected adnexal abnormality within 3 years of the initial scan. Women with adnexal abnormalities with solid elements had a 1 in 22 risk of developing epithelal ovarian cancer. The risk of borderline and Type I cancers was higher than Type II ovarian cancer where an ultrasound abnormality was detected [30].

For success of any screening programme, compliance with the strategy is essential. At the end of UKCTOCS, the compliance with both strategies was high (81% MMS vs 78% USS). The sensitivity was, as previously reported, higher in the multimodal arm (84% MMS vs 73% USS) [31]. There were very few complaints related to screen tests (2/10,000 screens in USS vs 0.86/10,000 screens MMS) despite 345,990 screens in the MMS and 327,775 screens in the USS arm (median of 8 in both) being carried out during the course of the trial. The "unnecessary" surgery undertaken in 50/10,000 screens (USS) vs 14/10,000 screens (MMS) translated to 4 operations per cancer detected in the MMS compared with 11 in the USS arm. The major complication rate in these women was 3.5% (USS) vs 3.1% (MMS) [31].

At the first UKCTOCS mortality analysis, there was a significant stage shift with 36.1% early stage (I/II) invasive ovarian cancer in the MMS arm versus 23.9% in the control arm ($p = 0.00013$) which was not observed in the USS arm (22.4% USS vs 23.9% control, $p = 0.642$). The stage shift was also significant in women with low volume (I/II/IIIa) disease (40.1% MMS vs 26% control, $p < 0.0001$) but not with USS screening (23.9% USS vs 26% control, $p = 0.57$) [31]. This was the first evidence of a stage shift in ovarian cancer screening. Compared with the control group, there was a trend towards a mortality benefit in both arms, with a 15% reduction in the MMS ($p = 0.10$) and 11% in the USS ($p = 0.21$) arm but this was not statistically significant. In addition, the mortality impact was only 8% in the first 7 years after randomisation but was 23% and 21% in years 7-14 post-randomisation in the MMS and USS arms, respectively (Table 1). As this was the last ovarian cancer trial to report, the unequivocal result was difficult to interpret in view of the continuing rise in the deaths in the control arm and leveling off in both the MMS and USS arms at the censorship of the 31st of December 2014.

As the mortality reduction observed in UKCTOCS was delayed in keeping with other cancer screening trials [32-36], the extent of the reduction was in line with that reported in breast cancer screening trials (15% - 25%), and the curves were separating at censorship, the follow up was extended until the 30th of June 2020. Over time, the age-standardised incidence and mortality rates for cancer and death from any cause increased such that at the end of the trial, rates in the control arm were similar to the UK population rates [36].

Over the last 15 years, there have been major advances in our understanding of ovarian cancer, on the origins of the disease, the precursor lesion identified for the first time but also reclassification of both disease site (WHO 2014) [37, 38] and stage (FIGO 2014) [39] which all have an impact on the ability to detect the disease. Firstly, the definition of the disease changed during the course of the trial. At the time that the trial commenced, ovarian cancer was thought to arise from the ovaries where the current understanding is that the majority of high-grade serous cancers arise in the fallopian tube and involve the ovaries secondarily [10]. The previous entity of primary peritoneal cancers were re-classified as mostly high-grade serous cancer by 2020. In addition, the stage (FIGO 2014) re-classification was incorporated [36]. The Outcomes review committee reviewed all trial specific notes to ensure the final reporting of the trial was in line with the current understanding of both the disease biology and updated stage classification.

At a censorship of the 30th of June 2020, a median follow-up of 16.3 years (3.16 million women-years) and a complete follow-up in 95% of the women in each group, the final mortality results of UKCTOCS showed no impact of screening on mortality from ovarian and tubal cancer (Table 1). This was observed using both the primary analysis test, the Versatile test (described in 2016, agnostic to a specific form of the screening effect and chosen following a consultation with 11 international experts) [40] and the Cox Proportional Hazards test [36].

There were 2055 women with ovarian and tubal cancer (1805 with invasive cancer) (WHO 2014 classification) with an incidence of ovarian and tubal cancer comparable across the groups (incidence per 100,000): 67.7 MMS, 68.2 USS and 65.4 control. The proportion of the most aggressive Type II cancers was also comparable across the groups - 79.2% MMS, 82.2% USS, 76.4% control.

The MMS strategy identified 39% more cancers at an early stage (Stage I/II), while detecting 10% fewer late-stage cancers (Stage III/IV) compared to the no screening group. There was no difference however in the incidence of early stage cancers detected in the ultrasound group compared to the no screening group [36]. The reduction in Stage III or IV disease incidence in the MMS group was not sufficient to translate into lives saved. It is therefore important to note that in screening trials, specifying cancer mortality rather than detection of early stage disease as the primary outcome is important. Based on the results of UKCTOCS, a general population screening cannot be recommended (Figure 1).

What Have We Learnt Over the Past Two Decades

Four decades of international efforts unfortunately did not have an impact on saving lives of women with ovarian cancer through screening with CA125 and ultrasound as screening tools. This may be for a number of reasons. One is that the interpretation of CA125, especially in the earlier trials, could have been improved by using a longitudinal algorithm-based approach. In UKCTOCS, the Risk of Ovarian Cancer Algorithm (ROCA) was able to detect a higher proportion of women with early stage disease in the MMS arm compared with the control arm. The novel algorithm approaches include the more recently described Methods of Mean Trends (MMT) algorithm, developed in 2015. When applied to all the CA125 data in UKCTOCS, it showed a similar performance (at a specificity of 89.5%, sensitivity of 86.5%) to ROCA (sensitivity 87.1%; specificity 87.6%; AUC 0.915) [41]. Another reason may be that there may be a better biomarker than CA125 that could improve current strategies. Until the late 2000s, the focus has mainly been on exploring the performance of promising markers in the differential diagnosis setting – the preclinical samples from prospective studies/trials [42] had not been available until more recently [43]. The main challenge of using CA125 is its non-specific elevation in benign conditions including endometriosis. Since 2007, with the discovery of Human Epididymis HE4, efforts have been made to explore its performance both in differential diagnosis [44, 45] and more recently in screening [46, 47]. Nested case control studies from PLCO have shown that HE4 is the most promising marker after CA125 (sensitivity of CA125 of 86% vs 73% for HE4). Despite this encouraging data, the complete sample set from the MMS of UKCTOCS did not show that HE4 adds to CA125 as a first line test. The MMT algorithm, incorporating multiple markers (CA125, HE4, CA72.4, TP53 autoantibodies), showed that CA125-MMT performed the best and that HE4 added little in the detection of invasive ovarian cancer within one year of diagnosis [47]. A further reason may be that CA125 is not elevated in around 15% of ovarian cancers and therefore the current strategies do not have the capability in detecting these cancers. Data from the MD Anderson, Australian Ovarian Cancer Study (AOCS) and UKCTOCS demonstrated that TP53 autoantibody profile can detect 16% of the screen-negative cancers a year prior to diagnosis [48]. Therefore, a combination of the TP53 autoantibody profile with CA125 may increase the sensitivity of screening. However, UKCTOCS data showed that in ovarian cancer screening of postmenopausal women, longitudinal CA125, HE4, CA72-4 and anti-TP53 autoantibodies do not improve on the longitudinal serum CA125 as a first-line test [47]. Epigenetic profiling may have a role in aiding earlier diagnosis and aid detection of screen-negative cancers [49].

Although UKCTOCS showed that the incidence of Stage I invasive ovarian cancer was higher in the MMS group compared with the control group, this did not translate to mortality benefit. The higher mortality in Stage I disease shown in UKCTOCS may be as the MMS strategy detects the most aggressive cancers [36]. The entire premise of screening in view of our more recent understanding of the disease (over the last two decades) is to detect high-grade serous cancers (HGSC) in early stage to have an impact on mortality. However, SEER from 2019 shows that survival in Stage I HGCS is worse than in Stage III/IV HGSC [12]. This indicates that our thinking needs to change as to where in the natural history of these cancers we need to detect for screening to have an impact on mortality from the disease.

Neither UKCTOCS nor PLCO showed a mortality benefit with screening. There were differences between the two trials. In PLCO, where serum CA-125 was interpreted using an absolute cut-off, women underwent a primary screening with evaluation and follow-up of positive results at the discretion of their physicians [8, 50]. In UKCTOCS, there was central coordination of all trial activities with close monitoring of the management of screen results and further referral, longitudinal algorithm approach to interpreting CA125 and the same team of clinicians looking after the women for the duration of the trial. However, despite these differences, the stage shift with MMS screening in UKCTOCS failed to show an impact on mortality. The detailed analysis of the treatment women received across the arms may shed some light and provide an opportunity to learn lessons that could be utilised in future trials. At present, in the general population, we cannot recommend ultrasound or CA125 screening (whether as a single cut-off or using an algorithm-based approach).

Screening for Ovarian Cancer in Women at High Risk

Women at high risk are those with a family history/mutations in the high penetrance genes BRCA1 and BRCA2 (>10% lifetime risk) [14]. BRCA1 and BRCA 2 mutation carriers have a 31-87% risk of developing breast cancer and a 15-40% risk of developing ovarian cancer [14]. The risk of ovarian cancer is lower in women with Lynch syndrome (approximately 2-15%), which varies based on the gene mutation with highest risk in MLH1 and MSH2 carriers [51].

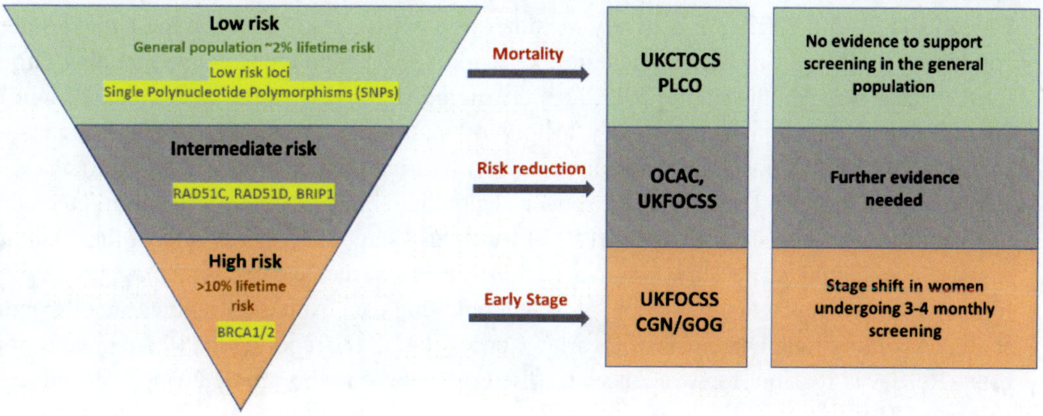

Figure 1. Screening recommendations based on general population trials or studies in women at high risk of ovarian cancer.

Current recommendations for women at high risk of ovarian cancer (based on family history or mutations in BRCA1/2) is risk reducing surgery where both ovaries and tubes are removed (risk reducing salpingo-oophorectomy, RRSO). The initial study by Rebbeck *et al.*, published in NEJM in 2002, investigated whether the risk of breast and ovarian cancer associated with BRCA1/2 mutations was reduced by bilateral prophylactic oophorectomy. This retrospective, case control study identified 551 women with germ line BRCA1/BRCA2 mutations from registries and studied the occurrence of breast and ovarian cancers for a follow-up of over 8 years. They concluded that the 259 women who had undergone bilateral prophylactic oophorectomy, when compared with the 292 matched controls who had not undergone the prophylactic procedure, had developed a lower number of ovarian and breast cancers [52]. The risk reduction was 96% for ovarian cancer and 53% for breast cancer. A more recent meta-analysis to clarify the role of risk reducing oophorectomy in BRCA1 and BRCA2 mutation carriers in reducing ovarian cancer mortality was conducted based on three prospective studies, which also demonstrated a significant risk reduction in ovarian risk by 80% (HR 0.19, 95%CI 0.13-0.27, $p < 0.00001$) [53]. The timing of risk reducing surgery adds further challenges as some women will not have completed their families or may have concerns regarding going into menopause prematurely. As in the general population, screening has been explored in the high risk women over the past three decades. Data from the United Kingdom Familial Ovarian Cancer Screening Study (UKFOCSS) Phase I suggested that annual screening in this group of women is not effective [54]. Phase II of the study which included a 4 monthly approach, using the ROCA, with prompt surgical intervention is recommended over annual screening to detect cancers early enough for a shift in stage [54]. The UKFOCSS Phase II confirmed that more frequent screening is able to detect women with early-stage disease where cytoreduction is possible in 92% of the women diagnosed within a year of the screen [55].

In UKFOCSS Phase II, 4,348 women with an estimated lifetime ovarian cancer risk of greater than 10% underwent ovarian cancer screening using serum CA125 using the ROCA every 4 months (with annual TVS if ROCA was normal or performed sooner in women with non-normal ROCA). Thirteen patients were diagnosed with ovarian cancer with 5 of these diagnosed with early-stage cancer. Sensitivity, positive predictive value, and negative predictive value of this screening protocol for detecting ovarian cancer within 1 year were 94.7%, 10.8%, and 100%, respectively. Another prospective study based in the United States, combining the data from Cancer Genetics Network (CGN) and Gynecology Oncology Group (GOG) trials was published in 2017 [56]. It included 3,692 women who were known to have *BRCA1/2* mutation and/or family history of multiple breast and/or ovarian cancers. It showed that a ROCA-based screening approach with serum CA125 testing every 3 months with transvaginal ultrasound annually or sooner depending on CA125 test results, detected 6 incidental ovarian cancers, of which 3 (50%) were early stage [56]. The results of these studies suggest a potential stage shift when a ROCA-based ovarian cancer screening protocol is followed in high-risk women. In view of the encouraging data from these studies, an NHS pilot study, 'Avoiding Late Diagnosis of Ovarian Cancer' (ALDO), reported in 2023 that screening using ROCA is feasible for women with a BRCA mutation who are deferring risk reducing surgery [57].

Risk reducing salpingo-oophorectomy (RRSO) still remains the current standard of care for ovarian cancer risk management in BRCA1/2 mutation carriers. However, concerns remain about premature menopause in women undergoing RRSO. Furthermore, several factors affect the uptake of the procedure [58]. Several more recent studies [59, 60] are exploring an early salpingectomy and delayed oophorectomy approach to delay the effects of premature menopause. In the United Kingdom, the multicentre, prospective cohort study - Preventing Ovarian Cancer by Early Excision of Tubes and Late Ovarian Removal (PROTECTOR) [60] study for premenopausal women who are at increased risk of developing ovarian cancer either because of a genetic mutation in BRCA1/2 genes or in moderate penetrance genes (RAD51C/RAD51D/BRIP1) [61, 62] or a strong family history of ovarian and breast cancer or ovarian cancer alone is underway. It has three arms: RRSO, 'risk reducing early salpingectomy with delayed oophorectomy' (RRESDO) and 'controls' (no surgery). Participants are able to select which arm of the study they wish to participate in. However, it is not known what proportion of women would potentially develop ovarian cancer were they to choose the RRESDO arm and what the long-term consequences on ovarian function would be. Hence this approach is still best used and evaluated as part of a clinical trial.

Can Genetics or Epidemiological Data Improve Screening Efforts?

In parallel to the efforts above, there have been major advances in our understanding of the genetic predisposition to ovarian cancer. Major international efforts through the Ovarian Cancer Association Consortium (OCAC) [63-69] have identified >35 low risk loci which, individually confer very little increase in risk, but in combination indicate an increase in risk of 2.8% [70]. Using genetic information alone (polygenic risk scores, PRS) may not be sufficient for risk stratified screening. Data from UKCTOCS showed that using a PRS based on 15 SNPs may identify women at 2.9% risk if in the highest quintile of risk [71]. Reproductive risk factors can augment the risk stratification efforts. Using the OCAC data, Pearce *at al* reported that in women without family history of ovarian cancer, PRS combined with information on oral contraceptive pill (OCP) use, history of endometriosis, and parity, can identify women at a gradient of risk from 0.35% to 8.78% [72]. If we consider that women in the general population have a lifetime risk of 2%, [73] this means that some women would be at lower risk than the general population and some are at higher risk, where risk reducing approaches include risk reducing surgery. Therefore, future screening strategies may be based on risk stratification where some women would not need to undergo screening as they would be at lower risk than the general population, some would be at 'intermediate' risk where screening would be recommended, and some would be at 'high' risk where risk reducing surgery may be discussed.

Current Dilemmas and Controversies

Despite increasing knowledge about the origins of ovarian cancer, there are still several dilemmas in management of this disease. As outlined earlier in this article ovarian cancers are divided into two main groups.[10] Type I cancers which are considered to be slow growing, less aggressive, and are usually diagnosed at an earlier stage at presentation. Type II ovarian cancers, mainly high-grade serous cancers are considered to be highly aggressive, rapidly evolving and generally tend to present at a higher stage. Though this can direct us towards the cancers that need to be identified to make a mortality impact with screening, clinically it is also well-known that Type I tumors can be diagnosed at a higher stage and are less chemosensitive [74-76] to the traditional drugs, thus also carrying a poorer prognosis. As evidence gathers on ovarian cancer originating in the fallopian tube, more clinicians are considering whether an early salpingectomy at the time of hysterectomy for benign reasons or other elective surgery would reduce the risk of developing ovarian cancer [77]. A systematic review undertaken in 2017, concluded that there is insufficient evidence for this practice. However, this practice has become increasing popular with a recent study in the United States showing that the rate at which opportunistic salpingectomy was being performed gradually increased from 2.4% (2001) to 5.7% (2010) (2.4-fold increase; $p < 0.001$), [78] predicting a 7.0% rate of opportunistic salpingectomy in 2015. However, in 2010, the rate of opportunistic salpingectomy began to increase substantially and reached 58.4% by 2015 (10.2-fold increase; $p < 0.001$). Early salpingectomy, despite the lack of long term data which is yet to accrue, has already started changing practice.

Some of the lessons learnt and questions that remain yet to be answered are: (1) early stage detection should not be the primary outcome in future trials but need to have ovarian cancer mortality as the primary outcome; [36, 79] (2) should women with mutations in moderate penetrance genes be advised to have prophylactic surgery; (3) opportunistic salpingectomy - whether to wait for the trial evidence or implement on national scale whilst accumulating trial evidence [80]; (4) Multiple Cancer Early Detection (MCED) tests - there is an impetus to use these tests to advance diagnosis at an early stage across many cancers despite the challenges these pose as to the further investigations for each cancer type [81]. The sensitivity of the tests from the preliminary data is over 80% however only 17% are detected at an early stage [82]; (5) frequency of screening in the general population - all trials have tested an annual strategy but with the recent DNA-based pan-cancer screening strategies, there may be an opportunity to collect blood every six months to screen for multiple cancers in women over 50 [83], and combine these results with or without CA125 to assess the performance in ovarian cancer screening.

In the last decade, based on mathematical modelling, we have learned that it takes close to 10 years for ovarian cancer to develop, with 4 years spent as *in situ*, stage I, or stage II cancers and approximately 1 year as stage III or IV cancers before they become clinically apparent [84]. In addition, the serous cancers are around 3cm when they progress to advanced stage (stage III or IV). To detect these cancers with screening and achieve a sensitivity of 50%, these cancers would have to be around 1.3 cm in diameter, and for 80% sensitivity, significantly smaller (less than 0.4cm in diameter). To have an effect on mortality (50% reduction), the annual screening test would have to detect the tumors when only 0.5cm in diameter [84]. We do not currently have the tests/imaging that could detect ovarian or tubal cancer when this small.

The Future

The precursor lesion, serous tubal intraepithelial carcinoma (STIC) with a p53 signature [11] allows identification of the lesion at the fimbrial end of the fallopian tube at a histological level. We do not yet have a blood biomarker which could reflect the presence in the circulation that could be used in the context of screening akin to cervical screening. Recently reported CancerSEEK panel [85] includes ctDNA to detect ovarian cancer. It showed a very high sensitivity for the detection of ovarian cancer. DETECT-A (Detecting cancers Earlier Through Elective Mutation-Based blood Collection and Testing) study of 10,000 women aged 65-75 utilised a multimodal multi-cancer strategy incorporating the early version of Cancer Seek blood test as first-line and diagnostic PET-CT as the second-line test. There are challenges with using PET CT as a second line test as it may not be sensitive enough to detect adnexal lesions/ovarian cancer, especially not in younger women who have physiologically active ovaries. The MCED tests are being explored in the NHS pilot the GRAIL Galleri test (based on the CancerSEEK test) to detect multiple cancers (up to 50) at early stage in 165,000 individuals, recently rolled out by NHS in the UK [86]. The performance of the NHS Galleri test in a range of cancers will only become available over the next few years.

Other strategies utilise the advances in epigenetics with an encouraging performance of the targeted methylation of plasma cell-free DNA (cfDNA) [82] test and the use of a micro-RNA signature in the OCaMIR test [87].

Conclusion

General population screening for ovarian cancer cannot currently be recommended. Any new approaches trialed in prospective RCTs are at least a decade away. The early detection of ovarian cancer in low-risk women is a question that remains to be answered. We urgently need better tests which will detect the most aggressive disease - which may not be at an early stage but still early in the natural history of the disease to make an impact on mortality. ALDO data shows that screening using an algorithm-based approach is feasible in women at high risk who are considering deferring risk reducing surgery.

References

[1] CRUK. *Ovarian cancer statistics: Ovarian cancer mortality*. (2018). https://www.cancerresearchuk.org/health-professional/cancer-statistics/statistics-by-cancer-type/ovarian-cancer#heading-One (accessed 22/12/2021.

[2] CRUK. *Ovarian cancer statistics: Ovarian cancer survival*. (2017). https://www.cancerresearchuk.org/health-professional/cancer-statistics/statistics-by-cancer-type/ovarian-cancer#heading-Two (accessed 22/12/2021.

[3] CRUK. *Ovarian cancer statistics: Ovarian cancer survival by stage at diagnosis*. (2017). https://www.cancerresearchuk.org/health-professional/cancer-statistics/statistics-by-cancer-type/ovarian-cancer/survival#heading-Three (accessed 22/12/2021.

[4] Campbell, S., Bhan, V., Royston, P., Whitehead, M. I., and Collins, W. P. (1989). Transabdominal ultrasound screening for early ovarian cancer. *BMJ*, **299**(6712), 1363-7.

[5] Jacobs, I. J., Skates, S. J., MacDonald, N., et al. (1999). Screening for ovarian cancer: a pilot randomised controlled trial. *Lancet*, **353**(9160), 1207-10.

[6] van Nagell, J. R., Jr., DePriest, P. D., Ueland, F. R., et al. (2007). Ovarian cancer screening with annual transvaginal sonography: findings of 25,000 women screened. *Cancer*, **109**(9), 1887-96.

[7] Kobayashi, H., Yamada, Y., Sado, T., et al. (2008). A randomized study of screening for ovarian cancer: a multicenter study in Japan. *Int J Gynecol Cancer*, **18**(3), 414-20.

[8] Buys, S. S., Partridge, E., Black, A., et al. (2011). Effect of screening on ovarian cancer mortality: the Prostate, Lung, Colorectal and Ovarian (PLCO) Cancer Screening Randomized Controlled Trial. *JAMA*, **305**(22), 2295-303.

[9] Pinsky, P. F., Yu, K., Kramer, B. S., et al. (2016). Extended mortality results for ovarian cancer screening in the PLCO trial with median 15years follow-up. *Gynecol Oncol*, **143**(2), 270-5.

[10] Kurman, R. J., and Shih, Ie M. (2010). The origin and pathogenesis of epithelial ovarian cancer: a proposed unifying theory. *Am J Surg Pathol*, **34**(3), 433-43.

[11] Shih, I. M., Wang, Y., and Wang, T. L. (2021). The Origin of Ovarian Cancer Species and Precancerous Landscape. *Am J Pathol*, **191**(1), 26-39.

[12] Peres, L. C., Cushing-Haugen, K. L., Kobel, M., et al. (2019). Invasive Epithelial Ovarian Cancer Survival by Histotype and Disease Stage. *J Natl Cancer Inst*, **111**(1), 60-8.

[13] CRUK. *Ovarian cancer statistics: ovarian cancer risk*. 2018. https://www.cancerresearchuk.org/health-professional/cancer-statistics/statistics-by-cancer-type/ovarian-cancer/risk-factors#heading-Zero (accessed 23/12/2021.

[14] Antoniou, A., Pharoah, P. D., Narod, S., et al. (2003). Average risks of breast and ovarian cancer associated with BRCA1 or BRCA2 mutations detected in case Series unselected for family history: a combined analysis of 22 studies. *Am J Hum Genet*, **72**(5), 1117-30.

[15] Einhorn, N., Bast, R., Knapp, R., Nilsson, B., Zurawski, V., Jr., and Sjovall, K. (2000). Long-term follow-up of the Stockholm screening study on ovarian cancer. *Gynecol Oncol*, **79**(3), 466-70.

[16] Partridge, E., Kreimer, A. R., Greenlee, R. T., et al. (2009). Results from four rounds of ovarian cancer screening in a randomized trial. *Obstet Gynecol*, **113**(4), 775-82.

[17] Temkin, S. M., Miller, E. A., Samimi, G., Berg, C. D., Pinsky, P., and Minasian, L. (2017). Outcomes from ovarian cancer screening in the PLCO trial: Histologic heterogeneity impacts detection, overdiagnosis and survival. *Eur J Cancer*, **87**, 182-8.

[18] ACS. American Cancer Society: *Can Ovarian Cancer Be Found Early?* (2021). https://www.cancer.org/cancer/ovarian-cancer/detection-diagnosis-staging/detection.html (accessed 23/12/2021.

[19] Force, U. S. P. S. T., Grossman, D. C., Curry, S. J., et al. (2018). Screening for Ovarian Cancer: US Preventive Services Task Force Recommendation Statement. *JAMA*, **319**(6), 588-94.

[20] Menon, U., Gentry-Maharaj, A., Ryan, A., et al. (2008). Recruitment to multicentre trials--lessons from UKCTOCS: descriptive study. *BMJ*, **337**, a2079.

[21] Burnell, M., Gentry-Maharaj, A., Ryan, A., et al. (2011). Impact on mortality and cancer incidence rates of using random invitation from population registers for recruitment to trials. *Trials*, **12**, 61.

[22] Skates, S. J., Menon, U., MacDonald, N., et al. (2003). Calculation of the risk of ovarian cancer from serial CA-125 values for preclinical detection in postmenopausal women. *J Clin Oncol*, **21**(10 Suppl), 206s-10s.

[23] Menon, U., Skates, S. J., Lewis, S., et al. (2005). Prospective study using the risk of ovarian cancer algorithm to screen for ovarian cancer. *J Clin Oncol*, **23**(31), 7919-26.

[24] Menon, U., Gentry-Maharaj, A., Hallett, R., et al. (2009). Sensitivity and specificity of multimodal and ultrasound screening for ovarian cancer, and stage distribution of detected cancers: results of the prevalence screen of the UK Collaborative Trial of Ovarian Cancer Screening (UKCTOCS). *Lancet Oncol*, **10**(4), 327-40.

[25] Gentry-Maharaj, A., Sharma, A., Burnell, M., et al. (2013). Acceptance of transvaginal sonography by postmenopausal women participating in the United Kingdom Collaborative Trial of Ovarian Cancer Screening. *Ultrasound Obstet Gynecol*, **41**(1), 73-9.

[26] Sharma, A., Burnell, M., Gentry-Maharaj, A., et al. (2016). Quality assurance and its impact on ovarian visualization rates in the multicenter United Kingdom Collaborative Trial of Ovarian Cancer Screening (UKCTOCS). *Ultrasound Obstet Gynecol*, **47**(2), 228-35.

[27] Menon, U., Ryan, A., Kalsi, J., et al. (2015). Risk Algorithm Using Serial Biomarker Measurements Doubles the Number of Screen-Detected Cancers Compared With a Single-Threshold Rule in the United Kingdom Collaborative Trial of Ovarian Cancer Screening. *J Clin Oncol*, **33**(18), 2062-71.

[28] Kalsi, J., Gentry-Maharaj, A., Ryan, A., et al. (2021). Performance Characteristics of the Ultrasound Strategy during Incidence Screening in the UK Collaborative Trial of Ovarian Cancer Screening (UKCTOCS). *Cancers (Basel)*, **13**(4).

[29] Sharma, A., Gentry-Maharaj, A., Burnell, M., et al. (2012). Assessing the malignant potential of ovarian inclusion cysts in postmenopausal women within the UK Collaborative Trial of Ovarian Cancer Screening (UKCTOCS): a prospective cohort study. *BJOG*, **119**(2), 207-19.

[30] Sharma, A., Apostolidou, S., Burnell, M., et al. (2012). Risk of epithelial ovarian cancer in asymptomatic women with ultrasound-detected ovarian masses: a prospective cohort study within the UK collaborative trial of ovarian cancer screening (UKCTOCS). *Ultrasound Obstet Gynecol*, **40**(3), 338-44.

[31] Jacobs, I. J., Menon, U., Ryan, A., et al. (2016). Ovarian cancer screening and mortality in the UK Collaborative Trial of Ovarian Cancer Screening (UKCTOCS): a randomised controlled trial. *Lancet*, **387**(10022), 945-56.

[32] Tabar, L., Vitak, B., Chen, T. H., et al. (2011). Swedish two-county trial: impact of mammographic screening on breast cancer mortality during 3 decades. *Radiology*, **260**(3), 658-63.

[33] Atkin, W., Wooldrage, K., Parkin, D. M., et al. (2017). Long term effects of once-only flexible sigmoidoscopy screening after 17 years of follow-up: the UK Flexible Sigmoidoscopy Screening randomised controlled trial. *Lancet*, **389**(10076), 1299-311.

[34] National Lung Screening Trial Research, T., Aberle, D. R., Adams, A. M., et al. (2011). Reduced lung-cancer mortality with low-dose computed tomographic screening. *N Engl J Med*, **365**(5), 395-409.

[35] Schroder, F. H., Hugosson, J., Roobol, M. J., et al. (2014). Screening and prostate cancer mortality: results of the European Randomised Study of Screening for Prostate Cancer (ERSPC) at 13 years of follow-up. *Lancet*, **384**(9959), 2027-35.

[36] Menon, U., Gentry-Maharaj, A., Burnell, M., et al. (2021). Ovarian cancer population screening and mortality after long-term follow-up in the UK Collaborative Trial of Ovarian Cancer Screening (UKCTOCS): a randomised controlled trial. *Lancet*, **397**(10290), 2182-93.

[37] Meinhold-Heerlein, I., Fotopoulou, C., Harter, P., et al. (2016). The new WHO classification of ovarian, fallopian tube, and primary peritoneal cancer and its clinical implications. *Arch Gynecol Obstet*, **293**(4), 695-700.

[38] Daya, D., Cheung, A. N., and Khunamornpong, S. (2014). Tumors of the peritoneum: epithelial tumors of Müllerian type. In: Kurman RJ CM, Herrington CS, Young RH, eds, ed. *WHO classification of tumors of female reproductive organs*. 4th ed. Lyon: International Agency for Research on Cancer, 92-3.

[39] Prat, J., and Oncology, FCoG. (2015). Staging Classification for Cancer of the Ovary, Fallopian Tube, and Peritoneum: Abridged Republication of Guidelines From the International Federation of Gynecology and Obstetrics (FIGO). *Obstet Gynecol*, **126**(1), 171-4.

[40] Burnell, M., Gentry-Maharaj, A., Skates, S. J., et al. (2021). UKCTOCS update: applying insights of delayed effects in cancer screening trials to the long-term follow-up mortality analysis. *Trials*, **22**(1), 173.

[41] Blyuss, O., Burnell, M., Ryan, A., et al. (2018). Comparison of Longitudinal CA125 Algorithms as a First-Line Screen for Ovarian Cancer in the General Population. *Clin Cancer Res*, **24**(19), 4726-33.

[42] Pepe, M. S., Etzioni, R., Feng, Z., et al. (2001). Phases of biomarker development for early detection of cancer. *J Natl Cancer Inst*, **93**(14), 1054-61.

[43] Pepe, M. S., Li, C. I., and Feng, Z. (2015). Improving the quality of biomarker discovery research: the right samples and enough of them. *Cancer Epidemiol Biomarkers Prev*, **24**(6), 944-50.

[44] Karlsen, M. A., Hogdall, E. V., Christensen, I. J., et al. (2015). A novel diagnostic index combining HE4, CA125 and age may improve triage of women with suspected ovarian cancer - An international multicenter study in women with an ovarian mass. *Gynecol Oncol*, **138**(3), 640-6.

[45] Gentry-Maharaj, A., Burnell, M., Dilley, J., et al. (2020). Serum HE4 and diagnosis of ovarian cancer in postmenopausal women with adnexal masses. *Am J Obstet Gynecol*, **222**(1), 56 e1- e17.

[46] Cramer, D. W., Bast, R. C., Jr., Berg, C. D., et al. (2011). Ovarian cancer biomarker performance in prostate, lung, colorectal, and ovarian cancer screening trial specimens. *Cancer Prev Res (Phila)*, **4**(3), 365-74.

[47] Gentry-Maharaj, A., Blyuss, O., Ryan, A., et al. (2020). Multi-Marker Longitudinal Algorithms Incorporating HE4 and CA125 in Ovarian Cancer Screening of Postmenopausal Women. *Cancers (Basel)*, **12**(7).

[48] Yang, W. L., Gentry-Maharaj, A., Simmons, A., et al. (2017). Elevation of TP53 Autoantibody Before CA125 in Preclinical Invasive Epithelial Ovarian Cancer. *Clin Cancer Res*, **23**(19), 5912-22.

[49] Widschwendter, M., Zikan, M., Wahl, B., et al. (2017). The potential of circulating tumor DNA methylation analysis for the early detection and management of ovarian cancer. *Genome Med*, **9**(1), 116.

[50] Menon, U., Gentry-Maharaj, A., and Jacobs, I. (2011). Ovarian cancer screening and mortality. *JAMA*, **306**(14), 1544, author reply -5.

[51] Bonadona, V., Bonaiti, B., Olschwang, S., et al. (2011). Cancer risks associated with germline mutations in MLH1, MSH2, and MSH6 genes in Lynch syndrome. *JAMA*, **305**(22), 2304-10.

[52] Rebbeck, T. R., Lynch, H. T., Neuhausen, S. L., et al. (2002). Prophylactic oophorectomy in carriers of BRCA1 or BRCA2 mutations. *N Engl J Med*, **346**(21), 1616-22.

[53] Marchetti, C., De Felice, F., Palaia, I., et al. (2014). Risk-reducing salpingo-oophorectomy: a meta-analysis on impact on ovarian cancer risk and all cause mortality in BRCA 1 and BRCA 2 mutation carriers. *BMC Womens Health*, **14**, 150.

[54] Rosenthal, A. N., Fraser, L., Manchanda, R., et al. (2013). Results of annual screening in phase I of the United Kingdom familial ovarian cancer screening study highlight the need for strict adherence to screening schedule. *J Clin Oncol*, **31**(1), 49-57.

[55] Rosenthal, A. N., Fraser, L. S. M., Philpott, S., et al. (2017). Evidence of Stage Shift in Women Diagnosed With Ovarian Cancer During Phase II of the United Kingdom Familial Ovarian Cancer Screening Study. *J Clin Oncol*, **35**(13), 1411-20.

[56] Skates, S. J., Greene, M. H., Buys, S. S., et al. (2017). Early Detection of Ovarian Cancer using the Risk of Ovarian Cancer Algorithm with Frequent CA125 Testing in Women at Increased Familial Risk - Combined Results from Two Screening Trials. *Clin Cancer Res*, **23**(14), 3628-37.

[57] Philpott S, Raikou M, Manchanda R, Lockley M, Singh N, Scott M, Evans DG, Adlard J, Ahmed M, Edmondson R, Woodward ER, Lamnisos A, Balega J, Brady AF, Sharma A, Izatt L, Kulkarni A, Tripathi V, Solomons JS, Hayes K, Hanson H, Snape K, Side L, Skates S, McGuire A, Rosenthal AN. The avoiding late diagnosis of ovarian cancer (ALDO) project; a pilot national surveillance programme for women with pathogenic germline variants in BRCA1 and BRCA2. *J Med Genet*. 2023

May;60(5):440-449. doi: 10.1136/jmg-2022-108741. Epub 2022 Nov 1. PMID: 36319079; PMCID: PMC10176325.

[58] Manchanda, R., Burnell, M., Abdelraheim, A., et al. (2012). Factors influencing uptake and timing of risk reducing salpingo-oophorectomy in women at risk of familial ovarian cancer: a competing risk time to event analysis. *BJOG*, **119**(5), 527-36.

[59] Steenbeek, M. P., Harmsen, M. G., Hoogerbrugge, N., et al. (2021). Association of Salpingectomy With Delayed Oophorectomy Versus Salpingo-oophorectomy With Quality of Life in BRCA1/2 Pathogenic Variant Carriers: A Nonrandomized Controlled Trial. *JAMA Oncol*, **7**(8), 1203-12.

[60] Gaba, F., Robbani, S., Singh, N., et al. (2021). Preventing Ovarian Cancer through early Excision of Tubes and late Ovarian Removal (PROTECTOR): protocol for a prospective non-randomised multi-center trial. *Int J Gynecol Cancer*, **31**(2), 286-91.

[61] Song, H., Dicks, E., Ramus, S. J., et al. (2015). Contribution of Germline Mutations in the RAD51B, RAD51C, and RAD51D Genes to Ovarian Cancer in the Population. *J Clin Oncol*, **33**(26), 2901-7.

[62] Ramus, S. J., Song, H., Dicks, E., et al. (2015). Germline Mutations in the BRIP1, BARD1, PALB2, and NBN Genes in Women With Ovarian Cancer. *J Natl Cancer Inst*, **107**(11).

[63] OCAC. *Ovarian Cancer Association Consortium (OCAC).* (2021). http://ocac.ccge.medschl.cam.ac.uk/ (accessed 22/12/2021.

[64] Bolton, K. L., Tyrer, J., Song, H., et al. (2010). Common variants at 19p13 are associated with susceptibility to ovarian cancer. *Nat Genet*, **42**(10), 880-4.

[65] Permuth-Wey, J., Lawrenson, K., Shen, H. C., et al. (2013). Identification and molecular characterization of a new ovarian cancer susceptibility locus at 17q21.31. *Nat Commun*, **4,** 1627.

[66] Phelan, C. M., Kuchenbaecker, K. B., Tyrer, J. P., et al. (2017). Identification of 12 new susceptibility loci for different histotypes of epithelial ovarian cancer. *Nat Genet*, **49**(5), 680-91.

[67] Song, H., Ramus, S. J., Tyrer, J., et al. (2009). A genome-wide association study identifies a new ovarian cancer susceptibility locus on 9p22.2. *Nat Genet*, **41**(9), 996-1000.

[68] Goode, E. L., Chenevix-Trench, G., Song, H., et al. (2010). A genome-wide association study identifies susceptibility loci for ovarian cancer at 2q31 and 8q24. *Nat Genet*, **42**(10), 874-9.

[69] Pharoah, P. D., Tsai, Y. Y., Ramus, S. J., et al. (2013). GWAS meta-analysis and replication identifies three new susceptibility loci for ovarian cancer. *Nat Genet*, **45**(4), 362-70, 70e1-2.

[70] UoC. *Major genetic study identifies 12 new genetic variants for ovarian cancer* (University of Cambridge). (2017). https://www.cam.ac.uk/research/news/major-genetic-study-identifies-12-new-genetic-variants-for-ovarian-cancer (accessed 23/12/2021.

[71] Yang, X., Leslie, G., Gentry-Maharaj, A., et al. (2018). Evaluation of polygenic risk scores for ovarian cancer risk prediction in a prospective cohort study. *J Med Genet*, **55**(8), 546-54.

[72] Pearce, C. L., Stram, D. O., Ness, R. B., et al. (2015). Population distribution of lifetime risk of ovarian cancer in the United States. *Cancer Epidemiol Biomarkers Prev*, **24**(4), 671-6.

[73] CRUK. *Ovarina cancer statistics: Ovarian cancer incidence*. (2018). https://www.cancerresearchuk.org/health-professional/cancer-statistics/statistics-by-cancer-type/ovarian-cancer#heading-Zero (accessed 22/12/2021.

[74] Perren, T. J. (2016). Mucinous epithelial ovarian carcinoma. *Ann Oncol*, **27 Suppl 1**, i53-i7.

[75] Colombo, N., Guthrie, D., Chiari, S., et al. (2003). International Collaborative Ovarian Neoplasm trial 1: a randomized trial of adjuvant chemotherapy in women with early-stage ovarian cancer. *J Natl Cancer Inst*, **95**(2), 125-32.

[76] Lorusso, D., and Pignata, S. (2017). Role of adjuvant chemotherapy in early-stage endometrioid and clear-cell ovarian cancer. *Ann Oncol*, **28**(12), 2909-11.

[77] Darelius, A., Lycke, M., Kindblom, J. M., Kristjansdottir, B., Sundfeldt, K., and Strandell, A. (2017). Efficacy of salpingectomy at hysterectomy to reduce the risk of epithelial ovarian cancer: a systematic review. *BJOG*, **124**(6), 880-9.

[78] Mandelbaum, R. S., Adams, C. L., Yoshihara, K., et al. (2020). The rapid adoption of opportunistic salpingectomy at the time of hysterectomy for benign gynecologic disease in the United States. *Am J Obstet Gynecol*, **223**(5), 721 e1- e18.

[79] Hackshaw, A., and Berg, C. D. (2021). An efficient randomised trial design for multi-cancer screening blood tests: nested enhanced mortality outcomes of screening trial. *Lancet Oncol*, **22**(10), 1360-2.

[80] Manchanda, R., Chandrasekaran, D., Saridogan, E., et al. (2016). Should Opportunistic Bilateral Salpingectomy (OBS) for Prevention of Ovarian Cancer Be Incorporated Into Routine Care or Offered in the Context of a Clinical Trial? *Int J Gynecol Cancer*, **26**(1), 31-3.

[81] Etzioni, R., Gulati, R., and Weiss, N. S. (2021). Multi-Cancer Early Detection: Learning from the past to Meet the Future. *J Natl Cancer Inst*.

[82] Klein, E. A., Richards, D., Cohn, A., et al. (2021). Clinical validation of a targeted methylation-based multi-cancer early detection test using an independent validation set. *Ann Oncol*, **32**(9), 1167-77.

[83] Bast, R. C., Han, C. Y., Lu, Z., and Lu, K. H. (2021). Next steps in the early detection of ovarian cancer. *Commun Med (London)*, **1**.

[84] Brown, P. O., and Palmer, C. (2009). The preclinical natural history of serous ovarian cancer: defining the target for early detection. *PLoS Med*, **6**(7), e1000114.

[85] Cohen, J. D., Li, L., Wang, Y., et al. (2018). Detection and localization of surgically resectable cancers with a multi-analyte blood test. *Science*, **359**(6378), 926-30.

[86] NHS. *NHS to pilot potentially revolutionary blood test that detects more than 50 cancers*. (2021). https://www.england.nhs.uk/2020/11/nhs-to-pilot-potentially-revolutionary-blood-test/(accessed 23/12/2021.

[87] Kandimalla, R., Wang, W., Yu, F., et al. (2021). OCaMIR-A Noninvasive, Diagnostic Signature for Early-Stage Ovarian Cancer: A Multi-cohort Retrospective and Prospective Study. *Clin Cancer Res*, **27**(15), 4277-86.

Chapter 3

The Role of Ultrasounds in the Diagnosis and Management of Adnexal Tumors

Natalie Nunes[1], MD, PhD, MRCOG and Davor Jurkovic[2,*], MD, PhD, FRCOG

[1]Department of Obstetrics and Gynaecology, West Middlesex University Hospital, Chelsea and Westminster Hospital Foundation Trust, London, UK

[2]Institute for Women's Health, University College Hospital, London, UK

Introduction

In modern clinical practices, adnexal tumors are detected more often with easier access to imaging both in acute and elective clinical settings.

Evaluation of an adnexal tumors commences with taking a detailed clinical history including presenting symptoms and past gynaecological, medical, surgical and family history. The aim of ultrasound examination is to determine the origin and nature of the lesion (benign, borderline, or malignant) and to help formulate a management plan.

Pattern Recognition is the method used by experienced ultrasound operators to characterize adnexal tumors based on a detailed assessment of their morphological characteristics in the context of clinical history and presenting symptoms. All evidence gathered so far shows that Pattern Recognition is the most accurate method to differentiate between benign and malignant tumors on ultrasound scans. (Meys et al., 2016; Nunes et al., 2018; Nunes et al., 2013; Timmerman et al., 2021; Valentin, 1999). However, the method is less accurate for the diagnosis of borderline ovarian tumors. (Yazbek et al., 2010; Yazbek et al., 2007)

In this chapter, we describe characteristics of common benign and malignant adnexal tumors following the principles of Pattern Recognition. When ultrasound scans are done by non-expert operators, there are several diagnostic models described in the literature which could be used to aid with the differential diagnosis between benign and malignant lesions. They are also discussed in the latter sections of this chapter.

* Corresponding Author's Email: davor.jurkovic@nhs.net.

In: Ovarian Cancer
Editors: Christos Iavazzo, Alexandros Fotiou and John Spiliotis
ISBN: 979-8-88697-633-5

Evaluation of Adnexal Tumors

Personal History

Patient's history helps clinicians to assess the impact of adnexal tumors on women's health and the possibility of malignancy. Whilst taking the history, one should inquire about the symptoms, such as pain, abdominal distention, palpable mass, menstrual irregularities, or post-menopausal bleeding/irregular bleeding on hormone replacement therapy (HRT). Patient's age and menopausal status as well as the use of hormonal therapies should be recorded along with information about previous surgical procedures and medical co-morbidities. Any personal history of cancer is of obvious importance.

Family History

Family history of breast, bowel, ovarian cancer as well as syndromes or the results of genetic testing such as BRCA, Lynch Syndrome or Peutz-Jeghers syndrome (PJS) should be recorded.

Physical Examination

On physical examination, it is important to assess a woman's general health and inspect the abdomen for signs of distension and previous surgical scars. Palpation should be carried out to assess tenderness and detect palpable abdominal tumors and examine their mobility. A note should be taken of hirsutism, virilization, or muco-cutaneous spots which can be seen in women with PJS.

Ultrasound Examination

Women presented with adnexal tumors should undergo both transvaginal and transabdominal examinations. If a transvaginal scan cannot be carried out (in virgins or in cases of severe vaginal atrophy), women should be offered transrectal scans. Internal scans provide high resolution images which facilitate detailed studies of tumor morphology and vascularity. In addition, it is possible to assess tumor mobility, tenderness, and presence of peritoneal deposits. Abdominal scans allow for a complete examination of large tumors, ascites, omental deposits, liver, kidney, and lymph node involvement.

Cyst/Tumor Descriptions

Solid/Cystic and Contents

The first element of a tumor that is examined and described is whether it is solid, cystic or both. Solid tumors are generally of uniform echogenicity, and they feel hard and heavy on palpation.

The walls of cystic tumors often appear hyperechoic because of posterior acoustic enhancement. The cyst fluid can be anechoic, low level echogenic, mixed echogenic or ground glass in appearance. (Andreotti et al., 2020; Timmerman et al., 2000)

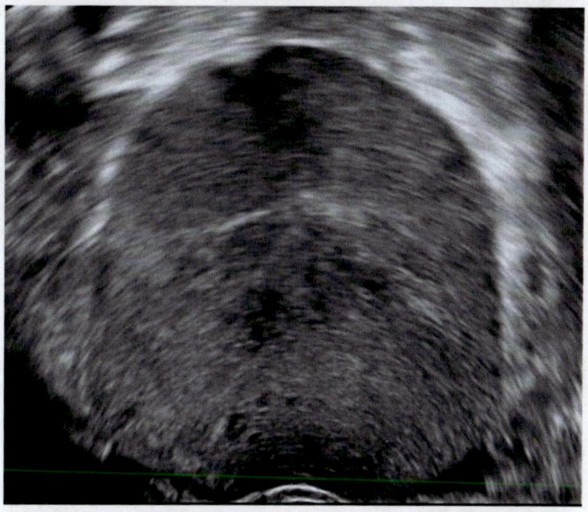

Figure 1. Solid tumor.

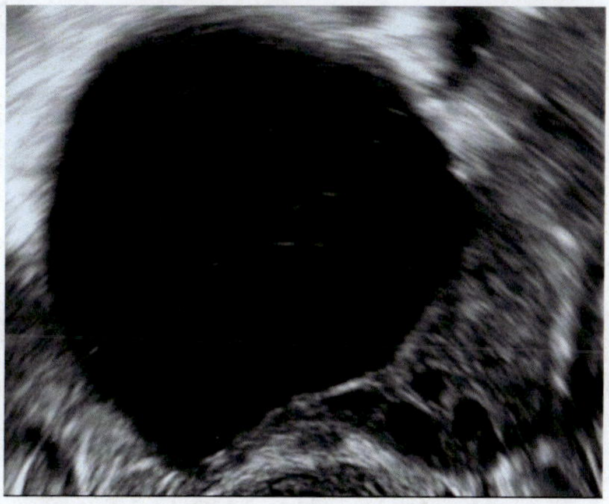

Figure 2. Cystic tumor.

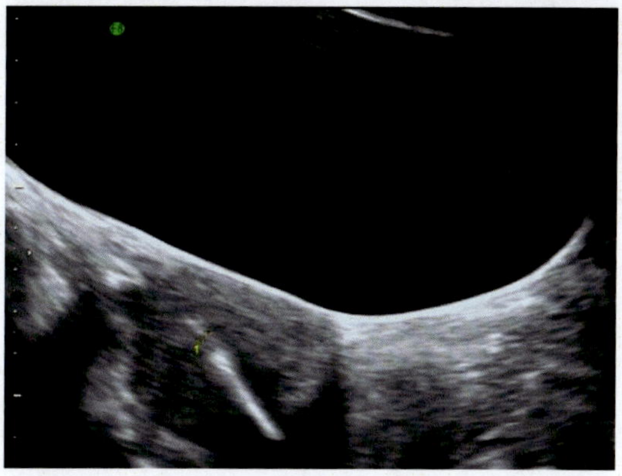

Figure 3. Anechoic cyst content.

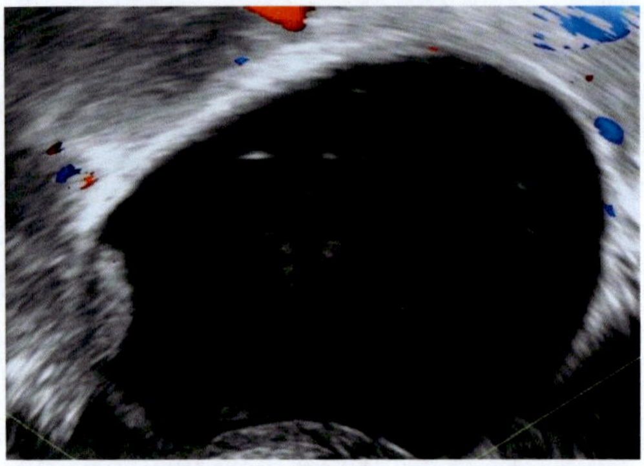

Figure 4. Low level echogenic cyst content.

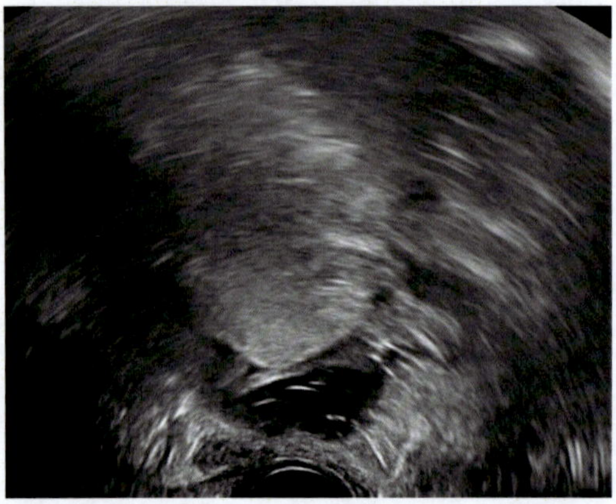

Figure 5. Mixed echogenic cyst content.

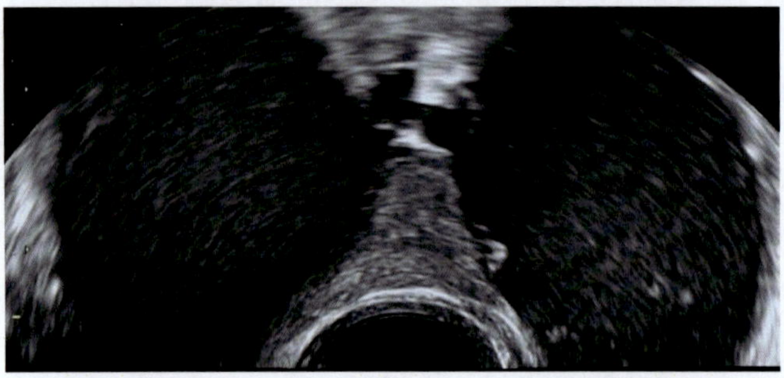

Figure 6. Ground glass cyst content.

Cystic tumors are further subdivided into unilocular (one cyst cavity), and multilocular (cyst cavity divided by septa). Cysts which contain a solid component are classified as cystic/solid.

Papillary Projections

These are raised areas on the inner surface of the cyst or septations measuring 3mm or more in height.

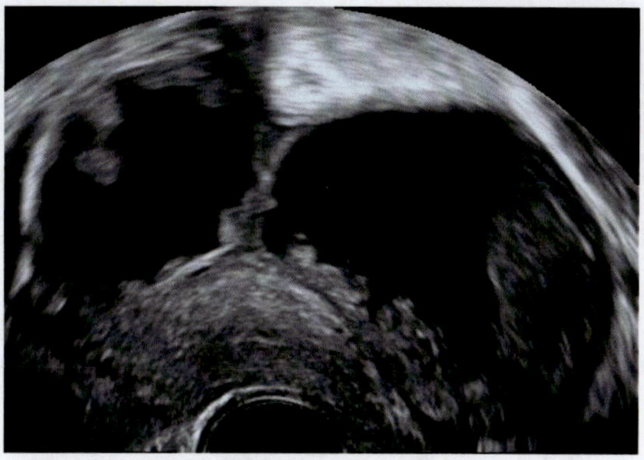

Figure 7. Papillary projections.

Vascularity

Tumor vascularity is assessed using color Doppler in a semi-quantitative way by using a subjective score of 1 (no vascularity demonstrated) to 4 (highly vascular). (ref) Pulsed Doppler flow velocity waveform analysis is of limited value in determining the nature of adnexal tumors.

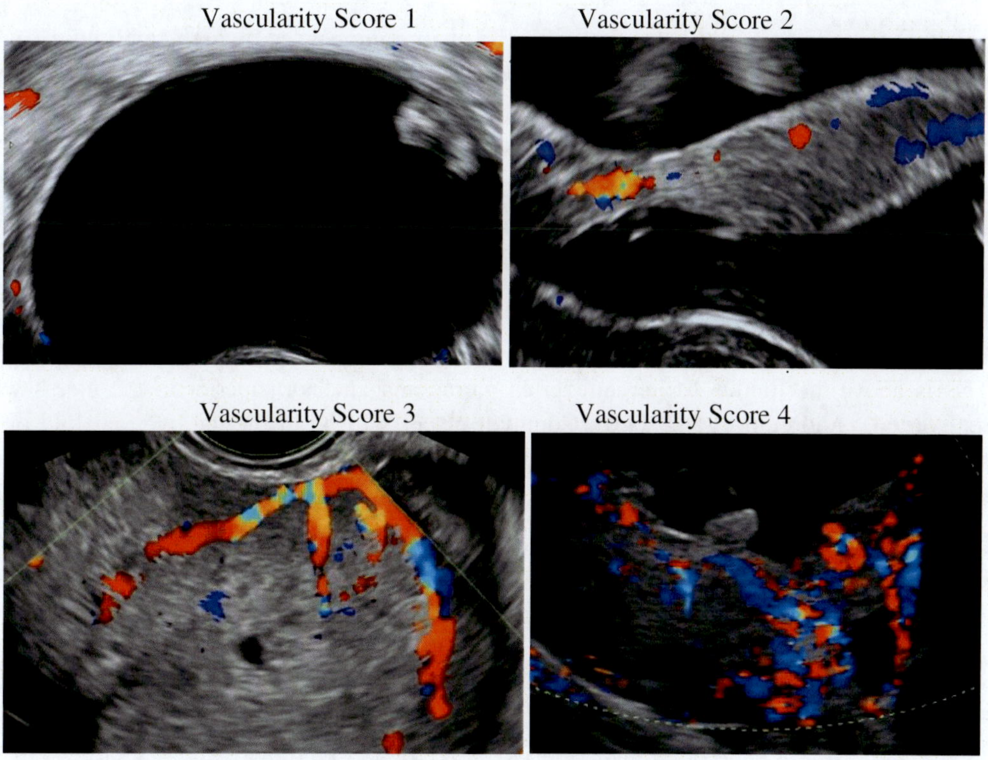

Figure 8. Vascularity scores.

Acoustic Shadowing

This is a physical phenomenon which occurs when ultrasound waves meet interface of tissues with very different acoustic impedance (e.g., soft tissue and bone). This causes almost complete reflection of ultrasound beam creating an impression of black shadow behind the interface. (Andreotti et al., 2020)

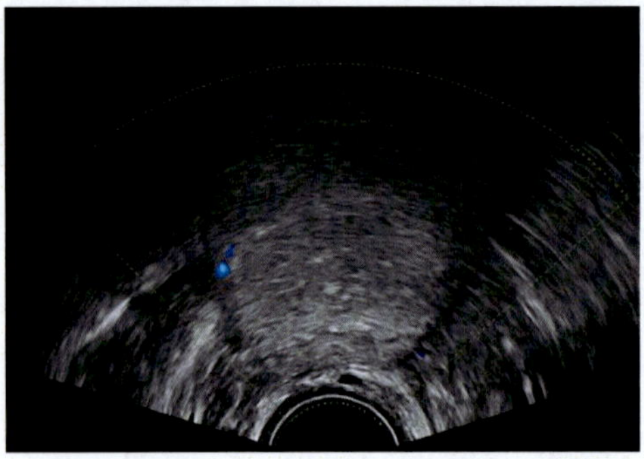

Figure 9. Acoustic shadowing.

Acoustic Streaming

This is the steady movement and flow of low density fluid caused by high amplitude acoustic waves. (Bjørnø, 2017) This feature is often seen in benign ovarian cystadenomas, but rarely in endometriomas which are filled with thick old blood. However, the streaming sign is not specific enough to discriminate accurately between ovarian endometriomas and other adnexal cysts. (Van Holsbeke et al., 2010)

Ascites

Free peritoneal fluid is labelled as ascites when it can be seen outside of the pouch of Douglas. This is above the fundus for an anteverted uterus and anterior/superior to the uterus when retroverted. (Andreotti et al., 2020). Common places will be in the uterovesical fold or the flanks and upper abdomen around the liver. The echogenicity and movement of the fluid should be noted as this could be anechoic (typical ascites), echogenic and mobile (infective, haemorrhagic or malignant) or echogenic and gelatinous (pseudomyxoma peritonii).

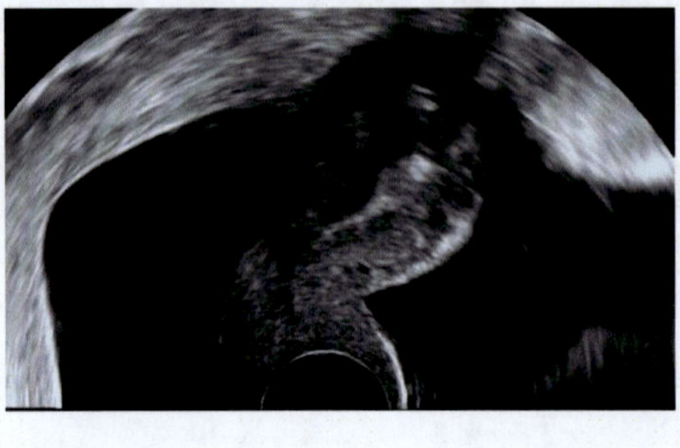

Figure 10. Ascites.

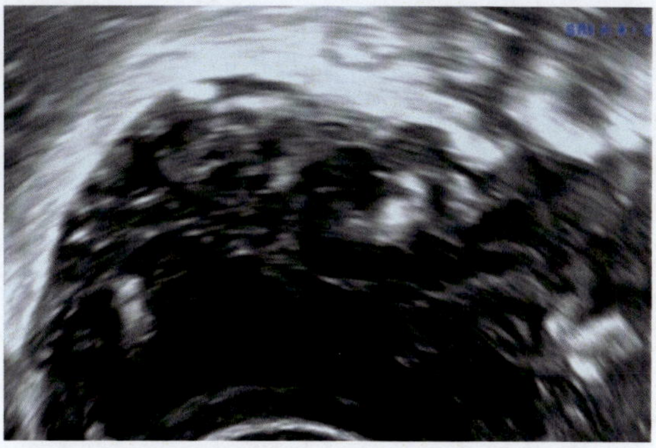

Figure 11. Pseudomyxoma peritonii.

Peritoneal Disease

Peritoneal deposits are best seen in the pouch of Douglas as raised areas on the peritoneum. In primary peritoneal disease, the entire peritoneum is often uniformly thickened rather than just a few raised deposits. (Levy et al., 2008; Qi et al., 2017)

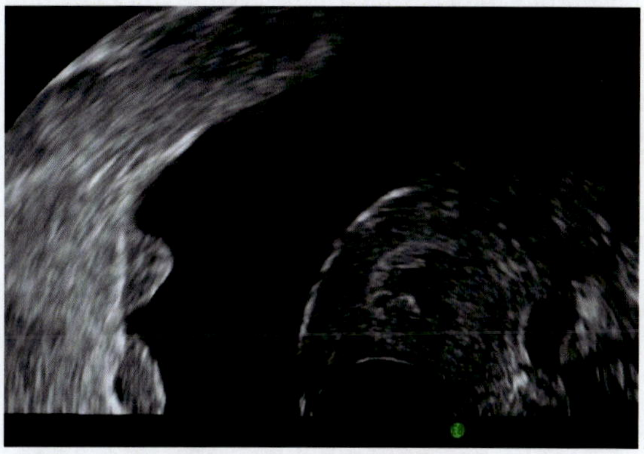

Figure 12. Peritoneal deposits.

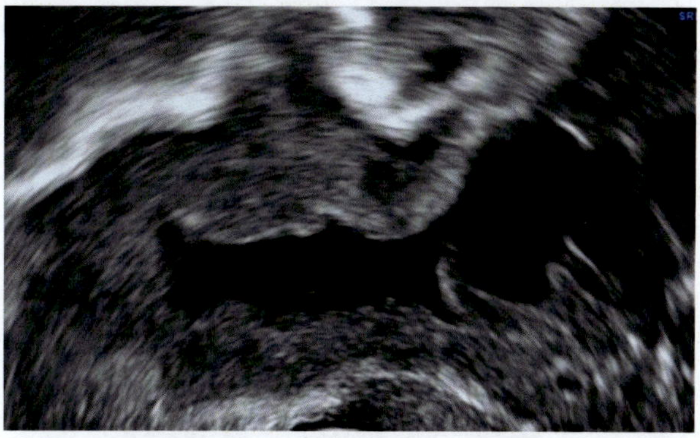

Figure 13. Primary peritoneal cancer.

Mobility

Mobility of the adnexal tumor is an important diagnostic feature. Masses that are fixed to the surrounding pelvic structures include tubo-ovarian abscess, endometriosis, loculated adhesions following previous pelvic surgery and invasive malignancies. Fixed lesions tend to be unusually low or high in the pelvis, there is a lack of sliding organs sign and their boundaries tend to be ill-defined.

Classification of Common Adnexal Tumors Using Pattern Recognition

Functional Cysts: Simple, Heamorrhagic and Corpora Lutea

Clinical Presentation

This depends on the type of functional cyst and whether a cyst accident has occurred such as rupture, haemorrhage or torsion.

Ultrasonographic Findings

Follicular cysts are simple unilocular cysts, hemorrhagic cysts contain echogenic fluid and may have clots which can resemble spiderweb or appear solid and irregular. (Valentin et al., 2013)

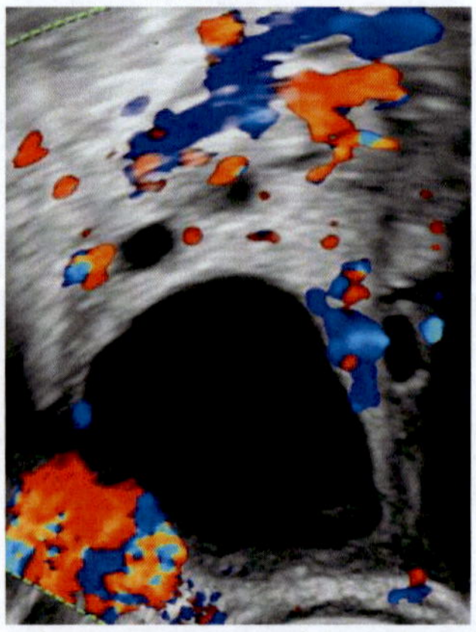

Figure 14. Simple cyst.

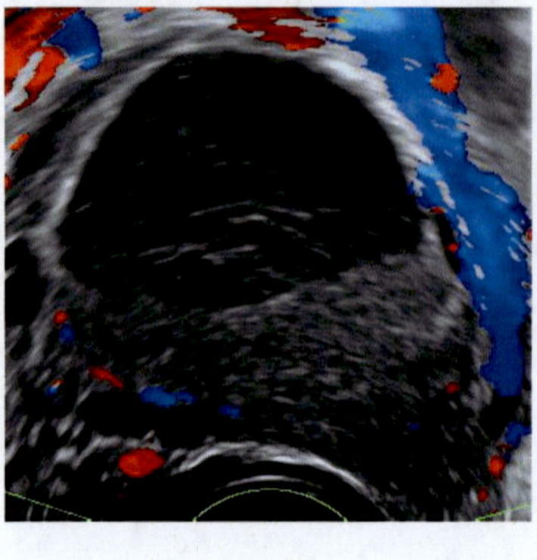

Figure 15. Hemorrhagic cyst.

Endometrioma

Clinical Presentation

Women with endometriosis may be asymptomatic or they may have a history of painful periods. They may also experience chronic pelvic pain, deep dyspareunia, dyschezia, hematuria, and/or change in bowel habits during her menstruation or subfertility.

Ultrasonographic Findings

A large study by Holsbeke et al. (2010) showed that endometriomas typically present themselves as unilocular (65%), avascular or poorly vascular (78%) cysts filled with hyperechoic 'ground glass' fluid (73%). (Holsbeke et al., 2010) Most patients are pre-menopausal (96%) and 35% experience pain during the ultrasound examination. This was much higher compared to other benign (19%) or malignant (45) adnexal tumors. Only 10% have papillary projections which was single in 70% of cases. During pregnancy, endometriomas typically decrease in size and change morphologically. (Pateman et al., 2014) The fluid changes to become hyperechoic with an irregular internal wall with highly vascular and prominent round papillary projections.

Other features of endometriosis can help confirm the diagnosis such as the presence of concomitant adenomyosis, 'kissing ovaries', extensive pelvic adhesions, peritoneal pseudocysts and endometriotic nodules on in recto-vaginal space, large bowel, bladder or pelvic ureters.

Malignant transformation in an endometrioma is relatively rare. The histological types which tend to arise from endometriosis are endometrioid and clear cell carcinomas. Endometrioid cancer developing from endometriomas tend to present themselves as unilocular cysts with prominent papillary projections arising from the cyst wall, whilst non-endometriosis cancer usually has large central solid component on ultrasound examination. (Moro et al., 2018; Testa et al., 2011)

- Ground glass contents
- Poorly vascular hyperechoic papillary projection
- 'Kissing ovaries'
- Negative acoustic streaming
- Normal overlying ovarian tissue
- Malignant endometrioid from endo

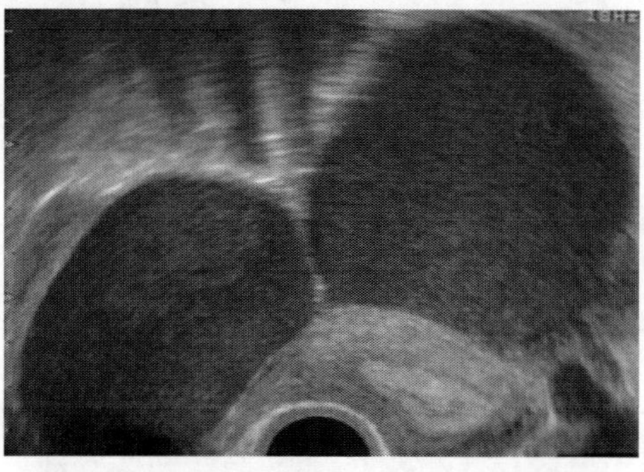

Figure 16. Endometrioma.

Germ Cell Tumors: Mature Cystic Teratoma (Dermoid Cyst)

Clinical Presentation

Benign dermoid cysts comprise 20% of ovarian tumors. (Maniar & Vang, 2019; Peterson et al., 1955). These often-asymptomatic slow growing tumors can be found in all age groups and in all sizes. (Hoo et al., 2010) Most women are asymptomatic, but sometimes torsion, rupture, infection, haemolytic anaemia, paraneoplastic encephalitis, and malignant transformation are present. (Maniar & Vang, 2019)

Ultrasonographic Findings

These tumors are avascular cysts with mixed echogenic content with pathognomonic features such as a Rokitansky nodule (81-86%), hair seen as a dot-dash sign (61%), floating fat (white ball) (93%) and calcified bone or teeth with marked acoustic shadowing (63%). (Sahin et al., 2017; Sayasneh et al., 2015; Valentin, 2004) Rokitansky nodules are echogenic inner-wall projections. (Patel et al., 1998; Sahin et al., 2017) Other significant features include fat-fluid or fluid-fluid levels, hair balls which may arise from the Rokitansky nodule and inability to move the fluid with acoustic streaming. Some of these cysts may not be visualised on an ultrasound scan at all due to their appearances being similar to surrounding echogenic bowel and the technique of palpation helps identify the cyst's presence.

- Mixed echogenicity
- Fluid levels
- Hair
- Acoustic shadowing
- Echogenic tubercle (Rokitansky nodule)
- Normal overlying ovarian tissue

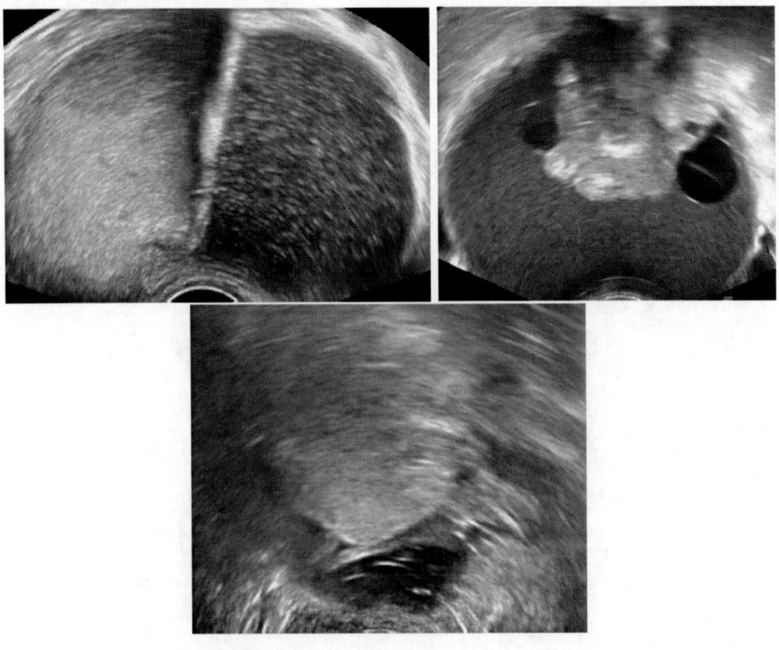

Figure 17. Mature cystic teratoma (dermoid cyst).

Germ Cell Tumors: Stuma Ovarii

Clinical Presentation

Dermoid cysts can have any type of tissue within it including thyroid tissue. Struma ovarii is a dermoid cyst comprised predominantly of thyroid tissue. (Maniar & Vang, 2019) Clinical presentation and complications are usually the same with the addition of possible thyroid enlargement, clinical thyrotoxicosis or a thyroid malignancy. (Yoo et al., 2008)

Ultrasonographic Findings

Struma ovarii it more likely to be multilocular, multilocular-solid or solid compared to dermoid cysts (Savelli et al., 2008). Yoo et al. found a third of tumors were diagnosed as struma ovarii or a dermoid cyst and another third were thought to be malignant. In his series there were 5/34 (14.7%) malignant struma ovarii tumors. Irregular walls were common (47-75%) and anechoic fluid was seen in (56-60%) tumors as opposed to the typical mixed echogenicity of a dermoid cyst. Benign struma ovarii had variable Doppler scores. (Weinberger et al., 2018)) Savelli et al. found the most characteristic feature was a 'struma pearl' which was a well circumscribed, smooth-surfaced, solid ball of tissue.

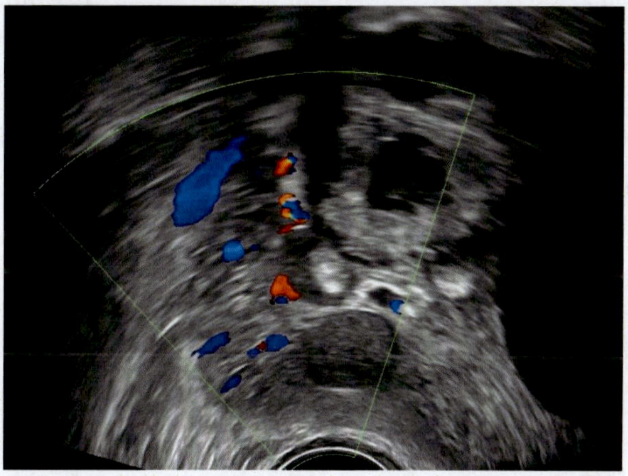

Figure 18. Stuma ovarii.

Sex-Chord Stromal Tumors: Fibroma/Fibrothecoma

Clinical Presentation

Women diagnosed with fibromas are typically asymptomatic, and their tumors are incidental findings on imaging done for other reasons. A small number of women may have associated ascites and a right pleural effusion (Meigs Syndrome). (Meigs, 1954), Fibrothecomas are three times less frequent than fibromas and the majority of them are found in postmenopausal women. (Bjorkholm & Pettersson, 1980)

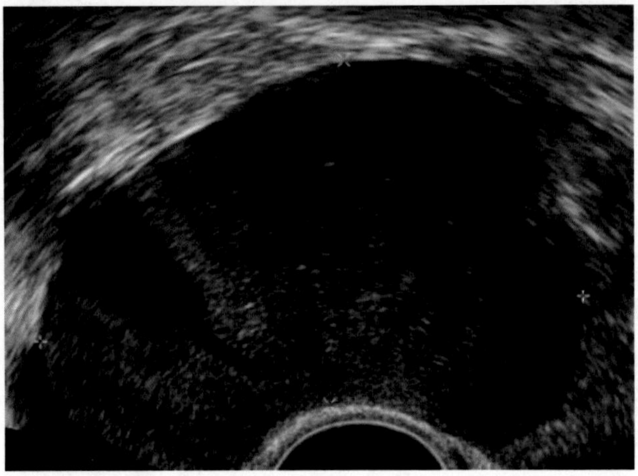

Figure 19. Fibroma.

Ultrasonographic Findings

Most are unilateral and solid (74% Fibromas [F], 80% of fibrothecomas [FT]) and typically large. (Paladini et al., 2009) Cystic tumors have few locules and no papillary projections. Largest solid components average 70mm [F] and 53mm [FT]. Acoustic shadowing was seen in a third of these patients which helps to confirm the benign nature of these tumors. (Chen et al., 2016). Half of them have some free fluid in the pouch of Douglas, but few have ascites and the color Doppler score is predominantly 2 (43% [F] and 40% [FT]) or 3 (47% [FT]). Using pattern recognition, 80% fibrothecomas were correctly identified versus 47% of fibromas. Differential diagnoses include pedunculated uterine fibroid, ovarian torsion, Brenner Tumor, lymphadenopathy, and gastrointestinal stromal tumors (GIST).

- Solid avascular/poorly vascular tumors
- Acoustic shadowing

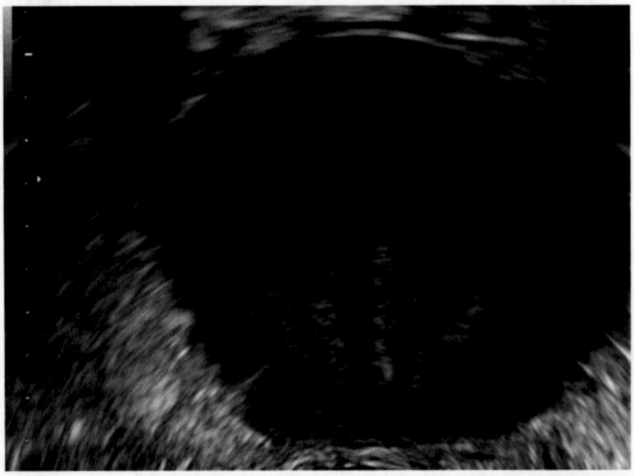

Figure 20. Fibrothecoma.

Sex-Chord Stromal Tumors: Granulosa Cell Tumors (GCT)/ Sertoli-Cell/Leydig-Cell

Clinical Presentation

Granulosa cell tumors are sex chord stromal tumors of low malignant potential. These women can be present with hyperestrogenic symptoms such as precocious puberty, galactorrhoea, breast enlargement, irregular menstrual bleeding, or postmenopausal bleeding.

Sertoli-cell tumors similarly are estrogen-producing and a patient can experience irregular bleeding. Most are benign and 75% or patients are ≤30 years of age. (Timmerman et al., 2021)

Leydig-cell tumors are male-hormone secreting tumors (testosterone, androstenedione) and 75% patients will experience virilization, such as clitoromegaly. Most are benign and the median age at presentation is 58 years of age.

Ultrasonographic Findings

GCT tumors are often slow growing and up to 80% can have a co-existing endometrial pathology with 10% having endometrial cancer. (Fox et al., 1975) Van Holsbeke et al. found 91% to be multilocular-solid or solid with 77% of multilocular cysts having 10 or more locules. (Van Holsbeke et al., 2008) The majority were larger than 50mm (96%) and half were over 100mm (52%). Cystic tumors had low level (44%) or mixed echogenic (38%) content. Tumors were vascular with 91% having a score of 3 or more and 22% had ascites present.

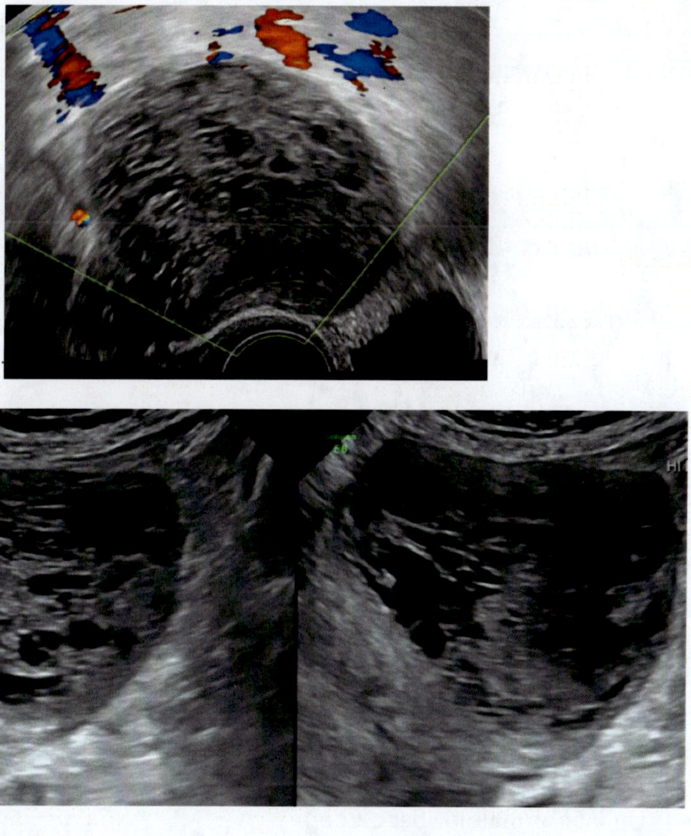

Figure 21. Granulosa cell tumor.

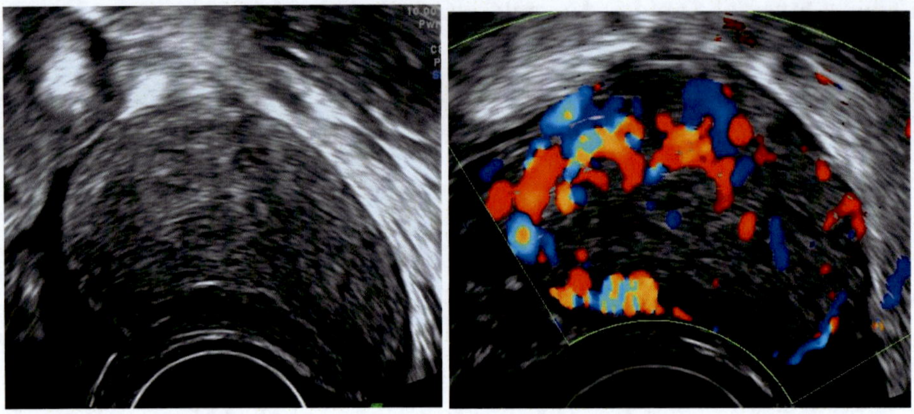

Figure 22. Sertoli cell tumor.

- Well circumscribed
- Large unilocular-solid
- Large multilocular–solid masses with many locules
- Solid tumors with heterogeneous echogenicity of the solid tissue
- Highly vascular
- Estrogen producing

Sertoli-cell tumors are typically solid and vascular like GCTs and with a median diameter of 90mm. (Demidov et al., 2008)

Leydig-cell tumors are also solid vascular tumors though smaller with a median diameter of 24mm.

Epithelial Tumors: Benign Cystadenoma/Cystadenofibroma

Clinical Presentation

These patients are typically in their 50s and the cyst is often unilateral (>80% cases).

Ultrasonographic Findings

Cystadenomas can be serous or mucinous. Serous accounts for two-thirds of benign ovarian epithelial tumors. (Seidman et al., 2019)

Serous cystadenomas are often unilocular or low level multilocular (<10 locules) with anechoic fluid and avascular papillary projections.

Serous cystadenofibromas have additional fibrotic papillary projections with 40% having acoustic shadowing. These are usually 50-80mm in diameter. (Timmerman et al., 2021)

Mucinous cystadenomas are typically multilocular (65%) with >10 locules with variable fluid echogenicity. There are often larger than their serous counterparts with a median diameter of 112mm.

- Unilocular/multilocular cyst
- Usually, unilateral

- May contain single or multiple papillary projections
- Often has evidence of fibrosis
- Normal adjacent ovarian tissue
- Typically, low vascularity on Doppler examination

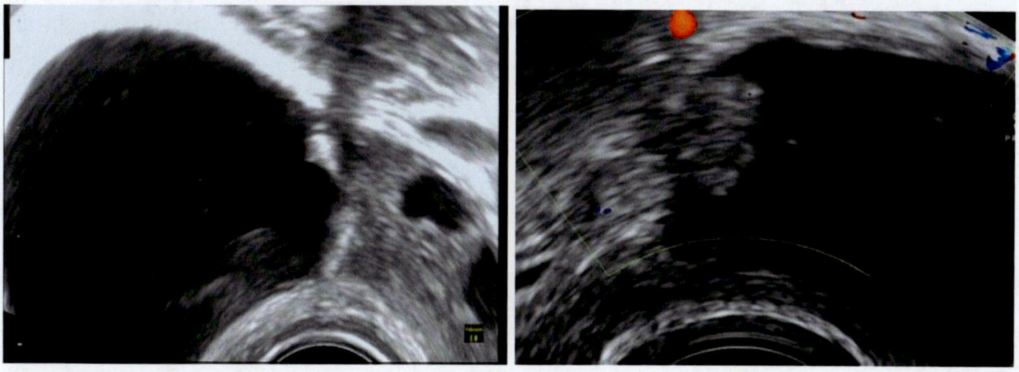

Figure 23. Cystadenoma/cystadenofibroma.

Epithelial Tumors: Brenner Tumors

Clinical Presentation

Patients range from 30 to 70 years of age though most are postmenopausal and asymptomatic. A few may be estrogen-producing. (Balasa et al., 1977) Most (83-99%) are benign.

Ultrasonographic Findings

Brenner tumors are usually small avascular solid calcified tumors with small cysts within, ranging in size from 20–80mm, though they may also be multilocular-solid. (Dierickx et al., 2012)

Epithelial Tumors: Borderline Ovarian Tumors (BOT)

Clinical Presentation

These patients often have tumors found incidentally, or they have vague lower abdominal symptoms. Most patients are aysmptomatic but some experience vague lower abdominal discomfort. BOTs, more often seen in pre-menopausal women, peak in the 5th decade versus primary invasive tumors which peak in the 6th and 7th decades. (Gotlieb et al., 2005)

Ultrasonographic Findings

BOTs have varying ultrasound appearances. They can get quite large despite a slower growth rate compared to invasive malignancies. They are usually well-circumscribed tumors with no evidence of invasion or ascites and they are often multilocular with papillary projections. (Valentin, 2004). Normal surrounding ovarian parenchyma is usually visible which has been referred to as a positive 'ovarian crescent sign'. (Franchi et al., 2013; Yazbek et al., 2006; Yazbek et al., 2007)

Serous BOTs (SBOTs) are bilateral in 35-40% cases and tend to have multiple papillary projections as do mucinous endocervical-type BOTs. Mucinous BOTs (MBOTs) tend to be more multilocular when compared to their benign counterparts. Classic honeycomb nodules (multilocular nodules) are seen in MBOTs of gastrointestinal type. Transitional cell (Brenner) BOTs are highly multilocular tumors and get very large (up to 23cm) and primarily only have symptoms of mass effect. They are rarely associated with a synchronous or metachronous bladder transitional cell carcinoma.

- All types:
  - Positive ovarian crescent sign
  - Absence of ascites and peritoneal tumor deposits
- Serous
  - Uni/multilocular, papillae
- Mucinous endocervical
  - Unilocular, papillae
- Mucinous gastrointestinal
  - Honeycomb nodule
  - Thick echogenic fluid

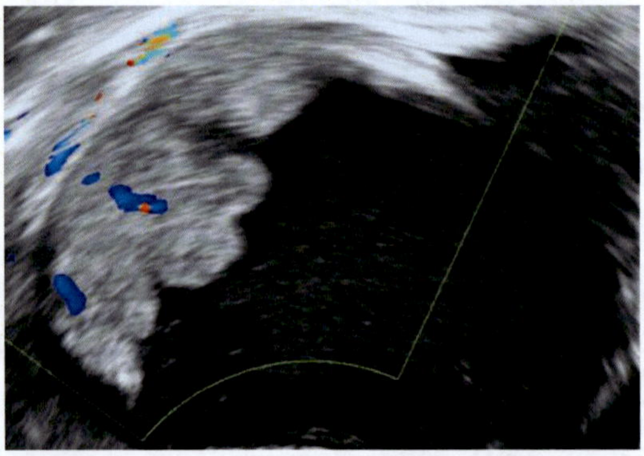

Figure 24. Serous borderline tumor.

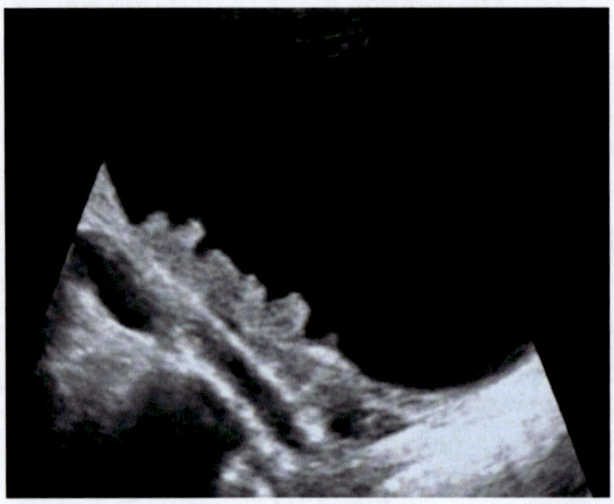

Figure 25. Mucinous endocervical borderline tumor.

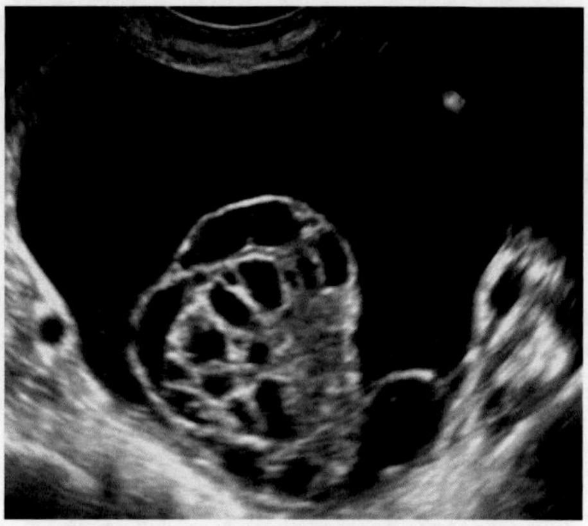

Figure 26. Mucinous gastrointestinal tumor.

Epithelial Tumors: Epithelial Adenocarcinoma

Clinical Presentation

These patients usually have vague symptoms of lower abdominal aching, bloating/distension, or vaginal bleeding. These women are typically postmenopausal.

Ultrasonographic Findings

Stage 1 primary invasive ovarian epithelial cancers versus stages 2–4 primary invasive ovarian epithelial cancers were larger, more likely to have papillary projections and were more often multilocular cysts. (Valentin et al., 2006) Advanced (Stage 2-4) tumors were more likely to be purely solid irregular tumors. On Doppler examination they tend to appear highly vascular. With increasing stage, ascites become more common.

- Predominately solid tumors with variable cystic component
- Often bilateral
- Poorly outlined boundaries
- Ipsilateral normal ovarian tissue not visible
- Evidence of necrosis
- Highly vascular on colour Doppler examination
- Immobile on palpation
- Ascites
- Tumor deposits
- Omental cake
- Involvement of other abdominal organs

Non-epithelial Malignant Tumors: Dysgerminomas, Immature Teratomas

Accounting for 10% malignant ovarian tumors, non-epithelial malignancies include malignant ovarian germ cell tumors (MOGCTs), sex cord-stromal tumors (SCSTs) and ovarian sarcomas. (Baker-Rand & Edey, 2021; Ray-Coquard et al., 2018)

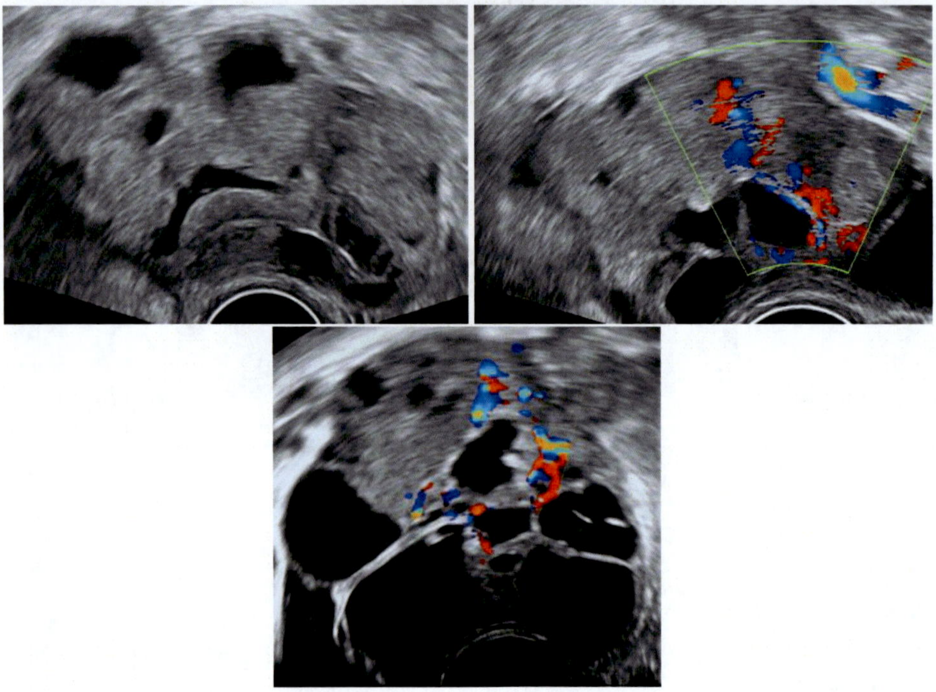

Figure 27. Epithelial adenocarcinoma.

Clinical Presentation

Dysgerminomas are uncommon malignant germ cell tumors with most occurring in women in their second and third decade. (Maniar & Vang, 2019) Women may be asymptomatic or may experience rapid abdominal distention due to rapid tumor growth. Patients may experience menstrual irregularities such as secondary amenorrhoea. Tumors may be hCG producing, mimicking a pregnancy and lactate dehydrogenase (LDH) levels may be raised.

Immature teratomas were found in women also in their second and third decade. In one series, half the women had a history of a benign mature teratoma in the past. Abdullahi (Abdullahi-Idle et al., 2020)

Ultrasonographic Findings

Dysgerminomas are large (median 118mm), solid (95%), highly vascular (score 3-4 [93%]) and lobulated. (Guerriero et al., 2011)

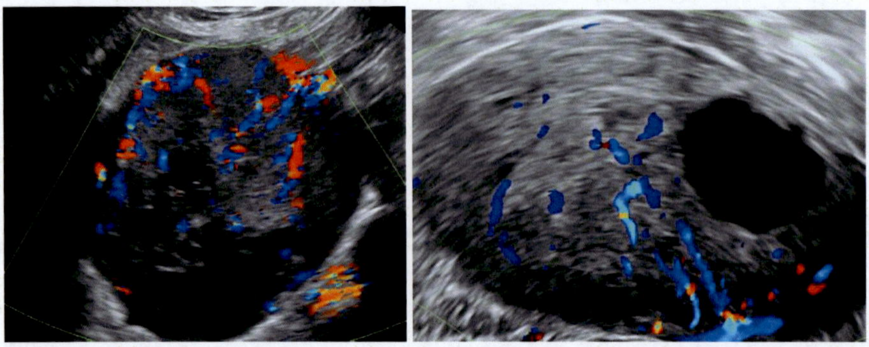

Figure 28. Dysgerminoma.

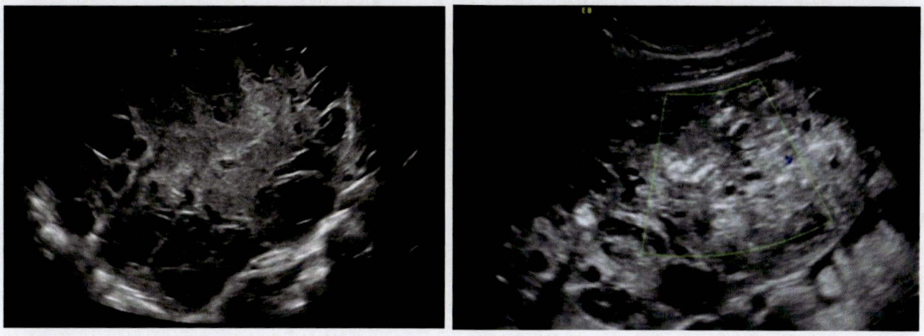

Figure 29. Immature teratoma.

*Immature teratomas*_were typically large (median 115mm), rapid growing, unilateral, unilocular-solid tumor. The solid component has been sound to be microcystic with evidence of fibrosis. Raised serum a-fetoprotein (aFP) levels were found in 42% of cases.

Metastatic

Clinical Presentation

These patients would often have a history of a previous malignancy. Most commonly found were intestine, stomach, breast and hematopoietic malignancies. (Lerwill & Young, 2019) Their symptoms were not dissimilar to those with a primary ovarian malignancy and usually constitutional or due to mass effect.

Ultrasonographic Findings

Over half (56%) of metastatic tumors are solid and highly vascular (score 3-4). (Valentin et al., 2006) They are well circumscribed and do not demonstrate local invasion as primary ovarian tumors do.

Ovarian metastases from lymphoma and stomach, breast and uterine primaries are usually solid. Colorectal and biliary tract metastases demonstrate varied morphological patterns with many being irregular and multilocular. (Testa et al., 2007)

- Well circumscribed
- Often bilateral
- Highly vascular

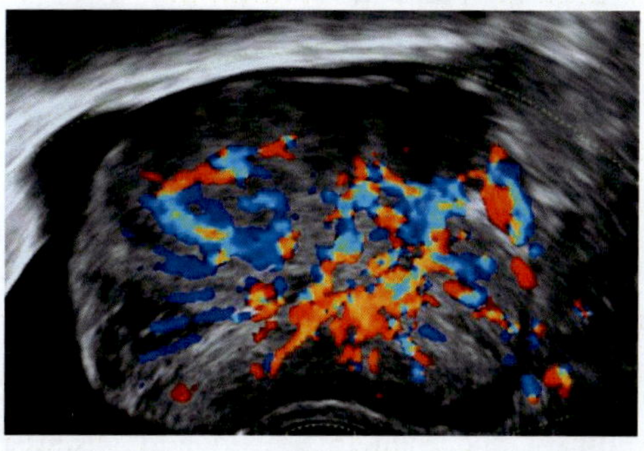

Figure 30. Metastatic ovarian tumor.

Non-ovarian: Tubal Structure

Clinical Presentation

This is variable and depends on whether it is an acute infective episode or a non-urgent incidental finding or part of fertility investigations.

Ultrasonographic Findings

Fimbrial cysts are typically small unilocular cysts which are usually seen near the ovaries. They are avascular and mobile.

Hydrosalpinges are caused by past pelvic infection resulting in chronic obstruction and dilation of the tube. They are sausage-shaped with incomplete septations and small papillary projections that are called "beads of a string". (Sayasneh et al., 2015)

- Sausage/snake shaped
- Incomplete septations
- 'Beads on a string'

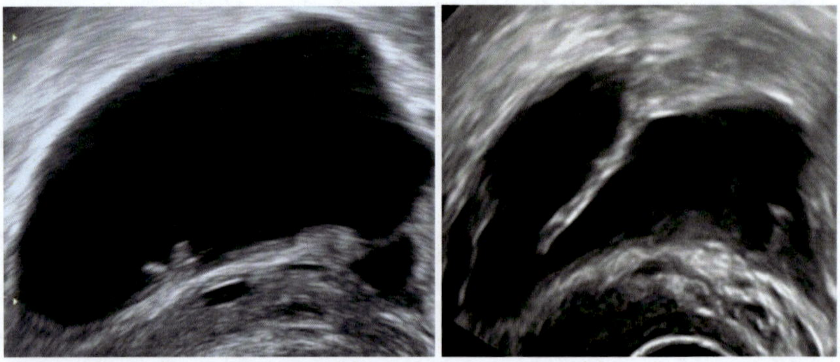

Figure 31. Hydrosalpinx.

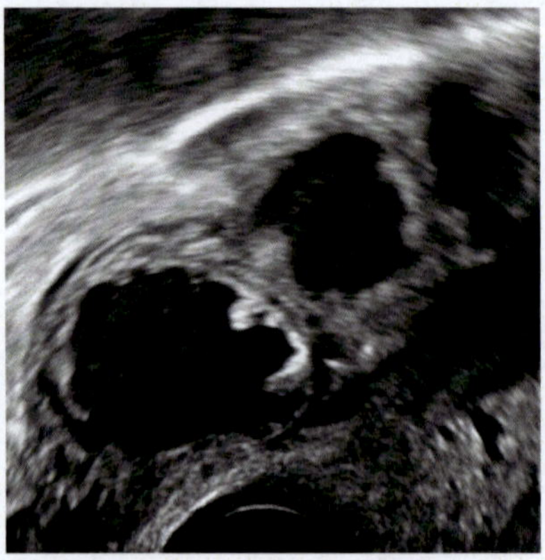

Figure 32. Early pelvic inflammatory disease.

In early pelvic inflammatory disease (PID) ultrasound features are subtle. First the fallopian tube becomes more prominent and then thickened and vascular. Later features include a pyosalpinx which show a ovoid or pear-shaped, dilated thick-walled tube with thickened endosalpingeal folds and echogenic fluid. (Timor-Tritsch et al., 1998) In cross section, this may demonstrate the "cog-wheel sign" and bright echogenic foci which can sometimes be confused for the hair in a dermoid cyst, which is in fact gas within the abscess. (Horrow, 2004)

- Ovoid or pear-shaped
- Thickened walls
- Echogenic fluid
- "Cog-wheel sign"
- Bright echogenic foci - gas

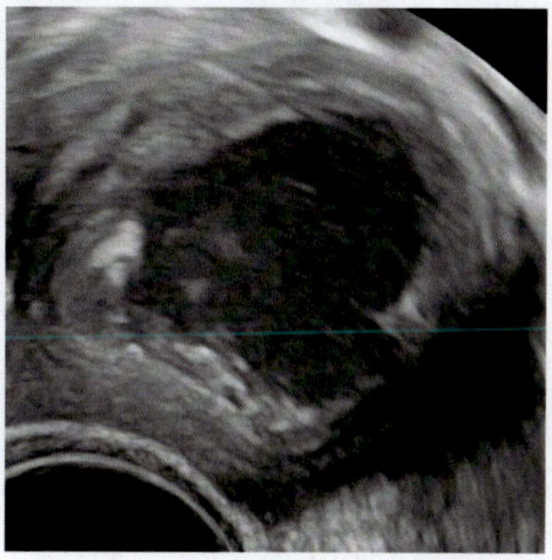

Figure 33. Tuboovarian abscess.

Non-ovarian: Tubal Cancer

Clinical Presentation

Constitutional and vague lower abdominal symptoms may prompt the examination that detects a tubal cancel but over half (62%) have been found to be asymptomatic. Patients are typically aged 55-60 years and tumors are typically unilateral.

Ultrasonographic Findings

A highly vascular ovoid or sausage-shaped predominantly solid, unilocular-solid or multi-locular solid tumors. (Ludovisi et al., 2014) Adjacent but separate normal ovary is usually found.

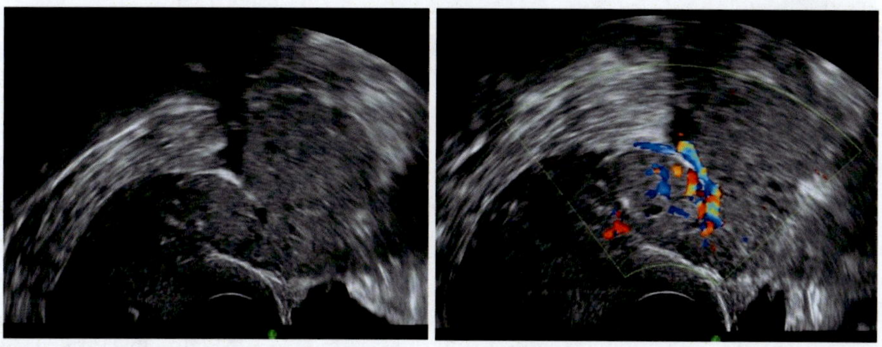

Figure 34. Tubal cancer.

Non-ovarian: Peritoneal Pseudocyst

Clinical Presentation

These patients almost always have a history of previous surgery, previous pelvic inflammatory disease (PID), endometriosis or other inflammatory condition in the pelvis such as inflammatory bowel disease, diverticulitis, or appendicitis. They cysts may be found in women with chronic pelvic pain, or they may be completely asymptomatic.

Ultrasonographic Findings

These cystic structures take the shape of the pelvic or may be very bizarrely shaped. Identifiable structures may be found within, such as the ovary and they may be unilocular or multilocular. These cysts will not move on palpation but a septation may 'flap' which is the "flapping sail sign". (Savelli et al., 2004; Ying et al., 2007)

- Take the shape of the pelvis, bizarre shapes
- Immobile
- Bizarre contents such as ovary in the middle
- Flapping sail sign
- History of endometriosis, pelvic infections, or past surgery

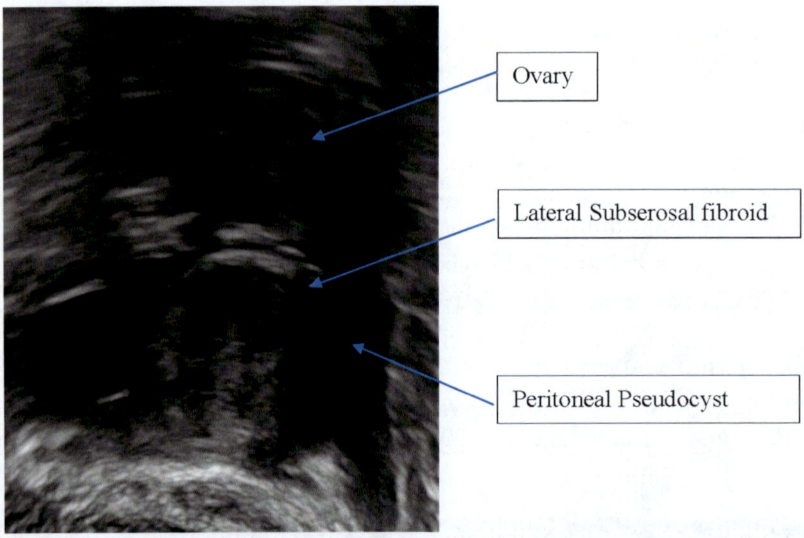

Figure 35. Peritoneal pseudocyst.

Alternative Diagnostic Tools

RMI

The Risk of Malignancy Index is a score calculated based on the menopausal status, a score calculated based on 5 ultrasound features and the serum CA-125 value in U/mL. (Geomini et al., 2009; Jacobs et al., 1990) A score of >200 suggests an increased risk of malignancy.

USS x M x CA-125 (U/mL)
USS - USS score (0, 1 or 3 for Bilateral, ascites, multilocular, solid, metastases)
M - Menopausal status (Pre-menopausal = 1, Postmenopausal = 3)

This is widely used but has some shortcomings. Once a woman is postmenopausal (score of 3) and has anything other than a simple cyst, she would often get an elevated score resulting in her being offered surgery and increasing her anxiety. (Nunes, 2017; Nunes et al., 2017)

International Ovarian Tumor Analysis (IOTA) Logistic Regression Models LR1 and LR2

These models are based on several ultrasound scan features along with personal history. (Testa et al., 2014; Timmerman et al., 2005) LR1 uses all 12 features while LR2 uses only six.

Table 1. IOTA LR1 and LR2

(1)	Personal history of ovarian cancer (yes=1, no=0)
(2)	Current hormonal therapy (yes=1, no=0)
(3)	Age in years
(4)	Maximum diameter of lesion (mm)
(5)	Pain during examination (yes=1, no=0)
(6)	Ascites present (yes=1, no=0)
(7)	Blood flow within solid papillary projections
(8)	Purely solid tumor (yes=1, no=0)
(9)	Maximum diameter of solid (mm) (max 50)
(10)	Irregular internal cyst wall (yes=1, no=0)
(11)	Acoustic shadows (yes=1, no=0)
(12)	Vascularity color score (1-4)

The probability of malignancy was calculated using the formula:

$y=1/(1+\exp-z)$

where $z=-\ 6.7468+1.5985\ (1)-0.9983\ (2)+0.0326\ (3)+0.00841\ (4)-0.8577\ (5)+1.5513\ (6)+1.1737\ (7)+0.9281\ (8)+0.0496\ (9)+1.1421\ (10)-2.3550\ (11)+0.4916\ (12)$

The probability y is dichotomized at a score of 0.1 to give a predictive diagnosis of cancer.

LR2 was calculated based on six of the above variables: (3), (6), (7), (9), (10) and (11). The formula to determine the probability of malignancy was:

$y=1/(1+\exp-z)$

where $z=-\ 5.3718+0.0354\ (3)+1.6159\ (6)+1.1768\ (7)+0.0697\ (9)+0.9586\ (10)-2.9486\ (11)$

The probability y is dichotomized at a score of 0.1 to give a predictive diagnosis of cancer.

LR1 And LR2 were shown to perform better than RMI with the area under the curve (AUC) of 0.930 (LR1), 0.918 (LR2) versus 0.875 (RMI).

In the less experienced ultrasound operator however, specificity was found to be reduced. (Nunes et al., 2013)

IOTA Simple Rules

The Simple Rules (SR) protocol was created to be based on ultrasound factors only. (Table 2) (Nunes et al., 2014; Timmerman et al., 2010; Timmerman et al., 2008)

Table 2. Simple rules

Malignant M-features	Benign B-features
1. Irregular solid tumor	1. Unilocular cyst
2. Ascites	2. Largest solid component is <7 mm in largest diameter
3. ≥ four papillary structures	3. Acoustic shadows
4. Irregular multilocular– solid tumor, largest diameter of ≥ 100 mm	4. Smooth multilocular tumor < 100 mm in largest diameter
5. Very high color content on color Doppler examination	5. No detectable blood flow on Doppler examination

If one or more benign features are present without any malignant features, then the tumor is defined as benign. If one or more malignant features are present without any benign features, then the tumor is defined as malignant. If no features are seen or if both malignant and benign features are observed, then the tumor is unclassified or indeterminate. The features were found to be absent in 11-24% patients in a meta-analysis. (Nunes et al., 2014) These patients would then need an alternative method of diagnosis.

When the tumor was classifiable, it was highly accurate with 93% sensitivity and 95% specificity. This was found to be particularly superior in asymptomatic post-menopausal women when an adnexal mass was found, when compared to the RMI protocol used by the Royal College of Obstetricians and Gynecologists. (Nunes et al., 2017)

ADNEX Model

The ADNEX model aims to distinguish between benign and borderline, FIGO Stage 1, FIGO Stage 2-4 and metastatic disease. (Berek et al., 2018) It uses three clinical predictors which are age, CA-125 and the centre. There are six additional ultrasound predictors which are maximum lesion diameter, % of solid tissue, >10 cyst locules, number of papillary projections, acoustic shadows, and ascites. The AUC was 0.943 (0.934 to 0.952) on the validation data. When using a cut-off of 10%, the sensitivity for malignancy was 96.5% and specificity 71.3%. (Van Calster et al., 2014; Van Calster et al., 2015)

O-RADS

The Ovarian-Adnexal Reporting and Data System (O-RADS) ultrasound risk stratification and management system was designed to determine if an adnexal mass is benign or malignant by categorizing its risk of malignancy, and to provide each of the six risk categories, a management recommendation plan. (Andreotti et al., 2020; Cao et al., 2021)

Table 3. O-RADS (Andreotti et al., 2020)

O-RADS Score/Category	Characterisation	Management
O-RADS 0	Incomplete evaluation	Repeat
O-RADS 1	The physiologic category (normal premenopausal ovary	Nothing
O-RADS 2	Almost certainly benign category (<1% risk of malignancy)	Depending on size and menopausal status: nothing, 8-12 week follow-up or one-year follow-up
O-RADS 3	Tumors with low risk of malignancy (1% to <10%)	Expert ultrasound operator or MRI
O-RADS 4	Tumors with intermediate risk of malignancy (10% to <50%)	Expert ultrasound operator or MRI Under Gynaecological oncologist
O-RADS 5	Tumors with high risk of malignancy (≥ 50%)	Under Gynaecological oncologist

The model is one used primarily in the United States of America, and it has pattern recognition at its core. Pattern recognition helps to detect and categorise the O-RADS 1 and O-RADS 2 tumors and when O-RADS 3 and O-RADS 4 are encountered, re-examination by an expert ultrasound operation is the first recommendation.

Conclusion

Ovarian/adnexal tumors are common findings, and the role of the ultrasound operator is to determine if the tumor is benign, borderline, or malignant. Pattern Recognition performs superiorly for all tumor types. Tumors and their typical appearances have been shown. When such expertise is not available, or there is uncertainty, there are many tools which can be utilised to classify the ovarian/adnexal tumors.

References

Abdullahi-Idle, S., Hayes, K., & Ross, J. A. (2020). Ultrasound features of immature ovarian teratomas- Case series and review of literature. *Ultrasound*, *28*(2), 82-90.

Andreotti, R. F., Timmerman, D., Strachowski, L. M., Froyman, W., Benacerraf, B. R., Bennett, G. L., ... Glanc, P. (2020). O-RADS US risk stratification and management system: A consensus guideline from the ACR ovarian-Adnexal Reporting and Data System committee. *Radiology*, *294*(1), 168-185. https://doi.org/10.1148/radiol.2019191150

Baker-Rand, H., & Edey, K. (2021). Nonepithelial ovarian cancers. *The Obstetrican and Gynaecologist*, *23*, 177-186. https://doi.org/10.1111/tog.12755

Balasa, R. W., Adcock, L. L., Prem, K. A., & Dehner, L. P. (1977). The Brenner tumor: a clinicopathologic review. *Obstetrics and gynecology*, *50*(1), 120-128.

Berek, J. S., Kehoe, S. T., Kumar, L., & Friedlander, M. (2018). Cancer of the ovary, fallopian tube, and peritoneum. Figo Cancer Report 2018. *International Journal of Gynecology and Obstetrics*, *143*, 59-78. https://doi.org/10.1002/ijgo.12614

Bjorkholm, E., & Pettersson, F. (1980). Granulosa-cell and theca-cell tumors. The clinical picture and long-term outcome for the Radiumhemmet series. *Acta Obstetricia et Gynecologica Scandinavica*, *59*(16), 361-365.

Bjørnø, L. (2017). Chapter 13 - Finite-Amplitude Waves. In T. H. Neighbors & D. Bradley (Eds.), *Applied Underwater Acoustics* (pp. 857-888). Elsevier. https://doi.org/https://doi.org/10.1016/B978-0-12-811240-3.00013-8

Cao, L., Wei, M., Liu, Y., Fu, J., Zhang, H., Huang, J., ... Zhou, J. (2021). Validation of American College of Radiology Ovarian-Adnexal Reporting and Data System Ultrasound (O-RADS US): Analysis on 1054 adnexal masses. *Gynecologic Oncology*, *162*(1), 107-112. https://doi.org/https://doi.org/10.1016/j.ygyno.2021.04.031

Chen, H., Liu, Y., Shen, L. f., Jiang, M. j., Yang, Z. f., & Fang, G. p. (2016). Ovarian thecoma-fibroma groups: clinical and sonographic features with pathological comparison. *Journal of Ovarian Research*, *9*(1), 1-7. https://doi.org/10.1186/s13048-016-0291-2

Demidov, V. N., Lipatenkova, J., Vikhareva, O., Holsbeke, V. C., Timmerman, D., & Valentin, L. (2008). Imaging of gynecological disease (2): clinical and ultrasound characteristics of Sertoli cell tumors, Sertoli-Leydig cell tumors and Leydig cell tumors. *Ultrasound in obstetrics & gynecology : the official journal of the International Society of Ultrasound in Obstetrics and Gynecology*, *31*(1), 85-91. https://doi.org/10.1002/uog.5227

Dierickx, I., Valentin, L., Holsbeke, V. C., Jacomen, G., Lissoni, A. A., Licameli, A., ... Timmerman, D. (2012). Imaging in gynecological disease (7): clinical and ultrasound features of Brenner tumors of the ovary. *Ultrasound in obstetrics & gynecology : the official journal of the International Society of Ultrasound in Obstetrics and Gynecology*, *40*(6), 706-713. https://doi.org/10.1002/uog.11149

Fox, H., Agrawal, K., & Langley, F. A. (1975). A clinicopathologic study of 92 cases of granulosa cell tumor of the ovary with special reference to the factors influencing prognosis. *Cancer*.

Franchi, D., Boveri, S., Fruscio, R., Fischerova, D., Guerriero, S., Moruzzi, M. C., ... Testa, A. C. (2013). Imaging in gynecological disease (8): ultrasound characteristics of recurrent borderline ovarian tumors. *Ultrasound in obstetrics & gynecology : the official journal of the International Society of Ultrasound in Obstetrics and Gynecology*, *41*(4), 452-458. https://doi.org/10.1002/uog.12276

Geomini, P., Kruitwagen, R., Bremer, G. L. L., Cnossen, J., & Mol, B. W. (2009). The accuracy of risk scores in predicting ovarian malignancy: a systematic review. *Obstetrics and gynecology*, *113*(2 Pt 1), 384-394. https://doi.org/10.1097/aog.0b013e318195ad17

Gotlieb, W. H., Chetrit, A., Menczer, J., Hirsh-Yechezkel, G., Lubin, F., Friedman, E., ... Ben-Baruch, G. (2005). Demographic and genetic characteristics of patients with borderline ovarian tumors as compared to early stage invasive ovarian cancer. *Gynecologic Oncology*, *97*(3), 780-783. https://doi.org/10.1016/j.ygyno.2005.02.022

Guerriero, S., Testa, A. C., Timmerman, D., Holsbeke, V. C., Ajossa, S., Fischerova, D., ... Valentin, L. (2011). Imaging of gynecological disease (6): clinical and ultrasound characteristics of ovarian dysgerminoma. *Ultrasound in obstetrics & gynecology : the official journal of the International Society of Ultrasound in Obstetrics and Gynecology*, *37*(5), 596-602. https://doi.org/10.1002/uog.8958

Holsbeke, V. C., Calster, V. B., Guerriero, S., Savelli, L., Paladini, D., Lissoni, A. A., ... Timmerman, D. (2010). Endometriomas: their ultrasound characteristics. *Ultrasound in Obstetrics & Gynecology*. https://doi.org/10.1002/uog.7668

Hoo, W. L., Yazbek, J., Holland, T., Mavrelos, D., Tong, E. N. C., & Jurkovic, D. (2010). Expectant management of ultrasonically diagnosed ovarian dermoid cysts: Is it possible to predict outcome? *Ultrasound in Obstetrics and Gynecology*, *36*(2), 235-240. https://doi.org/10.1002/uog.7610

Horrow, M. M. (2004). Ultrasound of Pelvic Inflammatory Disease. *Ultrasound Quarterly*, *20*(4).

Jacobs, I., Oram, D., Fairnks, J., Tuer, J., Frost, C., & Grudzinskas, J. G. (1990). A risk of malignancy index incorporating CA 125, ultrasound and menopausal status for the accurate preoperative diagnosis of ovarian cancer. *BJOG: An International Journal of Obstetrics & Gynaecology*, *97*(10), 922-929. https://doi.org/10.1111/j.1471-0528.1990.tb02448.x

Lerwill, M. F., & Young, R. H. (2019). Metastatic Tumors of the Ovary. In R. J. Kurman, L. H. Ellenson, & B. M. Ronnett (Eds.), *Blaustein's Pathology of the Female Genital Tract* (Seventh ed.). Springer Nature.

Levy, A. D., Arnáiz, J., Shaw, J. C., & Sobin, L. H. (2008). From the archives of the AFIP Primary peritoneal tumors: imaging features with pathologic correlation. *Radiographics*, *28*(2), 583-607. https://doi.org/10.1148/rg.282075175

Ludovisi, M., Blasis, D. I., Virgilio, B., Fischerova, D., Franchi, D., Pascual, M. A., ... Testa, A. C. (2014). Imaging in gynecological disease (9): clinical and ultrasound characteristics of tubal cancer. *Ultrasound in obstetrics & gynecology : the official journal of the International Society of Ultrasound in Obstetrics and Gynecology*, *43*(3), 328-335. https://doi.org/10.1002/uog.12570

Maniar, K. P., & Vang, R. (2019). Germ Cell Tumors of the Ovary. In R. J. Kurman & L. H. R. Ellenson, Brigitte M. (Eds.), *Blausteins Pathology of the Female Genital Tract* (Seventh ed., pp. 1047-1124). Springer Nature Switzerland. https://doi.org/10.1007/978-3-319-46334-6 (Springer)

Meigs, J. V. (1954). Fibroma of the ovary with ascites and hydrothorax—Meigs' syndrome. *American Journal of Obstetrics and Gynecology*, *67*(5), 962-987.

Meys, E. M. J., Kaijser, J., Kruitwagen, R. F. P. M., Slangen, B. F. M., Van Calster, B., Aertgeerts, B., ... Van Gorp, T. (2016). Subjective assessment versus ultrasound models to diagnose ovarian cancer: A systematic review and meta-analysis. *European Journal of Cancer*, *58*, 17-29. https://doi.org/10.1016/j.ejca.2016.01.007

Moro, F., Magoga, G., Pasciuto, T., Mascilini, F., Moruzzi, M. C., Fischerova, D., ... Testa, A. C. (2018). Imaging in gynecological disease (13): clinical and ultrasound characteristics of endometrioid ovarian cancer. *Ultrasound in obstetrics & gynecology*, *52*(4), 535-543. https://doi.org/10.1002/uog.19026

Nunes, N. (2017). *MD Thesis: Novel Approaches to Ultrasound Based Evaluation and Management of Adnexal Masses* READCUBE. http://scholar.google.com/scholar?q=MD Thesis&btnG=&hl=en&num=20&as_sdt=0%2C22

Nunes, N., Ambler, G., Foo, X., Naftalin, J., Derdelis, G., Widschwendter, M., & Jurkovic, D. (2017). Comparison of two protocols for the management of asymptomatic postmenopausal women with adnexal tumours-a randomised controlled trial of RMI/RCOG vs Simple Rules. *British Journal of Cancer*, *116*(5). https://doi.org/10.1038/bjc.2017.17

Nunes, N., Ambler, G., Foo, X., Naftalin, J., Widschwendter, M., & Jurkovic, D. (2014). Use of IOTA simple rules for diagnosis of ovarian cancer: Meta-analysis. *Ultrasound in Obstetrics and Gynecology*, *44*(5). https://doi.org/10.1002/uog.13437

Nunes, N., Ambler, G., Foo, X., Widschwendter, M., & Jurkovic, D. (2018). Prospective evaluation of IOTA logistic regression models LR1 and LR2 in comparison with subjective pattern recognition for diagnosis of ovarian cancer in an outpatient setting. *Ultrasound in Obstetrics and Gynecology*, *51*(6). https://doi.org/10.1002/uog.18918

Nunes, N., Ambler, G., Hoo, W. L., Naftalin, J., Foo, X., Widschwendter, M., & Jurkovic, D. (2013). A prospective validation of the IOTA logistic regression models (LR1 and LR2) in comparison to subjective pattern recognition for the diagnosis of ovarian cancer. *International Journal of Gynecological Cancer*, *23*(9). https://doi.org/10.1097/IGC.0b013e3182a6171a

Paladini, D., Testa, A., Holsbeke, V. C., Mancari, R., Timmerman, D., & Valentin, L. (2009). Imaging in gynecological disease (5): clinical and ultrasound characteristics in fibroma and fibrothecoma of the ovary. *Ultrasound in obstetrics & gynecology : the official journal of the International Society of Ultrasound in Obstetrics and Gynecology*, *34*(2), 188-195. https://doi.org/10.1002/uog.6394

Patel, M. D., Feldstein, V. A., Lipson, S. D., Chen, D. C., & Filly, R. A. (1998). Cystic teratomas of the ovary: Diagnostic value of sonography. *American Journal of Roentgenology*, *171*(4), 1061-1065. https://doi.org/10.2214/ajr.171.4.9762997

Pateman, K., Moro, F., Mavrelos, D., Foo, X., Hoo, W. L., & Jurkovic, D. (2014). Natural history of ovarian endometrioma in pregnancy. *BMC Women's Health*, *14*(1), 1-6. https://doi.org/10.1186/1472-6874-14-128

Peterson, W. F., Prevost, E. C., Edmunds, F. T., Hundley, J. M., & Morris, F. K. (1955). Benign Cystic Teratomas of the Ovary: A Clinico-statistical Study of 1,007 Cases With a Review of the Literature. *American Journal of Obstetrics and Gynecology*, *70*(2), 368-382. https://doi.org/10.1016/S0002-9378(16)37681-5

Qi, Z., Zhang, Y., Dai, Q., Xia, Y., & Jiang, Y. (2017). Peritoneal Carcinomatosis in Primary Ovarian Cancer: Ultrasound Detection and Comparison with Computed Tomography. *Ultrasound Med Biol*, *43*(9), 1811-1819. https://doi.org/10.1016/j.ultrasmedbio.2017.02.016

Ray-Coquard, I., Morice, P., Lorusso, D., Prat, J., Oaknin, A., Pautier, P., & Colombo, N. (2018). Non-epithelial ovarian cancer: ESMO Clinical Practice Guidelines for diagnosis, treatment and follow-up. *Annals of Oncology*, *29*(October), iv1-iv18. https://doi.org/10.1093/annonc/mdy001

Sahin, H., Abdullazade, S., & Sanci, M. (2017). Mature cystic teratoma of the ovary: a cutting edge overview on imaging features. *Insights into Imaging*, *8*(2), 227-241. https://doi.org/10.1007/s13244-016-0539-9

Savelli, L., De Iaco, P., Ghi, T., Bovicelli, L., Rosati, F., & Cacciatore, B. (2004). Transvaginal sonographic appearance of peritoneal pseudocysts. *Ultrasound in Obstetrics and Gynecology*, *23*(3), 284-288. https://doi.org/10.1002/uog.986

Savelli, L., Testa, A. C., Timmerman, D., Paladini, D., Ljungberg, O., & Valentin, L. (2008). Imaging of gynecological disease (4): clinical and ultrasound characteristics of struma ovarii. *Ultrasound in Obstetrics & Gynecology*, *32*(2), 210-219. https://doi.org/10.1002/uog.5396

Sayasneh, A., Ekechi, C., Ferrara, L., Kaijser, J., Stalder, C., Sur, S., ... Bourne, T. (2015). The characteristic ultrasound features of specific types of ovarian pathology (review). *International journal of oncology*, *46*(2), 445-458. https://doi.org/10.3892/ijo.2014.2764

Seidman, J. D., Ronnett, B. M., Shih, I.-M., Cho, K. R., & Kurman, R. J. (2019). Epithelial Tumors of the Ovary. In R. J. Kurman, L. H. Ellenson, & B. M. Ronnett (Eds.), *Blaustein's Pathology of the Female Genital Tract* (Seventh ed.). Springer Nature.

Testa, A., Kaijser, J., Wynants, L., Fischerova, D., Holsbeke, V. C., Franchi, D., ... Timmerman, D. (2014). Strategies to diagnose ovarian cancer: new evidence from phase 3 of the multicentre international IOTA study. *British journal of cancer*, *111*(4), 680-688. https://doi.org/10.1038/bjc.2014.333

Testa, A. C., Ferrandina, G., Timmerman, D., Savelli, L., Ludovisi, M., Holsbeke, V. C., ... Valentin, L. (2007). Imaging in gynecological disease (1): ultrasound features of metastases in the ovaries differ depending on the origin of the primary tumor. *Ultrasound in obstetrics & gynecology : the official journal of the International Society of Ultrasound in Obstetrics and Gynecology*, *29*(5), 505-511. https://doi.org/10.1002/uog.4020

Testa, A. C., Timmerman, D., Holsbeke, V. C., Zannoni, G. F., Fransis, S., Moerman, P., ... Ferrandina, G. (2011). Ovarian cancer arising in endometrioid cysts: ultrasound findings. *Ultrasound in Obstetrics & Gynecology*, *38*(1), 99-106. https://doi.org/10.1002/uog.8970

Timmerman, D., Ameye, L., Fischerova, D., Epstein, E., Melis, G. B., Guerriero, S., ... Valentin, L. (2010). Simple ultrasound rules to distinguish between benign and malignant adnexal masses before surgery: prospective validation by IOTA group. *BMJ (Clinical research ed.)*, *341*. https://doi.org/10.1136/bmj.c6839

Timmerman, D., Planchamp, F., Bourne, T., Landolfo, C., du Bois, A., Chiva, L., ... Fotopoulou, C. (2021). ESGO/ISUOG/IOTA/ESGE Consensus Statement on preoperative diagnosis of ovarian tumors. *Ultrasound in Obstetrics and Gynecology*. https://doi.org/10.1002/uog.23635

Timmerman, D., Testa, A. C., Bourne, T., Ameye, L., Jurkovic, D., Holsbeke, V. C., ... Valentin, L. (2008). Simple ultrasound-based rules for the diagnosis of ovarian cancer. *Ultrasound in obstetrics & gynecology : the official journal of the International Society of Ultrasound in Obstetrics and Gynecology*, *31*(6), 681-690. https://doi.org/10.1002/uog.5365

Timmerman, D., Testa, A. C., Bourne, T., Ferrazzi, E., Ameye, L., Konstantinovic, M. L., ... Valentin, L. (2005). Logistic Regression Model to Distinguish Between the Benign and Malignant Adnexal Mass Before Surgery: A Multicenter Study by the International Ovarian Tumor Analysis Group. *Journal of Clinical Oncology*, *23*(34), 8794-8801. https://doi.org/10.1200/jco.2005.01.7632

Timmerman, D., Valentin, L., Bourne, T. H., Collins, W. P., Verrelst, H., & Vergote, I. (2000). Terms, definitions and measurements to describe the sonographic features of adnexal tumors: a consensus opinion from the International Ovarian Tumor Analysis (IOTA) group. *Ultrasound in Obstetrics & Gynecology*, *16*(5), 500-505. https://doi.org/10.1046/j.1469-0705.2000.00287.x

Timor-Tritsch, I. E., Lerner, J. P., Monteagudo, A., Murphy, K. E., & Heller, D. S. (1998). Transvaginal sonographic markers of tubal inflammatory disease. *Ultrasound in Obstetrics & Gynecology*, *12*(1), 56-66. https://doi.org/https://doi.org/10.1046/j.1469-0705.1998.12010056.x

Valentin, L. (1999). Pattern recognition of pelvic masses by gray-scale ultrasound imaging: The contribution of Doppler ultrasound. *Ultrasound in Obstetrics and Gynecology, 14*(5), 338-347. https://doi.org/10.1046/j.1469-0705.1999.14050338.x

Valentin, L. (2004). Use of morphology to characterize and manage common adnexal masses. *Best practice & research. Clinical obstetrics & gynaecology, 18*(1), 71-89. https://doi.org/10.1016/j.bpobgyn.2003.10.002

Valentin, L., Ameye, L., Franchi, D., Guerriero, S., Jurkovic, D., Savelli, L., ... Timmerman, D. (2013). Risk of malignancy in unilocular cysts: a study of 1148 adnexal masses classified as unilocular cysts at transvaginal ultrasound and review of the literature. *Ultrasound in obstetrics & gynecology : the official journal of the International Society of Ultrasound in Obstetrics and Gynecology, 41*(1), 80-89. https://doi.org/10.1002/uog.12308

Valentin, L., Ameye, L., Testa, A., Lécuru, F., Bernard, J.-P., Paladini, D., ... Timmerman, D. (2006). Ultrasound characteristics of different types of adnexal malignancies. *Gynecologic Oncology, 102*(1), 41-48. https://doi.org/https://doi.org/10.1016/j.ygyno.2005.11.015

Van Calster, B., Hoorde, K., Valentin, L., Testa, A. C., Fischerova, D., Holsbeke, C., ... Group, I. (2014). Evaluating the risk of ovarian cancer before surgery using the ADNEX model to differentiate between benign, borderline, early and advanced stage invasive, and secondary metastatic tumours: prospective multicentre diagnostic study. *BMJ (Clinical research ed.), 349*. https://doi.org/10.1136/bmj.g5920

Van Calster, B., Hoorde, V. K., Froyman, W., Kaijser, J., Wynants, L., Landolfo, C., ... Timmerman, D. (2015). Practical guidance for applying the ADNEX model from the IOTA group to discriminate between different subtypes of adnexal tumors. *Facts, views & vision in ObGyn, 7*(1), 32-41.

Van Holsbeke, C., Domali, E., Holland, T. K., Achten, R., Testa, A. C., Valentin, L., ... Timmerman, D. (2008). Imaging of gynecological disease (3): clinical and ultrasound characteristics of granulosa cell tumors of the ovary. *Ultrasound in Obstetrics & Gynecology, 31*(4), 450-456. https://doi.org/10.1002/uog.5279

Van Holsbeke, C., Zhang, J., Van Belle, V., Paladini, D., Guerriero, S., Czekierdowski, A., ... Timmerman, D. (2010). Acoustic streaming cannot discriminate reliably between endometriomas and other types of adnexal lesion: a multicenter study of 633 adnexal masses [https://doi.org/10.1002/uog.7537]. *Ultrasound in Obstetrics & Gynecology, 35*(3), 349-353. https://doi.org/https://doi.org/10.1002/uog.7537

Weinberger, V., Kadlecová, J., Minář, L., Felsinger, M., Anton, M., Ovesná, P., ... Zikán, M. (2018). Struma ovarii - ultrasound features of a rare tumor mimicking ovarian cancer. *Medical Ultrasonography, 20*(3), 355-361. https://doi.org/10.11152/mu-1526

Yazbek, J., Ameye, L., Testa, A. C., Valentin, L., Timmerman, D., Holland, T. K., ... Jurkovic, D. (2010). Confidence of expert ultrasound operators in making a diagnosis of adnexal tumor: effect on diagnostic accuracy and interobserver agreement. *Ultrasound in obstetrics & gynecology : the official journal of the International Society of Ultrasound in Obstetrics and Gynecology, 35*(1), 89-93. https://doi.org/10.1002/uog.7335

Yazbek, J., Aslam, N., Tailor, A., Hillaby, K., Raju, K. S., & Jurkovic, D. (2006). A comparative study of the risk of malignancy index and the ovarian crescent sign for the diagnosis of invasive ovarian cancer. *Ultrasound in Obstetrics & Gynecology, 28*(3), 320-324. https://doi.org/10.1002/uog.2842

Yazbek, J., Raju, K. S., Ben-Nagi, J., Holland, T., Hillaby, K., & Jurkovic, D. (2007). Accuracy of ultrasound subjective 'pattern recognition' for the diagnosis of borderline ovarian tumors. *Ultrasound in Obstetrics & Gynecology, 29*(5), 489-495. https://doi.org/10.1002/uog.4002

Ying, W., Y. Li, Y. Z., & Xie, X. (2007). Cyst distortion: a new sonographic sign of peritoneal pseudocyst with regular morphology. *Ultrasound in Obstetrics and Gynecology, 29*(2), 239-240. https://doi.org/10.1002/uog.3926

Yoo, S.-C., Chang, K.-H., Lyu, M.-O., Chang, S.-J., Ryu, H.-S., & Kim, H.-S. (2008). Clinical characteristics of struma ovarii. *Journal of Gynecologic Oncology, 19*(2), 135-135. https://doi.org/10.3802/jgo.2008.19.2.135

Chapter 4

Preoperative Biomarkers to Predict Resectability of Patients with Ovarian Cancer

Valerio Mais[1,*], MD, PhD
Michele Peiretti[1], MD, PhD
Daniela Fanni[2], MD, PhD
Maria Luisa Fais[1], MD
Giulia Carboni[1], MD
Giuseppe Deo[1], MD
Giuseppina Fais[1], MD
and Stefano Angioni[1], MD, PhD
[1]Department of Surgical Sciences, Division of Gynecology and Obstetrics, University of Cagliari, Cagliari, Italy
[2]Department of Medical Sciences and Public Health, Division of Pathology, University of Cagliari, Cagliari, Italy

Introduction

This chapter aims to analyze state-of-the-art methods of using circulating levels of tumor markers in the preoperative assessment of the resectability of advanced-stage ovarian cancer. First, we highlighted how the prognosis of the tumor depends on the resectability of the tumor. Subsequently, we observed that the resectability of the tumor depends on the surgical ability of the center where the patient is operated on, in addition to the characteristics of the tumor itself and the individual patient. Finally, we examined the different predictive models proposed by various authors over time to predict the resectability of the tumor before planning a laparotomy to obtain optimal cytoreduction. Then, we analyzed the reliability of the various models that incorporate tumor biomarkers.

* Corresponding Author's Email: gineca.vmais@tiscali.it.

In: Ovarian Cancer
Editors: Christos Iavazzo, Alexandros Fotiou and John Spiliotis
ISBN: 979-8-88697-633-5

Ovarian Cancer

Epidemiology

Ovarian cancers account for 15-20% of all ovarian masses and in 90% of cases they are diagnosed in women over the age of 40 [1, 2]. The incidence of ovarian cancer varies according to the geographic area, with higher percentages in Europe and North America [2].

Histology

Ovarian cancer can arise from the surface epithelium, follicles or cortical stroma and oocytes [1]. Epithelial cancers represent 90% of ovarian cancers. They are derived from the ovarian surface epithelium of mesothelial origin. They are classified according to the cell type: serous, mucinous, endometrioid, clear cell, or transitional [1].

High-grade serous carcinoma is the most common histotype of ovarian cancer, and in the majority of cases, it occurs at an advanced stage. Bilateral involvement of the ovaries is observed in approximately 70% of cases (Figure 1), and cancers limited to the ovaries at the time of diagnosis are very rare [3, 4]. The average size of this neoplasm is often smaller than that observed in other ovarian carcinomas but high-grade serous carcinoma usually shows a greater propensity for extraovarian dissemination and extensive involvement of the omentum (Figure 2). Histologically, these are papillary and solid growth neoplasms with associated glandular-like formations. The cancer cells usually show a marked pleomorphism, with intermediate to mononuclear giant cells with prominent nucleoli. Their mitotic activity is generally high [5, 6].

Transitional carcinoma represents a variant of serous carcinoma characterized histologically by the presence of solid nests and papillary formations lined with urothelial-like cells with marked cytonuclear atypia, evident nucleoli and a clear granular cytoplasm [3].

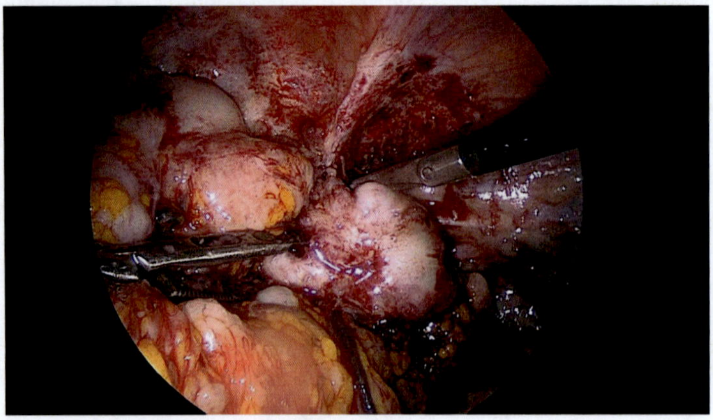

Figure 1. Bilateral involvement of the ovaries in high-grade serous carcinoma.

Low-grade serous carcinoma accounts for less than 5% of ovarian cancers. Histologically, these tumors show papillary structures lined with tumor cells with small and uniform nuclei associated with a variably hyalinized stroma in the context of which psammomatous bodies are observed. “Low-grade” nuclear characteristics and a low mitotic index are fundamental parameters for distinguishing between low- and high-grade serous carcinoma [2, 5, 6].

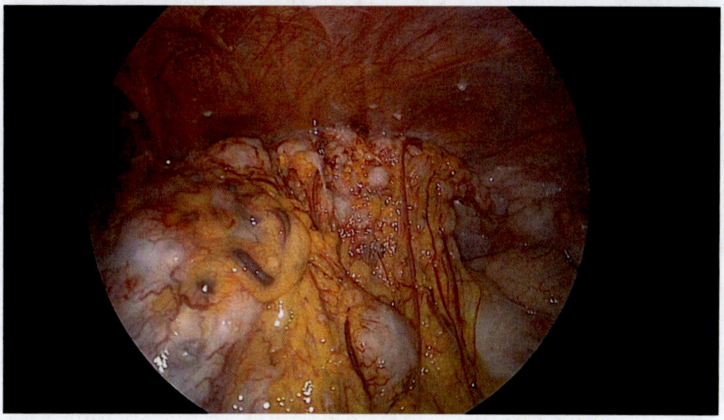

Figure 2. Extensive involvement of the omentum in high-grade serous carcinoma.

Mucinous tumors account for 10-15% of all ovarian tumors and they are mostly benign or borderline [3, 7, 8]. Primary mucinous ovarian cancers are very rare, and once the possibility of ovarian metastasis is excluded, especially from the gastrointestinal tract, only 3-4% of all ovarian cancers can be considered primary mucinous carcinomas [7, 8]. These neoplastic cells resemble cells in the gastric, intestinal or endocervical epithelium, although the majority of these carcinomas present themselves with gastric or small intestinal differentiation [7, 8]. The presence of a large mass and one-sidedness of the neoplasm are currently the main parameters to differentiate primitive mucinous ovarian cancer from metastasis (Figure 3). Furthermore, primary mucinous cancers are usually confined to the ovary and do not involve the ovarian surface [8]. Mucinous carcinomas are typically heterogeneous lesions where benign areas, borderline areas, areas of intraepithelial carcinoma and frankly invasive areas coexist in the context of the same neoplasm. Consequently, extensive macroscopic sampling is essential to formulate a correct diagnosis [8].

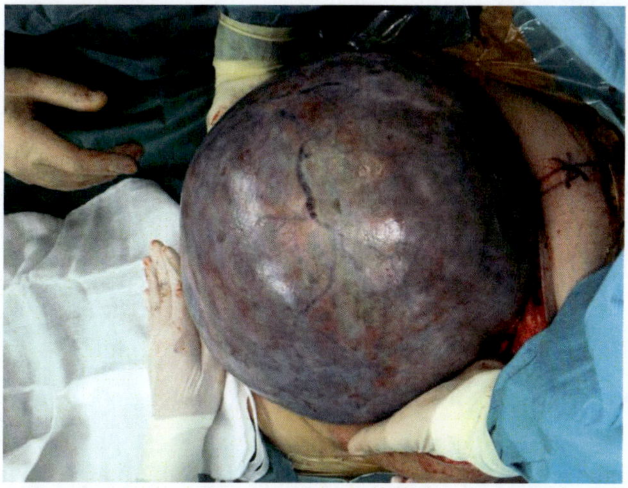

Figure 3. Primitive mucinous ovarian cancer.

Endometrioid ovarian cancers resemble their uterine counterparts; they represent 10% of all ovarian cancers, arise in women in the perimenopausal period and are often diagnosed at an early stage [3]. Histologically, these are low-grade adenocarcinomas that are frequently associated with outbreaks of ovarian or pelvic endometriosis and with areas of endometrioid adenofibroma or borderline endometrioid tumor [3, 9]. According to recent studies, even carcinomas defined as "seromucinous" represent variants of endometrioid carcinoma with mucinous differentiation [3, 10].

Clear cell carcinoma represents 10% of ovarian cancers, and usually occur in FIGO Stage I or II [3]. A close association with endometriosis has also been demonstrated for these neoplasms, and moreover, it has been shown that patients have a favorable prognosis in cases with an association with endometriosis [3, 11]. Upon microscopic examination, the main feature of these neoplasms is the presence of clear cytoplasmic cells associated with hobnail-type cells with eccentric and round nuclei [3, 12]. In any case, the diagnosis of clear cell carcinoma cannot be based exclusively on finding these characteristic cells that can also be observed in other histotypes. The main diagnostic parameters are the presence of multiple papillary formations, dense eosinophilic-hyaline material that expand from the center of the papillae, and hyaline blood cells [3, 12]. Although clear cell carcinomas are considered to be high-grade carcinomas, Stage IA patients have a relatively favorable outcome with five-year survival rates of 80-90%. Conversely, advanced cancers are associated with a poor prognosis [3, 12, 13].

Prognosis

The main prognostic factor in ovarian cancer is the stage of the disease at the time of diagnosis. The overall 5-year survival of patients with malignant epithelial tumors of the ovary is approximately 50%. The 5-year survival in Stage I is 70-90%, in Stage II it is 50-60%, in Stage III it is 20-40% and in Stage IV it is 10%. If the cancer is confined to the ovary, 5-year survival reaches 90% [14].

The prognostic factors with recognized importance in the early stages of the disease are the histological degree of differentiation (especially in Stage I); the substage (with particular attention to preoperative rupture of the cyst); the patient's age; the histological subtype; extracapsular growth; and the presence of ascites [15].

In the advanced stages of the disease, factors associated with a poor prognosis are mucinous histology, which in the advanced stages is often associated with a reduced probability of a response to first-line therapy with platinum; clear cell histology, which is characterized by a reduced sensitivity to platinum treatments; and residual disease after primary surgery [16-18].

Resectability

Cytoreductive Surgery

First instance cytoreductive surgery, primary debulking surgery or PDS is the most important step in the treatment of patients with advanced ovarian cancer. The procedures to be performed always include total extra fascial hysterectomy with bilateral adnexectomy; total omentectomy; appendectomy (only in mucinous carcinomas); removal of all of the pelvic and aortic bulky lymph nodes; and the removal of all macroscopically visible disease. Sometimes, to perform adequate surgical treatment, these patients must also undergo the removal of parts of the gastrointestinal system or the spleen and diaphragm, which are often involved in the disease (Figure 4). Numerous studies and recent meta-analyses have definitively confirmed that postsurgical tumor residue is an independent prognostic factor [17, 18]. Overall survival and disease-free survival correlate with residual cancer after primary surgery. The definition of optimal cytoreduction has changed several times over the years, and today, most authors consider cytoreduction with macroscopically absent residual tumor to be optimal [18, 19]. To achieve optimal cytoreduction, extensive upper abdominal surgery should be performed if necessary [20].

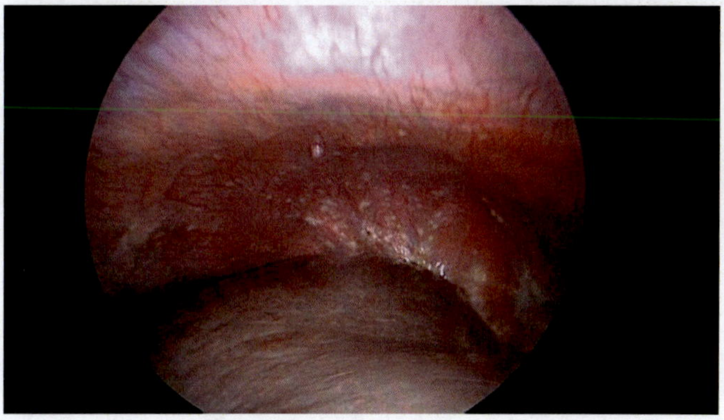

Figure 4. Diaphragmatic involvement in high-grade serous carcinoma.

Neoadjuvant Chemotherapy Followed by Interval Debulking Surgery

If complete primary debulking surgery (PDS) is impossible, surgical therapy can be used later after the start of chemotherapy treatment. This therapeutic strategy is defined as "neoadjuvant chemotherapy (NACT) followed by interval debulking surgery (IDS)." This strategy has the main objective of reducing the neoplastic mass in advanced tumors to decrease the risk of perioperative complications. In the past, a randomized study by the EORTC concluded that interval surgery performed after 3 cycles of platinum-based chemotherapy was able to increase survival [21]. In contrast, the GOG 152 study did not show an advantage in performing interval surgery in patients undergoing suboptimal cytoreduction when the first surgical approach was performed by an experienced oncologist gynecologist who had performed the maximum surgical resection [22]. Two phase III randomized studies (EORTC-55971 and CHORUS trial) have recently been published that do not show substantial differences in terms of OS and PFS between primary surgery and interval surgery. However, the considerable bias in the studies in question, including the low percentage of reported optimal cytoreduction as well as the heterogeneity of the surgical background of the centers involved, makes it difficult to draw definitive conclusions [23, 24].

Complete Resection of All Visible Disease Is the Goal of Surgical Treatment

The performance of incomplete surgery (first surgery or interval surgery) must be discouraged. Primary surgery is recommended in patients amenable to complete surgical resection with macroscopically absent residual disease and with an acceptable complication rate. The contradictions for abdominal cytoreduction are diffuse and deep infiltration of the mesentery root, diffuse carcinomatosis of the small intestine, infiltration of the hepatic hilum, and multiple hepatic intraparenchymal localizations of disease [21-24].

Ovarian cancer surgery should be reserved for expert centers of oncological gynecology and surgeons with adequate experience; in fact, some studies have shown an increase in survival and the primary cytoreduction rate in patients with ovarian cancer operated on in reference centers [25]. The patient's condition (ASA status) and the extent of the disease affect the ability to achieve optimal cytoreduction [26]. However, this result is strongly influenced by surgical effort [26]. The models for predicting optimal surgical outcomes based only on the characteristics of the tumor and the patient are therefore also dependent on the available level of surgical practice; therefore, their usefulness in patient selection for a primary nontraditional approach to ovarian cancer must be assessed with caution [25, 26].

Preoperative Assessment of Resectability

As previously stated, complete resection of all visible disease is the aim of surgery for the treatment of ovarian cancer, and incomplete surgery should be avoided. For this reason, the efforts of many researchers has focused on the identification of clinical, radiological and laboratory preoperative parameters that could reliably predict which patients could be operated on with a good probability of obtaining optimal cytoreduction [27-30].

Preoperative Imaging

Computed Tomography (CT)

Some authors have proposed predictive models of the possibility of achieving optimal debulking based on the interpretation of images obtained with computed tomography [31-35]. Depending on the authors, the models include the measurement/evaluation of peritoneal thickening, peritoneal implants, ascites, the involvement of the small and large intestine, involvement of the omentum, involvement of the mesentery, involvement of the suprarenal para-aortic lymph nodes, involvement of the diaphragm, liver and splenic lesions, and involvement of the root of the superior mesenteric artery [31-35]. Unfortunately, few studies have shown a high predictive value after undergoing external validation [28, 29].

Magnetic Resonance Imaging (MRI)

Preoperative assessment of resectability based only on CT images is often incomplete because CT may not show small metastatic lesions and cannot clearly distinguish malignant from benign lesions [28, 29]. MRI can offer more detailed images and better identify relationships between various structures and surrounding tissues [28, 29]. Some authors have therefore proposed predictive models based on images obtained with preoperative MRI examinations [36-38]. For models based on CT and MRI images, scores are assigned based on the evaluation of peritoneal thickening, peritoneal implants, ascites, involvement of the small and large intestine, involvement of the omentum, involvement of the mesentery, involvement of the suprarenal para-aortic lymph nodes, involvement of the diaphragm, liver and splenic lesions, and involvement of the root of the superior mesenteric artery [36-38]. Michielsen et al. described improved sensitivity and specificity of MRI compared to CT in predicting the risk of suboptimal debulking [38].

Positron Emission Tomography (PET)/CT

PET/CT identifies tissues with increased metabolism, such as tumor tissues. For this reason, predictive models of suboptimal debulking based on interpretations of PET images have been proposed [39-42]. These models have included PET/CT findings of the diaphragm, ascites, peritoneal carcinomatosis, small bowel mesentery implants, involvement of the hepatic hilum, and involvement of the mesenteric root [39-42]. The sensitivity and specificity of PET in predicting suboptimal cytoreduction varies, depending on the authors, from 51% to 100% for the first and from 88% to 100% for the second [39-42].

Laparoscopic Assessment

Rationale

The rationale behind applying diagnostic laparoscopy before performing primary laparotomy cytoreduction is based on several reflections. Unnecessary laparotomies should be avoided because they would not result in optimal cytoreduction. After laparoscopy, it is possible to proceed immediately with neoadjuvant chemotherapy if the patient is not a candidate for optimal first-instance cytoreductive surgery. However, it is also possible to obtain tissue samples for histological typing of ovarian cancer by laparoscopy.

First Attempts

The first study that retrospectively compared the use of laparoscopy before the start of a possible laparotomy in patients with ovarian cancer judged unresectable after preoperative radiological evaluation dates back to 1998 [43].

A Laparoscopic Score to Predict Optimal Primary Cytoreduction

Subsequent studies by Fagotti et al. [44-47] led to the proposal and progressive validation of the predictive index value (PIV) based on objective parameters obtainable with laparoscopy performed before any primary cytoreduction. The laparoscopic parameters used to derive the PIV were the extent of peritoneal carcinomatosis, the extent of diaphragmatic involvement, mesenteric infiltration, omental pathology, intestinal infiltration, stomach infiltration and liver metastases.

Validation of the Laparoscopic Score

A systematic review published in 2019 concluded that although there were some concerns about the heterogeneity of the studies included in the review, laparoscopic assessment may be an effective diagnostic tool in predicting the risk of residual gross disease after laparotomy for primary cytoreductive surgery [48].

Biomarkers

CA-125

CA-125 (Cancer Antigen 125) is a high molecular weight glycoprotein recognized by a monoclonal antibody (OC 125) obtained in 1981 by immunizing BALB/c mice with a papillary ovarian serous cyst adenocarcinoma cell line (OVCA 433) [49]. CA-125 is expressed by epithelial ovarian tumors as well as by other tissues of Mullerian origin [49]. Serum levels of CA-125 were initially described as typically elevated in more than 80% of patients with ovarian cancer and as being capable of reflecting the clinical evolution of neoplastic disease [49]. However, limitations related to the uncritical use of this biomarker also emerged later, since it can be elevated even in nonneoplastic conditions [49].

HE4

Human epididymal protein 4 (human epididymis protein 4, HE4) is also known as "epididymal secretory protein E4" and it belongs to the family of protease inhibitors called "whey acidic protein four-disulfide core domain (WFDC) proteins." It was initially described as a specific protein of the human epididymis and proposed as a marker of this tissue, assuming its involvement in the sperm maturation process. The genomic sequence coding for the WFDC family of proteins is present at the level of chromosome 20 [50, 51]. It was subsequently shown that this protein is also expressed by the vas deferens, respiratory epithelium, salivary glands, and distal tubule of the kidney and by the normal glandular epithelium of the female genital system but not by the superficial ovarian tissue. The genomic sequence encoding the WFDC family of proteins was then also found to be amplified in various pathological situations, such as carcinoma of the colon, stomach, pancreas, oral cavity, breast, endometrium and ovary. A role of this protein in carcinogenesis and tumor progression has therefore been hypothesized, more precisely in the migration and adhesion of ovarian cancer cells [52, 53].

Over the years, HE4 has acquired increasing clinical relevance thanks to its ability to differentiate benign adnexal masses from ovarian tumors more accurately than CA-125. Moore's group in 2012 showed that HE4 is less frequently elevated in benign pathologies than CA-125 (8% vs. 29%), with better specificity, especially in premenopausal women [54]. In healthy women, serum HE4 values vary up to a maximum of 150 pmol/L. This wide range is linked to the fact that HE4 values are influenced by age, BMI, smoking habit and respiratory diseases, such as asthma and chronic obstructive pulmonary disease (COPD), as well as by the presence of renal insufficiency, which is the main cause of false-positives with values that can exceed 1000 pmol/L [55-57].

Serum values of HE4 do not appear to be influenced by the phases of the ovarian cycle or by hormonal therapies, which is why HE4 can be measured at any phase of the menstrual cycle (unlike the CA-125 marker) and during the use of oral contraceptives [58]. Finally, the concentrations of HE4 do not change during the various trimesters of pregnancy relative to the condition of nongestation [55].

HE4 in Combination with CA-125 to Identify the Presence of Ovarian Cancer

Immunohistochemical studies have shown an overexpression of HE4 in 100% of ovarian carcinomas of endometrioid histotype, in 93% of ovarian carcinomas of serous histotype and in 50% of clear cell carcinomas [59]. HE4 is therefore elevated in epithelial ovarian cancers with the exception of the mucinous histotype. In 2008, Moore et al. [60] showed that HE4, when used as the only biomarker, has a sensitivity of almost 73%, greater than that of CA-125, in identifying the presence of ovarian cancer. The same authors also demonstrated that when used in combination, the two markers achieve a better ability to predict the malignancy of an adnexal mass [60]. In 2009, these authors developed an algorithm for calculating the "ROMA risk score" (risk of ovarian malignancy algorithm), which combines the levels of the two biomarkers (HE4 and CA-125) and simultaneously takes into account the patient's menopausal status [61]. The diagnostic capacity of the "ROMA Risk Score" was evaluated by the authors in two different multicenter clinical trials published in 2009 and 2011, characterized by two different incidences of ovarian neoplasms in the populations of women studied [61, 62]. The sensitivity of the "ROMA risk score" was 94% (with a specificity of 75%) in distinguishing benign from malignant pathologies [61, 62].

Preoperative Biomarkers to Predict Resectability

CA-125 and Primary Debulking Surgery

In 2010, a meta-analysis collected data from 14 previous publications concerning a total of 2192 patients [63]. The aim of the meta-analysis was to verify the ability of CA-125 levels measured before surgery to predict the possibility of optimal primary surgical cytoreduction [63]. Analysis of the data showed that preoperative levels of CA-125 do not allow accurate prediction of ovarian cancer resectability [63]. However, preoperative CA-125 levels above 500 U/mL were strongly associated with a high risk of suboptimal cytoreduction [63]. The conclusions of the meta-analysis published in 2010 were subsequently confirmed by other authors. Bachmann et al. [64] recently reported that the rate of optimal cytoreductions was higher in patients with CA-125 values below 500 U/mL. Furthermore, considering only patients in whom optimal primary cytoreduction was achieved, the prognosis in terms of both overall survival (OS) and progression-free survival (PFS) was better in patients who had preoperative CA-125 levels below 500 U/mL [64]. In 2017, Suidan et al. [35] included preoperative CA-125 levels greater than or less than 500 U/mL in their model for predicting the likelihood of optimal primary cytoreduction based on computed tomography images.

CA-125 and Interval Debulking Surgery

Pelissier et al. [65] published in 2014 the results of a retrospective study conducted in patients with advanced ovarian cancer that showed that CA-125 levels below 75 U/mL after the third course of chemotherapy were associated with an increased likelihood of achieving complete cytoreduction at interval debulking surgery. Matsuhashi et al. [66] reported in 2017 that low CA-125 levels after NACT (less than 35 U/mL) were associated with a greater chance for patients to have optimal interval debulking surgery and a longer PFS than those with high CA-125 levels (greater than 100 U/mL). In another retrospective study, however, complete interval debulking surgery was associated with a 90% reduction in CA-125 levels during neoadjuvant chemotherapy [67].

CA-125 and Secondary Cytoreduction for Recurrent Ovarian Cancer

Monitoring CA-125 levels in posttreatment asymptomatic patients allows for choosing the best time to perform secondary cytoreduction with the highest probability of achieving complete resectability [68]. Each week of delay following the first elevation of the marker levels corresponds to an additional 3% chance of failing to achieve optimal cytoreduction [68].

HE4 and Primary Debulking Surgery

As of 2013, some authors began to publish data suggesting that high plasma HE4 levels prior to surgery correlated with a lower chance of achieving optimal primary cytoreduction [69, 70]. In 2018, a meta-analysis of previous observational studies that collected a total of 1065 women with ovarian cancer found that the sensitivity of HE4 in predicting optimal cytoreduction was 0.81 with a specificity of 0.70 [71]. The authors therefore suggested that the plasma concentrations of the HE4 marker could represent a good method to predict the possibility of optimal debulking in women with ovarian cancer, even if the data collected up to that point came from studies that showed considerable heterogeneity [71].

HE4 and Interval Debulking Surgery

In 2016, Shen and Li [72] suggested that using a cutoff of 353 pmol/L, the assessment of HE4 levels was better than the assessment of CA-125 levels in predicting the possibility of achieving optimal primary cytoreduction in patients with ovarian cancer. In the same publication, the same authors also suggested that the assessment of HE4 levels had a better sensitivity than the assessment of CA-125 levels in predicting the possibility of optimal cytoreduction in cases of interval debulking surgery after neoadjuvant chemotherapy [72]. In this case, the cutoff proposed by the authors was 154 pmol/L before interval debulking surgery [72]. This suggestion was confirmed by Plotti et al. [73] in 2017. For these last authors, however, the cutoff of HE4 levels better able to indicate the possibility of obtaining optimal cytoreduction during interval debulking surgery was 226 pmol/L after neoadjuvant chemotherapy [73].

HE4 and Secondary Cytoreduction for Recurrent Ovarian Cancer

The first authors who evaluated the predictive role of HE4 in identifying cases that could achieve optimal debulking at the time of secondary cytoreduction for first ovarian cancer recurrence proposed a cutoff of 250 pMk, resulting in a sensitivity of 52% with a specificity of 93.8% [74]. In 2015, Angioli et al. [75] included preoperative levels of HE4 in a new predictive model for assessing the risk of optimal debulking in cases of secondary cytoreductive surgery in patients with ovarian cancer recurrence. The predictive model also included preoperative levels of CA-125, ascites and residual tumor at the end of primary cytoreduction [75]. This predictive model, in the hands of the authors, reached a sensitivity of 82% with a sensitivity of 83% [75]. However, this model still needs external validation.

The Value of CA125 and HE4 to Predict the Resectability of Ovarian Cancer According to the Latest Guidelines

Regarding CA-125, ovarian tumor resectability prediction based on the cutoff of 500 U/mL showed a sensitivity ranging from 52% to 80% for a specificity ranging from 40% to 89%. For this reason, it is not recommended to use serum levels of CA-125 for evaluation of the resectability of ovarian cancer [76]. Furthermore, the low level of evidence of the identified publications and the absence of uniform cutoffs of HE4 levels for evaluating the resectability of ovarian cancer do not allow us to recommend the use of this marker in the preoperative evaluation of candidate patients for cytoreduction [76].

Conclusion

The definition of optimal cytoreduction has changed several times over the years; today, most authors consider cytoreduction with macroscopically absent residual tumor to be optimal. Surgery is recommended in patients amenable to complete surgical resection with macroscopically absent residual disease. To avoid unnecessary laparotomy surgery, the identification of preoperative parameters that can predict which patients with advanced ovarian cancer might achieve complete surgical resection of the neoplastic disease is of fundamental importance.

Various models have been proposed based on both preoperative imaging and laparoscopic evaluation of the involvement of all peritoneal organs, and for many of them, external validation is still awaited.

Several authors have proposed the use of tumor biomarkers in predictive models of the resectability of advanced ovarian cancer, but the low level of evidence reached by their research does not allow us to affirm that biomarkers can be used effectively for this purpose.

References

[1] Torre, L. A., Trabert, B., DeSantis, C. E., Miller, K. D., Samimi, G., Runowicz, C. D., Gaudet, M. M., Jemal, A., & Siegel, R. L. Ovarian cancer statistics, 2018. *CA Cancer J Clin* 2018; 68:284–296.

[2] Islami F., Ward, E. M., Sung, H., Cronin, K. A., Tangka, F. K. L>, Sherman, R. L., Zhao, J., Anderson, R. N., Henley, S. J., Yabroff, K. R., Jemal, A., Benard, V. B. Annual report to the nation on the status of cancer, part 1: National cancer statistics. *JNCI J Natl Cancer Inst* 2021; 113:1648-1669.

[3] Prat, J., D'Angelo, E., & Espinosa, I. Ovarian carcinomas: at least five different diseases with distinct histological features and molecular genetics. *Hum Pathol* 2018; 80:11-27.

[4] Kurman R. J. and Shih Ie M. The Dualistic Model of Ovarian Carcinogenesis: Revisited, Revised, and Expanded. *Am J Pathol* 2016; 186:733-747.

[5] Gilks CB and Prat J. Ovarian carcinoma pathology and genetics: recent advances. *Hum Pathol*, 2009; 40:1213-1223.

[6] Prat, J. Ovarian carcinomas: five distinct diseases with different origins, genetic alterations, and clinicopathological features. *Virchows Arch* 2012; 460:237-249.

[7] Lee K. R. and Scully R. E. Mucinous tumors of the ovary: a clinicopathologic study of 196 borderline tumors (of intestinal type) and carcinomas, including an evaluation of 11 cases with 'pseudomyxoma peritonei.' *Am J Surg Pathol* 2000; 24:1447-1464.

[8] Rodriguez IM and Prat J. Mucinous tumors of the ovary: a clinicopathologic analysis of 75 borderline tumors (of intestinal type) and carcinomas. *Am J Surg Pathol* 2002; 26:139-152.

[9] Sainz de la Cuesta, R., Eichhorn, J. H., Rice, L. W., Fuller, Jr, A. F., Nikrui, N., & Goff, B. A. Histologic transformation of benign endometriosis to early epithelial ovarian cancer. *Gynecol Oncol* 1996; 60:238-244.

[10] Kurman R. J. and Shih Ie M. Seromucinous Tumors of the Ovary. What's in a Name? *Int J Gynecol Pathol,* 2016; 35:78-81.

[11] Ferrandina, G., Palluzzi, E., Fanfani, F., Gentileschi, S., Valentini, A. L., Mattoli, M. V., Pennacchia, I., Scambia, G., & Zannoni, G. Endometriosis-associated clear cell carcinoma arising in caesarean section scar: a case report and review of the literature. *World J Surg Oncol* 2016; 14:300.

[12] Improta, G., Pettinato, A., Høgdall, E., Santeusanio, G., Vatrano, S., Fraggetta, F., & Zannoni, G. F. Ovarian Clear Cell Carcinoma: From Morphology to Molecular Biology. *Appl Immunohistochem Mol Morphol* 2019; 27:631-636.

[13] Zannoni, G. F., Improta, G., & Fraggetta, F. PIK3CA in ovarian clear cell carcinoma. *Hum Pathol*, 2014. 45:2514.

[14] Heintz A. P., F. Odicino, P. Maisonneuve, U. Beller, J. L. Benedet, W. T. Creasman, H. Y. Ngan, S. PecorelliCarcinoma of the ovary. *J Epidemiol Biostat*, 2001; 6:107-138.

[15] Vergote, I., De Brabanter, J., Fyles, A., Bertelsen, K., Einhorn, N., Sevelda, P., Gore, M. E., Kærn, J., Verrelst, H., Sjövall, K., Timmerman, D., Vandewalle, J., Van Gramberen, M., & Tropé, C. G. Prognostic importance of degree of differentiation and cyst rupture in stage I invasive epithelial ovarian carcinoma. *Lancet* 2001; 357:176-182.

[16] Pisano C, Greggi, S., Tambaro, R., Losito, S., Iodice, F., Di Maio, M., Ferrari, E., Falanga, M., Formato, R., Iaffaioli, V. R., Pignata, S. Activity of chemotherapy in mucinous epithelial ovarian cancer: a retrospective study. *Anticancer Res* 2005; 25:3501-3505.

[17] Bristow, R. E., Tomacruz, R. S., Armstrong, D. K., Trimble, E. L., & Montz, F. J. Survival effect of maximal cytoreductive surgery for advanced ovarian carcinoma during the platinum era: a meta-analysis. *J Clin Oncol* 2002; 20:1248-1259.

[18] Allen D. G., A. P. Heintz, F. W. Touw. A meta-analysis of residual disease and survival in stage III and IV carcinoma of the ovary. *Eur J Gynaecol Oncol* 1995; 16:349-356.

[19] Chang, S. J., Hodeib, M., Chang, J., & Bristow, R. E. Survival impact of complete cytoreduction to no gross residual disease for advanced-stage ovarian cancer: a meta-analysis. *Gynecol Oncol* 2013; 130:493-498.

[20] Eisenhauer, E. L., Abu-Rustum, N. R., Sonoda, Y., Levine, D. A., Poynor, E. A., Aghajanian, C., Jarnagin, W. R., DeMatteo, R. P., D'Angelica, M. I., Barakat, R. R., & Chi, D. S. The addition of extensive upper abdominal surgery to achieve optimal cytoreduction improves survival in patients with stages IIIC-IV epithelial ovarian cancer. *Gynecol Oncol* 2006; 103:1083-1090.

[21] van der Burg, M. E. L., van Lent, M., Buyse, M., Kobierska, A., Colombo, N., Favalli, G., Lacave, A. J., Nardi, M., Renard, J., & Pecorelli, S. The effect of debulking surgery after induction chemotherapy

on the prognosis in advanced epithelial ovarian cancer. Gynecological Cancer Cooperative Group of the European Organization for Research and Treatment of Cancer. *N Engl J Med* 1995; 332:629-634.

[22] Rose P. G., Stacy Nerenstone, Mark F Brady, Daniel Clarke-Pearson, George Olt, Stephen C Rubin, David H Moore, James M Small, Gynecologic Oncology Group. Secondary surgical cytoreduction for advanced ovarian carcinoma. *N Engl J Med* 2004; 351:2489-2497.

[23] Vergote, I., Tropé, C. G., Amant, F., Kristensen, G. B., Ehlen, T., Johnson, N., Verheijen, R. H. M., van der Burg, M. E. L., Lacave, A. J., Panici, P. B., Kenter, G. G., Casado, A., Mendiola, C., Coens, C., Verleye, L., Stuart, G. C. E., Pecorelli, S., & Reed, N. S. Neoadjuvant chemotherapy or primary surgery in stage IIIC or IV ovarian cancer. *N Engl J Med* 2010; 363:943-953.

[24] Kehoe, S., Hook, J., Nankivell, M., Jayson, G. C., Kitchener, H., Lopes, T., Luesley, D., Perren, T., Bannoo, S., Mascarenhas, M., Dobbs, S., Essapen, S., Twigg, J., Herod, J., McCluggage, G., Parmar, M., & Swart, A. M. Primary chemotherapy versus primary surgery for newly diagnosed advanced ovarian cancer (CHORUS): an open-label, randomised, controlled, non-inferiority trial. *Lancet* 2015; 386:249-257.

[25] Dahm-Kähler, P., Palmqvist, C., Staf, C., Holmberg, E., & Johannesson, L. Centralized primary care of advanced ovarian cancer improves complete cytoreduction and survival - A population-based cohort study. *Gynecol Oncol* 2016; 142:211-216.

[26] Aletti, G. D., Gostout, B. S., Podratz, K. C., & Cliby, W. A. Ovarian cancer surgical resectability: Relative impact of disease, patient status, and surgeon. *Gynecol Oncol* 2006; 100:33-37.

[27] Kang S. and Park S. Y. To predict or not to predict? The dilemma of predicting the risk of suboptimal cytoreduction in ovarian cancer. *Ann Oncol* 2011; 22(Suppl 8):viii23-viii28.

[28] Gómez-Hidalgo, N. R., Martinez-Cannon, B. A., Nick, A. M., Lu, K. H., Sood, A. K., Coleman, R. L., & Ramirez, P. T. Predictors of optimal cytoreduction in patients with newly diagnosed advanced-stage epithelial ovarian cancer: Time to incorporate laparoscopic assessment into the standard of care. *Gynecol Oncol* 2015; 137:553-558.

[29] Song Y. J. Prediction of optimal debulking surgery in ovarian cancer. *Gland Surg* 2021; 10:1173-1181.

[30] Engbersen, M. P., Lahaye, M. J., Lok, C. A. R., Koole, S. N., Sonke, G. S., Beets-Tan, R. G. H., & Van Driel, W. J. Peroperative scoring systems for predicting the outcome of cytoreductive surgery in advanced-stage ovarian cancer - A systematic review. *Eur J Surg Oncol* 2021; 47:1856-1861.

[31] Nelson, B. E., Rosenfield, A. T., & Schwartz, P. E. Preoperative abdominopelvic computed tomographic prediction of optimal cytoreduction in epithelial ovarian carcinoma. *J Clin Oncol* 1993; 11:166–172.

[32] Bristow, R. E., Duska, L. R., Lambrou, N. C., Fishman, E. K., O'Neill, M. J., Trimble, E. L., & Montz, F. J. A model for predicting surgical outcome in patients with advanced ovarian carcinoma using computed tomography. *Cancer* 2000; 89:1532-1540.

[33] Dowdy, S. C., Mullany, S. A., Brandt, K. R., Huppert, B. J., & Cliby, W. A. The utility of computed tomography scans in predicting suboptimal cytoreductive surgery in women with advanced ovarian carcinoma. *Cancer* 2004; 101:346–352.

[34] Janco, J. M. T., Glaser, G., Kim, B., McGree, M. E., Weaver, A. L., Cliby, W. A., Dowdy, S. C., & Bakkum-Gamez, J. N. Development of a prediction model for residual disease in newly diagnosed advanced ovarian cancer. *Gynecol Oncol* 2015; 138:70-77.

[35] Suidan, R. S., Ramirez, P. T., Sarasohn, D. M., Teitcher, J. B., Iyer, R. B., Zhou, Q., Iasonos, A., Denesopolis, J., Zivanovic, O., Long Roche, K. C., Sonoda, Y., Coleman, R. L., Abu-Rustum, N. R., Hricak, H., & Chi, D. S. A multicenter assessment of the ability of preoperative computed tomography scan and CA-125 to predict gross residual disease at primary debulking for advanced epithelial ovarian cancer. *Gynecol Oncol* 2017; 145:27-31.

[36] Forstner, R., Hricak, H., Occhipinti, K. A., Powell, C. B., Frankel, S. D., & Stern, J. L. Ovarian cancer: staging with CT and MR imaging. *Radiology* 1995; 197:619-626.

[37] Espada, M., Garcia-Flores, J. R., Jimenez, M., Alvarez-Moreno, E., De Haro, M., Gonzalez-Cortijo, L., Hernandez-Cortes, G., Martinez-Vega, V., & Sainz De La Cuesta, R. Diffusionweighted magnetic resonance imaging evaluation of intra-abdominal sites of implants to predict likelihood of suboptimal cytoreductive surgery in patients with ovarian carcinoma. *Eur Radiol* 2013; 23:2636-2642.

[38] Michielsen, K., Dresen, R., Vanslembrouck, R., De Keyzer, F., Amant, F., Mussen, E., Leunen, K., Berteloot, P., Moerman, P., Vergote, I., & Vandecaveye, V. Diagnostic value of whole body diffusion-

weighted MRI compared to computed tomography for pre-operative assessment of patients suspected for ovarian cancer. *Eur J Cancer* 2017; 83:88-98.

[39] Hynninen, J., Kemppainen, J., Lavonius, M., Virtanen, J., Matomäki, J., Oksa, S., Carpén, O., Grénman, S., Seppänen, M., & Auranen, A. A prospective comparison of integrated FDG-PET/contrast-enhanced CT and contrast-enhanced CT for pretreatment imaging of advanced epithelial ovarian cancer. *Gynecol Oncol* 2013; 131:389–394.

[40] Fruscio, R., Sina, F., Dolci, C., Signorelli, M., Crivellaro, C., Dell'Anna, T., Cuzzocrea, M., Guerra, L., Milani, R., & Messa, C. Preoperative 18F-FDG PET/CT in the management of advanced epithelial ovarian cancer. *Gynecol Oncol* 2013; 131:689–693.

[41] Shim, S. H., Lee, S. J., Kim, S. O., Kim, S. N., Kim, D. Y., Lee, J. J., Kim, J. H., Kim, Y. M., Kim, Y. T., & Nam, J. H. Nomogram for predicting incomplete cytoreduction in advanced ovarian cancer patients. *Gynecol Oncol* 2015; 136:30-36.

[42] Alessi, A., Martinelli, F., Padovano, B., Serafini, G., Lorusso, D., Lorenzoni, A., Ditto, A., Lecce, F., Mira, M., Donfrancesco, C., Raspagliesi, F., & Crippa, F. FDG-PET/CT to predict optimal primary cytoreductive surgery in patients with advanced ovarian cancer: preliminary results. *Tumori* 2016; 102:103-107.

[43] Vergote, I., De Wever, I., Tjalma, W., Van Gramberen, M., Decloedt, J., & van Dam, P. Neoadjuvant chemotherapy or primary debulking surgery in advanced ovarian carcinoma: a retrospective analysis of 285 patients. *Gynecol Oncol* 1998; 71:431–436.

[44] Fagotti, A., Fanfani, F., Ludovisi, M., Lo Voi, R., Bifulco, G., Testa, A. C., & Scambia, G. Role of laparoscopy to assess the chance of optimal cytoreductive surgery in advanced ovarian cancer: a pilot study. *Gynecol Oncol* 2005; 96:729–735.

[45] Fagotti, A., Ferrandina, G., Fanfani, F., Ercoli, A., Lorusso, D., Rossi, M., & Scambia, G. A laparoscopy based score to predict surgical outcome in patients with advanced ovarian carcinoma: a pilot study. *Ann Surg Oncol* 2006; 13:1156–1161.

[46] Fagotti, A., Ferrandina, G., Fanfani, F., Garganese, G., Vizzielli, G., Carone, V., Salerno, M. G., & Scambia, G. Prospective validation of a laparoscopic predictive model for optimal cytoreduction in advanced ovarian carcinoma. *Am J Obstet Gynecol* 2008; 199:642.e1–642.e6.

[47] Fagotti, A., Vizzielli, G., De Iaco, P., Surico, D., Buda, A., Mandato, V. D., Petruzzelli, F., Ghezzi, F., Garzarelli, S., Mereu, L., Viganò, R., Tateo, S., Fanfani, F., & Scambia, G. A multicentric trial (Olympia-MITO13) on the accuracy of laparoscopy to assess peritoneal spread in ovarian cancer. *Am J Obstet Gynecol* 2013; 209:462.e1-462.e11).

[48] van de Vrie R., Marianne J. Rutten, Joyce Danielle Asseler, Mariska Mg Leeflang, Gemma G. Kenter, Ben Willem J. Mol, Marrije Buist. Laparoscopy for diagnosing resectability of disease in women with advanced ovarian cancer. *Cochrane Database Syst Rev* 2019; 3:CD009786.

[49] Jacobs I. and Bast R. C, Jr. The CA 125 tumor associated antigen: a review of the literature. *Hum Reprod* 1989; 4:1-12.

[50] Bouchard, D., Morisset, D., Bourbonnais, Y., & Tremblay, G. M. Proteins with whey-acidic-protein motifs and cancer. *Lancet Oncol* 2006; 7:167-174.

[51] Clauss, A., Lilja, H., & Lundwall, Å. A locus on human chromosome 20 contains several genes expressing protease inhibitor domains with homology to whey acidic protein. *Biochem J* 2002; 368:233-242.

[52] Lu, R., Sun, X., Xiao, R., Zhou, L., Gao, X., & Guo, L. Human epididymis protein 4 (HE4) plays a key role in ovarian cancer cell adhesion and motility. *Biochem Biophys Res Commun* 2012; 419:274-280.

[53] Galgano, M. T., Hampton, G. M., & Frierson, H. F. Comprehensive analysis of HE4 expression in normal and malignant human tissues. *Mod Pathol* 2006; 19:847-853.

[54] Moore, R. G., Miller, M. C., Steinhoff, M. M., Skates, S. J., Lu, K. H., Lambert-Messerlian, G., & Bast, R. C. Serum HE4 levels are less frequently elevated than CA125 in women with benign gynecologic disorders. *Am J Obstet Gynecol* 2012; 206: 351.e1-351.e8.

[55] Moore, R. G., Miller, M. C., Eklund, E. E., Lu, K. H., Bast, R. C., & Lambert-Messerlian, G. Serum levels of the ovarian cancer biomarker HE4 are decreased in pregnancy and increase with age. *Am J Obstet Gynecol* 2012; 206: 349.e1-349.e7.

[56] Bolstad, N., Øijordsbakken, M., Nustad, K., & Bjerner, J. Human epididymis protein 4 reference limits and natural variation in a Nordic reference population. *Tumour Biol* 2012; 33:141-148.

[57] Nagy, B., Krasznai, Z. T., Balla, H., Csobán, M., Antal-Szalmás, P., Hernádi, Z., & Kappelmayer, J. Elevated human epididymis protein 4 concentrations in chronic kidney disease. *Ann Clin Biochem* 2012; 49:377-380.

[58] Hallamaa, M., Suvitie, P., Huhtinen, K., Matomäki, J., Poutanen, M., & Perheentupa, A. Serum HE4 concentration is not dependent on menstrual cycle or hormonal treatment among endometriosis patients and healthy premenopausal women. *Gynecol Oncol* 2012; 125:667-672.

[59] Drapkin, R., von Horsten, H. H., Lin, Y., Mok, S. C., Crum, C. P., Welch, W. R., & Hecht, J. L. Human epididymis protein 4 (HE4) is a secreted glycoprotein that is overexpressed by serous and endometrioid ovarian carcinomas. *Cancer Res* 2005; 65:2162-2169.

[60] Moore R. G., Amy K. Brown, M. Craig Miller, Steven Skates, W. Jeffrey Allard, Thorsten Verch, Margaret Steinhoff, Geralyn Messerlian, Paul DiSilvestro, C. O. Granai, Robert C. Bast Jr. The use of multiple novel tumor biomarkers for the detection of ovarian carcinoma in patients with a pelvic mass. *Gynecol Oncol* 2008; 108:402-408.

[61] Moore R. G., D. Scott McMeekin, Amy K. Brown, Paul DiSilvestro, M. Craig Miller, W. Jeffrey Allard, Walter Gajewski, Robert Kurman, Robert C. Bast Jr, Steven J. Skates. A novel multiple marker bioassay utilizing HE4 and CA125 for the prediction of ovarian cancer in patients with a pelvic mass. *Gynecol Oncol* 2009; 112:40-46.

[62] Moore R. G., M. Craig Miller, Paul Disilvestro, Lisa M. Landrum, Walter Gajewski, John J. Ball, Steven J. Skates. Evaluation of the diagnostic accuracy of the risk of ovarian malignancy algorithm in women with a pelvic mass. *Obstet Gynecol* 2011; 118:280-288.

[63] Kang, S., Kim, T. J., Nam, B. H., Seo, S. S., Kim, B. G., Bae, D. S., & Park, S. Y. Preoperative serum CA125 levels and risk of suboptimal cytoreduction in ovarian cancer: a meta-analysis. *J Surg Oncol* 2010; 101:13-17.

[64] Bachmann, R., Brucker, S., Stäbler, A., Krämer, B., Ladurner, R., Königsrainer, A., Wallwiener, D., & Bachmann, C. Prognostic relevance of high pretreatment CA125 levels in primary serous ovarian cancer. *Mol Clin Oncol* 2021; 14:8.

[65] Pelissier, A., Bonneau, C., Chéreau, E., de La Motte Rouge, T., Fourchotte, V., Daraï, E., & Rouzier, R. CA125 kinetic parameters predict optimal cytoreduction in patients with advanced epithelial ovarian cancer treated with neoadjuvant chemotherapy. *Gynecol Oncol* 2014; 135:542-546.

[66] Matsuhashi, T., Takeshita, T., Yamamoto, A., Kawase, R., Yamada, T., Kurose, K., Doi, D., Konnai, K., Onose, R., & Kato, H. Serum CA 125 Level after Neoadjuvant Chemotherapy is Predictive of Prognosis and Debulking Surgery Outcomes in Advanced Epithelial Ovarian Cancer. *J Nippon Med Sch*. 2017; 84:170-176.

[67] Mahdi H, Kathryn A. Maurer, Benjamin Nutter, Peter G. Rose. The impact of percent reduction in CA-125 levels on prediction of the extent of interval cytoreduction and outcome in patients with advanced-stage cancer of Mullerian origin treated with neoadjuvant chemotherapy. *Int J Gynecol Cancer* 2015; 25:823-829.

[68] Fleming, N. D., Cass, I., Walsh, C. S., Karlan, B. Y., & Li, A. J. CA125 surveillance increases optimal resectability at secondary cytoreductive surgery for recurrent epithelial ovarian cancer. *Gynecol Oncol* 2011; 121: 249–252.

[69] Braicu, E. I., Fotopoulou, C., Van Gorp, T., Richter, R., Chekerov, R., Hall, C., Butz, H., Castillo-Tong, D. C., Mahner, S., Zeillinger, R., Concin, N., Vergote, I., & Sehouli, J. Preoperative HE4 expression in plasma predicts surgical outcome in primary ovarian cancer patients: Results from the OVCAD study. *Gynecol Oncol* 2013; 128:245-251.

[70] Angioli, R., Plotti, F., Capriglione, S., Aloisi, A., Montera, R., Luvero, D., Miranda, A., Cafà, E. V., Damiani, P., & Benedetti-Panici, P. Can the preoperative HE4 level predict optimal cytoreduction in patients with advanced ovarian carcinoma? *Gynecol Oncol* 2013; 128:579-583.

[71] Pergialiotis, V., Karampetsou, N., Bellos, I., Thomakos, N., & Daskalakis, G. The diagnostic accuracy of human epididymis factor 4 for the prediction of optimal debulking in patients with ovarian cancer: a meta-analysis of observational studies. *Int J Gynecol Cancer* 2018; 28:1471-1477.

[72] Shen Y and Li L. Serum HE4 superior to CA125 in predicting poorer surgical outcome of epithelial ovarian cancer. *Tumor Biol* 2016; 37:14765–14772.

[73] Plotti, F., Scaletta, G., Capriglione, S., Montera, R., Luvero, D., Lopez, S., Gatti, A., De Cicco Nardone, C., Terranova, C., & Angioli, R. The role of HE4, a novel biomarker, in predicting optimal cytoreduction after neoadjuvant chemotherapy in advanced ovarian cancer. *Int J Gynecol Cancer* 2017; 27: 696-702.

[74] Braicu, E. I., Chekerov, R., Richter, R., Pop, C., Nassir, M., Loefgren, H., Stamatian, F., Muallem, M. Z., Hall, C., Fotopoulou, C., Sehouli, J., & Pietzner, K. HE4 expression in plasma correlates with surgical outcome and overall survival in patients with first ovarian cancer relapse. *Ann Surg Oncol* 2014; 21:955-962.

[75] Angioli, R., Capriglione, S., Aloisi, A., Ricciardi, R., Scaletta, G., Lopez, S., Miranda, A., Di Pinto, A., Terranova, C., & Plotti, F. A Predictive Score for Secondary Cytoreductive Surgery in Recurrent Ovarian Cancer (SeC-Score): A Single-Centre, Controlled Study for Preoperative Patient Selection. *Ann Surg Oncol* 2015; 22:4217-4223.

[76] Bendifallah S., G. Body, E. Daraï, L. Ouldamer. [Diagnostic and prognostic value of tumor markers, scores (clinical and biological) algorithms, in front of an ovarian mass suspected of an epithelial ovarian cancer: Article drafted from the French Guidelines in oncology entitled "Initial management of patients with epithelial ovarian cancer" developed by FRANCOGYN, CNGOF, SFOG, GINECO-ARCAGY under the aegis of CNGOF and endorsed by INCa] *Gynecol Obstet Fertil Senol* 2019; 47:134-154.

Chapter 5

Computed Tomography (CT) and Magnetic Resonance Imaging (MRI) Findings in Ovarian Cancer

Skouras Ioannis[1], MD
Kokkali Kalliopi[2,*], MD
and Fotiou Alexandros[2], MD
[1]Department of Radiology, Metaxa Cancer Hospital of Piraeus, Piraeus, Greece
[2]Department of Gynecologic Oncology, Metaxa Cancer Hospital of Piraeus, Piraeus, Greece

Introduction

CT (computed tomography) and MRI (magnetic resonance imaging) are imaging techniques that have been widely used in the staging and follow up of patients with ovarian cancer. Preoperative imaging in ovarian cancer plays a crucial role in detection, characterization and staging of the disease.

Specifically preoperative imaging aims to:

- the confirmation and characterization of the primary ovarian mass as well as the exclusion of secondary ovarian disease.
- The assessment of tumor spread and of the tumor growth pattern, such as the extent of diaphragm involvement or pelvic sidewall infiltration.
- Recognition of possible surgical complications, such as bowel obstruction, hydronephrosis, venous thrombosis
- The prediction of non- resectability of the disease (tumor growth and localization) and the selection of candidates for optimal debulking surgery versus candidates for neoadjuvant chemotherapy
- the evaluation of the suitability for image-guided biopsy, particularly for neoadjuvant candidates or for patients with secondary disease in order to exclude metastatic spread from the gastrointestinal tract [1].

---

* Corresponding Author's Email: popi.koc@gmail.com.

In: Ovarian Cancer
Editors: Christos Iavazzo, Alexandros Fotiou and John Spiliotis
ISBN: 979-8-88697-633-5

Concerning the confirmation and characterization of the primary ovarian tumor, MRI has been proved to be a useful second-line tool in providing better tissue characterization and origin information, especially for large adnexal masses that have not been previously determined in an ultrasound. In many large multicenter studies, an MRI was shown to be superior in comparison with both CT and ultrasound in detecting malignancy in indeterminate ovarian tumors. The more common MRI findings are indicative of malignancies in vegetation in a cystic tumor and necrosis in a solid mass. Other findings indicative of malignancy could be papillary projections and septations. They are usually gadolinium-enhanced.

The extensive use of Multidetector Computed Tomography (CT) and the advantage of providing the required information in a short period of time make this imaging technique the technique of choice for preoperative staging of patients with ovarian cancer. The pattern of tumor growth as well as disease burden can be sufficiently assessed by computed tomography. Abdominal areas that are possibly infiltrated by the tumor, such as diaphragm, pelvic sidewall and retroperitoneal space can be accurately identified on CT imaging. Moreover, it can be used for the identification of tumor deposits in areas that are difficult to debulk at surgery. Such areas are the surface of the diaphragm, the mesenteric root, the lesser sac, and the paraaortic nodes above the renal vessels. Cancer deposits in these areas make the disease non-resectable and the patient into a candidate for neoadjuvant chemotherapy and interval cytoreductive surgery. A CT of the thorax is also considered to be a useful diagnostic tool in evaluation of lung parenchyma and pleural surfaces or in detecting possible bulky lymph nodes in the cardiophrenic region and mediastinum in advanced ovarian cancer. Furthermore, with the use of multidetector CT there is a large improvement in detection of peritoneal implants. However, the limitation of CT in depicting peritoneal metastases < 1 cm is still present. The staging accuracy may be improved using positron emission tomography (PET/CT) due to its benefit in identifying smaller peritoneal and serosal deposits as well as metastatic lesions outside the abdomen. However, its use in preoperative evaluation of ovarian cancer has not been well established [2, 3].

A structured imaging report for preoperative staging of ovarian cancer either by CT or MRI should include the description of the following structures:

- Size and morphology of the ovarian mass or masses, including the features demonstrating malignancy
- If there is unilateral or bilateral disease
- Endometrial thickness of uterus, invasion of the bladder or bowel, pelvic side-wall infiltrations.
- Implications of bowel obstruction (Figure 1), hydronephrosis, venous thrombosis.
- Ascites in the abdominal cavity and its amount (Figure 2).
- Omental deposits (Figure 3)
- The localization of peritoneal or serosal implants outside the pelvis and their size.
- Small intestine mesentery involvement and its contraction to intestine loops
- The involvement of supracolic ligaments such as gastrohepatic, gastrosplenic, splenocolic
- Sites of bulky (diameter >1 cm) or morphologically suspicious lymph nodes.
- Lymph nodes in cardiophrenic area with a short axis diameter of >5 mm.
- Surface, subcapsular or parenchymal liver and spleen metastases

- Abdominal wall invasion
- Pleural effusion
- The stage of disease according to the FIGO/TNM classification [1].

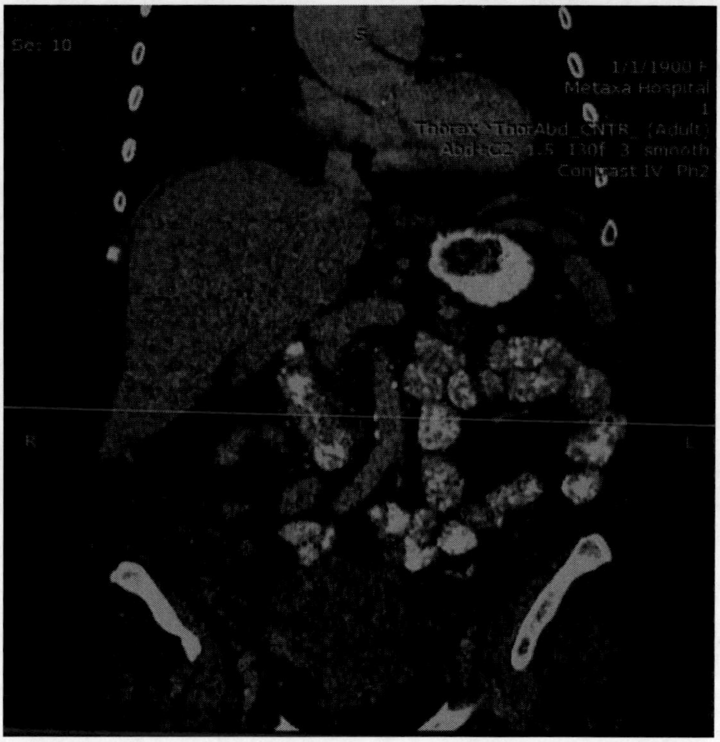

Figure 1. A large mass of the right ovary with solid and cystic components causing sigmoid colon invasion without bowel obstruction.

As mentioned previously, attention should be paid to sites that are not easily resectable in primary debulking surgery. The major factor that affects the resectability of disease seems to be peritoneal carcinomatosis localized in different sites such as the small intestine (resection of a large part of the small bowel could lead to short bowel syndrome), the mesentery, the stomach, the duodenum, the pancreas, the parenchymal of the liver (central or multisegmental), the hepatic hilum, the coeliac trunk, mesenteric and coeliac lymph nodes [4].

There are also objective models to quantify the peritoneal carcinomatosis and to predict optimal debulking feasibility in ovarian cancer patients. The most frequently used scoring system is the peritoneal cancer index (PCI). It is used to evaluate the extent of peritoneal cancer throughout the peritoneal cavity. This scoring system represents a diagnostic and prognostic tool that was originally developed for advanced colorectal cancer and for intraoperative assessment by oncosurgeons to determine better cytoreductive outcome. However, it can also be applied in ovarian cancer preoperatively by using any of imaging modalities.

The peritoneal cavity is divided into 13 well defined sites. The size of the largest tumor nodule is measured in each of the 13 regions. If no tumor is detected, a score of "0" is given to that region. A score of "1" is given if the largest tumor nodule is smaller than 0.5 cm. For nodules measuring between 0.5 cm and 5 cm, the score is "2." A score of "3" is given for disease larger than 5 cm.

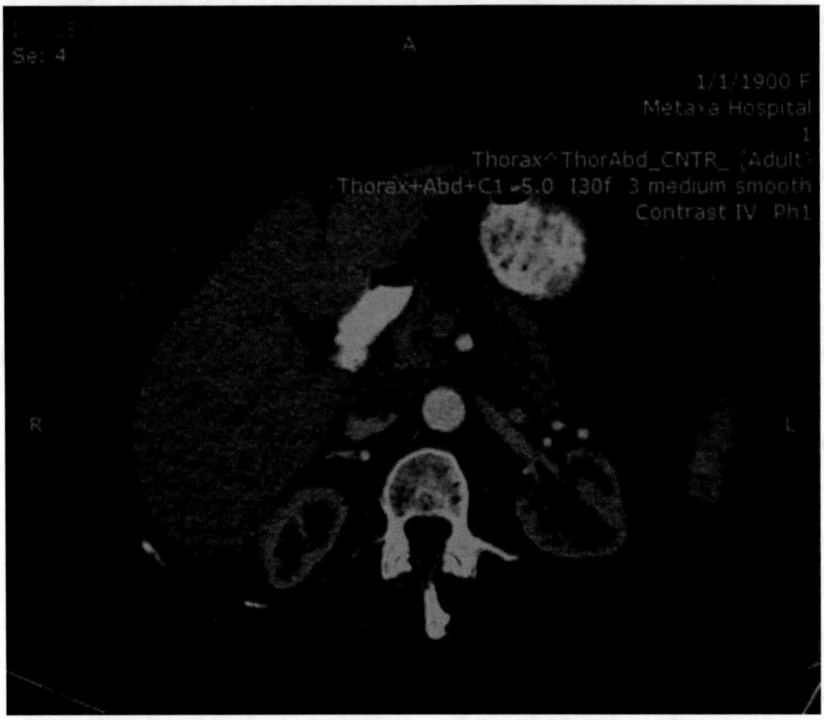

Figure 2. Free peri-hepatic ascites due to peritoneal carcinomatosis.

If layering or confluences of multiple small tumor nodules are present, the score is also "3." The PCI score is calculated by adding the scores of all 13 regions together with a maximum of 39 (13×3) (Image 4) [5].

The PCI score helps us in categorization of the volume of peritoneal carcinomatosis in small volume (PCI 0-9), moderate volume (PCI 10-20) and large volume (PCI > 20).

This categorization contributes to the prediction of non-resectability of disease and triage of the patients in candidates for optimal cytoreductive surgery and candidates for neoadjuvant chemotherapy. Moreover, PCI score has been proven to be an independent prognostic indicator for long-term outcome if the patients have a low volume peritoneal cancer index [6, 7].

Multidisciplinary team approach (MDT) has totally altered the management of patients with ovarian cancer over the last few years. According to this approach, an optimized individualized treatment modality should be provided for every patient with newly diagnosed ovarian cancer. This treatment decision depends on many different factors. First of all, one factor is the aforementioned non-resectability of the disease due to localization and tumor growth that make resection technically not feasible. The inoperability is another factor that includes the inability of the patient to tolerate the extent of the surgical manipulations that would be necessary for optimal tumor debulking. Last but not least, insufficiency of the surgeon and institution that cannot provide the appropriate skills and equipment respectively to perform complete resection is another factor that should be taken into consideration by the MDT. Preoperative imaging can affect all the aforementioned parameters and help in making a MDT decision [8].

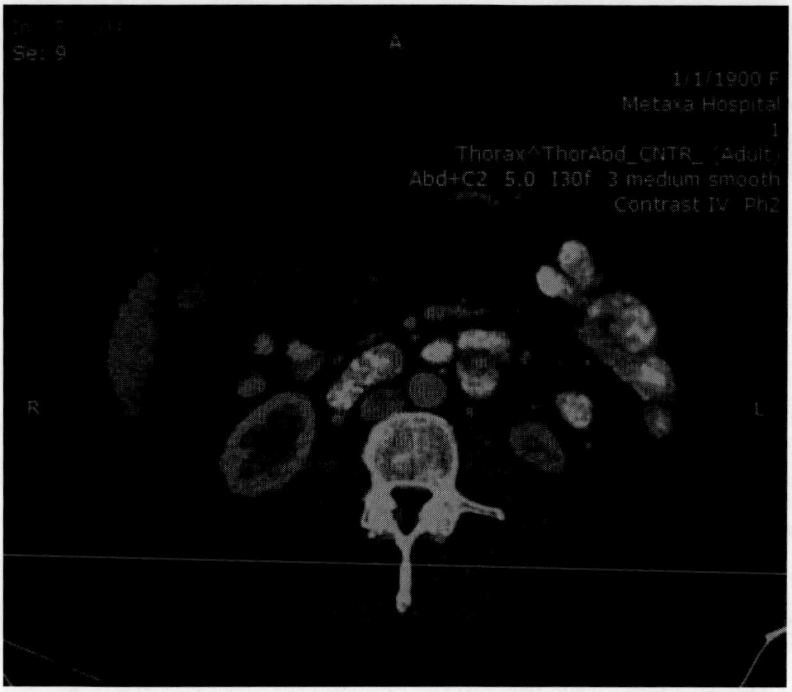

Figure 3. Free peri-hepatic ascites and nodular invasion of the greater omentum due to peritoneal carcinomatosis.

Overall, contrast enhanced CT (CECT) of the pelvis, upper abdomen and thorax cannot only offer essential information about the extent of the disease, but also identify the bulky disease in a rapid and easy way. However, this imaging technique seems not to be efficient at the detection of subcentimetric disease on bowel serosa and its mesentery [1, 9].

A novel staging modality, functional MRI, seems to have more accuracy in detecting peritoneal implants in contrast to CECT and PET-CT. Functional MRI includes dynamic contrast enhanced MRI (DCE MRI) and Diffusion weighted MRI (DW MRI) and combines multiple morphological images of high contrast resolution resulting in identification of small volume carcinomatosis on bowel serosa and its mesentery. This promising method has several disadvantages, though. The most important disadvantages of the method are low availability, little experience in both acquisition and interpretation, high cost, long examination time. There is also a small number of publications concerning this new technique found in the review of literature [10-12].

Conclusion

- An ultrasound seems to remain the first-line imaging modality for the characterization of the primary adnexal tumor.
- MRI (DCE, DW) is considered to be the second-line test for sonographically indeterminate tumors.
- MRI, CT, PET-CT are proved to be sufficient methods in identifying the extent of disease and tumor spread.

- Preoperative imaging displays hing specificity in identification of bulky disease and selection of the patients who can be candidates for primary cytoreduction.
- Preoperative imaging displays low sensitivity in depicting small volume peritoneal carcinomatosis in very important anatomical areas for cytoreductive surgery.
- Radiomics is a new era that may potentially enhance the diagnostic accuracy of imaging in ovarian cancer in the future.

References

[1] Forstner, R., Sala, E., Kinkel, K., & Spencer, J. A., ESUR guidelines: ovarian cancer staging and follow-up. *Eur. Radiol.*, 2010. 20(12): p. 2773-80.

[2] Penny, S. M., Ovarian Cancer: An Overview. *Radiol. Technol.*, 2020. 91(6): p. 561-575.

[3] Forstner, R., Early detection of ovarian cancer. *Eur. Radiol.*, 2020. 30(10): p. 5370-5373.

[4] Colombo, N., et al., ESMO-ESGO consensus conference recommendations on ovarian cancer: pathology and molecular biology, early and advanced stages, borderline tumours and recurrent disease. *Ann. Oncol.*, 2019. 30(5): p. 672-705.

[5] Sugarbaker, P. H., Management of peritoneal metastases - Basic concepts. *J. Buon*, 2015. 20 Suppl 1: p. S2-11.

[6] Laghi, Andrea, Davide Bellini, Marco Rengo, Fabio Accarpio, Damiano Caruso, Daniele Biacchi, Angelo Di Giorgio, and Paolo Sammartino., Diagnostic performance of computed tomography and magnetic resonance imaging for detecting peritoneal metastases: systematic review and meta-analysis. *Radiol. Med.*, 2017. 122(1): p. 1-15.

[7] Abdalla Ahmed, Shimaa, Hisham Abou-Taleb, Noha Ali, and Dalia M. Badary., Accuracy of radiologic-laparoscopic peritoneal carcinomatosis categorization in the prediction of surgical outcome. *Br. J. Radiol.*, 2019. 92(1100): p. 20190163.

[8] du Bois, A., T. Baert, and I. Vergote, Role of Neoadjuvant Chemotherapy in Advanced Epithelial Ovarian Cancer. *J. Clin. Oncol.*, 2019. 37(27): p. 2398-2405.

[9] Dauwen, H., B. Van Calster, C. M. Deroose, K. Op de Beeck, F. Amant, P. Neven, P. Berteloot, K. Leunen, D. Timmerman, and I. Vergote., PET/CT in the staging of patients with a pelvic mass suspicious for ovarian cancer. *Gynecol. Oncol.*, 2013. 131(3): p. 694-700.

[10] Michielsen, K., Vergote, I., Op de beeck, K., Amant, F., Leunen, K., Moerman, P., Deroose, C., Souverijns, G., Dymarkowski, S., De Keyzer, F., & Vandecaveye, V., Whole-body MRI with diffusion-weighted sequence for staging of patients with suspected ovarian cancer: a clinical feasibility study in comparison to CT and FDG-PET/CT. *Eur. Radiol.*, 2014. 24(4): p. 889-901.

[11] Michielsen, K., et al., Diagnostic value of whole body diffusion-weighted MRI compared to computed tomography for pre-operative assessment of patients suspected for ovarian cancer. *Eur. J. Cancer*, 2017. 83: p. 88-98.

[12] Rizzo, S., et al., Pre-operative evaluation of epithelial ovarian cancer patients: Role of whole body diffusion weighted imaging MR and CT scans in the selection of patients suitable for primary debulking surgery. A single-centre study. *Eur. J. Radiol.*, 2020. 123: p. 108786.

Chapter 6

The Role of 18FDG PET/CT Scans in Ovarian Cancer Patients

Lydia Iordanidou*, MD, PhD

Department of Nuclear Medicine, Metaxa Cancer Hospital of Piraeus, Piraeus, Greece

Introduction

Ovarian carcinoma remains the most lethal of the gynecological cancers, with advanced disease (stage III/IV) constituting over 70% of cases at presentation and an associated 5-year survival is less than 30% [1]. Worldwide data shows that ovarian tumors are among those with high incidence (seventh largest) and are responsible for a high number of cancer-related deaths (eighth highest) [2, 3].

In FIGO staging fallopian tube, ovarian and peritoneal cancers are amalgamated into a single system Cancer of the ovary, fallopian tube, and peritoneum [4].

Most of the information regarding imaging use for staging and evaluation of recurrence applies to epithelial ovarian cancers (EOC). Two major subtypes of epithelial ovarian cancers are distinguished by molecular, genetic, and morphologic characteristics, type 1 being the relatively indolent low-grade serous, low-grade endometrioid, mucinous tumors, transitional (Brenner), and clear cell carcinomas and type 2 being aggressive neoplasms, including high-grade serous or endometrioid, undifferentiated cancer and carcinosarcomas [5]

Type I EOCs account for 25% of all EOCs, but cause just 10% of deaths; they are largely diagnosed at an early stage and have four histologic subtypes characterized by different mutations:

1) low-grade serous EOC (KRAS, BRAF, HER2),
2) endometrioid EOC (PTEN and PI3KCA),
3) mucinous EOC (KRAS), and
4) clear-cell EOC (PI3KCA).

They have high genomic stability and span a continuum ranging from a benign cyst to a borderline lesion to an invasive tumor [7].

* Corresponding Author's Email: lydiaior@otenet.gr.

In: Ovarian Cancer
Editors: Christos Iavazzo, Alexandros Fotiou and John Spiliotis
ISBN: 979-8-88697-633-5

Type 1 diseases are more indolent with a better survival pattern as compared to type 2, which have greater aberrant mutational status and a more inherently aggressive tumor biology, albeit more chemo-sensitive.

Type 1, Mucinous ovarian carcinomas once deemed relatively common are now considered rare. The actual origin of these tumors remains controversial type II EOC has a particularly poor prognosis (overall five-year survival rate <20%) as it is normally diagnosed at an advanced stage when peritoneal carcinomatosis has already occurred (Table 1), [6, 7].

Table 1. Dualistic classification of EOC

	Type I EOC	Type II EOC
Frequency	25% of EOCs	75% of EOCs
Mortality	10%	90%
Diagnosis	Usually Early stage	Usually Advanced stage (carcinomatosis)
Progression	Slow	Fast
Histologic subtypes	Low-grade serous Low-grade endometrioid Clear-cell Mucinous	High-grade serous High-grade endometrioid Undifferentiated carcinoma Carcinosarcoma

Table 2. EOC classified according to histologic subtype

Histologic Subtype	High-grade Serous	Low-grade Serous	Mucinous	Endometrioid	Clear-Cell
% of all EOCs diagnosed	71%	4%	3%	8%	9%
% of early stage EOCs diagnosed	Nearly 0%	17%	12%	33%	38%
% of advan. Stage EOCs diagnosed	88%	3%	2%	3%	4%

It is now estimated that mucinous tumors account for 3% or less of ovarian cancer malignancies. The origin of mucinous ovarian carcinoma (MOC) has long been controversial. It is now recognized that in the past, many mucinous tumors involving the ovary were in fact misdiagnosed metastases from diverse extra-ovarian sites, such as the colon, stomach, pancreas and uterus. After revisions to the diagnostic criteria, the rate of mucinous tumors appearing to arise from the ovary fell from ~10% to only 3–5% of all epithelial ovarian cancers [8].

The aggressive (type 2) ovarian cancers most often present in advanced stages, stages III and IV, after the disease has spread widely out of the pelvis (Table 2).

They account for 75% of all EOCs and are responsible for 90% of deaths. Ninety-six percent of type II EOCs have a P53 mutation, while between 30% and 50% have a BRCA1 or BRCA2 mutation (the percentage varies depending on the application of BRCA or BRCAness criteria [9-11].

The decision regarding initial treatment for ovarian cancer depends on accurate staging.

Radiological imaging, including ultrasound, CT, FDG-PET/CT, and MRI have been used to assess the resectability of tumors, the candidacy of patients for effective cytoreductive surgery, the need for postoperative chemotherapy if debulking is suboptimal, and the need for referral to a gynecologic oncologist.

CT scans have limited sensitivity, especially to detect small peritoneal lesions. MRI is more sensitive, especially in the pelvic region [12].

Molecular imaging is defined as the visualization, characterization and measurement of biological processes at the molecular and cellular levels in humans and other living systems.

Although CT remains the principal technique in staging OC, the addition of FDG-PET seems to provide a better staging definition. The combined use of CT and PET yields a diagnosis and staging in a fast and accurate way [13].

^{18}FDG PET/CT Scan

For mammalian cells, glucose is a major source of energy. In the presence of oxygen, a complete breakdown of glucose generates 36 molecules of ATP from one molecule of glucose. Hypoxia is a hallmark of cancer; therefore, cancer cells prefer the process of glycolysis, which generates only two molecules of ATP from one molecule of glucose, and therefore, cancer cells need more molecules of glucose in comparison with normal cells. Increased uptake of glucose by cancer cells is due to increased expression of glucose transporters, especially GLUT1 and GLUT3, that are hypoxia responsive, as well as other glucose transport proteins. However, overexpression of glucose transporters, promoting the process of carcinogenesis, and increasing aggressiveness and invasiveness of tumors, the tendency to metastasize, decreases metastasis-free survival, causes a significantly poorer overall survival, and predicts worse prognosis in patients [14].

^{18} FDG PET/CT diagnostic technique is based on evaluating tissue glucose metabolism by measuring accumulated FDG, a glucose analogue, which like glucose is taken up by cells with high glucose consumption. Unlike glucose, FDG cannot be further metabolized in cells and therefore accumulates and its distribution reflects glucose uptake in the body.

PET imaging provides a whole-body image in a non-invasive manner, allowing assessment of heterogeneity between and within patients as well as repeat scanning to monitor treatment response. If the tumor lesion is relatively large, intra-lesional differences in tracer uptake can be visualized, e.g., necrotic areas as 'cold' spots or areas with relatively higher tracer uptake.

There are known confounding factors of benign/physiological uptake by the ovaries in the various phases of the menstrual cycle these need to be taken care of when PET /CT scans are performed for the diagnosis of ovarian carcinoma. Potential false positive FDG uptake can be seen during ovulation and in relation to corpus luteal cystsin premenopausal women (Figure 1). Physiologic uptake in the ovary manifests as ovoid with smooth margins or sometimes a rim of activity with a photopenic center. At contrast enhanced CT, this may appear to be a small rim-enhancing cyst.

Patients with irregular cycles have low probability of intense uptake in the ovary. The mechanism of physiologic ovarian uptake has been postulated to be due to an inflammatory reaction involving cytokines during the ovulatory process to increase glucose uptake to meet the metabolic demands of the growing follicle and the ovulated oocyte [15, 16].

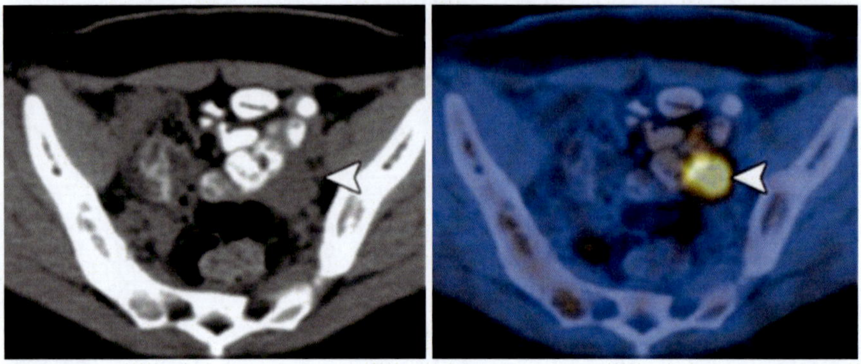

Figure 1. Corpus luteum cyst. CT scan (left) shows a hypoattenuating cystic lesion in the region of the left adnexa (arrowhead)fused PET/CT image (right) demonstrate increased FDG uptake in the lesion (arrowhead). This finding represents the left ovary, probably containing a corpus luteum cyst. Further information from the patient confirmed that this finding represented a menstrual cycle–related physiologic change, and subsequent ultrasonography revealed a corpus luteum cyst.

In premenopausal women, FDG PET scan should be performed just after menstruation to avoid physiologic FDG uptake. In postmenopausal ovaries, however, any ovarian uptake is pathologic. The presence of FDG uptake within the ovary of a postmenopausal woman therefore raises the question of OC [17, 18].

Potential false negative results can be seen in malignancies with a clear cell or mucinous histologic pattern that have been reported to have low-level FDG uptake [19]. Therefore, the sensitivity of FDG PET/CT for the detection of mucinous neoplasms has been shown to be relatively low.

Mucinous tumors have proportionally low tumor cellularity because they contain more clear gelatinous fluid (mucin), which can be intracellular or extracellular. In vitro studies have shown that FDG uptake directly correlates with the number of viable cancer cells; mucinous tumors have lower proportions of viable cancer cells therefore not demonstrate increased FDG avidity [20].

This increased glucose metabolism accounts for ^{18}F-FDG accumulation into cancer cells, which results in the positive signals (hot spots) in FDG-PET/CT scans. However, the mechanisms how ^{18}F-FDG is accumulated into cancer tissues are complex. These factors are divided into tumor-related (e.g., glucose metabolism, histological differentiation, vascular factor, tumor size and hypoxia) and non-tumor-related components (e.g., high serum glucose level and local inflammation).

Lesion uptake is measured by the SUV, which is calculated based on radioactivity in the lesion, the injected activity and the patient's body weight. If quantifying the average of all pixels within the region of interest (ROI), the result will be SUVavg, whereas with the maximum the result is expressed as: Estimation of lesion18F-FDG uptake.

Estimation of Lesion 18F-FDG Uptake

$$\frac{\text{SUVmax: SUV Mean ROI activity (mCi/mL)}}{\text{Injected activity (mCi)/body = weight (g)}}$$

Or lean body mass (LBM) or body surface area (BSA).

The maximum standardized uptake (SUVmax) value reflects the degree of glucose metabolism within the tumor, which represents the aggressiveness of the malignant lesion.

Quantitative PET/CT may be applied as a diagnostic or prognostic tool (i.e., single measurement) or for therapy response assessment (i.e., longitudinal studies). Metrics include standardized uptake values (SUV, general acronym) computed either using the body weight (SUV) or the lean body mass (SUL), metabolic active tumor volume (MATV or MTV) and total lesion glycolysis (TLG), defined as MATV × SUV mean. In fact, MATV is the volume inside auser- or algorithm-defined volume of interest (VOI) used to circumscribe the metabolically active tumor. Several techniques have been proposed to determine the limits of the VOI, threshold-based or algorithm-based [21], while TLG calculated by multiplying MATV by the mean SUV of all voxels in the MATV incorporates both 2-[18F]FDG uptake and size of the tumor, also known as whole metabolic burden of the tumor [22].

MATVs also allow extraction of heterogeneity features. However, radiomic features are greatly affected and sensitive to a few confounding factors, being image reconstruction settings an example, and this translates into challenges when aiming at its clinical implementation [23, 24].

It is therefore recommended to comply with harmonizing standards such as the EANM/EARL program, one of the international harmonization programs aiming at using ^{18}FDG PET/CT as a quantitative imaging biomarker [25].

Therapy assessment should be performed according to either the European Organisation for Research and Treatment of Cancer (EORTC) PET response criteria or PERCIST [26, 27].

It is important to effectively search for cancer deposits in the regions where this tumor spreads more frequently, namely, the peritoneum, the lymphatic system and the bloodstream. If ceCT can be done as part of the ^{18}FDG PET/CT, it may be evaluated by the multidisciplinary tumor board to avoid performing an additional separate diagnostic CT.

It is generally considered helpful to obtain multiphase contrast-enhanced CT imaging in patients with known/suspected ovarian cancer, especially for the evaluation of the liver, lymph nodes, mesentery, omentum, pleura and lungs [28].

Initial Diagnosis and Staging in Patients Presenting with a Pelvic Mass Suspicious for Ovarian Cancer

Pre-operative diagnostic work-up with computed tomography (CT), positron emission tomography (PET)-CT, or diffusion-weighted whole-body magnetic resonance imaging (MRI), should be used to assess the extent of disease [29].

PET/CT not routine indicated for characterizing adnexal lesions but may be considered if results will alter management [30, 31].

FDG-PET did not reveal much incremental benefit over ultrasound, MRI or all three modalities in combination for characterizing adnexal lesions.

While F18-FDG PET-CT has a limited role in assessment of the primary tumor, it is a particularly useful investigation for determining the lymph node and distant metastases, especially when it comes to extra abdominal spread [32, 33].

However, with the advent of FDG-PET/CT scanners in recent years, the role of PET imaging is being re-explored. PET/CT has been proven to provide incremental information in comparison with CT/MRI and play a role in the preoperative staging of carcinoma of the ovary.

Many publications have focused on the diagnostic efficacy of 18FDG PET/CT for ovarian cancer in patients presenting with a pelvic mass, aiming at optimal management decisions for identifying patients in whom surgical intervention is indicated (positive ^{18}FDGPET/CT).

Castellucci et al. [34] reported comparable sensitivity for 2-[18F]FDG PET/CT and TVUS (around 87–90%), but ^{18}FDG PET/CT presented better specificity.

PET/CT was particularly useful in stage IV patients where CT was prone to downstage patients by missing distant metastases.

In the study of Dauwen et al. FDG-PET/CT performed better than CT in diagnosing retroperitoneal LN metastases [35].

FDG-PET/CT was superior to conventional CT for the detection of carcinomatosis in subdiaphragmatic peritoneal surfaces and in the bowel mesentery and also for the detection of extra-abdominal disease [36].

In another prospective study of 97 patients presenting pelvic masses, Risum et al. reported high specificity of ^{18}FDG PET/ CT for detecting malignant disease, related to ovarian cancer as well as high sensitivity (92.5% and 100%, respectively) upstaging 25 of 66 FIGO stage III stage patients. [37].

Nam et al. [38] in 133 women obtained ^{18}FDG FDG PET/CT presented high accuracy (92%), better than pelvic power Doppler US (83%) and CT/MR (74%) in differentiating benign vs borderline/malignant adnexal masses. The authors also found that staging with 18FDG PET/CT was coincided with surgical staging in 78% of cases, indicating FDG PET/CT may be applied in the presurgical staging of patients in which ovarian cancer is suspected.

Kitajima et al. concluded overall advantage of PET/CT in tumor staging is generally more due to LN staging and in detecting unexpected distant metastases than in detecting local tumor spread in adjacent organs. [39].

In a meta-analysis of 882 patients, PET/CT was the most accurate imaging method for the detection of LNM in EOC patients [40].

In the study of Tardieu. A, a FRANCOGYN Group Study [41], PET-CT had high specificity for preoperative node evaluation in advanced EOC. In the case of advanced EOC management, considering the HAS 2018 recommendations [42] and following the LION study [43], specificity appeared to be the most important parameter for nodal assessment. Indeed, the fact that PET-CT had high specificity means that it was effective in confirming the absence of lymph node invasion on PET-CT in patients without lymph node metastasis. This allowed patients to avoid lymph node dissection, and thus reduced the morbidity associated with the surgical procedure. In this study with advanced EOC population, avoided pelvic and para-aortic surgery in 80% of patients.

Lymphatic dissemination to the pelvic and para-aortic lymph nodes is common, particularly in patients with advanced disease. Spread of disease through the lymphatic channels of the retroperitoneal lymph nodes and diaphragm may lead to dissemination into the supraclavicular or superior mediastinal lymph nodes and pleural space, or rarely, the internal mammary lymph nodes.

Lymph node metastasis is present in 10–20% of patients with presumed early-stage ovarian cancer, and it is present in 40–70% of patients with advanced-stage disease.

In a study of 30 women with advanced-stage (IIC–IV) epithelial ovarian cancer, pretreatment FDG-PET/CT was performed and detected supradiaphragmatic lymph node metastases (LNM) in one or more locations in 67% (20/30) of patients, whereas conventional CT found LNM only in 33% (10/30) of patients.

The patients with supradiaphragmatic LNM, had higher CA-125 levels, and more frequent peritoneal carcinomatosis ($p < 0.03$) compared to patients without supradiaphragmatic LNM in preoperative FDG-PET/CT [44].

As in other fields of oncology, it is a well-known fact that there is an overlap between the degree of FDG uptake in malignant, borderline–malignant and benign lesions. Thus, FDG PET/CT has a good diagnostic accuracy in discriminating ovarian cancer from benign tumors, this not being the case when trying to differentiate borderline–malignant from benign tumors because of its comparatively lower diagnostic accuracy in this context [45].

The false-negative patients appeared because of the absent or low 18FDG accumulation in early tumors and clear-cell, mucinous and cystic carcinomas (compared with serous carcinoma and epithelial carcinoma.

The false-positive results commonly appeared associated to 18FDG accumulation in benign conditions, such as cystadenomas, endometriomas and acute inflammatory processes, or in premenopausal ovaries deriving from cyclic functional activity changes.

However as mentioned before 70% of ovarian cancer have advanced disease (stage III/IV) at presentation and the utility of ^{18}FDG PET/CT in evaluating these patients is undeniable, especially with new generation TOF PET/CT scanners which provide higher spatial resolution, a higher count rate and preserved high sensitivity.

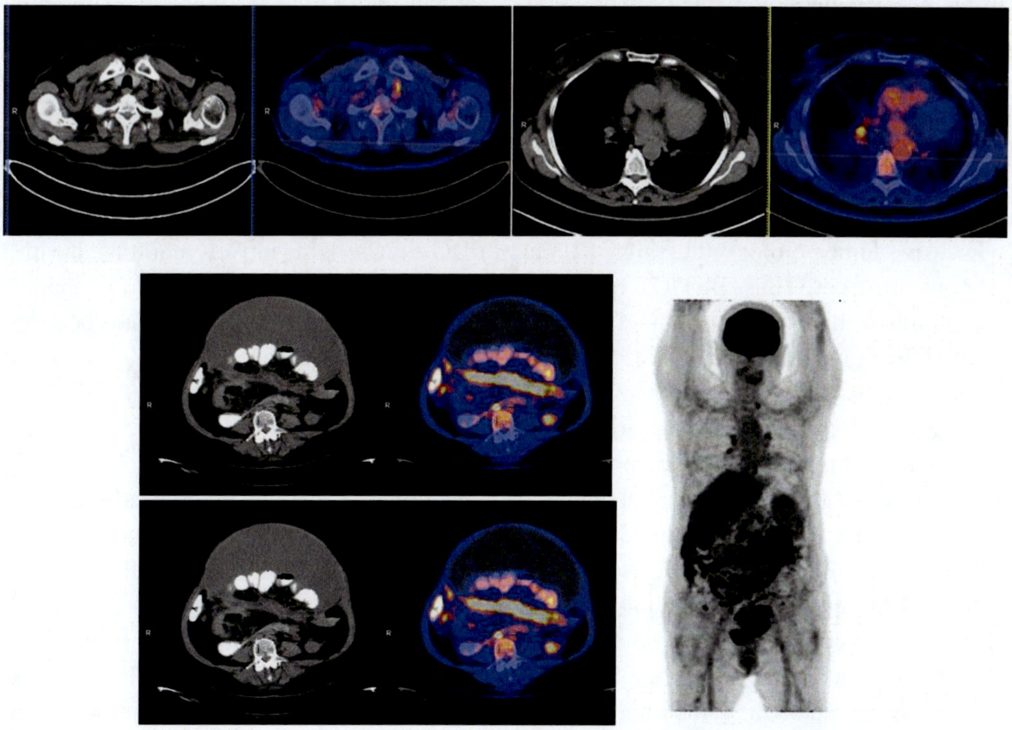

Figure 2. Representative stage IV F-18 FDG PET/CT images.

This translates also in better quantitative accuracy of lesion uptake and improves confidence in the clinical diagnosis [46]. Furthermore, it improves detectability of small lesions [47, 48] which has a major effect in EOC for tracing small peritoneal lesions and subcentimeter lymph nodes.

After several diagnostic biopsies of FDG-avid parasternal/supraclavicular lymph nodes we are today convinced that such lymph nodes represent stage IV disease in women with OC. Hence, the implementation of FDG-PET/CT may broaden our knowledge considerably on metastatic sites for OC that were not previously recognized (Figure 2).

Prognostic Value/Disease Prognostication

PET/CT has been found to be of some incremental value in prognostication and prediction of disease. There is broad evidence confirming the prognostic value^{18}FDG PET/CT in ovarian cancer, with many meta-analyses published in the last 10 years.

Recently, the prognostic role of 18F-FDG PET/CT through its metabolic parameters has been studied and PET imaging techniques could be used to explore the biological behaviour of tumors during therapy, however there is no consensus on their use [49].

Han S. et al. performed a meta-analysis on the prognostic value of 18F-FDG PET-derived volume-based parameters regarding metabolic tumor volume (MTV) and total lesion glycolysis (TLG) in patients with ovarian cancer.

MTV and TLG were significant prognostic factors despite the clinical heterogeneity and difference in methodology between the studies, patients with a high MTV or TLG have a higher risk of disease progression or death [50].

Several studies have evidenced significant associations between primary tumor SUVmax and pathology (serous/non-serous carcinoma).

Mucinous and clear cell ovarian cancer are Type 1 diseases which are more indolent with a better survival pattern as compared to type 2 and shows a significantly lower SUVmax than in serous carcinomas which have greater aberrant mutational status and a more inherently aggressive tumor biology thus high SUVmax FDG uptake is negatively correlated with the amount of mucin. Thus, PET/CT is limited particularly in hypocellular lesions of mucinous carcinoma with abundant mucin [51]. Mucinous neoplasms of the ovary may be benign, borderline, or malignant. The large majority are benign or borderline, accounting for 80% and 16%–17%, respectively.

Most high-grade serous carcinoma (HGSC) present at an advanced stage, while mucinous ovarian carcinoma (MOC) is diagnosed as stage 1 in 80% of the cases [52].

A 68-years old patient with known ascitic collection suspected by cytological examination for the presence of malignancy. PET/CT is ordered to delineate the underlying etiology.

MIP PET/CT and Transverse PET/CT images revealed an abdominal ascites, left hypermetabolic pelvic mass, multiple variable sized peritoneal nodules and tumor plaque deposits unevenly distributed in the peritoneal cavity with the largest 12.6 cm (Linear morphology) and most active one SUVmax:10.58 is seen in the mesentery. Also, there were multiple hypermetabolic lymph nodal groups (bilateral hilar, left supraclavicular, hepatic hilar and multiple small paraaortic lymph nodes). These findings strongly suggest potential malignancy with peritoneal carcinomatosis and lymph node metastases. Histopathologic examination post laparotomy confirmed high-grade serous ovarian carcinoma.

FDG uptake is negatively correlated with the amount of mucin. Thus, PET/CT is limited particularly in hypocellular lesions of mucinous carcinoma with abundant mucin.

Mucinous neoplasms of the ovary may be benign, borderline, or malignant. The large majority are benign or borderline, accounting for 80% and 16%–17%, respectively.

Prognosis is better in early disease, but worse in the advanced stage, compared to HGSC, which is mainly due to inadequate response to platinum-based chemotherapy.

Distinguishing primary MOC from metastatic mucinous carcinoma can be challenging but is essential.

18F PET/CT may increase the rate of detection of small metastases, particularly to the peritoneum or lymph nodes. These metastases may be too small to detect at CT but become apparent at PET/CT when metabolically active. Unfortunately, false negatives have been reported with mucinous carcinoma (Table 3).

Publications assessing the clinical utility of 18F-FDG PET/CT particularly in ovarian Clear Cell Carcinoma (CCC) patients are limited and mainly focused on patients with primary disease.

Ovarian CCC represents a great challenge due to its disease aggressiveness and chemotherapy resistance [53, 54] especially in recurrent ovarian CCC which is particularly chemoresistant [55].

Imaging with CT, fluorine 18 (^{18}F) fluorodeoxyglucose (FDG) PET/CT, and/or MRI may assist in initial treatment planning by allowing assessment of the resectability of tumors, the candidacy of patients for effective cytoreductive surgery, the need for neoadjuvant or postoperative chemotherapy if debulking is suboptimal, and the need for referral to a gynecologic oncologist (Table 3), [56].

In a study by Haruhisa Konishi, Ovarian Clear Cell Carcinoma (CCC) SUVmax was significantly higher in stage Ic than stage Ia, which indicated that biological characteristics such as glucose metabolism differed even within stage I. These results are considered to support the omission of adjuvant chemotherapy and fertility-sparing surgery for stage Ia CCC in the future from the perspective of glucose metabolism [57].

Table 3. CT, MRI, and 18 (18F) PET/CT in the setting of ovarian mucinous carcinoma

Modality	Strengths	Limitations
CT	May assist in initial treatment planning by allowing assessment of the resectability of tumors, the candidacy of patients for effective cytoreductive surgery, and the need for neoadjuvant or postoperative chemotherapy if debulking is suboptimal Detection of metastases to the peritoneum, omentum, mesentery, liver, spleen, lymph nodes, and lungs	Limited in detection of small (<5 mm) metastases, especially to bowel surface, mesentery, and peritoneum
MRI	Similar value to that of CT in initial treatment planning	Less widely available More expensive than CT Limited FOV compared with that of CT Decreased sensitivity for metastases
^{18}F PET/CT	In general, increased rate of detection of small metastases (when FDG avid), particularly to peritoneum or lymph nodes	False negatives may occur in mucinous neoplasms

According to a Japanese study with small cases (n = 11), positive FDG accumulation was shown in 54.5% of CCC patients and the median SUVmax was 3.52 before primary surgery [58].

A high glucose uptake could be compatible with an aggressive tumor as a sign of a glycolytic tumor and this can probably be exploited for the imaging of metabolically active tumors using 18F-FDG PET/CT.

Based on these assumptions, Perrone AM et al. [59] correlated 18F-FDG PET/CT metabolic parameters SUV_{max}, MTV and TLG with post relapse survival (PRS) and overall survival (OS) in Epithelial Ovarian Cancer (EOC) relapse. The study included 50 patients affected by EOC relapse who underwent ^{18}F-FDGPET/CT before surgery.

The authors found that one of these parameters, $SUV_{max,}$ is correlated with PRS and OS. SUVmax represents a prognostic factor (p = 0.024) of aggressiveness and the cut-off 13 represents a marker of poor prognosis (Figure 3).

In a retrospective study by Kim et al. the authors evaluated the prognostic value of quantitative metabolic parameters of 18F-FDG-PET/CT at the time of the first relapse in patients with EOC relapse. Results of this study showed that quantitative metabolic parameters measured with 18F-FDG-PET/CT at the time of first relapse were significant predictors of prognosis. SUVmax with a cut-off higher than 14 defines a worse course of the disease [60].

Peritoneal carcinomatosis (PC) is a common pathway of tumor dissemination in patients with ovarian cancer [61]. PC is a negative predictor of achieving complete tumor debulking, in which the success rate decreased significantly to 26% compared to 76% in patients without PC [62].

Therefore, it is important to select suitable patients for UDS and there is a need of an assessment tool that allow accurate disease evaluation in terms of disease resectability and likelihood of achieving complete tumor debulking.

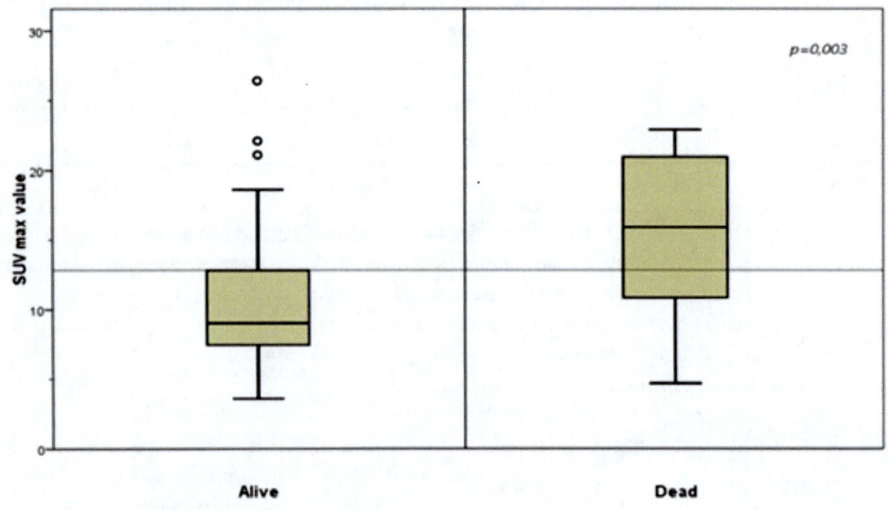

Figure 3. Standardized Uptake Values (SUVmax) value and Overall Survival. SUVmax greater than 13 represents a poor prognostic factor.

Previous studies had shown that 18F-fluorodeoxyglucose Positron Emission Tomography/ Computed Tomography (18F-FDG PET/CT) was promising in PC detection [63, 64].

A recent study by Tsoi TT et al. found that the number of metabolic active peritoneal sites impacted on the immediate surgical outcome, in that a higher number of metabolic active peritoneal sites was associated with increased risk of incomplete tumor debulking after surgery. Additionally, 18F-FDG PET/CT offered high accuracy in PC detection [65].

Several scores for laparotomic assessment of tumor/carcinomatosis extension have been described: the Sugarbaker score or the peritoneal cancer index (PCI) and The Aletti, Fagotti and Eisenkop scores, which attribute a score to several anatomical regions of the abdomen. The most widely used laparoscopic predictive models evaluating ovarian cancer's extension are the peritoneal carcinomatosis index, described by Sugarbaker, and the Fagotti score [66].

The use of scores is a method to compare results and determine in an objective way the treatment indicated for each patient; however, it is currently a challenge. The use of laparoscopic scores could reduce unnecessary laparotomies for those patients to whom the possibility of complete cytoreduction is scarce or non-existent. Neoadjuvant therapy and interval surgery are presented as valid alternatives for these patients [67].

In ovarian cancer in addition to the use of the area harboring the highest uptake, it is recommended to explore peritoneal index adapted PERCIST classification, where the target lesions would be based on one of the scores that have been developed for assessing the extension of peritoneal carcinomatosis.

Chong et al. evaluated PET/CT parameters to predict suboptimal cytoreduction and found a risk model for predicting suboptimal cytoreduction in advanced ovarian cancer. 51 patients underwent primary cytoreductive surgery for advanced ovarian cancer. A residual disease with maximal diameter > 1 cm was considered a suboptimal surgical result. The SUVmax values for nine abdominal regions, the sum of 9 regional SUVmax (WB1SUVmax) and WB2SUVmax (WB1SUVmax plus SUVmax of lymph nodes) were used for PET parameter (Figure 4). Multiple logistic regression analysis was used to determine the predictive value of PET and clinical parameters for risk model. The authors found that the presence of hypermetabolic lesions in the central, right upper, and left upper regions showed predictive value for suboptimal cytoreduction and the risk model could divide the risk groups of suboptimal cytoreduction. The DFS and OS in the high-risk group were significantly worse than those in the low-risk group [68].

In the study of Fagotti et al. [69] to assess the role of PET/CT to predict optimal cytoreduction in recurrent OC, the PET/CT estimated specificity and sensitivity of 56 and 93% and accuracy 79%, while positive predictive and negative predictive value was 77% and 83%, and they concluded that PET/CT can efficiently affect the plan of surgical treatment of patients with recurrent OC.

F-18 FDG PET/CT images were analyzed according to 9 regions covering the whole peritoneal cavity including pelvis. Each quadrant was considered as a possible implant site and was evaluated separately. The regions were numbered as follows; 0, central; 1, right upper; 2, epigastrium; 3, left upper; 4, left flank; 5, lower left; 6, pelvis; 7, right lower; and 8, right flank.

a. 18 FDG PET/CT images represents no evidence of peritoneal carcinomatosis in patients with ovary cancer.
b. F-18 FDG PET/CT shows ovary cancer patients with peritoneal carcinomatosis.

18F-FDG-PET/CT imaging was also proven a valuable tool in assessing the prognosis of ovarian cancer, through factors such as metabolic tumor volume, total lesion glycolysis and preoperative SUVmax being relevant in predicting the outcome of the disease or guiding the primary therapeutic approach during neoadjuvant chemotherapy [70].

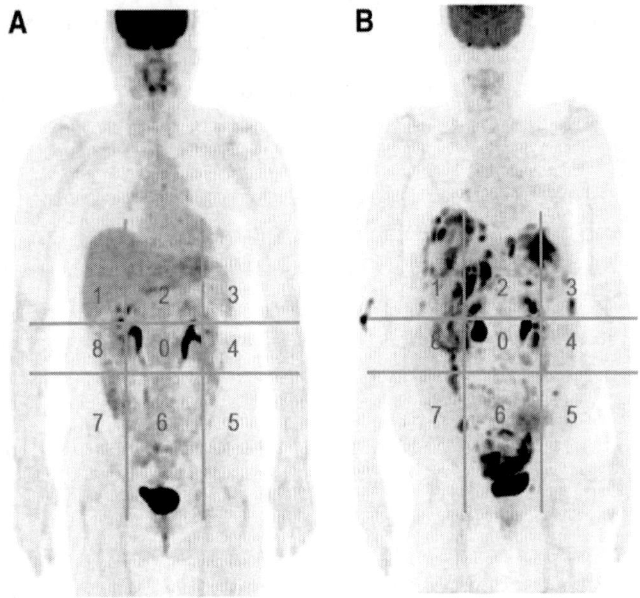

Figure 4. Representative F-18 FDG PET/CT images.

Vallius et al. examined the relationship between the reduction of maximum standardized uptake values (SUVmax) in 18F-FDG-PET/CT to histopathological changes obtained with neoadjuvant chemotherapy (NACT) in advanced epithelial ovarian cancer (EOC) They reported that patients with normalization of SUVmax after 3 courses had higher probabilities to benefit from additional 3 courses [71].

Risum et al. demonstrated that factors for predicting suboptimal cytoreduction include large bowel mesenteric deposits, which could be picked up on PET/CT with high sensitivity prior to surgery and thus help in prognostication [72]. However, the few studies done in this area cannot be very strong contenders to replace second-look laparotomy [73-75].

PET-CT scans and serum CA-125 levels could, be predictive factors in posttreatment overall survival. Chu et al. observed that patients with both elevated CA-125 and positive PET-CT scans had the worst survival out of their study group, and those with both negative had the best prognosis. An intermediate survivability was observed at those that had just one of them positive [76].

In the work of Levy et al. [77] in which 52 patients were assessed by CA125 elevation above the normal limit. It was evident that patients with a pattern of abrupt rise of CA125 had worse prognosis than patients with a progressive increase. Thus, beyond the estimation of kinetic values of CA125, helps in the selection of patients referred to perform a [18F]FDG-PET/CT to detect early disease recurrence.

Moreover, the literature refers those patients with a doubling time of CA125 shorter than 40 days have a significantly shorter survival than those whose doubling time is >40 days (10.6 months vs. 22.1 months), independently of the time to disease progression [78].

In a recent Chinese study, the authors focused on the PET/CT imaging in patients with first relapse. The majority of patients had FDG-avid recurrent lesions and the median SUVmax was 7.10 (range, 3.00–20.60). Further, they assessed the prognostic implications of PET/CT-based metabolic parameters and found that higher TLG along with platinum-resistant recurrence and peritoneal carcinomatosis, proved to be negative predicators of overall survival after multivariate analysis. [79]. Whether patients with higher TLG required more aggressive treatment warranted further assessment.

Therapy Assessment

There are few clinical trials evaluating the role of 2-[18F] FDG PET/CT in the assessment of therapy response.

The goal of the current standard of care of ovarian cancer is a cytoreductive (also called debulking) surgery and systemic chemotherapy (platinum-based). The definitions of platinum-sensitive and -resistant EOC based on time of disease recurrence (before or after six months of the end of chemotherapy) that currently determine the need for platinum retreatment will probably evolve as new treatments result in longer disease-free periods. Similarly, the concept of late recurrence (i.e., at least 18 months disease free), which could be addressed by new surgery if localized, will probably need to be reviewed. Finally, the increasing use of maintenance treatments capable of slowing disease progression will probably mean that the current surgical dogma of achieving zero residual disease will probably no longer apply in a few decades.

18F-FDG PET/CT can also be applied to determine the efficiency of the treatment often being a decisive factor in deciding the opportunity for treatment changes.

MIP whole-body PET and fused PET /CT images (Upper panel) revealed an implantation in the right anterior abdominal wall and small hypermetabolic nodules /infiltrates in the left paracolic region and in serosal surface of the rectosigmoid. She underwent new cycles of chemotherapy and was referred for a second PET/CT scan for response evaluation (lower panel). Compared to the previous PET/CT there is a decrease in metabolic activity as well as in the size of the known implantation in the right anterior abdominal wall and additionally there is an elimination of small peritoneal implants. The above findings are indicative of a partial response to prior therapy.

F18-FDG PET-CT is able to identify patients with a poor response to chemotherapy who would benefit from switching to the next line of treatment [80, 81].

This underlines the crucial aspect of the metabolic changes of tumors that should be assessed alongside the morphological ones, with nuclear medicine imaging through 18F-FDG PET-CT remaining the only viable tool for achieving both at the same time at present.

Therapy assessment with PET can rely on the EORTC PET response criteria, released in 1999 or on the PET Response Criteria in Solid Tumors (PERCIST) criteria which were introduced in 2009. Since EOC often presents as a bulky disease and is known to be a heterogeneous disease in terms of expression of various immunohistochemical markers, using volumetric PET metrics such as the metabolic active tumor volume (MATV) or the total lesion glycolysis (TLG) could be of added value.

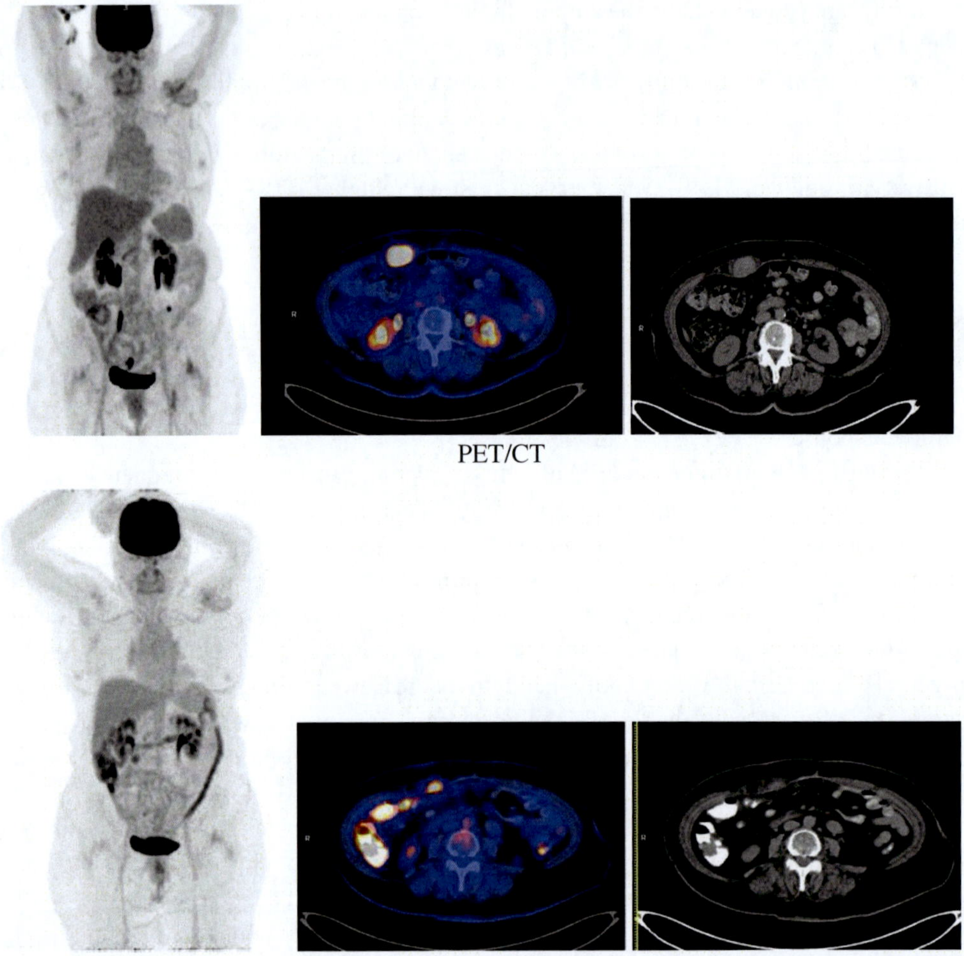

Figure 5. A 74-year-old female with high-grade serous ovarian carcinoma following surgical debulking and adjuvant chemotherapy. The patient was referred for PET/CT scan due to clinical suspicion for intra-abdominal recurrence, three years since initiation of treatment.

However, unlike PERCIST and EORTC criteria for which thresholds to discriminate between stable, progressive, or responding metabolic disease are known, optimal thresholds for MATV or TLG variation between baseline and post-treatment scans are yet to be determined.

Aide N et al. [82] examined 18F-FDG PET parameter changes after one cycle of treatment compared to baseline in patients receiving first-line neoadjuvant anti-angiogenic nintedanib combined to paclitaxel-carboplatin chemotherapy or chemotherapy plus placebo and evaluated the ability of 18F-FDG PET parameters to predict progression-free survival (PFS), overall survival (OS), and success of second-look surgery.

EORTC and PERCIST criteria were applied to classify patients as responders (partial metabolic response and complete metabolic response) or non-responders (stable metabolic disease and progressive metabolic disease). Variation in MATV/ TLG did not predict PFS or OS, and no optimal threshold could be found for MATV/TLG for predicting survival, but a statistically significant correlation was observed between ΔSULpeak and ΔCA-125 between baseline sample and that performed after the second cycle (Figure 5).

The authors conclude that 18F-FDG PET using EORTC or PERCIST criteria appeared to be a useful tool in ovarian cancer trials to analyze early tumor response and predict second-look surgery outcome and survival. An advantage of PERCIST over EORTC criteria is the correlation of ΔSULpeak and ΔCA-125, PET response preceding tumor markers response by 1 month.

Therapy monitoring by PET could help to optimize neoadjuvant therapy protocols and to avoid ineffective preoperative therapy in nonresponders, but this must be proven in a larger number of patients and in different neoadjuvant settings such as chemotherapy, radiation therapy, hormone therapy or a combination of these.

A retrospective study conducted by Caobelli et al. in 2016 [83] with 168 females undergoing restaging PET CT at least 6 months following primary surgery and completion of adjuvant treatment showed that a negative study was associated with a significantly longer progression-free survival and a higher overall survival rate after 4 years of follow up, compared with a positive PET CT at the end of treatment.

There is relatively less defined course in terms of therapeutic intervention with positive PET/CT results in this clinical setting when compared with other malignancies and more data is required to be able to make clinical recommendations for the use of ^{18}F-FDG PET CT in disease monitoring and surveillance of ovarian cancer [84, 85].

Relapse Detection

The early recurrence detection is crucial for planning of the optimal treatment aiming to have a better life quality with longer period free of disease.

Sequential assessment of CA 125 is used to evaluate the ovarian cancer response for treatment. Yet, normal levels of CA 125 cannot exclude the disease, and raised CA 125 levels could not differentiate localized from diffuse tumor recurrence [86-88]. Thus, imaging essentially play a major role to detect ovarian cancer recurrence.

Muñoz et al. [89] also observed that PET-CT with 18F-FDG was more accurate than CA125 alone in diagnosing early ovarian carcinoma recurrence (CA-125 was negative in 50% of the cases that were confirmed through PET-CT). Negative levels of CA-125 cannot exclude active disease, either as recurrence, residual disease or progression. Palomar et al. [90] also identified 53% of cases where CA-125 was below 30 UI/mL but had positive PET-CT 18F-FDG scans, indicating a potential role of PET-CT in monitoring, even in patients with negative serum CA-125. The cut-off value for CA-125 remains, however, a topic that is still debatable among studies.

Evaluating early recurrent disease in ovarian cancer is challenging. For those with high serum tumor markers and negative computed tomography (CT) or magnetic resonance imaging (MRI) findings, functional imaging with 18F-FDG positron emission tomography (PET)/CT helps evaluate early recurrent or small-volume disease [91, 92].

Although post contrast CT is used on a wide spectrum, its sensitivity for detection of minute peritoneal and serosal implants is limited and its ability to differentiate postoperative fibrosis from tumor recurrence is doubtful.

Pelvic MRI is beneficial for the assessment of the local disease recurrence, yet anatomical alterations which occurs postoperatively made MRI with very low specificity [93, 94].

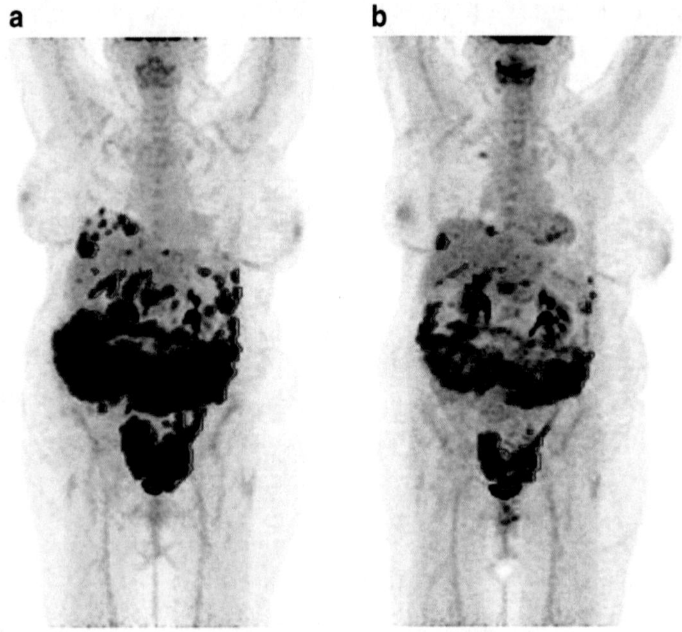

Figure 6. Example of metabolic active tumor volume (MATV) delineation in a patient with stage IIIc FIGO ovarian cancer enrolled in the CHIVA trial [82] in the chemotherapy plus placebo arm classified as partial metabolic responder according to EORCT PET response criteria and PERCIST. Note: the uptake visible in the right upper chest is related to a central venous catheter Early therapy assessment FDG PET/CT (b) was performed 20 days after base line scan (a), after the first cycle of treatment. Maximum intensity projections (MIP) of 2-[18F]FDG PET are present.

FDG PET, again combined with CT, is the most accurate technique to evaluate for suspected recurrent ovarian cancer.

18F-FDG PET/CT has been shown to be superior to CT and MRI in detection of recurrent ovarian cancer [95].

Cengiz A et al. retrospectively studied fifty-two patients (30-80 years old, mean: 58.5 ± 10.6 years) who had been histopathologically diagnosed with ovarian cancer. They underwent ^{18}F-FDG PET/CT imaging for re-staging due to elevation of CA-125 levels, 18F-FDG PET/CT findings were compared with histopathological, radiological and clinical follow-up results. They found the sensitivity, specificity, PPV, NPV and accuracy of 18F-FDG PET/CT in detecting ovarian cancer recurrence in patients with elevated CA-125 levels were calculated as 94%, 75%, 98%, 50% and 96%, respectively [96].

Sari et al. [97] investigated the role of ^{18}F-FDG PET/CT in recurrent ovarian cancer with high tumor markers or suspicious lesions on CT and they reported the sensitivity, specificity and accuracy of PET/CT as 96.1%, 100% and 97%, respectively.

However cystic or necrotic lesions and low-grade tumor OC may result in FN 18F-FDG PET/CT imaging findings.

According to a study of Bhosale et al. PET/CT detected recurrence in 58% of cases when CA125 was normal, while 31% of patients with normal CA 125 and negative CT had ovarian cancer recurrence confirmed by histology [98].

Furthermore, high values of CA125 cannot differentiate local recurrence from distant metastases [99].

It is the role of imaging, and especially PET/CT, to answer that question.

Several reports point to the superior performance of 18F-FDG PET/CT in the detection of recurrent ovarian cancer. 18F-FDG PET/CT is reported to have found positive lesions in many instances in which CT alone was negative [100] Furthermore, 18F-FDG PET was able to document the evidence of disease recurrence 6 mo before findings could be seen on CT [101].

A meta-analysis comparing techniques for detection of recurrence determined that PET/CT (sensitivity, 91%; specificity, 88%) performed better than CT (sensitivity, 79%; specificity, 84%) or MRI (sensitivity, 75%; specificity, 78%) [102].

According to Kitajima et al. [103] the main advantage of PET/CT in EOC is remote lymph node staging and detection of metastases rather than diagnosis of EOC itself.

Moreover, the presurgical staging of advanced disease with PET/CT has evidenced that up-staging from stage III to IV happens in a high proportion of cases [104]. In addition, FDG PET/CT improves the identification of stage III/IV patients for whom complete debulking is not possible.

A resent meta-analysis including 8 studies and 594 patients reported a joint sensitivity and specificity for metastasis of 0.72 (95% confidence interval [CI] = 0.61–0.81) and 0.93 (95% CI = 0.85–0.97), respectively [105].

The authors concluded that pre-treatment 18F-FDG PET/CT showed moderate sensitivity and high specificity for detecting metastasis in ovarian cancer. With its low false-positive rate, 18F-FDG PET/CT can help decide the selection of surgical approaches or alternative treatment options.

Indeed, 18F-FDG PET/CT may represent an alternative approach to characterize relapsed ovarian tumors. In the future, clinicians should consider the metabolic information provided by 18F-FDG PET/CT in the therapeutic choices for their patients.

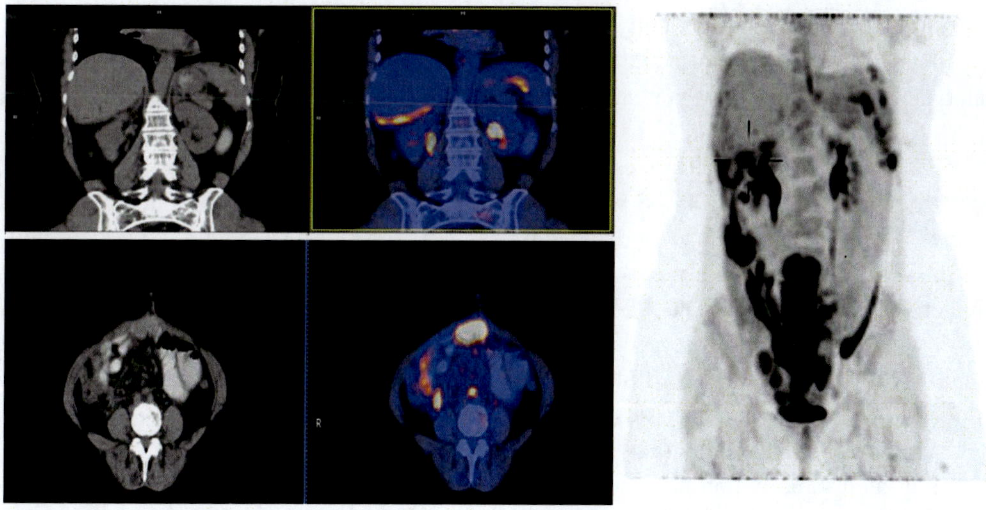

Figure 7. Female patient 52 years old having history of cancer ovary, 3 years after treatment with radical surgery and adjuvant chemotherapy. On routine work up, she had discovered elevated CA125 serum tumor marker 155 ng/ml. FDG PET MIP IMAGE (left), and fused PET/CT (right) images obtained for evaluation of disease recurrence, show multiple enhancing nodules of varying sizes scattered throughout the pelvic cavity, including the cul-de-sac. An additional hypermetabolic nodular tumor deposit is seen in the anterior abdomen, a characteristic finding of omental involvement and also in subhepatic and splenic regions. These findings strongly suggest peritoneal carcinomatosis.

Hypermetabolic tumor implants, especially in subdiaphragmatic or subhepatic locations, on the serosal surfaces of the bowel, or in small nodes, are more conspicuous with PET than with conventional imaging (Figure 7).

Conversely, lack of high-level tracer uptake in post-treatment findings (e.g., fat necrosis, seroma, reactive nodal enlargement) decreases the false-positive rate. In addition, with fusion PET/CT, the CT images provide high-resolution, measurable information on the extent of disease and the anatomic sites of involvement for treatment planning and follow-up.

There has been no publication focusing on the clinical utility of PET/CT-based metabolic variables in patients with recurrent ovarian CCC.

In a recent Chinese study [106], the authors focused on the PET/CT imaging in patients with first relapse. The majority of patients had FDG-avid recurrent lesions and the median SUVmax was 7.10 (range, 3.00–20.60). Further, they assessed the prognostic implications of PET/CT-based metabolic parameters and found that higher TLG along with platinum-resistant recurrence and peritoneal carcinomatosis, proved to be negative predicators of overall survival after multivariate analysis. Whether patients with higher TLG required more aggressive treatment warranted further assessment.

Impact of PET/CT on the Treatment Planning

PET/CT can have a superior role in the detection of ovarian carcinoma recurrence with a power of accurate localization of the lesions; thus, it can alter the treatment plan.

In the study of Fulham et al. [107] which was carried on 90 female patients with suspicion of ovarian carcinoma recurrence, PET–CT displayed a superior detection rate that was achieved by contrast CT which subsequently modified the treatment in 60% of cases.

PET/CT has the power to detect metastasis with increased metabolic activity even in non-enlarged lymph nodes; however, small or necrotic lymph nodes can have false-negative results [108].

Signorelli M et al. [109] investigated the role of 18F-FDG PET/CT in the pre-operative nodal metastases detection in 68 women with ovarian cancer grossly confined to the pelvis. Twelve women (17.6%) had nodal metastases. 18F-FDG PET/CT correctly identified 10 patients with nodal involvement. Sensitivity, specificity, accuracy, positive and negative-predictive value of 18F-FDG PET/CT in detecting nodal metastases were 83.3%, 98.2%, 95.6%, 90.9% and 96.5%, respectively. The authors conclude that high negative predictive value of 18F-FDG PET/CT allows avoidance of SAPL in the vast majority of women, minimizing operative and post-surgical complications.

Many studies have shown 2-[18F]FDG PET/CT has a better diagnostic performance in detecting metastatic lymph nodes compared with ceCT only. A meta-analysis by Yuan et al. [110] (including 882 patients from 18 studies) showed that 2-[18F]FDG PET/CT had better accuracy than both ceCT and MR in detecting metastatic lymphadenopathies, with sensitivity and specificity values of 73% and 96% for 2-[18F]FDG PET/CT, 42% and 95% for ceCT and 54% and 88% for MRI, respectively, with significant differences reached only in sensitivity.

These studies evidence that 2-[18F]FDG PET/CT may be a precise imaging test for selecting patients could benefit from systematic lymphadenectomy (Figure 8).

Thus, the high negative predictive value (NPV) may avoid lymphadenectomy in many cases, reducing to a minimum the surgical complications.

^{18}F-FDG-PET scan showing positive left para-aortic lymph nodes and one left Internal iliac lymph node indicating lymph node metastases, in keeping with FIGO Stage IIIC2.

A diagnostic laparotomy confirmed paraortic and internal iliac lymph nodes positive for metastases.

PET-CT has also proven itself to be more effective than conventional imaging in detecting distant, extra-abdominal metastases, particularly in the case of supradiaphragmatic lymph node involvement.

Nam et al. [111] also reported that PET/CT was able to identify 15.8% of cases of unexpected extra-abdominal lymph node extension and 3.8% of cases with other synchronous tumors.

In the study carried out by Simcock et al. [112], PET/CT had significantly changed the treatment plan of recurrent OC in 57% of the subjects.

In the work of Bilici A et al. PET/CT changed the management in 51.6% of 60 patients with suspected recurrent ovarian cancer who had previously undergone primary debulking surgery and had been treated with adjuvant chemotherapy. PET/CT led to the use of previously unplanned treatment procedures in 61.2% and the avoidance of previously planned therapeutic procedures in 38.8% patients [113].

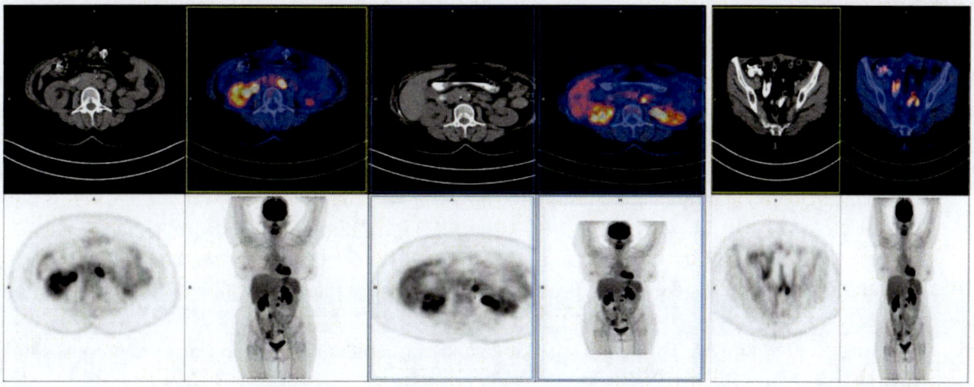

Figure 8. Patient 49 years old with previous high-grade, serous papillary ovarian carcinoma, stage IA, 3 years following radical surgery and R0 resection She was referred for surveillance posttreatment PET/CT with normal CA-125.

PET/CT is a helpful modality in the evaluation of ovarian cancer recurrence; it can detect and localize the recurrence with high accuracy, thus can influence and modify the treatment plan, and reduce the need for the look surgery.

Conclusion

Although ^{18}F-FDG PET/CT is most useful in relapse detection followed by its prognostic value, and there is less evidence for therapy assessment and low-quality evidence for initial diagnosis and staging in patients presenting with a pelvic mass, has assumed increasing importance in the management of patients with ovarian cancers in recent years. The role of PET/CT in the management of EOC may progress and become clearer in the coming years. The NCCN already recommends it for the diagnosis and monitoring of ovarian cancers.

This trend reflects a desire to obtain accurate staging, early disease detection, to influence optimal treatment selection and minimize morbidity and mortality.

We speculate the areas in which PET/CT may develop a role in the clinical management of ovarian carcinoma in the future are:

- a promising technique in monitoring response to therapy
- initial staging of the disease with better accuracy that would guide the correct therapeutic strategy
- and disease prognostication especially as a replacement of second-look laparotomy following completion of primary therapy.

In these areas, presently this is not used in routine clinics but might change with better results with the application of combined imaging approach and better quantification techniques, however it must be determined by results from more clinical studies, evidence-based approach, and the availability of newer salvage treatment modalities.

References

[1] Kim, S. J., Rosen, B., Fan, I., Ivanova, A., McLaughlin, J. R., Risch, H., Narod, S. A., & Kotsopoulos, J. Epidemiologic factors that predict long-term survival following a diagnosis of epithelial ovarian cancer. *Br J Cancer.* 2017;116:964–971.

[2] Coburn S. B., Bray F., Sherman M. E., Trabert B. International patternsand trends in ovarian cancer incidence, overall and by histologicsubtype. *Int J Cancer*. 2017;140:2451–60.

[3] Torre, L. A., Trabert, B., DeSantis, C. E., Miller, K. D., Samimi, G., Runowicz, C. D., Gaudet, M. M., Jemal, A., & Siegel, R. L. Ovarian cancer statistics, 2018. *CA Cancer J Clin*. 2018;68:284–96.

[4] Berek J. S., Kehoe S. T., Kumar L., Friedlander M. Cancer of the ovary, fallopian tube, and peritoneum. *Int J Gynaecol Obstet*. 2018 Oct; 143 Suppl 2():59-78.

[5] Kurman R. J. Shihle M. The origin and pathogenesis of epithelial ovarian cancer: a proposed unifying theory. *Am J Surg Pathol*. 2010; 34: 433-443.

[6] Dion, L., Carton, I., Jaillard, S., Nyangoh Timoh, K., Henno, S., Sardain, H., Foucher, F., Levêque, J., de la Motte Rouge, T., Brousse, S., & Lavoué, V. The Landscape and Therapeutic Implications of Molecular Profiles in Epithelial Ovarian Cancer *J. Çlin. Med*. 2020, 9, 2239.

[7] Terada K. Y., Ahn H. J., Kessel B. Differences in risk for type 1 and type 2 ovarian cancer in a large cancer screening trial. *J Gynecol Oncol*. 2016;27:e25.

[8] Cheasley, D., Wakefield, M. J., Ryland, G. L., Allan, P. E., Alsop, K., Amarasinghe, K. C., Ananda, S., Anglesio, M. S., Au-Yeung, G., Böhm, M., Bowtell, D. D. L., Brand, A., Chenevix-Trench, G., Christie, M., Chiew, Y.-E., Churchman, M., DeFazio, A., Demeo, R., Dudley, R., Fairweather, N., Fedele, C. G., Fereday, S., Fox, S. B., Gilks, C. B., Gourley, C., Hacker, N. F., Hadley, A. M., Hendley, J., Ho, G. Y., Hughes, S., Hunstman, D. G., Hunter, S. M., Jobling, T. W., Kalli, K. R., Kaufmann, S. H., Kennedy, C. J., Köbel, M., Page, C. Le, Li, J., Lupat, R., McNally, O. M., McAlpine, J. N., Mes-Masson, A. M., Mileshkin, L., Provencher, D. M., Pyman, J., Rahimi, K., Rowley, S. M., Salazar, C., Samimi, G., Saunders, H., Semple, T., Sharma, R., Sharpe, A. J., Stephens, A. N., Thio, N., Torres, M. C., Traficante, N., Xing, Z., Zethoven, M., Antill, Y. C., Scott, C. L., Campbell, I. G. and Gorringe, K. L. The molecular origin and taxonomy of mucinous ovarian carcinoma. *Nat Commun*. 2019 Sep 2; 10(1):3935.

[9] Cancer Genome Atlas Research Network. "Integrated genomic analyses of ovarian carcinoma." *Nature* vol. 474,7353 609-15. 29 Jun. 2011, doi:10.1038/nature10166.

[10] Gadducci, A., Fuso, L., Cosio, S., Landoni, F., Maggino, T., Perotto, S., Sartori, E., Testa, A., Galletto, L., & Zola, P. Are surveillance procedures of clinical benefit for patients treated for ovarian cancer? A retrospective Italian multicentric study. *Int J Gynecol Cancer.* 2009; 19: 367-374.

[11] Lutz, A. M., Willmann, J. K., Drescher, C. W., Ray, P., Cochran, F. V., Urban, N., & Gambhir, S. S. Early diagnosis of ovarian carcinoma: is a solution in sight? *Radiology*. 2011; 259: 329-345.

[12] Schmidt S, Meuli RA, Achtari C, Prior JO. Peritoneal carcinomatosis in primary ovarian cancer staging: comparison between MDCT, MRI, and 18F-FDG PET/CT. *Clin Nucl Med* 2015; 40: 371–377.

[13] S. Martinez-Roman, P. T. Ramirez, J. Oh, M. G. Viciedo, H. A. MacApinlac Combined positron emission tomography and computed tomography for the detection of recurrent ovarian mucinous adenocarcinoma *Gynecol Oncol*, 96 (2005), pp. 888-891.

[14] Monika Pliszka and Leszek Szablewski. Cancers 2021, 13, 4184. Expression of glucose transporters in diseases. In *Human Glucose Transporters in Health and Diseases*; Cambridge Scholary Publishing, Lady Stephenson Library: Newcastle upon Tyne, UK, 2019; pp. 63–227.

[15] Nishizawa S, Inubushi M, Okada H. Physiological 18F-FDG uptake in the ovaries and uterus of healthy female volunteers. *Eur J Nucl Med Mol Imaging* 2005;32(5):549–556.

[16] Espey LL. Ovulation as an inflammatory reaction: a hypothesis. *Biol Reprod* 1980;22(1):73–106.

[17] O. Dorigo, J. S. Berek. Personalizing CA125 levels for ovarian cancer screening. *Cancer Prevent Res*, 4 (2011), pp. 1356-1359.

[18] Amish Lakhanietbal. FDG PET/CT Pitfalls in *Gynecologic and Genitourinary Oncologic Imaging Radiographics* 2017; 37(2):577-594.

[19] Berger KL, Nicholson SA, Dehdashti F, Siegel BA. FDG PET evaluation of mucinous neoplasms: correlation of FDG uptake with histopathologic features. *AJR Am J Roentgenol* 2000;174(4):1005–1008.

[20] Higashi K, Clavo AC, Wahl RL. Does FDG uptake measure proliferative activity of human cancer cells? In vitro comparison with DNA flow cytometry and tritiated thymidine uptake. *J Nucl Med* 1993;34(3):414–419.

[21] Meyer, H. J.; Wienke, A.; Surov, A. Associations between GLUT expression and SUV values derived from FDG-PET in different tumors—A systematic review and meta-analysis. *PLoS ONE* 2019, 14, e217781.

[22] Xia, H.; Chen, J.; Gao, H.; Kong, S. N.; Deivasigamani, A.; Shi, M.; Xie, T.; Hui, K. M. Hypoxia-induced modulation of glucose transporters impacts 18F-fluorodeoxyglucose PET-CT imaging in hepatocellular carcinoma. *Eur. J Nucl. Med. Mol. Imaging* 2020, 47, 787–797.

[23] Ancey, P.-B.; Contat, C.; Meylan, E. Glucose transporters in cancer—From tumor cells to the tumor microenvironment. *FEBS J.* 2018, 16, 2926–2943.

[24] Yamada, K.; Brink, I.; Bissé, E.; Epting, R.; Engelhard, R. Factors influencing [F-18]-2-fluoro-2-deoxy-D-glucose (F-18 FDG) uptake in melanoma cells: The role of proliferative rate, viability, glucose transporter expression and hexokinase activity. *J. Dermatol*. 2005, 32, 316–334.

[25] Aide N, Lasnon C, Veit-Haibach P, Sera T, Sattler B, Boellaard R. EANM/EARL harmonization strategies in PET quantification: from daily practice to multicentre oncological studies. *Eur J Nucl Med Mol Imaging*. 2017 Aug;44(Suppl 1):17-31.

[26] Vanhoe, K.; Thomeer, M.; Derveaux, E.; Shkedy, Z.; Owokotomo, O. E., Adriaensen, P.; Mesotten, L. Correlations between the metabolic profile and 18F-FDG-Positron Emission Tomography-Computed Tomography parameters reveal the complexity of the metabolic reprogramming within lung cancer patients. *Sci. Rev*. 2019, 9, 16212.

[27] Baschnagel, A. M.; Wobb, J. L.; Dilworth, J. T.; Williams, L.; Eskandari, M.; Wu, D.; Pruetz, B. L.; Wilson, G. D. The association of 18F-FDG PET and glucose metabolism biomarkers GLUT1 and HK2 in p16 positive and negative head and neck squamous cell carcinoma. *Radiother. Oncol*. 2015, 117, 118–124.

[28] Delgado Bolton RC, Aide N, Colletti PM, Ferrero A, Paez D, Skanjeti A, Giammarile F. EANM guideline on the role of 2 [18F]FDG PET/CT in diagnosis, staging, prognostic value, therapy assessment and restaging of ovarian cancer, endorsed by the American College of Nuclear Medicine (ACNM), the Society of Nuclear Medicine and Molecular Imaging (SNMMI) and the International Atomic Energy Agency (IAEA) *Eur J Nucl Med Mol Imaging*. 2021 Sep;48(10):3286-3302.

[29] ESMO–ESGO consensus conferencerecommendations on ovarian cancer: pathology andmolecular biology, early and advanced stages, borderline tumours and recurrent disease. *Annals of Oncology* 30: 672–705, 2019.

[30] Nam EJ, Yun MJ, Oh YT, (Diagnosis and staging of primary ovarian cancer: Correlation between PET/CT, Doppler US, and CT or MRI. *Gynecol. Oncol*, 116(3), 389–394 (2010).

[31] Schröder W, Zimny M, Rudlowski C, Büll U, Rath W. The role of 18F-fluorodeoxyglucose positron emission tomography (18F-FDG PET) in diagnosis of ovarian cancer. *Int. J. Gynecol. Cancer* 9(2), 117–122 (1999).

[32] Kemppainen, J.; Hynninen, J.; Virtanen, J.; Seppänen, M. PET/CT for Evaluation of Ovarian Cancer. *Semin. Nucl. Med.* 2019, 49, 484–492.

[33] Fruscio, R.; Sina, F.; Dolci, C.; Signorelli, M.; Crivellaro, C.; Dell'Anna, T.; Cuzzocrea, M.; Guerra, L.; Milani, R.; Messa, C. Preoperative 18F-FDG PET/CT in the management of advanced epithelial ovarian cancer. *Gynecol. Oncol.* 2013, 131, 689–693.

[34] Castellucci, P., Perrone, A. M., Picchio, M., Ghi, T., Farsad, M., Nanni, C., Messa, C., Meriggiola, M. C., Pelusi, G., Al-Nahhas, A., Rubello, D., Fazio, F., & Fanti, S. Diagnostic accuracy of 18F-FDG PET/CT in characterizing ovarian lesions and staging ovarian cancer: correlation with transvaginal ultrasonography, computed tomography, and histology. *Nucl Med Commun.* 2007;28:589–95.

[35] Dauwen, H., Van Calster, B., Deroose, C. M., Op de Beeck, K., Amant, F., Neven, P., Berteloot, P., Leunen, K., Timmerman, D., & Vergote, I. PET/CT in the staging of patients with a pelvic mass suspicious for ovarian cancer. *Gynecol Oncol.* 2013;131(3):694–700.

[36] Hynninen, J., Kemppainen, J., Lavonius, M., Virtanen, J., Matomäki, J., Oksa, S., Carpén, O., Grénman, S., Seppänen, M., & Auranen, A. A prospective comparison of integrated FDG-PET/contrast-enhanced CT and contrast-enhanced CT for pretreatment imaging of advanced epithelial ovarian cancer. *Gynecol Oncol.* 2013 Nov;131(2):389-94.

[37] Risum, S., Hogdall, C., Loft, A., Berthelsen, A., Hogdall, E., Nedergaard, L., Lundvall, L., & Engelholm, S. The diagnostic value of PET/CT for primary ovarian cancer–a prospective study. *Gynecol Oncol.* 2007;105:145–9.

[38] Nam, E. J., Yun, M. J., Oh, Y. T., Kim, J. W., Kim, J. H., Kim, S., Jung, Y. W., Kim, S. W., & Kim, Y. T. Diagnosis and staging of primary ovarian cancer: correlation between PET/CT, Doppler US, and CT or MRI. *Gynecol Oncol.* 2010;116:389–94.

[39] Kitajima, K., Murakami, K., Yamasaki, E., Kaji, Y., Fukasawa, I., Inaba, N., & Sugimura, K. Diagnostic accuracy of integrated FDG-PET/contrast-enhanced CT in staging ovarian cancer: comparison with enhanced CT. Mal J Med HealthSci 13(2): 29-37, June 2017 37 *Eur J Nucl Med Mol Imaging*. 2008;35(10):1912–20.

[40] Yuan, Y., Gu, Z. X., Tao, X. F., Liu, S. Y. Computer tomography, magnetic resonance imaging, and positron emission tomography or positron emission tomography/computer tomography for detection of metastatic lymph nodes in patients with ovarian cancer: a meta-analysis *Eur J Radiol.* 2012 May;81(5):1002-6.

[41] Tardieu, A., Ouldamer, L., Margueritte, F., Rossard, L., Lacorre, A., Bourdel, N., Lades, G., Sallée, C., Monteil, J., & Gauthier, T. Assessment of Lymph Node Involvement with PET-CT in Advanced Epithelial Ovarian Cancer. A FRANCOGYN Group Study. *J. Clin. Med.* 2021, 10, 602.

[42] Ferron, G.; Narducci, F.; Pouget, N.; Touboul, C. [Surgery for advanced stage ovarian cancer: Article drafted from the French Guidelines in oncology entitled «Initial management of patients with epithelial ovarian cancer» developed by FRANCOGYN, CNGOF, SFOG, GINECO-ARCAGY under the aegis of CNGOF and endorsed by INCa]. *Gynecol. Obstet. Fertil. Senol.* 2019, 47, 197–213.

[43] Harter, P., Sehouli, J., Lorusso, D., Reuss, A., Vergote, I., Marth, C., Kim, J.-W., Raspagliesi, F., Lampe, B., Aletti, G., Meier, W., Cibula, D., Mustea, A., Mahner, S., Runnebaum, I. B., Schmalfeldt, B., Burges, A., Kimmig, R., Scambia, G., Greggi, S., Hilpert, F., Hasenburg, A., Hillemanns, P., Giorda, G., von Leffern, I., Schade-Brittinger, C., Wagner, U. and du Bois, A. A Randomized Trial of Lymphadenectomy in Patients with Advanced Ovarian Neoplasms. *N. Engl. J. Med.* 2019, 380, 822–832.

[44] Hynninen, J., Auranen, A., Carpén, O., Dean, K., Seppänen, M., Kemppainen, J., Lavonius, M., Lisinen, I., Virtanen, J., & Grénman, S. FDG PET/CT in staging of advanced epithelial ovarian cancer:

frequency of supradiaphragmatic lymph node metastasis challenges the traditional pattern of disease spread. *Gynecol Oncol.* 126 (1):64–8; 2012.

[45] Tanizaki Y, Kobayashi A, Shiro M, Ota N, Takano R, Mabuchi Y, Yagi, S., Minami, S., Terada, M., Ino, K. Diagnostic value of preoperative SUVmax on FDG-PET/ CT for the detection of ovarian cancer. *Int J Gynecol Cancer Soc.* 2014;24:454–60.

[46] Daube-Witherspoon ME, Surti S, Perkins AE, Karp JS (2014) Determination of accuracy and precision of lesion uptake measurements in human subjects with time-of-flight PET. *J Nucl Med* 55:602–607.

[47] Surti, S., Scheuermann, J., El Fakhri, G., Daube-Witherspoon, M. E., Lim, R., Abi-Hatem, N., Moussallem, E., Benard, F., Mankoff, D., & Karp, J. S. (2011) Impact of TOF PET on whole-body oncologic studies: a human observer detection and localization study. *J Nucl Med* 52:712–719.

[48] Conti, M., Bendriem, B. The new opportunities for high time resolution clinical TOF PET. *Clin Transl Imaging* 7, 139–147 (2019). https://doi.org/10.1007/s40336-019-00316-5.

[49] Li Q., Zhang J., Cheng W., Zhu C., Chen L., Xia F., Wang M., Yang F., Ma X. Prognostic value of maximum standard uptake value, metabolic tumor volume, and total lesion glycolysis of positron emission tomography/computed tomography in patients with nasopharyngeal carcinoma: A systematic review and meta-analysis. *Medicine* (Baltimore) 2017;96:8084.

[50] Han S., Kim H., Kim Y. J., Suh C. H., Woo S. Prognostic value of volume-based metabolic parameters of 18F-FDG PET/CT in ovarian cancer: a systematic review and meta-analysis. *Ann Nucl Med.* 2018 Dec;32(10):669-677.

[51] Abdelhafez, Y., Tawakol, A., Osama, A., Hamada, E., & El-Refaei, S. Role of 18F-FDG PET/CT in the detection of ovarian cancer recurrence in the setting of normal tumor markers. *The Egyptian Journal of Radiology and Nuclear Medicine* 47(2016)1787-1794.

[52] Seidman, J. D., Horkayne-Szakaly, I., Haiba, M., Boice, C. R., Kurman, R. J., & Ronnett, B. M. The histologic type and stage distribution of ovarian carcinomas of surface epithelial origin. *Int J Gynecol Pathol.* 2004 Jan; 23(1):41-44.

[53] del Carmen MG, Birrer M, Schorge JO. Clear cell carcinoma of the ovary: a review of the literature. *Gynecol Oncol.* 2012;126:481–90.

[54] Anglesio M. S., Carey M. S., Kobel M., Mackay H., Huntsman D. G. Clear cell carcinoma of the ovary: a report from the first ovarian clear cell symposium, June 24th, 2010. *Gynecol Oncol.* 2011;121:407–15.

[55] Crotzer D. R., Sun C. C., Coleman R. L., Wolf J. K., Levenback C. F., Gershenson D. M. Lack of effective systemic therapy for recurrent clear cell carcinoma of the ovary. *Gynecol Oncol.* 2007;105:404–8).

[56] Marko, J., Marko, K. I., Pachigolla, S. L., Crothers, B. A., Mattu, R., & Wolfman, D. J. Mucinous Neoplasms of the Ovary: Radiologic-Pathologic Correlation. *Radio Graphics* 2019; 39:982–997).

[57] Haruhisa Konishietal. Prognostic Significance of Fluorodeoxyglucose Positron Emission Tomography Maximum StandardizedUptake Value in Stage I Ovarian Clear Cell Carcinoma: A Retrospective Observational Study Open *Journal of Obstetrics and Gynecology*, 2016, 6, 136-143.

[58] Tanizaki Y., Kobayashi A., Shiro M., Ota, N., Takano, R., Mabuchi, Y., Yagi, S., Minami, S., Terada, M., Ino, K. Diagnostic value of preoperative SUVmax on FDG-PET/CT for the detection of ovarian cancer. *Int J Gynecol Cancer.* 2014;24:454–60.

[59] Perrone, A., Dondi, G., Lima, G., Castellucci, P., Tesei, M., Coluccelli, S., Gasparre, G., Porcelli, A., Nanni, C., Fanti, S., & De Iaco, P. Potential Prognostic Role of 18F-FDG PET/CT in Invasive Epithelial Ovarian Cancer Relapse. A Preliminary Study. *Cancers* (Basel). 2019;11(5):713. Published 2019 May 23. doi:10.3390/cancers11050713.

[60] Kim, C. Y., Jeong, S. Y., Chong, G. O., Son, S. H., Jung, J., Kim, D. H., Lee, S. W., Ahn, B. C., & Lee, J. Quantitative metabolic parameters measured on F-18 FDG PET/CT predict survival after relapse in patients with relapsed epithelial ovarian cancer. *Gynecol Oncol.* 2015 Mar; 136(3):498-504.

[61] Healy J. C., Reznek R. H. The peritoneum, mesenteries and omenta: normal anatomy and pathological processes. *Eur Radiol.* 1998; 8(6):886-900.

[62] Harter, P., Hahmann, M., Lueck, H. J., Poelcher, M., Wimberger, P., Ortmann, O., Canzler, U., Richter, B., Wagner, U., Hasenburg, A., Burges, A., Loibl, S., Meier, W., Huober, J., Fink, D., Schroeder, W., Muenstedt, K., Schmalfeldt, B., Emons, G., & du Bois, A. Surgery for recurrent ovarian cancer: role

of peritoneal carcinomatosis: exploratory analysis of the DESKTOP I Trial about risk factors, surgical implications, and prognostic value of peritoneal carcinomatosis. *Ann Surg Oncol*. 2009 May;16(5):1324-30.

[63] Klumpp BD, Schwenzer N, Aschoff P, Miller S, Kramer U, Claussen CD, Bruecher B, Koenigsrainer A, Pfannenberg C . Preoperative assessment of peritoneal carcinomatosis: intraindividual comparison of 18F-FDG PET/CT and MRI. *Abdom Imaging*. 2013 Feb; 38(1):64-71.

[64] Pfannenberg, C., Königsrainer, I., Aschoff, P., Öksüz, M. Ö., Zieker, D., Beckert, S., Symons, S., Nieselt, K., Glatzle, J., Weyhern, C. V., Brücher, B. L., Claussen, C. D., & Königsrainer, A. 18-FDG PET/CT to select patients with peritoneal carcinomatosis for cytoreductive surgery and hyperthermicintraperitoneal chemotherapy. *Ann Surg Oncol*. 2009 May; 16(5):1295-303.

[65] Tsoi TT, Chiu KWH, Chu MY, Ngan HYS, Lee EYP. Metabolic active peritoneal sites affect tumor debulking in ovarian and peritoneal cancers. *J Ovarian Res*. 2020;13(1):61.

[66] Greggi, S., Falcone, F., Scaffa, C., du Bois, A., Samartzis, E. P. P., Pujade-Lauraine, E., Cibula, D., Mądry, R., Korach, J., Gungorduk, K., McNeish, I. A., Zanagnolo, V., Marth, C., van Altena, A. M., Aravantinos, G., Sehouli, J., Vergote, I., & Gonzalez Martin, A. Evaluation of surgical resection in advanced ovarian, fallopian tube, and primary peritoneal cancer: Laparoscopic assessment. A European Network of Gynaecological Oncology Trial (ENGOT) group survey. *Int. J. Gynecol. Cancer* 2020, 30, 819–824.

[67] Van De Vrie, R., Rutten, M. J., Asseler, J. D., Leeflang, M. M., Kenter, G. G., Mol, B. W., Buist, M. Laparoscopy for diagnosing resectability of disease in women with advanced ovarian cancer. *Cochrane Database Syst Rev*. 2019.

[68] Chong, G. O., Jeong, S Y., Lee, Y. H., Lee, H. Y. "The ability of whole-body SUVmax in F-18 FDG PET/CT to predict suboptimal cytoreduction during primary debulking surgery for advanced ovarian cancer." *Journal of ovarian research* vol. 12,1 12. 4 Feb. 2019.

[69] Fagotti A, Fanfani F, Rositto C, Lorusso D, De Gaetano AM, Giordano A, Vizzielli G, Scambia G (2008) A treatment selection protocol for recurrent ovarian cancer patients: the role of FDG-PET/CT and staging laparoscopy. *Oncology* 75:152–158.

[70] Konishi, H.; Takehara, K.; Kojima, A.; Okame, S.; Yamamoto, Y.; Shiroyama, Y.; Yokoyama, T.; Nogawa, T.; Sugawara, Y. Maximum standardized uptake value of fluorodeoxyglucose positron emission tomography/computed tomography is a prognostic factor in ovarian clear cell adenocarcinoma. *Int. J. Gynecol. Cancer*. 2014, 24, 1190–1194.

[71] Vallius, T., Peter, A., Auranen, A., Carpén, O., Kemppainen, J., Matomäki, J., Oksa, S., Roering, P., Seppänen, M., Grénman, S., & Hynninen, J. 18F-FDG-PET/CT can identify histopathological non-responders to platinum-based neoadjuvant chemotherapy in advanced epithelial ovarian cancer. *Gynecol Oncol*. 2016;140:29–35.

[72] Risum, S., Høgdall, C., Loft, A., Berthelsen, A. K., Høgdall, E., Nedergaard, L., Lundvall, L., & Engelholm, S. A. Prediction of suboptimal primary cytoreduction in primary ovarian cancer with combined positron emission tomography/computed tomography – a prospective study. *Gynecol. Oncol.* 108(2), 265–270 (2008).

[73] Lee, M. C., Kim, S., Chung, J.-K., Kang, S. B., Kim, M. H., Jeong, J. M., & Lee, D. S. [18F] FDG PET as a substitute for second-look laparotomy in patients with advanced ovarian carcinoma. *Eur. J. Nucl. Med. Mol. Imaging* 31(2), 196–201 (2004).

[74] Smith GT, Hubner KF, McDonald T, Thie JA. Avoiding second-look surgery and reducing costs in managing patients with ovarian cancer by applying F-18-FDG PET. *Clin. Positron Imaging* 1(4), 263 (1998).

[75] Vallius, T., Hynninen, J., Kemppainen, J., Alves, V., Auranen, K., Matomäki, J., Oksa, S., Virtanen, J., Grénman, S., Auranen, A., & Seppänen, M. 18F-FDG-PET/CT based total metabolic tumor volume change during neoadjuvant chemotherapy predicts outcome in advanced epithelial ovarian cancer. *Eur. J. Nucl. Med. Mol. Imaging* 2018, 45, 1224–1232.

[76] Chu, L. C., Tsai, H. L., Wang, H., Crandall, J., Javadi, M. S., Wahl, R. L. Posttreatment FDG PET/CT in predicting survival of patients with ovarian carcinoma. *EJNMMI Res*. 2016, 6, 4–11.

[77] Levy, T., Weiser, R., Boaz, M., Ben Shem, E., Golan, A., & Menczer, J. The significance of the pattern of serum CA125 level ascent to above the normal range in epithelial ovarian, primary peritoneal and tubal carcinoma patients. *Gynecol Oncol* 2012;129:165–8.

[78] Han, L. Y., Karavasilis, V., Hagen, T. van, Nicum, S., Thomas, K., Harrison, M., Papadopoulos, P., Blake, P., Barton, D. P. J., Gore, M., & Kaye, S. B. Doubling time of serum CA125 is an independent prognostic factor for survival in patients with ovarian cancer relapsing after first-line chemotherapy. *Eur J Cancer* 2010;46: 1359–64.

[79] Ye, S., Liu, S., Xiang, L., Wu, X., & Yang, H. 18F-FDG PET/CT-based metabolic metrics in recurrent tumors of ovarian clear cell carcinoma and their prognostic implications. *BMC Cancer* 19, 226 (2019).

[80] Vallius, T., Peter, A., Auranen, A., Carpén, O., Kemppainen, J., Matomäki, J., Oksa, S., Roering, P., Seppänen, M., Grénman, S., & Hynninen, J. 18F-FDG-PET/CT can identify histopathological non-responders to platinum-based neoadjuvant chemotherapy in advanced epithelial ovarian cancer. *Gynecol. Oncol.* 2016, 140, 29–35.

[81] Young AIMN Working Group, Caobelli, F., Alongi, P., Evangelista, L., Picchio, M., Saladini, G., Rensi, M., Geatti, O., Castello, A., Laghai, I., Popescu, C. E., Dolci, C., Crivellaro, C., Seghezzi, S., Kirienko, M., De Biasi, V., Cocciolillo, F., & Quartuccio, N. Predictive value of 18F-FDG PET/CT in restaging patients affected by ovarian carcinoma: A multicentrestudy. *Eur. J. Nucl. Med. Mol. Imaging*. 2016, 43, 404–413.

[82] Aide, N., Fauchille, P., Coquan, E., Ferron, G., Combe, P., Meunier, J., Alexandre, J., Berton, D., Leary, A., De Rauglaudre, G., Bonichon, N., Pujade Lauraine, E., & Joly, F. Predicting tumor response and outcome of second-look surgery with (18)F-FDG PET/CT: insights from the GINECO CHIVA phase II trial of neoadjuvant chemotherapy plus nintedanibin stage IIIc-IV FIGO ovarian cancer. *Eur J Nucl Med Mol Imaging*. 2020.

[83] Young AIMN Working Group, Caobelli, F., Alongi, P., Evangelista, L., Picchio, M., Saladini, G., Rensi, M., Geatti, O., Castello, A., Laghai, I., Popescu, C. E., Dolci, C., Crivellaro, C., Seghezzi, S., Kirienko, M., De Biasi, V., Cocciolillo, F., & Quartuccio, N. Young AIMN Working Group Predictive value of 18F-FDG PET/CT in restaging patients affected by ovarian carcinoma: a multicentre study. *Eur J Nucl Med Mol Imaging* 2016; 43: 404–13.

[84] Markman M. Use of positron emission tomography scans in ovarian cancer: a diagnostic technique in search of an indication. *J. Clin. Oncol*. 23(30) 7385–7387 (2005).

[85] Rusu G, Achimaș-Cadariu P, Piciu A, Căinap SS, Căinap C, Piciu D. A Comparative Study between 18F-FDG PET/CT and Conventional Imaging in the Evaluation of Progressive Disease and Recurrence in Ovarian Carcinoma. *Healthcare* (Basel). 2021 Jun 3;9(6):666.

[86] Folk, M. Botsford, A. G. Musa Monitoring cancer antigen 125 levels in induction chemotherapy for epithelial ovarian carcinoma and predicting outcome of second-look procedure *Gynecol Oncol*, 57 (2) (1995), pp. 178-182.

[87] Patsner, J. W. Orr Jr, W. J. Mann Jr, P. T. Taylor, E. Partridge, T. Allmen Does serum CA-125 level prior to second-look laparotomy for invasive ovarian adenocarcinoma predict size of residual disease? *Gynecol Oncol*, 38 (3) (1990), pp. 373-376 S.C.

[88] Rubin, S. C., Hoskins, W. J., Hakes, T. B., Markman, M., Reichman, B. S., Chapman, D., & Lewis, J. L. Serum CA 125 levels and surgical findings in patients undergoing secondary operations for epithelial ovarian cancer *Am J Obstet Gynecol*, 160 (3) (1989), pp. 667-670.

[89] Muñoz, A. P., García, J. M. C., Rubio, M. D. P. T., Vicente, A. M. G., Pardo, F. J. P., Londoño, G. A. J., Castrejón, Á. S., Aguilar, E. A. Value of [18F]FDG-PET/CT and CA125, serum levels and kinetic parameters, in early detection of ovarian cancer recurrence. *Medicine* 2018, 97.

[90] Palomar, A., Nanni, C., Castellucci, P., Ambrosini, V., Montini, G. C., Allegri, V., Pettinato, C., Al-Nahhas, A., Soriano, A., Grassetto, G., Rubello, D., & Fanti, S. Value of FDG PET/CT in patients with treated ovarian cancer and raised CA125 serum levels. *Mol. Imaging Biol*. 2012, 14, 123–129.

[91] Sari, O., Kaya, B., Ozcan Kara, P., Kara Gedik, G., Celik, C., Ozbek, O., & Serdengecti, M. The role of FDG-PET/CT inovarian cancer patients with high tumor markers or suspicious lesion on contrast-enhanced CT in evaluation of recurrence and/or in determination of intraabdominal metastases. *Revista Espanola de Medicina Nuclear e Imagen Molecular*. 2012;31(1):3-8.

[92] Mat Nawi N, Mohamad I. Evaluation of recurrent ovarian cancer: An evolution. *International Journal of Human and Health Sciences* 2020;4(1):15-8.

[93] Gu, P., Pan, L. L., Wu, S. Q., Sun, L., & Huang, G. CA 125, PET alone, PET-CT, CT and MRI in diagnosing recurrent ovarian carcinoma: a systematic review and meta-analysis *Eur J Radiol*, 71 (2009), pp. 164-174.

[94] Low, R. N., Duggan, B., Barone, R. M., Saleh, F., & Song, S. Y. T. Treated ovarian cancer: MR imaging, laparotomy reassessment, and serum CA-125 values compared with clinical outcome at 1 year. *Radiology*, 235 (2005), pp. 918-926.

[95] Fulham, M. J., Carter, J., Baldey, A., Hicks, R. J., Ramshaw, J. E., & Gibson, M. The impact of PET-CT in suspected recurrent ovarian cancer: A prospective multi-centre study as part of the Australian PET Data Collection Project. *Gynecol Oncol*. 2009 Mar; 112(3):462-8.

[96] Cengiz A, Koç ZP, Özcan Kara P, Yürekli Y. The Role of ^{18}F-FDG PET/CT in Detecting Ovarian Cancer Recurrence in Patients with Elevated CA-125 Levels. *Mol Imaging Radionucl Ther*. 2019;28(1):8-14.

[97] Sari O, Kaya B, Kara PO, Gedik GK, Celik C, Ozbek O, Serdengecti M The role of FDG-PET/CT in ovarian cancer patients with high tumor markers or suspicious lesion on contrast-enhanced CT in evaluation of recurrence and/or in determination of intraabdominal metastases. *Rev Esp Med Nucl Imagen Mol*. 2012 Jan-Feb; 31(1):3-8.

[98] Bhosale, P., Peungjesada, S., Wei, W., Levenback, C. F., Schmeler, K., Rohren, E., Macapinlac, H. A., & Iyer, R. B. Clinical utility of positron emissioin tomography/computed tomography in the evaluation of suspected recurrent ovarian cancer in the setting of normal CA 125 levels. *Int J Gynecol Cancer* (2010) 6:936–44.

[99] Rubini, G., Altini, C., Notaristefano, A., Merenda, N., Rubini, D., Ianora, A. A. S., & Asabella, A. N. Role of 18F-FDG PET/CT in diagnosing peritoneal carcinomatosis in the restaging of patient with ovarian cancer as compared to contrast enhanced CT and tumor marker CA-12. *Rev Esp Med Nucl Imagem Mol* (2014) 33(1):22.

[100] Thrall MM, DeLoia JA, Gallion H, Avril N. Clinical use of combined positron emission tomography and computed tomography (FDG-PET/CT) in recurrent ovarian cancer. *Gynecol Oncol*. 2007;105:17–22.

[101] Zimny, M., Siggelkow, W., Schröder, W., Nowak, B., Biemann, S., Rath, W., & Buell, U. 2-[fluorine-18]-fluoro-2-deoxyd-glucose positron emission tomography in the diagnosis of recurrent ovarian cancer. *Gynecol Oncol*. 2001;83:310–315.

[102] Gu P, Pan LL, Wu SQ, Sun L, Huang G. CA 125, PET alone, PET-CT, CT and MRI in diagnosing recurrent ovarian carcinoma: a systematic review and meta-analysis. *Eur J Radiol* 2009; 71:164–17.

[103] Kitajima, K., Murakami, K., Sakamoto, S., Kaji, Y., Sugimura, K. Present and future of FDG-PET/CT in ovarian cancer. *Ann. Nucl. Med*. 2011, 25, 155–164.

[104] Risum, S., Høgdall, C., Loft, A., Berthelsen, A. K., Høgdall, E., Nedergaard, L., Lundvall, L., & Engelholm, S. A. Does the use of diagnostic PET/CT cause stage migration in patients with primary advanced ovarian cancer? *Gynecol Oncol*. 2010;116:395–8.

[105] Han S., Woo S, Suh C. H., Lee J. J. Performance of pre-treatment 18F-fluorodeoxyglucose positron emission tomography/computed tomography for detecting metastasis in ovarian cancer:a systematic review and meta-analysis. *J Gynecol Oncol*. 2018;29:e98.

[106] Ye, S., Liu, S., Xiang, L., Wu, X., & Yang, H. 18F-FDG PET/CT-based metabolic metrics in recurrent tumors of ovarian clear cell carcinoma and their prognostic implications. *BMC Cancer* 19, 226 (2019).

[107] Fulham MJ, Carter J, Baldey A, Hicks RJ, Ramshaw JE, Gibson M (2009) The impact of PET–CT in suspected recurrent ovarian cancer: a prospective multi-centre study as part of the Australian PET data collection project. *Gynecol Oncol* 112:462–468.

[108] Choi HJ, Roh JW, Seo SS, Lee S, Kim JY, Kim SK, Kang KW, Lee JS, Jeong JY, Park SY (2006) Comparison of the accuracy of magnetic resonance imaging and positron emission tomography/computed tomography in the presurgical detection of lymph node metastases in patients with uterine cervical carcinoma: a prospective study. *Cancer* 106(4):914–922.

[109] Signorelli, M., Guerra, L., Pirovano, C., Crivellaro, C., Fruscio, R., Buda, A., Cuzzucrea, M., Elisei, F., Ceppi, L., & Messa, C. Detection of nodal metastases by 18F-FDG PET/ CT in apparent early-stage ovarian cancer: a prospective study. *Gynecol Oncol.* 2013;131:395–9.

[110] Yuan Y, Gu ZX, Tao XF, Liu SY. Computer tomography, magnetic resonance imaging, and positron emission tomography or positron emission tomography/computer tomography for detection of metastatic lymph nodes in patients with ovarian cancer: a meta-analysis. *Eur J Radiol.* 2012.

[111] Nam E. J., Yun M. J., Oh Y. T., Kim J. W., Kim S., Jung Y. W., Kim S. W., Kim Y. T. Diagnosis and staging of primary ovarian cancer: Correlation between PET/CT, Doppler US, and CT or MRI. *Gynecol. Oncol.* 2010;116:389–394.

[112] Simcock B., Neesham D., Quinn M., Drummond E., Milner A., Hicks R. J. (2006) The impact of PET/CT in the management of recurrent ovarian cancer. *Gynecol Oncol* 103:271–276).

[113] Bilici A., Ustaalioglu B. B., Seker M., Canpolat N., Tekinsoy B., Salepci T., Gumus M. Clinical value of FDG PET/CT in the diagnosis of suspected recurrent ovarian cancer: is there an impact of FDG PET/CT on patient management? *Eur J Nucl Med Mol Imaging.* 2010 Jul;37(7):1259-69.

Chapter 7

The Pathogenesis of Ovarian Cancer

Victoria Psomiadou*, **MD**
Department of Gynecologic Oncology, Metaxa Cancer Hospital of Piraeus, Piraeus, Greece

Introduction

Ovarian cancer is the most lethal gynecological cancer. In 2020, over 313,959 women were diagnosed with ovarian cancer, almost 207,252 died from ovarian cancer, while GLOBOCAN estimates on their website that by 2040, OC incidence and death rate will rise by 47% and 59% accordingly. In the United States and Japan, ovarian cancer accounts for 2.5% and 3.1% of cancer diagnoses, respectively, and is the 9th leading cause of cancer-related deaths. While the rate of treatment of patients with disease limited to the ovaries exceeds 90%, patients with metastatic disease have a 5-year survival rate of 25%-30% [1].

Regarding the management, many surgical techniques have been developed and platinum-based chemotherapy is the golden standard, recently improved by the introduction of bevacizumab. Moreover, biological factors have significantly improved the free disease survival (PFS), but also the overall survival (OS), as shown by two studies in 2011. Although the prognosis is more favorable in patients with Stage I/II tumors, the majority of patients present are with advanced Stage (III/IV) disease. It has been suggested that most ovarian carcinomas originate from the ovarian epithelium postoperatively or from occluded cysts formed after rupture and remodeling of the follicles.

The basis of understanding any malignancy is determining its exact origin. A better understanding of carcinogenesis advocates a clearer understanding of the effects of the malignancy and, consequently, of its diagnosis, classification, treatment and prevention.

For many epithelial neoplasms, the cell of origin is clearly defined through identifiable precursor lesions. For example, colorectal adenocarcinoma results from dysplastic lesions within the colonic mucosa, and cervical cancer comes from human papillomavirus (HPV) - infected cells in the cervical region. Unlike these types of tumors, the origin of epithelial ovarian cancer (EOC) is not clearly defined. In addition, primary peritoneal cancer and primary fallopian tube cancer are usually grouped with the EOC, despite the clearly different anatomical regions [2].

---

* Corresponding Author's Email: psomiadouvictoria@gmail.com.

In: Ovarian Cancer
Editors: Christos Iavazzo, Alexandros Fotiou and John Spiliotis
ISBN: 979-8-88697-633-5

Many theories have been proposed regarding the cells of origin and the mechanisms of ovarian cancer carcinogenesis, which are traditionally based on epidemiological studies and pathological observation. These theories have largely assumed that the EOC stems from a single disease process. As technology advances and more sophisticated molecular techniques are developed, we now understand that EOC is a complex and heterogeneous disease process. Just as endometriosis is involved in the development of some endometrial adenocarcinomas, newer evidence suggests that the fallopian tube may play a critical role in the origin of what has traditionally been termed ovarian cancer.

Risk Factors

Factors associated with a lower risk of developing ovarian cancer include pregnancy, oral contraceptives, breastfeeding, fallopian tube ligation and hysterectomy. All of these factors are associated with ovulating less and it is believed that an ovulating more plays an important role in the development of ovarian cancer. In 1971, Fathalla first described the theory of "incessant ovulation." According to the hypothesis of incessant ovulation, each ovulation creates a "trauma," and the epithelial cells of the ovarian surface (Ovarian Surface Epithelium-OSE) are then repaired through increased proliferation, increasing the chance of DNA damage and carcinogenic mutations. Chicken studies have shown a high rate of metastatic ovarian adenocarcinomas in chickens that had been forced to produce an increased number of eggs without any ovulation breaks. OSE cells were thought to be damaged during the ovulation process and then encapsulate and form cortical cysts. These cysts were thought to then undergo metaplasia whereupon their epithelium transformed into mullerian-type, resulting in dysplastic and eventually ovarian cancer. This transformation can result from continuous exposure to growth factors secreted in the cyst that would normally be released in the peritoneal cavity after being secreted by cells on the surface of the ovaries. This theory is further supported by epidemiological data from human studies showing an association between ovulation and an increased risk of ovarian cancer. Women who have "breaks" in ovulation due to pregnancy and breastfeeding appeared to have a lower risk of disease. In addition, women who take oral contraceptive pills (OCPs) and therefore have fewer ovulation cycles have a reduced risk of ovarian cancer by almost 50% [3].

However, this hypothesis is inconsistent with the observation that patients with polycystic ovary syndrome who have reduced ovulation cycles also appear to have an increased risk of ovarian cancer. Thus, although it was initially suggested that the use of OCP reduced the risk of ovarian cancer by reducing the number of ovulation cycles. It appears that the end result is that the protective effect of OCP is similar to that of progesterone-only preparations that usually do not inhibit ovulation.

Due to the weaknesses identified in the case of incessant ovulation, another theory has been proposed as to how OSE turns into malignancy. The gonadotropin hypothesis states that overstimulation of OSE via follicle-stimulating hormone (FSH) and luteinizing hormone (LH) receptors leads to increased proliferation and a risk of malignancy. Pregnant women and ladies taking OCP maintain lower gonadotropin levels, possibly explaining the reduced risk for EOC. This might also explain the increased risk of EOC in infertile women, women with polycystic ovary syndrome and women with other kinds of primary infertility, who even have increased gonadotropin production. Increased gonadotropin production in perimenopausal women may additionally be to blame for the rise within the incidence of EOC that happens approximately 10 years after menopause. However, despite these theories, serum levels of FSH and LH haven't been related to disease risk in either premenopausal or postmenopausal women. Additionally, although animal studies have shown that exposure to gonadotropins promotes tumor growth, no studies are able to demonstrate malignant replacement of OSE or cortical cysts by exposure to gonadotropins [4].

Although these and further theories have been proposed to describe how ovarian mesothelioma could undergo metaplasia and dysplasia, perhaps the biggest gap in understanding the ovarian carcinogenesis process from the OSE is the identification of a true precancerous lesion of high-grade serous carcinoma. Although benign ovarian cystadenomas can develop into a borderline (and later low-grade) tumor, the progression of low-grade to high-grade serous cancer is extremely rare. Ovarian endometriosis has been found in endometrioid and some mixed histological types of ovarian cancers, but does not appear to be a causative agent of serous tumors.

Investigation on the Cell of Origin

As the complexity and heterogeneity of the origin of ovarian cancer became apparent, it was clear that there might not be one site or etiology for all sorts of EOCs. As an example, endometriosis has been associated more closely with several cases of endometrial and clear cell EOCs. Mucinous tumors are identified as often coming from the appendix or other gastrointestinal foci. Thus, the search for a precursor to high-grade serous carcinoma intensified.

Ovarian Carcinogenesis: Type 1 and Type 2

Ovarian tumors are often distinguished, in step with the degree of differentiation, based on the presence of nuclear atypia and also the presence or absence of stromal infiltration into three groups: benign, marginal malignancy and malignant tumors (carcinomas). Ovarian carcinomas are classified into serous, mucinous, endometrial, transcellular and transient epithelium, according to the kinds of epithelium of the feminine reproductive tract. The serous type is the most common and represents 70% of the EOC.

It has been suggested that ovarian carcinomas originate in the superficial ovarian epithelium (OSE) and subsequent metaplasia leads to the development of various cell types (serous, mucinous, endometrial, clear cell and transient epithelium) which form the morphological subtypes of epithelial ovarian carcinomas [5]. However, histopathological, molecular, and genetic studies led by Kurman and Shih have recently proposed a better model for ovarian carcinogenesis, which distinguishes two broad categories, characterized as type I, where ovarian precursors are clearly described, and type II, where such lesions have not been clearly described and where tumors develop de novo from the epithelium of the fallopian tubes and/or ovaries [5]. Type I tumors are further divided into: low-grade serous, mucinous, endometrioid, clear cell, and transient cell carcinomas, while Type II tumors include high-grade serous carcinomas, undifferentiated carcinomas, and ovarian carcinosarcomas. Type I tumors appear to behave more "lazily" and appear to be part of a morphological and molecular continuum starting with benign cystadenoma/adenofibroma tumors, which then develop into atypically proliferating or borderline tumors and eventually to malignancies. They are often confined to the ovary at diagnosis, with a stable genome and no TP53 mutations, although somatic mutations have often been detected in many genes. Each morphological subtype exhibits a characteristic molecular profile characterized by mutations targeting specific cell signaling pathways. And although clear cell carcinoma is referred to as a Type I tumor, it can actually belong to an intermediate category due to its mutations and behavior.

Type II tumors appear to be more aggressive, diagnosed at an advanced stage, and are genetically highly unstable. The majority carry TP53 mutations and almost half of the cases have a mutation, hypermethylation or dysfunction of the BRCA gene 1 and 2. Recently, an increasingly amount of evidence suggests that these tumors may have originated from the epithelium of the fallopian tube and/or the superficial epithelium of the ovaries. (See figure at: DOI: 10.1016/j.ajpath.2015.11.011).

Type 1

Endometrial Carcinoma (EC) and Clear Cell Carcinoma (CCC)

ECs account for 10% of all ovarian cancers. They occur most frequently within the perimenopausal age and at an early stage. These tumors are bilateral in 28% of cases, are related to endometrial carcinomas in 15-20% of cases and appear to arise from endometrial cysts. The origin of endometriosis has not yet been clarified; it's not clear if it's associated with a metastatic process or retrograde menstruation. Endometriosis is related to molecular abnormalities, including activation of the oncogenetic pathway, which allows endometrial tissue to be implanted, to survive and "invade" the ovaries and peritoneal tissue. Ligation may have a protective effect for endometrial and clear cell carcinoma, as this procedure prevents retrograde menstruation, but doesn't protect against high-grade serous carcinomas, because it doesn't prevent possible exfoliation of abnormal tubular cells.

High-grade ECs are morphologically indistinguishable from HGSCs, and frequently express the WT1 gene. ECs also are characterized by ARID1A mutations, CTNNB abnormalities, PTEN inactivation or PIK3CA mutations and frequently have a good prognosis. Additionally, they're immunoreactive to vimentin, cytokeratins 7 and 20, estrogen receptors (ER) and progesterone receptors.

Mutations within the β-catenin CTNNB1 gene, which is involved in cell proliferation and therefore the Wnt signaling pathway, are found in up to 30% of endometrial carcinomas, but are uncommon in other subtypes. This finding suggests that *β-catenin* and *wnt* pathway deregulation are important factors within the development of endometrial carcinomas. Additionally, somatic mutation of the PI3K gene (PIK3CA) has been reported in 20% of endometrial and clear cell carcinomas. More specifically, mutations within the *p110* subunit of phosphoinositide 3-kinases (PI3K), called *PIK3CA*, are often responsible for activating the PI3K-Akt/mammalian target of the rapamycin complex (mTOR) in mammals. A newer study reported that PIK3CA mutations occur only in high-grade endometrial or clear cell carcinomas. Microsatellite instability is observed in endometrial and clear cell carcinoma, but isn't detected in serous and mucinous tumors.

There is growing evidence that endometrial and clear cell carcinomas can arise from endometrial foci. The particular association between endometriosis and ovarian malignancy and its epidemiological model are widely studied. For both endometriosis and ovarian cancer, increased risks were related to infertility, premature and delayed menopause and atokia, and protective factors with fallopian tube ligation, hysterectomy, and OCPs during pregnancy.

Molecular variants that are characteristic of the inflammatory process in endometriosis may contribute via signaling processes and are related to the survival and development to malignant mutation of the ovarian surface epithelium. Ovarian endometriosis disrupts the balance of cytokine levels (interleukin-1, interleukin-6 and interleukin-8) by triggering cytokines related to immunoregulation and growth (e.g., tumor necrosis factor (TNF-) alpha) almost like those seen in ovarian malignancies. Endometriosis also drastically alters the hormonal environment and triggers the release of proteins (such as insulin-like growth factor (IGF)) on which ovarian cancer cells appear to depend. The tendency of endometrial cells to proliferate into clones, as a result of endogenous abnormalities and extensive inflammation observed in endometriosis, creates a continual flow of stimulatory signals, which causes progressive transcriptional changes, resulting in sustained proliferation. This also increases the speed of DNA repair and so the prospect of mutations accumulating in these cells.

Mutations of the phosphatase and tensin homologue (PTEN) in its tumor suppressor gene on chromosome 10 are often found in endometrial ovarian carcinomas. The identification of those PTEN mutations in endometriosis-lesions (20.6%) still as in endometrioid (20%) and clear cell ovarian carcinomas (8.3%) supports the idea that endometriosis could be a precursor of those forms of tumors [6].

In an experimental model of ovarian carcinoma of the ovary in mice, deletion of PTEN together with activation of the KRAS oncogene within the ovarian surface epithelium led to the formation of precursor endometriosis lesions, which developed into intrauterine infiltrates. KRAS may be a member of a family of proteins capable of regulating cell growth, survival and differentiation. Mutations within the KRAS gene are characteristic of low-grade ovarian tumors and are rare in Stages III and IV. Other mechanisms that may deregulate the KRAS gene in ovarian cancer are gene amplifications, which are found in approximately 11% of ovarian tumors and micro-RNA (miRNA) *Let-7* molecules. *Let-7* binds to a particular site within the three prime untranslated regions (3′-UTR) of KRAS mRNA and induces regulation of the latter.

The above results demonstrate that the expression of the K-RAS oncogene and also the inactivation of the PTEN tumor suppressor are an early event within the development of endometrioid carcinoma. Pathologically, the coexistence of ovarian cancer and endometriosis is commonly observed, with the latter being called "atypical endometriosis," which may be a supposedly precursor lesion involving nuclear cell atypia.

It has also recently been proven that the carcinogenesis of endometrial and clear cell carcinomas resulting from endometrial cysts is significantly affected by the microenvironment within which the tumor occurs. Since the contents of an endometrial cyst consist mainly of concentrated degraded blood, the concentration of iron is significantly high in endometrial cysts. Free iron is related to the development of cancer through the induction of oxidative stress. Epithelial cells within the endometriosis cyst are highly exposed to oxidative stress (reactive oxygen species (ROS)) and hypoxia and, therefore, are more at risk of cell and DNA damage while DNA repair is less effective.

Ovarian clear cell carcinomas (OCCCs) are rare tumors in Europe (4%) (2012) and the USA (5%) (2002), however, they're common in Japan (20%). OCCCs are usually considered chemoresistant tumors. Although OCCC is categorised as a Type I tumor, it should actually belong to an intermediate category. It's estimated that OCCC signature is initially induced by a stressful environment within the endometrial cyst and finally it is stabilized [1].

Mucinous Carcinoma (MC)

There are many theories about the origin of ovarian mucinous carcinoma. It's been widely accepted that a subset of mucinous carcinomas can develop in association with ovarian teratomas. However, in the majority of those tumors, no evidence of teratoma is found. Other theories about the origin of those tumors include mucinous metaplasia of the ovarian surface epithelium, endometriosis, and Brenner tumors. However, mucinous metaplasia of the superficial epithelium or ovarian occlusive cysts is extremely rare and only few such cases are reported. Mucinous carcinomas can develop in endometriosis; however, this seems to be relatively uncommon, except in cases of Mullerian endocervical tumors or mixed (seromucinous) borderline malignancies.

Regardless of the origin of the ovarian mucinous carcinoma, morphological changes from cystadenoma to mucinous borderline tumor (MBT) followed by intraepithelial carcinoma and invasive carcinoma are reported. Almost like low-grade serous carcinomas, mucinous carcinomas and associated MBTs and mucinous cystadenomas show the identical KRAS mutation, supporting the "adenoma-carcinoma" hypothesis and therefore the aspect that mucinous carcinomas develop gradually from mucinous cystedenomas and MBT. These findings suggest that the KRAS mutation is an early event regarding the pathogenesis of ovarian mucinous tumors. Additionally, these tumors are often immunoreactive to cytokeratin 7 and 20.

Most of primary mucinous carcinomas of the ovaries (and borderline malignancies) are the so-called intestinal (enteric or non-specific) type, unilateral and Stage I. Advanced neoplasms (III or IV) are extremely uncommon. It's now clear that ovarian mucinous tumors are related to peritoneal pseudomyxoma nearly always originating from the appendix. While many primary mucinous ovarian cancers involve goblet cells and sometimes even Paneth cells or neuroendocrine cells, the presence of goblet cells isn't necessarily a part of an intestinal-type mucinous tumor. In fact, many of them look more like gastric or pancreatic mucinous neoplasms [6].

Low-grade Serous Carcinoma (LGSC)

Low-grade serous carcinomas are genetically stable and are characterized by an occasional number of genetic mutations. Therefore, they develop slowly from certain precursor lesions and don't behave aggressively. They are much more uncommon than high-grade serous carcinomas and are thought to progress gradually from benign serous cystadenomas to serous borderline tumors (SBTs) and at last to low-grade serous carcinomas.

KRAS mutations at codons 12 and 13 occur in one-third of SBTs and in 33% of low-grade serous carcinomas. Similarly, BRAF mutations in codon 599 occur in 28% of SBTs and in 30% of low-grade serous carcinomas. Mutations in ERBB2 occur in less than 5% of those tumors. KRAS and BRAF mutations are detected in both SBT and epithelial cystadenomas related to SBTs. These findings suggest that KRAS and BRAF mutations are very early events in oncogenesis, before the development of SBTs. The KRAS, BRAF, and ERBB2 oncogenes are "upstream regulators" of *mitogen-activated protein kinase (MAPK)*, and mutations in these genes cause structural activation of the MAPK signal transition pathway, which successively results in uncontrolled cell proliferation.

There are several theories about the origin of serous tumors. The classical theory suggests that these tumors come from an *enclosed* ovarian epithelium formed by a fragmented epithelium that undergoes Müllerian metaplasia. It's been suggested that ovarian mesothelioma may get to an epithelial or mesenchymal phenotype, responding to signals related to ovulation. Exposure of the mesothelial cells of such an inclusion cyst to the microenvironment of the ovarian layer can result in Müllerian epithelial metaplasia. However, cases of these cysts turning into serous carcinomas are rare.

Another theory suggests that the tumors may have originated from a secondary Müllerian system, believed to represent fetal remnants of the Müllerian pores, located inside the ovarian hilum (hilus ovarii). These "Müllerian" epithelial cysts form serous tumors and their proliferation causes the elimination of the adjacent ovarian parenchyma. However, SBTs rarely occur at the ovarian hilum.

The latest theory suggests that low-grade serous carcinomas originate within the fallopian tube. Specifically, that the epithelial cells of the female internal reproductive organ are implanted within the epithelium of the ovaries, forming inclusion cysts, and transform to serous neoplasms. It is believed that chronic inflammation can cause the salpinx cells to proliferate, leading to clumps of cells falling off and implanting within the ovarian and peritoneal surfaces, finally leading to SBTs [7].

Type 2

High-grade Serous Carcinoma (HGSCs)

These tumors are instantly high-grade, develop rapidly and are often diagnosed at an advanced stage. HGSCs are the most common ovarian cancers (70%). At their molecular level, they are characterized by mutations within the proteins p53, BRCA, WT1 and p16 and high levels of ki67 and infrequently express estrogen receptors (ERs). Estrogen receptors are expressed in LGSC and EC, but are negative in most CCCs and MCs. More specifically, serous high-grade carcinomas are characterized by mutations within the TP53 gene in almost 80% of cases and a high Ki67 proliferation rate (between 50% and 75%). Additionally, overexpression of HER2/neu is found in 20-67%, activation of AKT in 12-30% and inactivation of p16 in 15% of cases. Additionally, an overexpression of the HLA-G Major Histocompatibility Complex, Class I, G is found in 61% of cases and an overexpression of apolipoprotein E (apoE) has been observed in 66% of cases, but is rare in low-grade serous carcinomas. Chromosomal rearrangements are rather more common in these kinds of tumors, possibly reflecting a high degree of genetic instability. Currently, up to 10-15% of ovarian cancers are thought to be inherited [8].

Mutations within the high-penetrance genes, BRCA1 and BRCA2, are related to 90% of inherited cases of ovarian cancer. The lifetime ovarian cancer risk of BRCA1 and BRCA2 mutants is approximately 40–50% and 20-30%, respectively. Specifically, women with inherited mutations BRCA1 and BRCA2 have a 17-44% overall chance of developing high-grade serous ovarian cancer and 69-72% of developing carcinoma.

The BRCA1/2 genes encode tumor suppressor proteins, with a functional role in maintaining DNA integrity. Pathogenic variants of the BRCA1/2 germline substantially increase a woman's lifetime risk of breast and ovarian cancer, combined with an increased risk of other cancers, like prostate, pancreatic and melanoma. These variants are inherited with autosomal dominance and therefore the prevalence within the general population ranges from 1/400 to 1/800, but can reach as high as 1/40 in Ashkenazi Jewish women. Women with pathogenic variants of BRCA1 and BRCA2 have a cumulative risk of ovarian cancer during their lifetime of 39%–44% and 11%–17%, respectively, a risk significantly increased compared to 1.4% of the typical ovarian cancer risk during a woman's lifetime [8]. The risk of ovarian cancer begins increase after the age of 40 in women with BRCA1 and after the age of 50 in women with the BRCA2 mutation. Given the histopathological similarity between high-grade serous carcinoma of the ovary, peritoneum and fallopian tubes, this increased risk affects all the above carcinomas [9].

In 2001, Piek et al. found mutations in female internal reproductive organ in women who had either BRCA mutations or a powerful case history of ovarian cancer and who underwent prophylactic bilateral tubal resection (BSO). These dysplastic and hyperplastic lesions resembled high-grade serous carcinoma, but without stromal infiltration. These malignancies were found within the peripheral part of the fallopian tube in 4-17% of women with BRCA mutations at the time of bilateral tubal resection (BSO), of which 57% to 100% were located within the distal part of the fallopian tube. Dysplastic lesions within the fallopian tube epithelium are called "serous intraepithelial carcinomas (STICs)." In 2003, the same group of authors hypothesized that hereditary serous carcinomas may originate within the uterine tube epithelium, which has fallen on the surface of the ovary or peritoneum, resulting in early malformation, named SCOUT (secretory cell out-growths), and consisting of a minimum of 30 consecutive, almost exclusively, secretory pseudostratified epithelial cells. An immunohistochemical analysis can confirm the diagnosis, which is characterized by a low ratio of PTEN and Ki67 and, in most cases, the absence of TP53 mutations [10]. (See figure at: DOI: 10.1002/cam4.2725).

TP53 signatures are the following early entities whose immunohistochemical definition includes a minimum of 12 consecutive p53-expressing secretory cells with a low proliferation rate (Ki67 <10%). They are small groups of cells with a strong expression of p53 and are observed mainly in fibria, no matter BRCA status. The production-activity of p53 has been shown to be low. However, when p53 signature proceeds to STIC, it acquires high reproductive activity with high Ki-67 or MIB1 expression and cytological atypia. Of particular interest is the fact that transient lesions between the p53 signature and therefore the STIC are frequently reported, with intermediate morphological features called serous intraepithelial tubular lesions (STILs). The presence of those transient lesions further suggests that the p53 signature may be a precursor to STIC. "Serial intraepithelial tubal lesions" (STILs), also called "transient intraepithelial tubal lesions" (TILTs) by some authors include p53 signatures, salpinx dysplasia, and even epithelial atypia. These are described as a bunch of tubal abnormalities, with different p53 signatures compared to STICs, within the process of carcinogenesis, SCOUTs are also possible to turn into benign lesions expressing p53 (p53 signature) with a low proliferation rate and low genetic instability. In these cases, benign lesions expressing p53 (STILs/TILTs) will occur, reminiscent of tubal dysplasia lesions, culminating within the onset of STICs. No STICs are detected in mucosal, endometrial carcinomas or carcinosarcomas. Thus, STICs appear to be associated with the development of serous carcinomas [11, 12].

It has been reported that the connection of the fallopian tube epithelium to the mesothelium of the fallopian tube serum, called "TPJ" (Tubal Peritoneum Junction), may be a potential site of carcinogenesis. This connection is particularly helical with mesothelial tabs extending from the peritoneal-fallopian tube connection at the outer ends of the fibria. The extensive and complex lymphatic system is in almost direct contact with the basic membrane of the fallopian tube epithelium, suggesting that even a minimally invasive carcinoma could easily invade this system and spread rapidly throughout the abdominal cavity. Thus, if small areas of STICs undergo malignant mutation, due to their location, they invade the adjacent ovary and the surrounding peritoneal pelvis. Prospective studies identify a 7-year window between the development of STICs and the development of ovarian cancer, which is rapidly followed by metastases [13]. (See figure at: DOI: 10.1002/cam4.2725).

On the other hand, serous carcinoma can actually have an ovarian origin. Koshiyama et al. studied 543 patients with ovarian epithelial carcinomas. Remarkably, 8 of the 9 patients with serous carcinomas without any ultrasound abnormalities at the last visit presented with Stage III tumors and the final pathological report after surgery showed that no malignancy was detected in adjacent lesions, indicating that serous carcinomas may arise de novo from the ovaries suddenly and evolve very quickly [14].

In 1994, Bell and Scully reported 14 cases of sporadic microcarcinomas in macroscopically normal ovaries. Most of them were serous carcinomas, indicating de novo carcinogenesis, while there were no cases of mucosal carcinomas [15]. In addition, a notable study by Flesken-Nikitin, et al. in mice, reported that ovarian hilum cells showed an increased transformation-potential after inactivation of tumor suppressor proteins p53 (Trp53) and retinoblastoma 1 (Rb1). These pathways often changed into high-grade serous carcinoma. In short, the ovarian superficial epithelium (OSE) at the fallopian tube (TPJ) contains a stem cell site that is responsible for its regeneration and is prone to malignant transformation. These stem cells in the ovarian hilum may have increased transformation-potential after inactivation of *Trp 53* and *Rb 1* proteins and may be the source of high-grade serous carcinoma.

In order to clarify the molecular mechanisms through which serous carcinoma develops from the fallopian tubes, several HGSC genomic analyses were performed, such as the Cancer Genome Atlas (TCGA). This analysis found that the TP53 mutation was very common (96%), as expected, and additional genes including NF1, BRCA1, BRCA2, RB1 and CDK12 also carried somatic mutations with relatively low levels but statistically significant frequencies. Thus, copies of somatic DNA with significant numbers of aberrations were detected, including CCNe1, MYC and MECOM, each particularly amplified in more than 20% of the tumors. Pathway analyses showed that the RB-related (67%) and RAS/PI3K (45%) signaling pathways were activated and homologous recombination (HRD) mechanism failure was observed in up to 49% of cases, through hypermethylation and silencing of the promoter site of BRCA1, as well as through its stem lines and its somatic mutations. These findings showed that the range of HGSC mutations made it completely different from other histological types of ovarian cancer, with extremely high TP53 mutations and frequent deficiency of the homologous recombination mechanism (HRD) [16].

In addition, to the pathogenic variants BRCA1/BRCA2 that are associated with an ovarian cancer (OC) risk of 17-44% by age 80, susceptibility gene test of RAD51C (lifetime OC risk = 11%), RAD51D (lifetime OC risk = 13%) and BRIP1 (lifetime OC risk = 5.8%) is now part of clinical practices. Genome-wide correlation studies (GWAS) have identified ~ 30 validated single nucleotide polymorphisms (SNPs) that modify the risk for OC. Newer risk-prediction models incorporating validated SNPs in a multidisciplinary risk score based on epidemiological/family history (FH)/hormonal data and moderate-high penetration susceptibility genes, can be used to predict the risk of life-threatening cancer, improving the accuracy of risk assessment and allowing stratification of the population in risk layers, allowing targeted prevention/screening for those patients at an increased risk [17].

Conclusion

- Ovarian epithelial cancer is the deadliest gynecological cancer.
- The five-year survival rate reaches 70-90% in Stage I, 50-60% in Stage II, 20-40% in Stage III and 10% in Stage IV.
- Factors associated with a lower risk of developing ovarian cancer include pregnancy, oral contraceptives, breastfeeding, fallopian tube ligation, and hysterectomy.
- Popular theories about the aggravating factors for the development of the disease refer to the increased number of ovulations and the increased exposure to gonadotropins.
- Ovarian epithelial carcinomas are classified into serous, mucinous, endometrial, clear cell and transitional cell carcinoma (TCC). Serous type represents 70%.
- Based on their precursor lesions, ovarian carcinomas are divided into Type I where ovarian lesions are clearly described, and Type II, where such lesions are not clearly described and where tumors grow de novo from the fallopian tube/or ovarian epithelium.
- Type I tumors are further divided into: low-grade serous, mucinous, endometrial, clear cell, and transient cell carcinomas, while Type II tumors include high-grade serous carcinomas, undifferentiated carcinomas, and carcinosarkomas.
- 10-15% of ovarian cancers are thought to be inherited and 90% of inherited cases of ovarian cancer are related to mutations in the high penetration genes, BRCA1 and BRCA2.
- The risk of ovarian cancer during the lifetime of BRCA1 and BRCA2 mutants is approximately 40–50% and 20-30% respectively. (See figure at: DOI: 10.1155/2013/852839).

References

[1] https://worldovariancancercoalition.org/wp-content/uploads/2020/10/2020-World-Ovarian-Cancer-Atlas_FINAL.pdf.

[2] Cook SA, Tinker AV. PARP Inhibitors and the Evolving Landscape of Ovarian Cancer Management: A Review. *Bio Drugs.* 2019 Jun;33(3):255-273. doi: 10.1007/s40259-019-00347-4. PMID: 30895466.

[3] Fathalla MF. Incessant ovulation-a factor in ovarian neoplasia *Lancet.* 1971;2(7716):163.

[4] Sherman-Baust CA, Kuhn E, Valle BL, Shih IeM, Kurman RJ, Wang TL, Amano T, Ko MS, Miyoshi I, Araki Y, Lehrmann E, Zhang Y, Becker KG, Morin PJ. A genetically engineered ovarian cancer mouse model based on fallopian tube transformation mimics human high-grade serous carcinoma development. *J Pathol.* 2014 Jul;233(3):228-37. doi: 10.1002/path.4353. PMID: 24652535; PMCID: PMC4149901.

[5] Kurman RJ, Shih IeM. The Dualistic Model of Ovarian Carcinogenesis: Revisited, Revised, and Expanded. *Am J Pathol.* 2016 Apr;186(4):733-47. doi: 10.1016/j.ajpath.2015.11.011. PMID: 27012190; PMCID: PMC5808151.

[6] Prat, J, "Ovarian carcinomas: five distinct diseases with different origins, genetic alterations, and clinicopathological features," *Virchows Archiv,* vol. 460, no. 3, pp. 237–249, 2012.

[7] Erickson BK, Conner MG, Landen CN Jr. The role of the fallopian tube in the origin of ovarian cancer. *Am J Obstet Gynecol.* 2013 Nov;209(5):409-14. doi: 10.1016/j.ajog.2013.04.019. Epub 2013 Apr 10. PMID: 23583217; PMCID: PMC3937451.

[8] Walker M, Jacobson M, Sobel M. Management of ovarian cancer risk in women with BRCA1/2 pathogenic variants. *CMAJ.* 2019 Aug 12;191(32):E886-E893. doi: 10.1503/cmaj.190281. PMID: 31405835; PMCID: PMC6690830.

[9] Darelius A, Lycke M, Kindblom JM, Kristjansdottir B, Sundfeldt K, Strandell A. Efficacy of salpingectomy at hysterectomy to reduce the risk of epithelial ovarian cancer: a systematic review. *BJOG.* 2017 May;124(6):880-889. doi: 10.1111/1471-0528.14601. PMID: 28190289.

[10] Piek JM, Verheijen RH, Kenemans P, Massuger LF, Bulten H, van Diest PJ. BRCA1/2-related ovarian cancers are of tubal origin: a hypothesis. *Gynecol Oncol.* 2003 Aug;90(2):491. doi: 10.1016/s0090-8258(03)00365-2. PMID: 12893227.

[11] Gaba F, Robbani S, Singh N, McCluggage WG, Wilkinson N, Ganesan R, Bryson G, Rowlands G, Tyson C, Arora R, Saridogan E, Hanson H, Burnell M, Legood R, Evans DG, Menon U, Manchanda R; PROTECTOR team. Preventing Ovarian Cancer through early Excision of Tubes and late Ovarian Removal (PROTECTOR): protocol for a prospective non-randomised multi-center trial. *Int J Gynecol Cancer.* 2021 Feb;31(2):286-291. doi: 10.1136/ijgc-2020-001541. Epub 2020 Sep 8. PMID: 32907814.

[12] Kyo S, Ishikawa N, Nakamura K, Nakayama K. The fallopian tube as origin of ovarian cancer: Change of diagnostic and preventive strategies. *Cancer Med.* 2020 Jan;9(2):421-431. doi: 10.1002/cam4.2725. Epub 2019 Nov 25. PMID: 31769234; PMCID: PMC6970023.

[13] Rescigno P, Cerillo I, Ruocco R, Condello C, De Placido S, Pensabene M. New hypothesis on pathogenesis of ovarian cancer lead to future tailored approaches. *Biomed Res Int.* 2013;2013:852839. doi: 10.1155/2013/852839. Epub 2013 Aug 25. PMID: 24063014; PMCID: PMC3766984.

[14] Koshiyama M, Matsumura N, Konishi I. Recent concepts of ovarian carcinogenesis: type I and type II. *Biomed Res Int.* 2014;2014:934261. doi: 10.1155/2014/934261. Epub 2014 Apr 23. PMID: 24868556; PMCID: PMC4017729.

[15] Scully C, Bell C, Porter K, Porter S. Views of dental patients about the education and practice of dentists. *Community Dent Oral Epidemiol.* 1994 Apr;22(2):112-3. doi: 10.1111/j.1600-0528.1994.tb01583.x. PMID: 8205775.

[16] Flesken-Nikitin A, Choi KC, Eng JP, Shmidt EN, Nikitin AY. Induction of carcinogenesis by concurrent inactivation of p53 and Rb1 in the mouse ovarian surface epithelium. *Cancer Res.* 2003 Jul 1;63(13):3459-63. PMID: 12839925.

[17] Gaba F, Blyuss O, Liu X, Goyal S, Lahoti N, Chandrasekaran D, Kurzer M, Kalsi J, Sanderson S, Lanceley A, Ahmed M, Side L, Gentry-Maharaj A, Wallis Y, Wallace A, Waller J, Luccarini C, Yang X, Dennis J, Dunning A, Lee A, Antoniou AC, Legood R, Menon U, Jacobs I, Manchanda R. Population Study of Ovarian Cancer Risk Prediction for Targeted Screening and Prevention. *Cancers* (Basel). 2020 May 15;12(5):1241. doi: 10.3390/cancers12051241. PMID: 32429029; PMCID: PMC7281662.

Chapter 8

Inherited Ovarian Cancer-Linked Syndromes and Management

Malcolm Scott[1]
Adam Rosenthal[1,*], PhD
and Terri McVeigh[2], PhD
[1]University College London Hospitals NHS Foundation Trust
and UCL Elizabeth Garrett Anderson Institute for Women's Health, London, UK
[2]Cancer Genetics Unit, The Royal Marsden NHS Foundation Trust, London, UK

Introduction

Ovarian cancer (OC) still poses a significant challenge for screening, diagnosis and treatment; OC has a 5-year survival rate of 42.6% in the UK, (CRUK). Around 10-15% of epithelial OCs are thought to be hereditary. The ultimate goal of identifying women with a hereditary predisposition to OC is to prevent them developing the disease and thereby reducing the impact on patients and their families, whilst reducing healthcare costs.

Identifying women either with or at risk of inherited OC has a number of benefits. Firstly, a patient with OC who carries a *BRCA1/BRCA2* pathogenic variant has better therapeutic options and medium-term survival due to poly(ADP-ribose) polymerase (PARP) inhibitors. (Bolton et al.). There is increasing evidence to suggest that women with cancer demonstrating deficient homologous recombination repair (HRR) due to variants in other HRR genes such as *RAD51C, RAD51D* and *BRIP1* may also benefit from targeted treatments. Secondly, women at risk of inherited OC can consider the option of prevention via risk-reducing surgery. Thirdly, blood relatives of a patient diagnosed with a constitutional (germline) pathogenic variant predisposing to inherited OC can access cascade testing and benefit from prevention if found to carry the familial pathogenic variant. Finally, there is also a role for pre-implantation genetic diagnosis (PGD) to allow women to select embryos which do not carry their cancer-causing pathogenic variant, through assisted reproduction technology. The authors acknowledge that fertility treatment carries significant challenges both technically and psychologically and its cost alone may prevent it being a viable option for all women with constitutional variants.

---

* Corresponding Author's Email: adam.rosenthal@ucl.ac.uk.

In: Ovarian Cancer
Editors: Christos Iavazzo, Alexandros Fotiou and John Spiliotis
ISBN: 979-8-88697-633-5

This chapter discusses appropriate management of women with inherited increased OC risk. These women are usually healthy, but surgical prevention will expose them to the morbidity of risk-reducing surgery; so, this must be considered carefully. It is important to select the correct operation, thereby minimising the risk of complications. In general terms a total laparoscopic hysterectomy (TLH) with bilateral salpingo-oophorectomy (BSO) is only indicated in Lynch Syndrome (LS) due to the concomitant increased risk of endometrial cancer. For women with pathogenic variants in *BRCA1*, *BRCA2* and 'moderate penetrance' genes, laparoscopic BSO is usually all that is required. Surveillance is an option only for those deferring or declining surgery, and careful counselling around its limitations is paramount.

From a genetic point of view, the OC risk associated with constitutional pathogenic variants is inherited in an autosomal dominant pattern. It is important to remember that even though many inherited pathogenic variants cause predominantly female cancers, the pathogenic variants are also carried and passed on equally by men as well as women. These pathogenic variants also exhibit incomplete penetrance, meaning that not all variant-carriers will develop cancer. Ovarian cancer susceptibility genes are mostly involved in DNA repair, particularly Homologous Recombination Repair. Pathogenic variants (as opposed to benign variants) disrupt the gene product's (protein) function. Although dominantly inherited, variants in DNA repair genes act recessively at the cellular level, such that both alleles need to be inactivated to cause cancer, in line with Knudson's 'Two-hit hypothesis.' Homologous Recombination Repair deficiency results in failure to correct errors arising during DNA replication, leading to an accumulation of somatic variants and genomic instability; a hallmark of cancer.

Identifying Women at Risk of Inherited Ovarian Cancer

To determine whether a patient carries a pathogenic variant, constitutional genetic testing is recommended. Each healthcare system will have a different threshold for genetics referral and gene testing. There is a downward trend of this threshold as the cost of gene testing falls. In primary and secondary care doctors need to think about inherited risk when a patient is diagnosed with breast cancer, ovarian cancer or a Lynch Syndrome associated cancer, listed in table below. Table 1 below is an example of the referral criteria used in the UK.

Each country will have specific clinical genetics referral criteria. For the purposes of inherited ovarian cancer these criteria can be split into two broad areas. Firstly, when a patient has a personal history of cancer plus or minus family history and secondly, in a patient without cancer, but either a confirmed cancer-predisposing pathogenic variant in a family member or a strong family history of relevant cancers as described above. When a heritable cancer risk factor is suspected it is most informative to first test the family member/members affected by the suspected inherited cancer.

Over the last few years, it has been recognised that the above traditional family history-based model of genetic testing misses around 50% of variant-carriers (Manchanda R, Burnell M et al.). Another approach has now been developed in parallel, for women diagnosed with OC. So called 'mainstreaming' involves offering newly-diagnosed OC patients the option of genetic testing on the basis that it may influence their treatment options. For example, carriers of constitutional pathogenic variants in *BRCA1/BRCA2* may be offered PARP-inhibitor therapy. Mainstreaming testing is usually offered by the treating surgeon or oncologist, with the clinical geneticist only involved if the patient is found to carry a variant, or if the family history warrants further specialist evaluation. Following identification of a pathogenic causative variant, onward referral to Clinical Genetics ensures that cascade testing of blood-relatives is offered and that the patient themselves is given further information (e.g., about managing their other cancer risks) and support relevant to their mutation status.

Table 1. Example of a cancer genetics referral criteria. Adapted from North East Thames Regional Genetics Service: Cancer Genetics Referral Criteria

<table>
<tr><td rowspan="2">Patient has breast or ovarian cancer</td><td colspan="2">Manchester Scoring System</td></tr>
<tr><td>Cancer and age at diagnosis</td><td>Score</td></tr>
<tr><td rowspan="13">• Breast cancer diagnosed aged 30 years or younger
• Triple positive breast cancer aged 35 years or younger
• Bilateral breast cancer, both diagnoses <50 years
• Triple negative breast cancer diagnosed <60 years
• Breast cancer <45 and a first degree relative with breast cancer <45 years
• Breast cancer and a Manchester score* of 15 or greater
• Ovarian cancer
• Male breast cancer
• Ashkenazi Jewish ancestry and breast cancer at any age
• Patient is unaffected with cancer but all affected family members are deceased, AND Manchester Score* of 17 or greater</td><td>Female breast cancer <30</td><td>11</td></tr>
<tr><td>Female breast cancer 30-39</td><td>8</td></tr>
<tr><td>Female breast cancer 40-49</td><td>6</td></tr>
<tr><td>Female breast cancer 50-59</td><td>4</td></tr>
<tr><td>Female breast cancer >59</td><td>2</td></tr>
<tr><td>Male breast cancer <60</td><td>13</td></tr>
<tr><td>Male breast cancer >59</td><td>10</td></tr>
<tr><td>Ovarian cancer <60</td><td>13</td></tr>
<tr><td>Ovarian cancer >59</td><td>10</td></tr>
<tr><td>Pancreatic cancer</td><td>1</td></tr>
<tr><td>Prostate cancer <60</td><td>2</td></tr>
<tr><td>Prostate cancer >59</td><td>1</td></tr>
<tr><td>Each side of the family to be calculated separately</td><td></td></tr>
<tr><td colspan="3">Colorectal Cancer</td></tr>
<tr><td colspan="3">• Loss of proteins on mismatch repair immunohistochemistry (MMR IHC). If loss of MLH1 and PMS2, first carry out MLH1 promoter hypermethylation studies and refer if not hypermethylated.
• Patient diagnosed with bowel cancer younger than 50 years
• Patient diagnosed with two Lynch syndrome-related cancers** where one is either colorectal or endometrial cancer
• Patient diagnosed with bowel cancer and family reaches Amsterdam Criteria***
• Patient diagnosed with a non-colorectal Lynch syndrome-related cancer** younger than 50 years e.g., endometrial or ovarian cancer (MMR IHC testing to first be performed locally, if possible)
• Patient is unaffected with cancer but all affected family members are deceased, AND they have a first degree relative with bowel cancer younger than 30 years, OR they have two first degree relatives diagnosed with a Lynch syndrome related cancer** younger than 60 years, OR family reaches Amsterdam Criteria***</td></tr>
</table>

* Manchester Score: a calculation based on the numbers of breast, ovarian, prostate and pancreatic cancer cases in a family, with variable scores awarded to each cancer depending on the type and age at diagnosis. Higher scores correlate with a priori probability of identifying an underlying pathogenic variant in BRCA1 or BRCA2

**Lynch-related cancers comprise: colorectal, endometrial, endocervical, ovarian, pancreatic, ureteric, transitional cell cancer of renal pelvis, gastric, hepatobiliary tract, small bowel, glioblastoma, pancreatic, prostate, multiple sebaceous adenomata, multiple sebaceous epitheliomas, multiple keratoacanthomas, and sebaceous carcinoma.

*** Amsterdam Criteria: >3 closely related family members diagnosed with Lynch-related cancers over >2 generations with >1 case diagnosed The clinical geneticist/genetic counsellor will take a thorough family history to determine what, if any, gene test may be warranted. It is important to remember when counselling women that referral to clinical genetics does not guarantee that a genetic test will be indicated. The family history of cancer should ideally be confirmed with death certificates and/or histopathology reports, and if available the results of genetic tests of any affected family members. The family history should ideally include both age of onset and histological type of cancer (e.g., high-grade serous OC).

In the UK, the National Institute for Health and Care Excellence (NICE) has acknowledged that endometrial cancer can be the sentinel cancer in Lynch Syndrome by publishing new guidance on testing women newly diagnoses with endometrial cancer for Lynch Syndrome. NICE now recommends that all women diagnosed with endometrial cancer should have immunohistochemistry (IHC) testing of the tumor to identify those with a mismatch repair (MMR) deficiency. When the deficiency is loss of MLH1 and PMS2 proteins, then *MLH1* promotor hypermethylation testing of the tumor DNA should be done in the first instance, given that the significant majority of MLH1/PMS2 deficient endometrial cancers will be accounted for by this mechanism. Only when *MLH1* promotor hypermethylation is not detected in the tumor should a constitutional genetic test be offered to confirm LS. A constitutional genetic test to determine if LS is the underlying cause of MMR deficiency should be offered when the IHC shows abnormal loss of MSH2 and/or MSH6 or isolated PMS2 protein expression. (ref NICE)

How to Determine Level of Risk

The question that needs to be answered is 'does the variant and / or family history confer a high enough OC risk to warrant risk-reducing surgery.' Historically in the UK, the threshold used was a minimum 10% lifetime risk. More recently in the UK setting, Manchanda et al. showed that risk-reducing surgery is cost effective when applied to women with a lifetime risk of 4-5% (Manchanda et al.). The cost and availability of surgery must be considered when deciding the level of OC risk at which to offer risk-reducing surgery.

A woman known to carry a high-risk pathogenic alteration, such as those in *BRCA1, BRCA2, MLH1, MSH2*, or *MSH6*, is usually considered to be at sufficiently high risk of OC to offer risk-reducing surgery irrespective of her family history. The timing of this depends on the specific variant, her reproductive choices, and the side effects of premature menopause. As table 2 shows, most high-risk pathogenic variants, except for those variants in *MSH6*, meet the 4-5% cost-effectiveness threshold for risk-reducing surgery by the age of 50. When considering prophylactic ovarian surgery in women with Lynch Syndrome, it is important to remember that these women also have a 40-60% lifetime risk of developing endometrial cancer (Barrow et al.) and this will be the more pressing risk to consider for the timing of surgery for these women.

Table 2. Cumulative risk (%) of ovarian cancer associated with high-risk pathogenic variants in different genes (Kuchenbaecker et al.)

Gene	Cumulative Ovarian cancer risk to age 50 years associated with pathogenic variants	Cumulative Ovarian cancer risk to age 80 years (*to age 75 years) associated with pathogenic variants
BRCA 1	20% (95% CI = 16% to 36%)#	44% (95% CI = 36% to 53.7%)#
BRCA 2	6.5% (95% CI = 3.7%% to 11.5%)#	17% (95% CI = 11% to 25%)#
MLH1	6.10% (95% CI = 3.8% to 9.8%)	11% (95% CI = 7.4% to 19.7%)*
MSH2	10.50% (95% CI = 6.9% to 15.7%)	17.40% (95% CI = 11.8% to 31.2%)*
MSH6	2.30% (95% CI = 0.4% to 24.6%)	10.80% (95% CI = 3.7% to 38.6%)*

Table 3. Cumulative risk (%) of ovarian cancer in associated with variants in "moderate risk" ovarian cancer susceptibility genes

Gene	Cumulative risk % to age 50 years	Cumulative risk % to age 80 years
RAD51C	1% (95% CI = 0.6% to 2%)	11% (95% CI = 6% to 21%) (Yang et al. RAD51C and D paper)
RAD51D	0.8% (95% CI = 0.5% to 2%)	13% (95% CI = 7% to 23%) (Yang et al.)
PALB2	0.6% (95% CI = 0.3% to 1.3%)	4.8% (95% CI = 2.5% to 9.7%) (Yang et al. – PALB2 paper)
BRIP1		5.8% (95% CI = 3.6% to 9.1%) (Ramus et al.)

There are other genes in which pathogenic variants confer a moderately increased risk of ovarian cancer, such as *BRIP1, RAD51C, RAD51D* and *PALB2* – with associated risks of the order of 2-4-fold that of population level risk. For these women, family history and personal protective factors should be considered when determining the overall level of risk. Table 3 shows the cumulative lifetime risks associated with variants in moderate risk genes. The risk to the age of 50 years is much lower than risks associated with variants in in *BRCA1, BRCA2, MLH1, MSH2 or MSH6*, therefore it is reasonable to consider delaying risk reducing surgery until closer to the age of the natural menopause to reduce the morbidity of a premature menopause. Risks associated with pathogenic variants in *BRIP1* confer a risk of later-onset ovarian cancer, with the median age of diagnosis being 61 years.

It should also be noted that, as constitutional pathogenic variants in these genes are rarer than those in the high-risk genes, fewer cases have been reported in the literature. Consequently, the confidence intervals around risk estimates are relatively wide (see Table 3).

Worryingly, according to a recent analysis of the Prospective Registry Of Multiplex Testing (PROMPT) an online database of individuals with constitutional pathogenic variants, some women are undergoing RRSO following identification of constitutional pathogenic variants in genes that confer a risk of other cancers, but that have not been proven to be associated with ovarian cancer predisposition, such as *CHEK2* (Domchek, Robson et al.).

The authors recommend discussing moderate-penetrant gene carriers with a Clinical Geneticist in order to confirm the age-specific risk as well as lifetime risk of OC before going ahead with RRSO.

Some women may have a strong family history of OC but uninformative constitutional genetic testing. In this scenario they may still be deemed to have an OC risk high enough to offer risk-reducing surgery. In such cases, it is crucial to confirm the family history. In order for surgery to be justifiable, it would usually be necessary to confirm two cases of non-mucinous OC in the family. Where available it is advisable to use a multidisciplinary approach when deciding on whether a patient's risk has met the threshold for risk-reducing surgery. This should include a clinical geneticist, genetic counsellor, gynaecologist and where necessary, a clinical psychologist.

When determining risk, it is also important to remember that there are protective reproductive factors which reduce the risk of OC in the general population. These include multiparity, breastfeeding, and use of the oral contraceptive pill. There is growing evidence that COCP use reduces the risk of ovarian cancer in BRCA carriers specifically (Huber et al.). These factors are unlikely to provide sufficient protection to change the recommendation to undergo RRSO in BRCA-carriers, but it is possible that they might have an influence on the age at which some would have the surgery. The relative importance of reproductive factors affecting OC risk is greater when calculating risk in women carrying pathogenic variants in moderate-penetrant genes. As such women may have an *a priori* lifetime risk of e.g., 5-10%, it is possible that extensive pill-use and multiparity might reduce an individual's risk to a level at which risk-reducing surgery might not be recommended.

Risk prediction models such as CanRisk (ref) are being developed to incorporate multiple risk factors including mutation status, family history, and reproductive factors known to influence OC risk. These have shown promise but need to be validated before they can be used in clinical practice with regards to OC risk-estimation. They aim to provide individualised risk prediction to patients, thus helping them make more informed choices with regard to their management.

BRCA1 and *BRCA2*

Pathogenic variants in *BRCA1* are associated with the highest known risk of OC, with variants in *BRCA2* a close second. *BRCA1* and *BRCA2* are tumor suppressor genes. Biallelic inactivation (i.e., inactivation of both copies) of either *BRCA1* or *BRCA2* typically leads to deficient homologous recombination repair, and failure of repair of DNA damage.

It is important to consider important differences between *BRCA1* and *BRCA2* to determine optimal patient management. Variants in either gene confer a lifetime risk high enough to warrant risk-reducing ovarian surgery, but variants in *BRCA1* are associated with an earlier onset of disease and higher absolute OC risk and therefore such carriers need to be managed slightly different than carriers of pathogenic variants in *BRCA2*. The age at which the cumulative risk of OC goes above 5%, is in the early 40s for variants in *BRCA1* and in the early 50s for variants in *BRCA2*. (Andrews et al.) If there is no family history of early onset OC, then risk-reducing surgery can be considered from the age 35 years for carriers of variants in *BRCA1*, but may be deferred to after 40 years for carriers of variants in *BRCA2*. These ages may be reduced pragmatically to 5 years before the age of onset of the youngest OC diagnosis in the family. For example, if a *BRCA1*-carrier has a confirmed case of ovarian cancer at the age of 37 years in her family, then it is reasonable to offer her RRSO from the age of 32 onwards. This assumes that there may be shared genetic or environmental factors which drive early-onset OC in her family, and that OC takes a few years to grow from a single cell to a point where it causes symptoms.

The Table below quantifies the age-related OC risk associated with pathogenic variants in *BRCA1* and *BRCA2* and is useful when counselling women about their current and short to medium term (as opposed to lifetime) risk as shown in Table 4 below. It is crucial that women understand their risk of developing OC in the next few years is much lower than their lifetime risk and therefore delaying surgery until closer to the age of natural menopause may be an option some women may wish to consider.

Risk-reducing BSO is the surgical option of choice for women who carry a constitutional pathogenic variant in *BRCA1/BRCA2* and is the only proven way to reduce OC cancer risk and all-cause mortality (Marchetti et al.).

Table 4. Estimated ovarian cancer incidence (%) and ratio in carriers of pathogenic variants in *BRCA1* and *BRCA2*. (Adapted from Antoniou et al. Average Risks of Breast and Ovarian Cancer Associated with BRCA1 or BRCA2 Mutations Detected in Case Series Unselected for Family History: A Combined Analysis of 22 Studies)

Age	*BRCA1*	*BRCA2*
20-24 years	0.001 (1:100000)	0.001 (1:100000)
25-29 years	0.002 (1:50000)	0.002 (1:50000)
30-34 years	0.18 (9:5000)	0.004 (1:25000)
35-39 years	0.28 (7:2500)	0.01 (1:10000)
40-44 years	0.87 (87:10000)	0.08 (1:1250)
45-49 years	1.49 (149:10000)	0.14 (7:5000)
50-54 years	0.96 (6:625)	0.60 (3:500)
55-59 years	1.19 (119:10000)	0.75 (3:400)

Some women may request a total hysterectomy in addition to removal of the tubes and ovaries. This is not advocated, unless there is a separate gynaecological indication, as variants in *BRCA1/BRCA2* are not thought to increase the risk of endometrial cancer (EC) sufficiently to justify the increased morbidity, cost and risks of hysterectomy compared to RRSO alone. The meta-analysis by Nahshon et al. found a small increased risk of EC in *BRCA1/BRCA2*-carriers with an absolute risk of 0.54%; twice that of the general population. They also report that the rare uterine serous papillary cancer (USPC) is up to ten times more common in *BRCA1/BRCA2*-carriers versus the general population. However, although the prognosis of USPC is poor, it remains a rare cancer even in *BRCA1/BRCA2*-carriers, with an absolute risk of just 0.29%. In view of this, it is the practice at the authors' institutions only to offer hysterectomy if there is a histologically proven case of USPC in the relevant side of a patient's family. Women should be advised that if they have any unscheduled vaginal bleeding once they have recovered from RRSO, they should contact their GP/family doctor to have this investigated.

It has been previously stated that premenopausal RRSO reduced the risk of subsequent breast cancer (Domchek, Friebel et al.), but further research has called this into question due to multiple sources of bias. (Mavaddat et al.). The systematic review done by Stjepanovic et al. aimed to reduce these biases and did show breast cancer risk was reduced in *BRCA1*-carriers who had a premenopausal RRSO. The effect in women who carry pathogenic variants in *BRCA2* remains unclear and needs a larger cohort and longer follow-up to estimate any benefit of premenopausal RRSO in reducing breast cancer risk (Stjepanovic et al.). The authors recommend caution and individualised counselling of patients when deciding on when to have a RRSO as a breast cancer risk-reduction strategy; currently this strategy should not replace breast surveillance nor risk-reducing mastectomy as proven successful interventions.

Women who decline or delay risk-reducing surgery may consider surveillance, but only if they have been extensively counselled about its limitations; it cannot prevent OC, nor does it routinely diagnose OC at stages which would be expected to be cured. The only surveillance technique shown to consistently down-stage OC in clinical trials of BRCA-carriers is the Risk of Ovarian Cancer Algorithm (ROCA) test. This algorithm analyses rate of change of CA125 over time, taking into account a woman's menopausal status, age, and *a priori* ovarian cancer risk (general population risk vs. high-risk population), to indicate her current likelihood of having OC. Overall, two US trials (Skates et al.) and one UK trial (Rosenthal et al.) diagnosed 47% of all BRCA-carriers' OCs at stages 3a or lower. This compares to 100% of all OCs in BRCA-carriers being diagnosed at stage 3b or worse in women no longer on surveillance in the UK trial. As would be expected, this downstaging by surveillance resulted in a very high (95%) complete cytoreduction rate, a lower requirement for neo-adjuvant chemotherapy, and modest levels of surgical effort compared to those women who developed OC when no longer on surveillance (Rosenthal et al.). Whilst these findings would be anticipated to translate into improved survival, this remains speculative, due to the non-randomised nature of these trials. They do however suggest that surveillance using the ROCA test may be a reasonable 'damage-limitation' option for women who choose to decline or defer RRSO. The UK National Health Service (NHS) has recently completed a pilot national surveillance program for BRCA-carriers using the ROCA test and results have recently been presented at the European Society of Gynaecological Oncology conference (Philpott et al.). These indicate that surveillance performance is maintained in a 'real world' (as opposed to clinical trial) setting. If surveillance becomes part of the standard management of women declining or deferring RRSO, it is crucial that at every contact or correspondence they are reminded that RRSO remains the only way to reduce OC mortality; surveillance should not be used as a reason to defer surgery indefinitely.

Lynch Syndrome

Lynch syndrome (LS) is an inherited condition which predisposes women to a number of gynaecological and non-gynaecological cancers; the most prevalent being endometrial and colon cancer, but there is also a 6-12% cumulative lifetime risk of OC (depending on underlying genotype) (Helder-Woolderink et al.). LS accounts for 10-15% of inherited ovarian cancers, and is most commonly caused by a heterozygous constitutional pathogenic variant in one of the mismatch repair (MMR) genes *MLH1*, *MSH2*, *MSH6, PMS2*, and rarely by constitutional deletion of the 3' end of the *EpCAM* gene, or by constitutional hypermethylation of the *MLH1* promoter. An *EpCAM* deletion causes LS by silencing of *MSH2* (Tutlewska et al.) and should be managed in the same way as a patient with a *MSH2* pathogenic variant. In the context of discussing the risk of inherited ovarian cancer, it is important to note that the risk of ovarian cancer does not appear to be markedly increased in Lynch Syndrome caused by pathogenic variants in *PMS2*.

As with ovarian cancer risk-management in women with inherited pathogenic BRCA variants, the main gynaecological risk-reduction strategy in women with Lynch Syndrome is surgery. In LS this includes total hysterectomy and BSO (preferably via the laparoscopic route) (Crosbie et al.), due to the increased risk of endometrial cancer (EC). The ovaries may be conserved in premenopausal women with LS carrying *PMS2* alterations, as these do not appear to increase the risk of OC.

Clearly, hysterectomy and BSO has significant implications for the health of the patient, especially if they are premenopausal. Current data suggests there is no survival advantage if this surgery is undertaken before age 40 years (Dominguez-Valentin et al.). However, surgery can be considered before this age in specific circumstances e.g., when there is a family history of EC or OC occurring under the age of 45 years or when the patient is already post-menopausal despite their young age.

Ideally, surveillance for endometrial cancer (EC) and OC might allow women with LS to delay risk-reducing surgery until after natural menopause, thus minimising the negative impact of such surgery. However, evidence of the efficacy of EC and OC screening in women with LS is lacking. Consequently, the Manchester International Consensus of Lynch Syndrome specialists does not recommend that invasive surveillance should be routinely offered to women with Lynch Syndrome, acknowledging the lack of robust evidence (Crosbie et al.). The consensus recommends that further research in the area of gynaecological cancer surveillance in women with LS could help guide future surveillance programmes.

Women who wish to delay or decline this surgery, acknowledging there is no proven alternative, may opt for surveillance even though there is a lack of robust evidence for it. Ovarian surveillance typically entails a yearly transvaginal ultrasound and CA125 blood test. When counselling women about their level of risk of developing OC or EC, a useful resource is the Prospective Lynch Syndrome Database (PLSD) (REF). This allows the user to input the patient's specific mismatch repair gene alteration, along with their age and the cancer type for which risk-information is required (e.g., endometrium or ovaries). The database then provides percentage risk estimates for these cancers in 10-year age-groups, along with graphs showing how the risk increases over time (including confidence intervals). This is a useful way to illustrate to patients their level of risk, helping them to make an informed choice as to whether they would like to undergo risk-reducing surgery or surveillance.

It is important to note that pathogenic *PMS2* variants do not appear to increase OC risk in the same way as Lynch Syndrome caused by pathogenic variants in other MMR genes (Broeke et al.). Therefore, OC surveillance is not recommended and such women should consider retention of their ovaries at the time of risk-reducing surgery, depending on the age at which such surgery is performed, given that most women undergoing hysterectomy with ovarian conservation in their late 40s will experience ovarian failure soon afterwards (Moorman et al.).

There is evidence that the use of aspirin reduces the incidence of colon cancer in women with LS (Burn, Gerdes et al.), so it important to ensure patients are aware of this and are taking it unless they have contra-indications. The optimal dosing has yet to be defined and is currently under investigation in the CaPP3 research study (HRA website), but a dose of 75mg/day is known to be safe for the large majority of patients. It is not currently known whether aspirin reduces the risk of OC or EC in women with LS. Patients should be warned of the need to stop aspirin one week prior to major surgery including risk-reducing hysterectomy and BSO, in order to reduce the risk of peri-operative bleeding.

It is important to inform patients of the symptoms of OC and EC and to seek urgent medical assessment if these develop. At every contact with a patient it should also be re-iterated to them that risk-reducing surgery is the only proven way to reduce the risk of gynaecological cancer.

'Moderate Risk' Ovarian Cancer Susceptibility Genes - *BRIP1, PALB2, RAD51C, RAD51D*

Targeted resequencing of genes involved in the same cellular pathways (e.g., homologous recombination repair) as *BRCA1* and *BRCA2* have identified constitutional pathogenic variants in some of these genes in BRCA-negative families with multiple OC cases. Constitutional pathogenic variants in such genes are generally associated with a lifetime risk of OC that is increased compared to the general population (2-4-fold), but much lower than in carriers of variants in *BRCA1* and *BRCA2*. Consequently, they are often referred to as 'moderately penetrant' for OC. These genes are increasingly being included in breast/ovarian 'gene panel' testing. Panel-based testing facilitates simultaneous analysis of multiple different genes implicated in the risk of the cancer of interest. As described above, careful consideration is required when determining a patients' OC risk when they carry a variant in a moderate penetrance gene. If a patient's OC risk is deemed high enough for risk-reducing surgery, she would be managed in the same way as a BRCA carrier, but importantly, the age at which such surgery is recommended is different.

The cumulative risk by age 50 for carriers of variants in *RAD51C* and *RAD51D*, as shown above in Table 3, is not significantly higher than that of the general population. Cummings et al. demonstrated that the median age of ovarian cancer in carriers of pathogenic *BRIP1* variants was 65 years of age, although the age of onset, and cancer risk, may differ depending on the specific *BRIP1* genotype (Flaum et al.).

Pathogenic variants in *PALB2* are associated with more modestly increased ovarian cancer risks compared to the other moderate penetrant genes, and risk-reducing surgery should usually only be considered if there is a family history of ovarian cancer. In America the National Comprehensive Cancer Network (NCCN) have published guidance for managing ovarian cancer risk in carriers of variants in moderate penetrance genes. The NCCN recommend consideration of RRSO from age 45-50 in patients with pathogenic variants in *RAD51C*, *RAD51D* and *BRIP1* taking into account their family history. On the other hand the NCCN recommend that the ovarian cancer risk in carriers of *PALB2* pathogenic variants should be managed based upon family history. If considering risk-reducing surgery for women who carry variants in moderate penetrance genes, this can be delayed until nearer the age of the menopause, unless there is a family history suggesting earlier onset of OC.

OC surveillance is not currently recommended for patients who carry variants in moderate risk pathogenic variants and further research is required in this area.

Low Penetrance Ovarian Cancer Susceptibility Alleles

Several dozen ovarian cancer susceptibility loci have been identified through large-scale genome wide association studies, (Dareng et al.) many of which are not within genes, but rather in intergenic regions throughout the genome. The risk associated with individual variants (typically Single Nucleotide Polymorphisms, SNPs) at such loci is typically very low, but the cumulative effect of multiple co-inherited variants may significantly increase the lifetime risk of ovarian cancer. It is estimated that variation at these low penetrance loci may account for up to 6% of the heritability of epithelial ovarian cancer. A Polygenic Risk Score (PRS) can be calculated by adding the number (usually weighted depending on associated risks) of risk alleles for certain variants. There is a growing body of work to suggest that PRS may be useful in stratifying risks in carriers of moderate or highly penetrant variants, which may in turn influence when, if at all, risk-reducing surgery is undertaken. Further validation studies are required. At present, generation of PRS is undertaken on a research basis only, and is best interpreted in the context of other clinical risk factors (Torkamani et al.); risk-reducing surgery is not currently recommended based on PRS alone.

Surveillance

Ideally, surveillance for OC would allow high-risk women to delay risk-reducing surgery until after natural menopause, thus minimising the negative impact of such surgery. OC screening in the general population has not been shown to reduce mortality (Menon et al.). Inherited OC may demonstrate different histological types to the general population; high-grade serous (HGS) ovarian cancer predominates in those caused by a constitutional pathogenic variants in *BRCA1*/*BRCA2* and the moderate penetrance genes. The histology of Lynch syndrome ovarian cancers is usually of non-serous histological type, with endometrioid and clear cell carcinomas predominating (Helder-Woolderink et al.).

As HGS OC is associated with increased serum CA125 there was hope that this could be used in surveillance of high-risk women. Ultrasound and CA125 alone have not proved an effective method of surveillance, but the use of the Risk of Ovarian Cancer Algorithm (ROCA) test, which looks at baseline levels of CA125 and the subsequent changes thereafter has been shown to result in a reduction in the stage at diagnosis, as demonstrated in the UKFOCCS trial (Rosenthal et al.), thus improving the chance of having successful complete primary surgical resection of the cancer. These results are encouraging, but needs to be validated in a 'real world' setting. Furthermore, should women opt for surveillance, they need to understand that it cannot prevent OC and currently there is no evidence that it can reduce the high mortality rates associated with the disease.

The recommendations for LS surveillance differ from country to country as demonstrated in Table 5 below.

Table 5. International Lynch Syndrome surveillance guidelines. (Adapted from: Ryan et al. Should women with Lynch syndrome be offered gynaecological cancer surveillance?)

Guidelines	UK 2019	ESMO 2016	ASCO 2015	NCCN 2021
Symptom awareness education	Yes age 25	Yes	Yes	Yes
Gynaecological examination	Yes	Yes	Yes	-
Pelvic Ultrasound	No	Yes	Yes	No
CA125	No	Not stated	No	No
Endometrial biopsy	No	Annually from 30-35	Annually from 30-35	Every 1-2 years from age 30-35
Hysterectomy and BSO	Yes (no earlier than 35 and pre-op endometrial biopsy and ultrasound)	Yes	Yes	Yes
Research needed	Yes	-	-	-

If a patient with LS opts for surveillance, acknowledging the limitations, then the authors institution offers an annual hysteroscopy and endometrial biopsy, a pelvic ultrasound scan and CA125 blood test. Prospective data from this surveillance should be collected for the purposes of research.

Risk-Reducing Surgery

Risk reducing surgery to remove both ovaries and fallopian tubes remains the only proven way to reduce the risk of inherited OC. (Eleje et al. (BRCA) Schmeler et al. (LS)). As the surgery is to prevent rather than treat cancer, women should be counselled meticulously regarding possible complications; unlike cancer patients, who are often willing to accept high surgical risks in order to treat their disease, women undergoing RRSO are usually healthy and may be less willing to accept surgical risks. For this reason the authors believe in the minimum operation necessary to prevent the relevant cancer. A hysterectomy carries higher risk of complications and is associated with longer recovery and increased healthcare costs compared with a laparoscopic BSO. Therefore, it should only be offered to women with LS, or women with increased OC risk who have a valid gynaecological indication (e.g., large symptomatic fibroids).

The removal of the ovaries, especially in pre-menopausal women can have a significant impact on reproductive, physical and psychological health. These women do not have cancer, but rather are at high risk of developing cancer, making the decision to remove healthy reproductive organs a complex and challenging one. Careful counselling is required prior to surgery, this can be done by the gynaecologist, menopause specialist, and in complex or challenging cases, a referral to clinical psychology to assist the woman with her decision-making may be helpful.

Removing the ovaries has other important impacts other than just the obvious loss of fertility. The average age of the menopause in general is 51 years. Women who experience a premature menopause are at increased risk of all-cause mortality, osteoporosis and fractures, cardiovascular disease, type 2 diabetes and depression (Mishra et al.). More recently, premature menopause has been identified as a risk-factor for dementia (Georgakis et al.). In view of this, women with no personal history of breast cancer are recommended to take hormone replacement therapy (HRT) following premenopausal RRSO until they are 51 years. This is particularly relevant for carriers of pathogenic variants predisposing to high breast cancer risks. Some oncologists will agree to women with triple negative breast cancer having low-dose HRT but there remains a theoretical risk that a recurrence would be hormone receptor positive. This may impact the timing of the decision to have risk-reducing surgery. If a patient cannot have HRT, then alternative options are available to modify their cardiovascular risk and bone health. However, non-hormonal management of acute symptoms such as flushes, loss of libido and low mood is generally less effective than HRT. General advice should be given to women about a healthy, active lifestyle with balanced diet, and regular blood pressure, diabetes and cholesterol checks with their General Practitioner/family doctor. Bone health is maintained through impact, weight bearing exercise, monitored via regular bone mineral density scans and treatment with bisphosphonates where necessary. If a patient with prior breast cancer has very severe or debilitating menopause symptoms, then HRT could still be considered but the final decision should depend on discussions with her oncologist.

Other considerations when counselling women about risk-reducing surgery include but are not limited to:

1. Age-related risk – At what age her risk is high enough to consider surgery vs risk of side effects or surgical complications
2. Infertility and premature menopause
3. The need for HRT and possible contraindications to HRT, including previous breast cancer
4. The surgical risks, including in the context of prior pelvic/abdominal surgery and relevant medical comorbidities.
5. The patient may never develop OC even if they don't undergo risk-reducing surgery
6. The patient may feel different and/or experience worse quality of life even with HRT
7. There is limited long term evidence of HRT efficacy in preventing osteoporosis, cardiovascular disease and dementia specifically in women at high risk of OC
8. Further surgery and/or other treatment would be required if OC is identified following histopathological analysis of the resected tubes and ovaries.

Surgical-Pathological Considerations

Firstly, peritoneal washing for cytological examination should be obtained by instillation of normal saline into the peritoneal cavity BEFORE starting the bilateral salpingo-oophorectomy (BSO). The BSO should include the full length of the fallopian tubes, taking care to avoid diathermy damage to the fimbrial end of the tube as this can mask an occult cancer. The histology request form should state that the patient is at increased risk of ovarian cancer and to ask for the SEEFIM (Sectioning and Extensively Examining the FIMbriated End) protocol, discussed below. It is also important to mention if the patient has previously had breast or other cancers. Right and left sided specimens should be sent in separate containers/pots in case an occult cancer is identified, to facilitate the potential for unilateral para-aortic lymphadenectomy at subsequent surgical staging. If a peritoneal or omental biopsy is indicated, then these should be examined in their entirety.

Women taking tamoxifen for breast cancer treatment, should be advised not to discontinue this prior to surgery, unless the risk of venous thromboembolism (VTE) associated with Tamoxifen outweighs the risk of interrupting treatment (NICE 2019). The authors recommend taking an endometrial biopsy at the time of RRSO in women on Tamoxifen, as such surgery provides an ideal opportunity to check the health of the endometrium in a population at increased risk of endometrial cancer due to their tamoxifen treatment. (NICE 2019). And finally, thromboprophylaxis should be considered for all women undergoing risk-reducing surgery and anti embolism stockings applied. RRSO is usually done as a day case, the authors' institution recommends a one-off injection of low molecular weight heparin (LMWH) as thromboprophylaxis 6 hours post-operatively. Women having a risk-reducing TLH and BSO should continue LMWH as long as they remain in hospital.

Histological Sampling to Reduce Risk of Missing STIC/Cancer

It is very important to ensure that a thorough histological examination of the fallopian tubes and ovaries is undertaken by a specialist gynaecological pathologist who is aware of the patient's genetic status. This is because occult OC or serous tubal intraepithelial carcinoma (STIC) lesions, which are pre-cursor lesions to high-grade serous OC, may be found even with a normal pre-operative pelvic ultrasound and CA125. STICs and early ovarian cancers may be only 1mm in size. Therefore the 'SEE-FIM' protocol is recommended (Medeiros et al.). This protocol uses narrower slicing intervals of 2mm to ensure a more complete assessment of the entire fallopian tube is achieved compared with conventional histological assessment. Using this strategy reduces the risk of missing an occult cancer, which would result in the patient receiving inadequate treatment and a worse prognosis. Women should be counselled that even if they have successful surgery and thorough histopathological assessment, they may still carry a very small residual risk of primary peritoneal cancer (PPC) and should contact their general practitioner if they develop any worrying symptoms in the future. However, recent evidence supports that true PPC is probably very rare in patients who have undergone a risk-reducing BSO in a specialist gynaecological oncology centre and no STIC lesion is identified by the SEE-FIM protocol (Crosbie, Flaum et al.).

Future Management Possibilities

As has been described in this chapter there is lack of evidence in many areas of care for women at increased risk of OC especially around surveillance. There is hope that risk-prediction models can revolutionise the guidance given to women, rather than just depending on genotype and family history. It may be possible that women with high-risk pathogenic variants, but multiple protective factors, may not reach the threshold for risk-reducing surgery. Conversely there could be women without an identified highly-penetrant gene pathogenic variant with multiple other unidentified genetic or environmental/lifestyle risk factors who would reach the surgical threshold.

The fallopian tube is now believed to be the origin of HGS OC (Piek et al., SOONG et al., Mederios et al.) and therefore research is ongoing into the option of early salpingectomy and delayed oophorectomy for women with increased OC risk (Gaba et al.). This option is attractive as it reduces the negative impact of a premature menopause. The hope is that this research will show improved post-surgical quality of life associated with effective risk-reduction.

Conclusion

The management of women with an inherited risk of OC is complex, but with careful assessment of risk, counselling and risk-reducing surgery, there is a clear opportunity to prevent OC and save lives. There is still work to do to optimise OC surveillance, and improve the accuracy of risk-prediction. These tools could enable many women to safely delay risk-reducing surgery until the age of natural menopause, thus reducing the morbidity such surgery causes.

Acknowledgments

Adam Rosenthal was supported by the NIHR Biomedical Research Centre at University College London Hospitals National Health Service Foundation Trust and University College London.

Malcolm Scott was supported by the Margaret Spittle Cancer Research Fellowship.

References

Ovarian Cancer Statistics | Cancer Research UK

Barrow E, Hill J, Evans DG. Cancer risk in Lynch Syndrome. *Fam Cancer.* 2013 Jun;12(2):229-40. doi: 10.1007/s10689-013-9615-1. PMID: 23604856.

Bolton KL, Georgia Chenevix-Trench, Cindy Goh, Siegal Sadetzki, Susan J Ramus, Beth Y Karlan, Diether Lambrechts, Evelyn Despierre, Daniel Barrowdale, Lesley McGuffog, Sue Healey, Douglas F Easton, Olga Sinilnikova, Javier Benítez, María J García, Susan Neuhausen, Mitchell H Gail, Patricia Hartge, Susan Peock, Debra Frost, D Gareth Evans, Rosalind Eeles, Andrew K Godwin, Mary B Daly, Ava Kwong, Edmond S K Ma, Conxi Lázaro, Ignacio Blanco, Marco Montagna, Emma D'Andrea, Maria Ornella Nicoletto, Sharon E Johnatty, Susanne Krüger Kjær, Allan Jensen, Estrid Høgdall, Ellen L Goode, Brooke L Fridley, Jennifer T Loud, Mark H Greene, Phuong L Mai, Angela Chetrit, Flora Lubin, Galit Hirsh-Yechezkel, Gord Glendon, Irene L Andrulis, Amanda E Toland, Leigha Senter, Martin E Gore, Charlie Gourley, Caroline O Michie, Honglin Song, Jonathan Tyrer, Alice S Whittemore, Valerie McGuire, Weiva Sieh, Ulf Kristoffersson, Håkan Olsson, Åke Borg, Douglas A Levine, Linda Steele, Mary S Beattie, Salina Chan, Robert L Nussbaum, Kirsten B Moysich, Jenny Gross, Ilana Cass, Christine

Walsh, Andrew J Li, Ronald Leuchter, Ora Gordon, Montserrat Garcia-Closas, Simon A Gayther, Stephen J Chanock, Antonis C Antoniou, Paul D P Pharoah, EMBRACE; kConFab Investigators; Cancer Genome Atlas Research Network, Association between BRCA1 and BRCA2 mutations and survival in women with invasive epithelial ovarian cancer. *JAMA*. 2012;307(4):382-390. doi:10.1001/jama.2012.20.

Domchek SM, Robson ME. Update on Genetic Testing in Gynecologic Cancer. *J Clin Oncol.* 2019;37(27):2501-2509. doi:10.1200/JCO.19.00363.

Huber D, Seitz S, Kast K, Emons G, Ortmann O. Use of oral contraceptives in BRCA mutation carriers and risk for ovarian and breast cancer: a systematic review. Arch Gynecol Obstet. 2020 Apr;301(4):875-884. doi: 10.1007/s00404-020-05458-w. Epub 2020 Mar 5. Erratum in: *Arch Gynecol Obstet.* 2021 Oct 7;: PMID: 32140806; PMCID: PMC8494665.

Kuchenbaecker, K. B., Hopper, J. L., Barnes, D. R., Phillips, K.-A., Mooij, T. M., Roos-Blom, M.-J., Jervis, S., van Leeuwen, F. E., Milne, R. L., Andrieu, N., Goldgar, D. E., Terry, M. B., Rookus, M. A., Easton, D. F., Antoniou, A. C., and the BRCA1 and BRCA2 Cohort Consortium, McGuffog, L., Evans, D. G., Barrowdale, D., … Olsson, H. Risks of Breast, Ovarian, and Contralateral Breast Cancer for *BRCA1* and *BRCA2* Mutation Carriers. *JAMA*. 2017;317(23):2402–2416. doi:10.1001/jama.2017.7112.

Manchanda R, Burnell M, Gaba F, Desai R, Wardle J, Gessler S, Side L, Sanderson S, Loggenberg K, Brady AF, Dorkins H, Wallis Y, Chapman C, Jacobs C, Legood R, Beller U, Tomlinson I, Menon U, Jacobs I. Randomised trial of population-based BRCA testing in Ashkenazi Jews: long-term outcomes. *BJOG*. 2020 Feb;127(3):364-375. doi: 10.1111/1471-0528.15905. Epub 2019 Sep 10. PMID: 31507061.

Manchanda R, Menon U. Setting the Threshold for Surgical Prevention in Women at Increased Risk of Ovarian Cancer. *Int J Gynecol Cancer*. 2018 Jan;28(1):34-42. doi: 10.1097/IGC.0000000000001147. PMID: 29252925.

North East Thames Regional Genetics Service - North Central London GP Website (northcentrallondonccg.nhs.uk).

Ramus, S. J., Song, H., Dicks, E., Tyrer, J. P., Rosenthal, A. N., Intermaggio, M. P., Fraser, L., Gentry-Maharaj, A., Hayward, J., Philpott, S., Anderson, C., Edlund, C. K., Conti, D., Harrington, P., Barrowdale, D., Bowtell, D. D., Alsop, K., Mitchell, G., Cicek, M. S., … Gayther, S. A. Germline Mutations in the BRIP1, BARD1, PALB2, and NBN Genes in Women With Ovarian Cancer. *JNCI J Natl Cancer Inst* [Internet]. 2015 Nov;107(11).

Testing strategies for Lynch syndrome in people with endometrial cancer Diagnostics guidance [DG42] Published: 28 October 2020 NICE.

Yang X, Song H, Leslie G, Engel C, Hahnen E, Auber B, Horvath J., Kast, K., Niederacher, D., Turnbull, C., Houlstron, R., Hanson, H., Loveday, C., Dolinsky, J. S., LaDyca, H., Ramus, S. J., Menon, U., Rosenthal A. N., Jacobs, I., Gayther, S. A., Dicks, E., Nevanlinna, H., Aittomaki, K., Pelttari, L. M., Ehrencrona, H., Borg, A., Kvist, A., Rivera, B., Hansen, T. V. O., Djursby, M., Lee, A., Dennis, J., Bowtell, D. D., Traficante, N., Diez, O., Balmana, J., Gruber, S. B., Chenevix-Trench, G., kConFab Investigators, Jensen, A., Kjaer, S. K., Hogdall, E., Castera, L., Garber, J., Janavicius, R., Osorio, A., Golmard, L., Vega, A., Couch, F. J., Robson, M., Growald, J., Domchek, S. M., CUlver, J. O., de la Hoya, M., Easton, D. F., Foulkes, W. D., Tischkowitz, M., Meindl, A., Schmutzler, R. K., Pharoah, P. D., P., Antoniou, A. C. Ovarian and Breast Cancer Risks Associated With Pathogenic Variants in RAD51C and RAD51D. *J Natl Cancer Inst* [Internet]. 2020;112(12):1242–50.

Yang, X., Leslie, G., Doroszuk, A., Schneider, S., Allen, J., Decker, B., Dunning, A. M., Redman, J., Scarth, J., Plaskocinska, I., Luccarini, C., Shah, M., Pooley, K., Dorling, L., Lee, A., Adank, M. A., Adlard, J., Aittomäki, K., Andrulis, I. L., … Tischkowitz, M. "Cancer Risks Associated With Germline *PALB2* Pathogenic Variants: An International Study of 524 Families." *Journal of clinical oncology: official journal of the American Society of Clinical Oncology* vol. 38,7 (2020): 674-685. doi:10.1200/JCO.19.01907.

Welcome to CanRisk

Andrews L, Mutch DG. Hereditary Ovarian Cancer and Risk Reduction. *Best Pract Res Clin Obstet Gynaecol.* 2017 May;41:31-48. doi: 10.1016/j.bpobgyn.2016.10.017. Epub 2017 Jan 17. PMID: 28254144.

Antoniou, A, Pharoah, PDP, Narod, S, Risch, HA, Eyfjord, JE, Hopper, JL, Loman, N, Olsson, H, Johannsson, O, Borg, Å, Pasini, B, Radice, P, Manoukian, S, Eccles, DM, Tang, N, Olah, E, Anton-Culver, H, Warner, E, Lubinski, J, ... Easton, DF. "Average risks of breast and ovarian cancer associated with BRCA1 or BRCA2 mutations detected in case Series unselected for family history: a combined analysis of 22 studies." *American journal of human genetics* vol. 72,5 (2003): 1117-30. doi:10.1086/375033.

Broeke, SW, van der Klift, HM, Tops, CMJ, Aretz, S, Bernstein, I, Buchanan, DD, de la Chapelle, A, Capella, G, Clendenning, M, Engel, C, Gallinger, S, Gomez Garcia, E, Figueiredo, JC, Haile, R, Hampel, HL, Hest, L. van, Hopper, JL, Hoogerbrugge, N, von Knebel Doeberitz, M, ... Win, AK Cancer Risks for PMS2-Associated Lynch Syndrome. *J. Clin. Oncol.* 2018, 36, 2961–2968.

Burn, J, Gerdes, AM, Macrae, F, Mecklin, JP, Moeslein, G, Olschwang, S, Eccles, D, Evans, DG, Maher, ER, Bertario, L, Bisgaard, ML, Dunlop, MG, Ho, JW, Hodgson, SV, Lindblom, A, Lubinski, J, Morrison, PJ, Murday, V, Ramesar, R, ... Bishop, DT. Long-term effect of aspirin on cancer risk in carriers of hereditary colorectal cancer: an analysis from the CAPP2 randomised controlled trial. *Lancet*. 2011;378(9809):2081-2087. doi:10.1016/S0140-6736(11)61049-0.

CaPP3 - *Health Research Authority* (hra.nhs.uk).

Crosbie EJ, Flaum N, Harkness EF, Clayton RD, Holland C, Martin-Hirsch P, Wood N, Keating P, Woodward ER, Lalloo F, Donnai P, Edmondson RJ, Evans DG. Specialist oncological surgery for removal of the ovaries and fallopian tubes in BRCA1 and BRCA2 pathogenic variant carriers may reduce primary peritoneal cancer risk to very low levels. *Int J Cancer*. 2021 Mar 1;148(5):1155-1163. doi: 10.1002/ijc.33378. Epub 2020 Nov 11. PMID: 33152107; PMCID: PMC7839461.

Crosbie, EJ, Ryan, NAJ, Arends, MJ, Bosse, T, Burn, J, Cornes, JM, Crawford, R, Eccles, D, Frayling, IM, Ghaem-Maghami, S, Hampel, H, Kauff, ND, Kitchener, HC, Kitson, SJ, Manchanda, R, McMahon, RFT, Monahan, KJ, Menon, U, Møller, P, ... Evans, DG. Manchester International Consensus Group. The Manchester International Consensus Group recommendations for the management of gynaecological cancers in Lynch syndrome. *Genet Med* 2019;21:2390-400. doi: 10.1038/s41436-019-0489-y pmid: 30918358.

Cummings S, Roman SS, Saam J, Bernhisel R, Brown K, Lancaster JM, Usha L. Age of ovarian cancer diagnosis among BRIP1, RAD51C, and RAD51D mutation carriers identified through multi-gene panel testing. *J Ovarian Res*. 2021 Apr 29;14(1):61. doi: 10.1186/s13048-021-00809-w. PMID: 33926482; PMCID: PMC8086272.

Dareng, EO, Tyrer, JP, Barnes, DR, Jones, MR, Yang, X, Aben, KKH, Adank, MA, Agata, S, Andrulis, IL, Anton-Culver, H, Antonenkova, NN, Aravantinos, G, Arun, BK, Augustinsson, A, Balmaña, J, Bandera, EV, Barkardottir, RB, Barrowdale, D, Beckmann, MW, ... Pharoah, PDP. Polygenic risk modelling for prediction of epithelial ovarian cancer risk. *Eur J Hum Genet* 30, 349–362 (2022). https://doi.org/10.1038/s41431-021-00987-7.

Domchek SM, Tara M Friebel, Christian F Singer, D Gareth Evans, Henry T Lynch, Claudine Isaacs, Judy E Garber, Susan L Neuhausen, Ellen Matloff, Rosalind Eeles, Gabriella Pichert, Laura Van t'veer, Nadine Tung, Jeffrey N Weitzel, Fergus J Couch, Wendy S Rubinstein, Patricia A Ganz, Mary B Daly, Olufunmilayo I Olopade, Gail Tomlinson, Joellen Schildkraut, Joanne L Blum, Timothy R Rebbeck. Association of risk-reducing surgery in BRCA1 or BRCA2 mutation carriers with cancer risk and mortality. *JAMA*. 2010;304(9):967-975. doi:10.1001/jama.2010.1237.

Dominguez-Valentin, M, Crosbie, EJ, Engel, C, Aretz, S, Macrae, F, Winship, I, Capella, G, Thomas, H, Nakken, S, Hovig, E, Nielsen, M, Sijmons, RH, Bertario, L, Bonanni, B, Tibiletti, MG, Cavestro, GM, Mints, M, Gluck, N, Katz, L, ... Møller, P. Risk-reducing hysterectomy and bilateral salpingo-oophorectomy in female heterozygotes of pathogenic mismatch repair variants: a Prospective Lynch Syndrome Database report. *Genet Med* 23, 705–712 (2021). https://doi.org/10.1038/s41436-020-01029-1.

Eleje, GU, Eke, AC, Ezebialu, IU, Ikechebelu, JI, Ugwu, EO, & Okonkwo, OO. "Risk-reducing bilateral salpingo-oophorectomy in women with BRCA1 or BRCA2 mutations." *The Cochrane database of systematic reviews* vol. 8,8 CD012464. 24 Aug. 2018, doi:10.1002/14651858.CD012464.pub2.

Flaum N, van Veen EM, Smith O, Amico S, Newman WG, Crosbie EJ, Edmondson R, Smith MJ, Evans DG. Dominant-negative pathogenic variant BRIP1 c.1045G>C is a high-risk allele for non-mucinous epithelial ovarian cancer: A case-control study. *Clin Genet*. 2022 Jan;101(1):48-54. doi: 10.1111/cge.14068. Epub 2021 Oct 7. PMID: 34585738.

Gaba, F, Robbani, S, Singh, N, McCluggage, WG, Wilkinson, N, Ganesan, R, Bryson, G, Rowlands, G, Tyson, C, Arora, R, Saridogan, E, Hanson, H, Burnell, M, Legood, R, Evans, DG, Menon, U, & Manchanda, R. Preventing Ovarian Cancer through early Excision of Tubes and late Ovarian Removal (PROTECTOR): protocol for a prospective non-randomised multi-center trial *International Journal of Gynecologic Cancer* 2021;31:286-291.

Georgakis MK, Beskou-Kontou T, Theodoridis I, Skalkidou A, Petridou ET. Surgical menopause in association with cognitive function and risk of dementia: A systematic review and meta-analysis. *Psychoneuroendocrinology*. 2019 Aug;106:9-19. doi: 10.1016/j.psyneuen.2019.03.013. Epub 2019 Mar 19. PMID: 30928686.

Helder-Woolderink JM, Blok EA, Vasen HF, Hollema H, Mourits MJ, De Bock GH. Ovarian cancer in Lynch syndrome; a systematic review. *Eur J Cancer*. 2016 Mar;55:65-73. doi: 10.1016/j.ejca.2015. 12.005. Epub 2016 Jan 13. PMID: 26773421.

Marchetti, C., De Felice, F., Palaia, I., Perniola, G., Musella, A., Musio, D., Muzii, L., Tombolini, V., & Panici, P. B. Risk-reducing salpingo-oophorectomy: a meta-analysis on impact on ovarian cancer risk and all-cause mortality in BRCA 1 and BRCA 2 mutation carriers. *BMC Womens Health*. 2014;14:150. Published 2014 Dec 12. doi:10.1186/s12905-014-0150-5.

Mavaddat N, Peock S, Frost D, Ellis S, Platte R, Fineberg E, Evans DG, Izatt L, Eeles RA, Adlard J, Davidson R, Eccles D, Cole T, Cook J, Brewer C, Tischkowitz M, Douglas F, Hodgson S, Walker L, Porteous ME, Morrison PJ, Side LE, Kennedy MJ, Houghton C, Donaldson A, Rogers MT, Dorkins H, Miedzybrodzka Z, Gregory H, Eason J, Barwell J, McCann E, Murray A, Antoniou AC, Easton DF; EMBRACE. Cancer risks for BRCA1 and BRCA2 mutation carriers: results from prospective analysis of EMBRACE. *J Natl Cancer Inst*. 2013 Jun 5;105(11):812-22. doi: 10.1093/jnci/djt095. Epub 2013 Apr 29. PMID: 23628597.

Mavaddat, N, Antoniou, AC, Mooij, TM, Hooning, MJ, Heemskerk-Gerritsen, BA, Noguès, C, Gauthier-Villars, M, Caron, O, Gesta, P, Pujol, P, Lortholary, A, Barrowdale, D, Frost, D, Evans, DG., … Easton, DF. Risk-reducing salpingo-oophorectomy, natural menopause, and breast cancer risk: an international prospective cohort of BRCA1 and BRCA2 mutation carriers [published correction appears in Breast Cancer Res. 2020 Feb 26;22(1):25]. *Breast Cancer Res*. 2020;22(1):8. Published 2020 Jan 16. doi:10.1186/s13058-020-1247-4.

Medeiros, F, Muto, MG, Lee, Y, Elvin, JA, Callahan, MJ, Feltmate, C, Garber, JE, Cramer, DW, & Crum, CP. The tubal fimbria is a preferred site for early adenocarcinoma in women with familial ovarian cancer syndrome. *Am J Surg Pathol*. (2006) 30:230–6. doi: 10.1097/01.pas.0000180854.28831.77.

Menon, U, Gentry-Maharaj, A, Burnell, M, Singh, N, Ryan, A, Karpinskyj, C, Carlino, G, Taylor, J, Massingham, SK, Raikou, M, Kalsi, JK, Woolas, R, Manchanda, R, Arora, R, Casey, L, Dawnay, A, Dobbs, S, Leeson, S, Mould, T, … Parmar, M. Ovarian cancer population screening and mortality after long-term follow-up in the UK Collaborative Trial of Ovarian Cancer Screening (UKCTOCS): a randomised controlled trial. *Lancet*. 2021;397(10290):2182-2193. doi:10.1016/S0140-6736(21)00731-5.

Mishra GD, Pandeya N, Dobson AJ, Chung HF, Anderson D, Kuh D, Sandin S, Giles GG, Bruinsma F, Hayashi K, Lee JS, Mizunuma H, Cade JE, Burley V, Greenwood DC, Goodman A, Simonsen MK, Adami HO, Demakakos P, Weiderpass E. Early menarche, nulliparity and the risk for premature and early natural menopause. *Hum Reprod*. 2017 Mar 1;32(3):679-686. doi: 10.1093/humrep/dew350. PMID: 28119483; PMCID: PMC5850221.

Moorman PG, Myers ER, Schildkraut JM, Iversen ES, Wang F, Warren N. Effect of hysterectomy with ovarian preservation on ovarian function. *Obstet Gynecol*. 2011 Dec;118(6):1271-1279. doi: 10.1097/AOG. 0b013e318236fd12. PMID: 22067716; PMCID: PMC3223258.

Nahshon C, Segev Y, Gemer O, Bar Noy T, Schmidt M, Ostrovsky L, Lavie O. Should the risk for uterine cancer influence decision making for prophylactic hysterectomy in BRCA1/2 mutated patients- a systematic review and meta-analysis. *Gynecol Oncol*. 2021 Mar;160(3):755-762. doi: 10.1016/j.ygyno. 2020.11.034. Epub 2020 Dec 10. PMID: 33309051.

Philpott, S, Raikou, M, Manchanda, R, Evans, G, Edmondson, R, Menon, U, Ahmed, M, Woodward, E, Lamnisos, A, Lockley, M, Scott, M, Singh, N, Skates, S, Mcguire, A, & Rosenthal, A. 423 Results of the avoiding late diagnosis of ovarian cancer (ALDO) project; a pilot national surveillance program for BRCA mutation-carriers *International Journal of Gynaecologic Cancer* 2021;31:A373-A374.

Piek JM, van Diest PJ, Zweemer RP, Jansen JW, Poort-Keesom RJ, Menko FH, Gille, JJP, Jongsma, APM, Pals, G, Kenemans, P, & Verheijen, RHM. Dysplastic changes in prophylactically removed Fallopian tubes of women predisposed to developing ovarian cancer. *J Pathol.* (2001) 195:451–6. doi: 10.1002/path.1000.

Prospective Lynch Syndrome Database (PLSD) - cumulative risk for cancer by age, genetic variant, and gender in carriers subject to colonoscopy https://sigven78.shinyapps.io/plsd_v4/.

Rosenthal, AN, Fraser, LSM, Philpott, S, Manchanda, R, Burnell, M, Badman, P, Hadwin, R, Rizzuto, I, Benjamin, E, Singh, N, Evans, DG, Eccles, DM, Ryan, A, Liston, R, Dawnay, A, Ford, J, Gunu, R, Mackay, J, Skates, SJ, ... on behalf of the United Kingdom Familial Ovarian Cancer Screening Study collaborators. Evidence of Stage Shift in Women Diagnosed With Ovarian Cancer During Phase II of the United Kingdom Familial Ovarian Cancer Screening Study [published correction appears in J Clin Oncol. 2017 Aug 10;35(23):2722]. *J Clin Oncol.* 2017;35(13):1411-1420. doi:10.1200/JCO.2016.69. 9330.

Ryan N, Snowsill T, McKenzie E, Monahan KJ, Nebgen D. Should women with Lynch syndrome be offered gynaecological cancer surveillance? *BMJ.* 2021 Sep 2;374:n2020. doi: 10.1136/bmj.n2020. PMID: 34475027.

Schmeler KM, Lynch HT, Chen LM, Munsell MF, Soliman PT, Clark MB, Daniels MS, White KG, Boyd-Rogers SG, Conrad PG, Yang KY, Rubin MM, Sun CC, Slomovitz BM, Gershenson DM, Lu KH. Prophylactic surgery to reduce the risk of gynecologic cancers in the Lynch syndrome. *N Engl J Med.* 2006 Jan 19;354(3):261-9. doi: 10.1056/NEJMoa052627. PMID: 16421367.

Skates SJ, Mark H Greene, Saundra S Buys, Phuong L Mai, Powel Brown, Marion Piedmonte, Gustavo Rodriguez, John O Schorge, Mark Sherman, Mary B Daly, Thomas Rutherford, Wendy R Brewster, David M O'Malley, Edward Partridge, John Boggess, Charles W Drescher, Claudine Isaacs, Andrew Berchuck, Susan Domchek, Susan A Davidson, Robert Edwards, Steven A Elg, Katie Wakeley, Kelly-Anne Phillips, Deborah Armstrong, Ira Horowitz, Carol J Fabian, Joan Walker, Patrick M Sluss, William Welch, Lori Minasian, Nora K Horick 1, Carol H Kasten, Susan Nayfield, David Alberts, Dianne M Finkelstein, Karen H Lu 4 Early Detection of Ovarian Cancer using the Risk of Ovarian Cancer Algorithm with Frequent CA125 Testing in Women at Increased Familial Risk - Combined Results from Two Screening Trials. *Clin Cancer Res.* 2017;23(14):3628-3637. doi:10.1158/1078-0432.CCR-15-2750.

Song H, Dicks EM, Tyrer J, Intermaggio M, Chenevix-Trench G, Bowtell DD, Traficante, N, Group, A, Brenton, J, Goranova, T, Hosking, K, Piskorz, A, van Oudenhove, E, Doherty, J, Harris, HR, Rossing, MA, Duerst, M, Dork, T, Bogdanova, NV, ... Pharoah, P. Population-based targeted sequencing of 54 candidate genes identifies PALB2 as a susceptibility gene for high-grade serous ovarian cancer. *J Med Genet* [Internet]. 2021 May;58(5):305–13.

Soong TR, Howitt BE, Miron A, Horowitz NS, Campbell F, Feltmate CM, Muto, MG, Berkowitz, RS, Nucci, MR, Xian, W, & Crum, CP. Evidence for lineage continuity between early serous proliferations (ESPs) in the Fallopian tube and disseminated high-grade serous carcinomas. *J Pathol.* (2018) 246:344–51. doi: 10.1002/path.5145.

Stjepanovic N, Villacampa G, Nead KT, Torres-Esquius S, Melis GG, Nathanson KL, Teule A, Brunet J, Y Cajal TR, Llort G, Dienstmann R, Rue M, Domchek SM, Balmaña J. Association of premenopausal risk-reducing salpingo-oophorectomy with breast cancer risk in BRCA1/2 mutation carriers: Maximising bias-reduction. *Eur J Cancer.* 2020 Jun;132:53-60. doi: 10.1016/j.ejca.2020.03.009. Epub 2020 Apr 20. PMID: 32325420.

Tamoxifen - managing adverse effects: scenario: Tamoxifen - prescribing information. Excellence. National Institute for Health and Care. s.l.: NICE; 2019.

Torkamani A, Wineinger NE, Topol EJ. The personal and clinical utility of polygenic risk scores. *Nat Rev Genet.* 2018;19(9):581–590. doi:10.1038/s41576-018-0018-x.

Tutlewska K, Lubinski J, Kurzawski G. Germline deletions in the EPCAM gene as a cause of Lynch syndrome - literature review. *Hered Cancer Clin Pract.* 2013;11(1):9. Published 2013 Aug 12. doi:10.1186/1897-4287-11-9.

Chapter 9

Pathology of Epithelial Ovarian Tumors

Helen J. Trihia*, MD, PhD

Department of Pathology, Metaxa Cancer Hospital, Piraeus, Greece

Abstract

One of the most difficult and challenging subjects in the field of gynecological oncology is the classification and understanding of the pathogenesis of epithelial ovarian tumours. The pathogenesis of these tumours, the variation of the morphologic types, as well as the accumulating data concerning treatment and prognosis, tend to be a source of frustration to gynaecological oncologists, pathologists and all scientists involved with the various therapeutic approaches. The clinical and pathological characteristics as well as special pathological and immunohistochemical features are presented, illustrated with several photos, in order to clarify the special features of each neoplasm. This chapter aims to provide the most up-to-date research on epithelial ovarian tumours, including the recent data on pathogenesis and the current strategies for diagnosis and prognosis. The WHO Blue Books, here the WHO Classification of the Female Genital Tumours; WHO Classification of Tumours series, 5th ed.; vol. 4, which forms the basis of this chapter, are of increasing importance to pathologists, to practitioners of other clinical disciplines involved in cancer management. As important are the base for uniform standards in diagnosis, so that the patients can benefit from multicentre clinical trials.

Ovarian Carcinoma

- Second most common female genital tract malignancy in developed countries.
- Second leading cause of death among gynaecological cancers.
- Most cases advanced (stage III-IV) at diagnosis.
- Overall prognosis is poor (approximately 35% with a 5 year survival).
- Heterogeneous group of neoplasms.
- Clinically often considered as one disease.
- Pathogenesis was, until recently, largely unknown.
- Different morphological types have different underlying pathogenesis, molecular events, natural behavior and prognoses.

* Corresponding Author's Email: eltrix@otenet.gr.

In: Ovarian Cancer
Editors: Christos Iavazzo, Alexandros Fotiou and John Spiliotis
ISBN: 979-8-88697-633-5

- Many studies/clinical trials lump all types together.
- Studies/clinical trials must include good pathological reviews.

Ovarian Tumourigenesis: A Proposed Model Based on Morphological and Molecular Genetic Analysis

- Ovarian cancer tumours develop from three main cell types in the ovaries: epithelial, germ cells and stromal cells.
- Epithelial tumours account for almost 90% of all ovarian tumours.
- Type I are usually low grade, slowly growing tumours which arise in a stepwise manner from borderline neoplasms or some other precursor which usually exhibit somatic mutations in genes encoding protein kinases and other signalling molecules.
- Type II are usually high grade, rapidly growing neoplasms. Approximately half of high grade serous ovarian cancers harbor defects in homologous recombination.
- Tends not to replace morphologic subtypes but are concerned with mechanisms of tumour development.
- Parallels with type I and type II uterine cancer.
- Arguments against use of type I and type II schemes.
- Perpetuates error of lumping together unrelated tumour types.
- Best not to use (similar arguments in uterus)

Type I Ovarian Carcinomas

- Low grade serous
- Mucinous
- Endometrioid carcinoma
- Malignant Brenner tumour
- Clear cell carcinoma

Type II Ovarian Carcinomas

- High grade serous
- Carcinosarcoma
- Undifferentiated carcinoma

To Discuss

- Morphological types of ovarian *epithelial* neoplasms (benign, borderline and malignant).
- Pathogenesis of different types.
- Grading.

- Problematic areas in determining type.
- Proposed new classification of ovarian carcinomas.
- Theory of origin of high grade serous carcinoma from fallopian tube.

General Introduction

Surface epithelial-stromal ovarian tumours are composed of epithelial elements traditionally believed to originate from the ovarian surface epithelium (or its derivatives, epithelial inclusion glands and cysts) and a stromal component derived from ovarian stroma. Nowadays, we know that a subset of ovarian serous carcinoma is of tubal origin. Exceptions to the foregoing are tumours (particularly clear cell and endometrioid tumours) that arise from the epithelium of endometriosis or an adenofibroma. Furthermore, occasional mucinous tumours arise from the mucinous component of a teratoma and the rare squamous carcinoma from the squamous component of a teratoma or metaplastic squamous epithelium within an endometriotic cyst.

The classification of female genital tumours has evolved significantly over the last decade in light of new and often key molecular discoveries that have influenced the categorization of a number of these neoplasms. Distinctive molecular alterations are now known for many female genital tumours and have proved to be helpful for their correct categorization. Therefore, as in other organ systems, the morphological classification continues to advance into an integrated morphological-molecular classification that will have an impact on diagnosis and treatment. The classification of female genital tumours is intended for worldwide use, and there are many areas where, for various reasons, the application of immunohistochemistry or molecular pathology is limited. Additionally, standard aspects of conventional pathology remain the bedrock of interpretation and classification of female genital tract (FGT) neoplasms in routine practice, and to emphasize this point, the essential diagnostic criteria for this entity are based on these characteristics. *Terminology is the common language used by pathologists and treating physicians for optimal patient care and should be consistently applied.* Therefore, before making a change in terminology, it is important to consider the impact of that change. On the other hand, some important revisions have been made since the 4th edition of the WHO Classification. For example, serous borderline tumours with micropapillary architecture are now included within the broad group of serous borderline tumours, and the term 'non-invasive low-grade serous carcinoma' is not recommended for them. Low-grade and high-grade serous ovarian carcinomas are considered distinct tumour types rather than a spectrum, because they have different origins, as well as different morphology and molecular and genetic signatures. The previous (4th) WHO classification first divided ovarian serous carcinoma into low-grade and high-grade carcinomas, which represent two completely different tumour types (with different morphology, pathogenesis, molecular events and prognosis) rather than low-grade and high-grade forms of the same neoplasm. It is now well established that a significant majority of so-called HGSCS arise from the distal fibrial end of the fallopian tube from a precursor lesion known as serous tubal intraepithelial carcinoma, whereas almost all low-grade serous carcinomas (LGSCs) arise within the ovary from benign and borderline serous tumours.

Seromucinous carcinoma was included in the previous classification and was defined as a carcinoma composed predominantly of serous and endocervical-type mucinous epithelium, often with foci containing clear cells and areas of endometrioid and squamous differentiation.

It has been removed from the classification because it is a poorly reproducible diagnosis and there is significant overlap with other tumour types, especially endometrioid carcinoma. Immunohistochemical and molecular studies have also suggested that most of these tumours represent unusual morphological patterns of endometrioid carcinoma; therefore seromucinous carcinoma is now considered a subtype of endometrioid carcinoma.

Increasingly, immunohistochemistry (and molecular testing) is used to classify ovarian carcinomas, although morphology remains the mainstay in diagnosis. Previously there was poor interobserver agreement among pathologists in the classification of ovarian carcinomas, but the classification is now highly reproducible using modern diagnostic criteria supplemented (when necessary) by immunohistochemistry.

There have been temporal changes linked to changes in the classification of borderline ovarian tumours, which, since ICD-O-3 in 1990, are now grouped as non-malignant.

The surface epithelial-stromal tumours of the ovary are traditionally subclassified by their (a) epithelial cell types; (b) the relative amounts of their epithelial and stromal components; (c) location of their epithelial elements: surface (exophytic), cystic (endophytic), or both; and (d) their growth patterns and nuclear features.

Benign tumours have absent or minimal cellular stratification or atypia and no invasion.

Borderline tumours (tumours of low malignant potential) have epithelial stratification and atypia but no invasion (with the exception of microinvasion), which are subdivided primarily into those of usual type (atypical but not malignant epithelium) and those with intraepithelial carcinoma. Borderline tumours may contain foci of microinvasion; maximal allowable dimensions of the invasive tumour has varied, most commonly been <5 mm or <10 mm^2. Aside from Brenner tumours that typically contain a predominant stromal component, when the stroma of a tumour occupies an area greater than that of the glands, the suffix 'fibroma' is added (e.g., serous adenofibroma), and when more than a rare cyst >1cm in diameter is present, the prefix 'cyst' is used (e.g., serous cystadenofibroma).

Admixtures of neoplasia may be encountered in surface epithelial tumours, including those with two or more types of neoplastic epithelium or variable combinations of benign, borderline and/or carcinomatous components. Thus, careful gross examination and thorough histological sampling of these tumours are necessary for accurate classification.

The classification of ovarian neoplasms in the (last) 5th edition of the WHO Classification of tumours is largely unchanged from the previous 4th edition. One addition to the current classification is mesonephric-like carcinoma. The category of mixed carcinoma has also been reintroduced in the current classification although it is stressed that mixed carcinomas in the ovary are very uncommon and that most carcinomas, that look mixed from a morphological point of view, in fact represent a single neoplastic type with areas morphologically mimicking another tumour type.

5th Who Classification (2020) of Ovarian Epithelial Tumours

- Serous
- Mucinous
- Endometrioid
- Clear cell
- Seromucinous

- Brenner
- Other

More analytically:

Epithelial Tumors

- *Serous tumors*
  - Serous cystadenoma, adenofibroma and surface papilloma
  - Serous borderline tumor
  - Serous borderline tumor, micropapillary variant
  - Low grade serous carcinoma
  - High grade serous carcinoma
- *Mucinous tumors*
  - Mucinous cystadenoma and adenofibroma
  - Mucinous borderline tumor
  - Mucinous carcinoma
- *Endometrioid tumors*
  - Endometrioid cystadenoma and adenofibroma
  - Endometrioid borderline tumor
  - Endometrioid carcinoma
- *Clear cell tumors*
  - Clear cell cystadenoma and adenofibroma
  - Clear cell borderline tumor
  - Clear cell carcinoma
- *Seromucinous tumors*
  - Seromucinous cystadenoma and adenofibroma
  - Seromucinous borderline tumor
- *Brenner tumors*
  - Brenner tumor
  - Borderline Brenner tumor
  - Malignant Brenner tumor
- *Other carcinomas*
  - Mesonephric-like adenocarcinoma
  - Undifferentiated and dedifferentiated carcinoma
  - Carcinosarcoma
  - Mixed carcinoma

Differences from Previous Studies

- Increase in serous
- Marked decrease in mucinous
- Reversal of endometrioid and clear cell ratio

Typing of Ovarian Carcinomas

- At present, of limited therapeutic significance
- Treatment more dependent on *stage* and *grade*
- NEW ERA OF DIFFERENT THERAPY FOR DIFFERENT OVARIAN CANCER TYPES (surgery, traditional chemotherapy, targeted therapies)
- Ongoing trials regarding alternative therapeutic agents in clear cell, mucinous and low grade serous carcinoma (chemoresistant neoplasms)

Other Reasons for Typing

- Carcinoma grading (differs between different types)
- Personal and family history risk
- Clear cell and mucinous histology (although rare) are independent predictors of poor outcome in advanced stage
- Need for lymphadenectomy in Stage I ovarian carcinoma

Recent Population-Based (Washington/British Columbia)

- 68-71% serous
- 3% mucinous
- 9-11% endometrioid
- 12-13% clear cell
- 1% transitional
- 6% mixed

Low Stage (I/II) Versus High Stage (III/IV)

I/II III/IV

- Serous 36% 88%
- Clear cell 26% 5%
- Endometrioid 27% 3%
- Mucinous 8% 1%

Grading of Ovarian Carcinoma

- No universal grading system
- Several in use (FIGO, WHO, Shimizu/Silverberg) but inconsistently applied
- Some systems are universal; some apply different criteria for different types

Grading systems proposed by FIGO, WHO and the GOC are based on architectural features sometimes combined with nuclear features. A two-tier grading system is now generally used for serous carcinoma.

Serous Tumours

Serous Cystadenoma, Adenofibroma and Surface Papilloma of the Ovary

- *Definition.* Serous cystadenoma, adenofibroma and surface papilloma of the ovary, are benign, partially or completely cystic lesions measuring > 1 cm in size and composed of cells resembling fallopian tube epithelium or cuboidal non-ciliated epithelium resembling ovarian surface epithelium (< 1 cm signifies a cortical inclusion cyst). Adenofibromas and cystadenofibromas are composed predominantly of fibrous stroma, with glands and cysts forming a minor component.
- *Clinical findings.* They are present over a broad age range and are generally asymptomatic, or symptoms related to an ovarian mass.
- *Gross appearance.* Macroscopically, tumours vary widely in size (3-10cm, up to 30cm). Cystadenomas exhibit smooth outer and inner surfaces and are filled with watery fluid.
- *Microscopic appearance.* Usually small, uni- to multilocular cysts lined by a single layer of tall, columnar, ciliated cells resembling normal tubal epithelium or cuboidal non-ciliated epithelium resembling ovarian surface epithelium, in varying proportions. Serous cystadenomas are predominantly cystic. Adenofibromas and cystadenofibromas are composed mainly of fibrous stroma, with glands and cysts forming a minor component. If < 10% of the total tumor volume shows epithelial proliferation within the cysts that would otherwise qualify as a serous borderline tumor, designated as serous cystadenoma with focal epithelial proliferation.
- *Prognosis.* Serous cystadenomas, adenofibromas and surface papillomas are benign, but they may recur after incomplete excision. Focal epithelial proliferation on the ovarian surface, where it is exposed to the peritoneal cavity, may potentially be associated with recurrent disease.

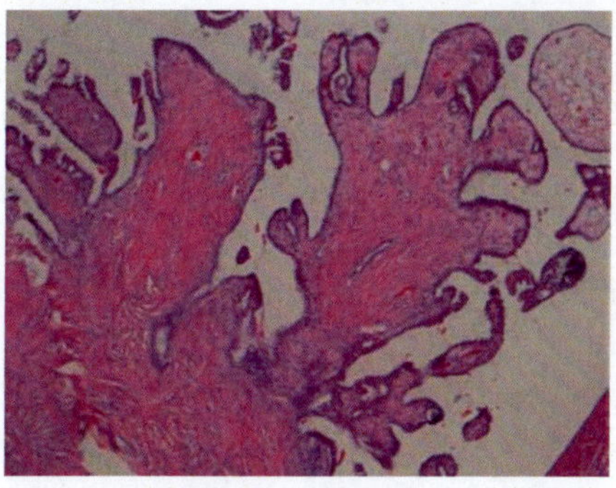

Figure 1. H&E. Histological section of a serous cystadenoma, lined by bland, tubal-type epithelium with occasional ciliated cells.

Serous Borderline Tumour of the Ovary

- *Definition.* Ovarian serous borderline tumor (SBT) is a low grade epithelial neoplasm, generally in younger women with a favorable prognosis when diagnosed at an early stage.
  - Defined as a non-obligate precursor to low grade serous carcinoma (LGSC).
  - As a borderline tumor, it can give rise to extra-ovarian abdominoperitoneal or lymph node implants.
- *Clinical findings & epidemiology.* The median age is in the fifth decade, with a range from the second to ninth decades; i.e., younger than high grade serous carcinoma (HGSC). Up to 15% of ovarian serous neoplasms are of the borderline type and they are frequently bilateral (up to 33%). These are symptoms attributable to an ovarian mass.
- *Gross appearance.* Macroscopically, tumours are generally >5cm and may be intracystic (and lined by excrescences) and/or exophytic with surface involvement.
- *Microscopic appearance.* Typical SBT is characterized by hierarchical branching papillae with variable amounts of stoma in the cores. The epithelium is stratified with tufting and cell detachment. The micropapillary/cribriform subtype has elongated micropapillae without stromal cores (at least 5 times longer than wide) that directly emanate from large papillae (the so-called Medusa head appearance) and/or small punched out cribriform spaces. An area of pure micropapillary/cribriform growth measuring =>5mm is required for the tumour to be classified as a micropapillary/cribriform subtype. The nuclear features should not be high-grade and mitoses are rare. Stromal microinvasion is defined as invasion <5mm in greatest dimension in any single focus. No desmoplasia should be present. These cells may sometimes be within lymphatic spaces. This pattern is diagnosed as SBT with microinvasion. If the morphology resembles low-grade serous carcinoma (LGSC) and invasion measures <5mm in greatest dimension, in any single focus, the tumour should be classified as microinvasive LGSC, and extensive sampling should be performed to exclude the larger foci of invasion. The term 'implant' is used in the context of extra-ovarian disease associated with the SBT of the ovary. Implants of serous borderline, are by definition, non-invasive. If there is invasion, a diagnosis of LGSC should be made. Non-invasive implants, that display hierarchically branching papillae or detached clusters of cells, not associated with stroma, are designated as epithelial implants. Desmoplastic implants consist of single cells or clusters of cells, embedded in a reactive-appearing (granulation tissue, or fasciitis-like) or desmoplastic stroma that predominates over the epithelial component and appears tacked on to the peritoneal surface. Invasive implants (i.e., extraovarian LGSC) exhibit a variety of patterns. In most cases the epithelial component predominates and there is destructive invasion of underlying structures (e.g., invasion into myometrium or muscularis propria of bowel) or obliteration of normal omental architecture by invasive tumour. Rare implants cannot be classified as either non-invasive or invasive, because of ambiguous morphology, and are designated as indeterminate. Lymph node involvement by SBT is not equivalent to metastatic carcinoma, but should be staged as N1 disease.

- *Prognosis.* Patients with FIGO Stage I SBT show no significant difference in overall survival compared with the general population; in contrast, women with advanced disease have decreased rate of survival. A reported 4-7% of women with SBT develop subsequent carcinoma, usually low-grade, but rarely high-grade. Risk factors for subsequent development of carcinoma include micropapillary/cribriform subtype, advanced stage, bilaterality, ovarian surface involvement and residual disease after surgery. The presence of invasive implants (LGSC) is the most important adverse prognostic factor. Lymph node involvement is not considered an adverse prognostic factor. In most studies, stromal microinvasion has not negatively affected the outcome.

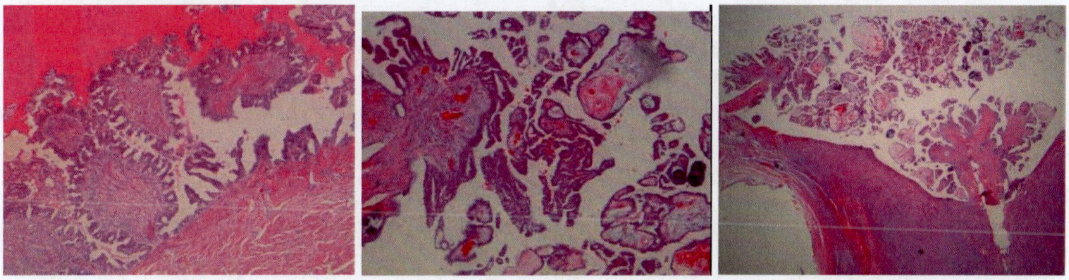

(a) (b) (c)

Figure 2a, b, c. H&E. Serous borderline tumour. Papillae are architecturally complex, with hierarchical branching, lined by stratified epithelium with detached small clusters of cells. Prominent microcalcifications in (b) and (c).

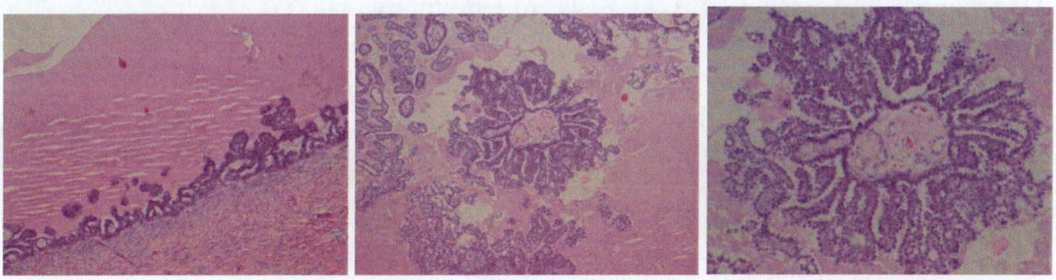

(d) (e) (f)

Figure 3d, e, f. H&E. Micropapillary serous borderline tumour. Micropapillary architecture is prominent. Elongated micropapillae directly emanate from a large papilla, producing the so-called Medusa head appearance (in (e), (f): higher magnification of (e)).

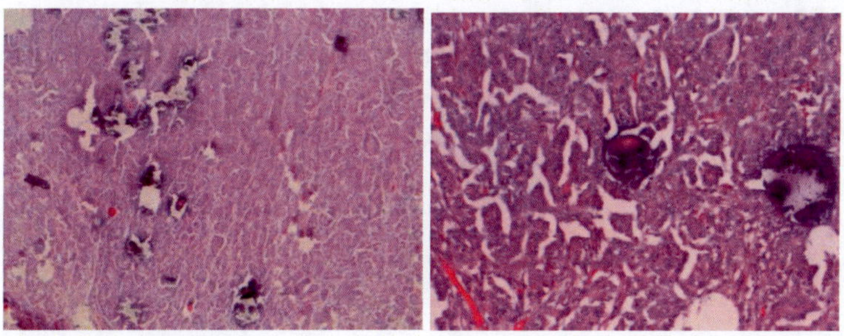

(g) (h)

Figure 4g, h. H&E. Microinvasive low grade serous carcinoma in SBT. Prominent micropapillary pattern with microcalcifications.

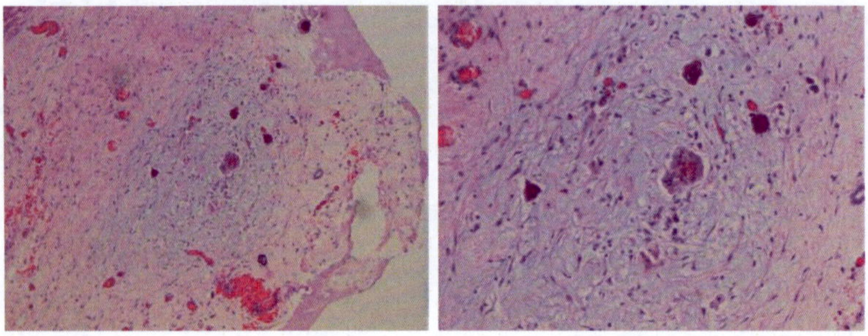

(i) (j)

Figure 5i, k. H&E. Non-invasive implants associated with ovarian serous borderline tumour. Individual epithelial cells and microcalcifications are present within loose myxoid desmoplastic stroma.

Ovarian Serous Carcinoma (OSC)

- Most common ovarian carcinoma.
- Often advanced stage at diagnosis.
- Traditionally graded as grade I,II,III (well-, moderately- , and poorly differentiated).
- Several grading systems in use.

Ovarian Serous Carcinoma (OSC)-Recent Developments

- Two distinct tumour types (called low grade and high grade OSC).
- Not two grades of same neoplasm.
- Different neoplasms with different underlying pathogenesis, molecular events, behavior, prognosis.
- High grade much more common than low grade.
- Use instead of traditional grading schemes.

Pathogenesis (Low Grade Serous)

- Low grade arises from pre-existing benign and borderline tumours (not all cases).
- Micropapillary variant of borderline tumour may be an intermediate stage in the development of low grade serous carcinoma.
- Well-defined adenoma-carcinoma sequence.

Pathogenesis (High Grade Serous)

- Thought to arise directly from epithelium of distal fallopian tube.
- Well-defined precursor lesion (postulated to be serous tubal intraepithelial carcinoma)-rapid development- doesn't arise from borderline tumour.

Morphology

- Classification as high grade or low grade serous is reproducible (MD Anderson system).
- Distinction based mostly on nuclear atypia (not on architecture) in the worst area of the tumour.
- Low grade serous-uniform nuclei with mild atypia; <12 mitoses per 10 HPFs; usually approximately 2 mitoses per 10 HPFs; no necrosis or multinucleation.
- High grade serous- moderate to marked atypia; >12 mitoses per 10 HPFs; often necrosis and multinucleate cells.

Corellation between Grading Systems

- Almost all grade II and III in old systems are high grade.
- Grade I in old systems may be low grade or high grade.

Low Grade Serous Carcinoma of the Ovary

- *Definition.* Epithelial carcinoma of serous cell lineage, usually with distinctive patterns of invasion and low grade cytologic atypia.
- *Clinical findings & epidemiology.* Abdominal pain/swelling. Incidental finding. Most patients present with advanced stage disease. Can manifest as recurrence following diagnosis of serous borderline tumour.
  - Mean age: fifth to sixth decades
  - Presents ~10 years earlier than patients with high grade serous carcinoma

  3.5% of all ovarian carcinomas; 5% of all serous tumours. A small subset of patients have a prior history of serous borderline tumour (SBT). Both tumors can coexist in up to 85% of cases in variable combinations. Can be synchronous, metachronous, ipsilateral or contralateral.
  - May rarely progress to high grade serous carcinoma, sarcomatoid carcinoma or carcinosarcoma.
- *Gross appearance.* Often bilateral ovarian masses, solid or solid and cystic with calcifications.
- *Microscopic appearance.* LGSCs exhibit a variety of patterns and several patterns of invasion are present in an individual tumour. The nuclei exhibit mild to moderate atypia, with < 3-fold variation in nuclear size, occasionally with a central nucleolus. Mitotic figures are present, usually 1-2 mitoses/mm^2. Psammoma bodies are often present. Necrosis is rare. These tumours frequently co-exist with SBT. Tumours are typically diffusely positive for Ker7, PAX8, ER and WT1; p16 expression is patchy and p53 exhibits wild type immunoreactivity.
- *Prognosis.* Excellent with surgical excision alone if confined to the ovary. Extraovarian spread at presentation associated with poor outcome. 5 and 10 year survival rate in advanced stage is 80% and 50%, respectively. Better prognosis than high grade serous carcinoma when matched by stage.

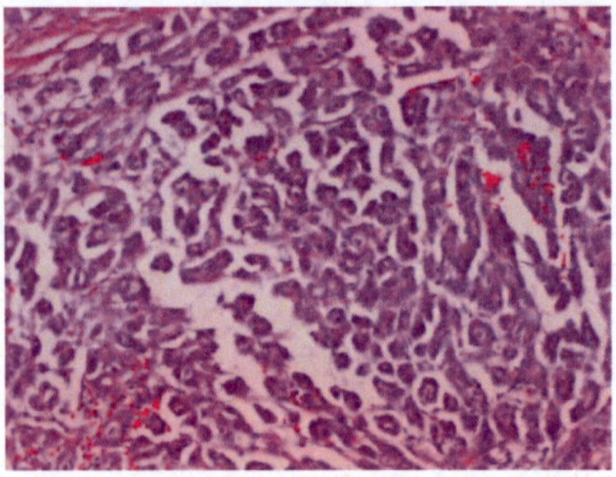

Figure 6. H&E. Low-grade serous carcinoma. Small papillae containing cells with uniform nuclei and inconspicuous mitotic activity.

High Grade Serous Carcinoma

- *Definition*. Epithelial carcinoma of serous cell lineage with papillary, glandular and solid growth patterns and high grade cytologic atypia.
- *Clinical findings*. Mean age: 63 years. Symptoms:
  - Abdominal distension / bloating / pain
  - Nausea
  - Anorexia / early satiety
  - Back pain
  - Urinary incontinence
  - Advanced disease at presentation in ~80% of cases
- *Epidemiology & Pathogenesis*. HGSC accounts for the majority of ovarian carcinoma diagnoses (approximately 70%), and related deaths with higher incidence in white populations. Age >60 years, a family history of breast/ovarian carcinoma, and infertility, are risk factors, whereas multiparity, breast feeding, oral contraceptive use, late menarche, and early menopause, are protective factors. Hereditary predisposition in 15-20% of cases involving BRCA genes. Associated with homologous recombination defects. Nearly every tumour harbours an aberant TP53 mutation.
- *Gross appearance*. Often bilateral, solid and cystic ovarian masses, large and exophytic. Variable in size; exophytic with solid or papillary growth; solid areas, tan to white with necrosis and hemorrhage; serous/bloody fluid filled cysts. Fallopian tube can be grossly involved at fimbriated end. There is often extensive extraovarian involvement.
- *Microscopic appearance*. There is a variety of growth patterns. Solid growth of columnar to cuboidal cells with eosinophilic cytoplasm and slit-like spaces (fusion of papillae). Hierarchical papillary branching, glandular and cribriform patterns are common. Significant nuclear atypia. Nuclei are large and markedly atypical (nuclear size variability >3-fold, including large, bizarre and multinucleated forms), with high mitotic activity, typically > 5mitoses/mm^2 (equating > 12 mitoses/10 HPF), including atypical mitoses. On low power, occasional tumours have an architecture resembling that of serous borderline tumour and do not demonstrate overt destructive invasion, but are diagnosed as HGSC on the basis of the nuclear features. Homologous

recombination-deficient tumours frequently display variant architecture, which includes SET (solid, endometrial-like, transitional) patterns (more common in BRCA1 mutations). These tumours often display geographical necrosis and a prominent lymphocytic infiltrate. Psammoma bodies are variable. Serous tubal intraepithelial carcinoma (STIC) (90% fimbria, 10% ampulla/isthmus) exhibits similar histologic features; may be bilateral (10-20%) and multifocal. Approximately 90% of tumours demonstrate nuclear expression of WT1 and approximately 95% exhibit an abnormal pattern of p53 expression, 3 patterns, a) mutation-type labeling, represented by strong diffuse staining in at least of 80% of cells, b) no expression (with an intact internal control), or c) (rarely) diffuse cytoplasmic staining, with intensity similar to that of internal nuclear controls (loss of function mutation disrupting nuclear localization domain). High Ki67 proliferation index (>75%). CK7, CA125 and PAX8 are typically positive and ER is frequently expressed, p16 demonstrates strong diffuse immunoreactivity in >=50% of tumours. CK20, CEA, HNF1β, and Napsin A, are typically negative in these tumours.

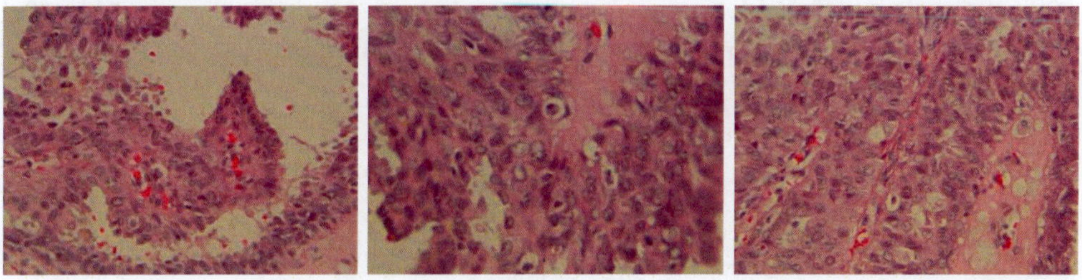

(a) (b) (c)

Figure 7a, b, c. H&E. High grade serous carcinoma. Papillary structures containing cells with pleomorphic nuclei and prominent mitoses.

- *Prognosis.* Most important is the stage, ~40% overall 5 year survival. In advanced stage disease, the amount of residual tumor present after staging and debulking is the most important factor. Low Ki67 proliferation index is associated with platinum resistance and decreased survival. CD3+ or CD8+ tumor infiltrating lymphocytes confer favorable prognosis. Poly (ADP-ribose) polymerase (PARP) inhibitors with best response in patients with BRCA1/BRCA2 mutations or other homologous recombination deficiency and platinum sensitivity.

Molecular (Low Grade Serous)

- KRAS or BRAF mutations in approx. 2/3 (early in evolution- mutations found in benign and borderline tumours; identical mutations in borderline and malignant areas in same tumour).
- ERBB2 mutations.
- KRAS and BRAF mutations are mutually exclusive; equivalent effect on tumourigenesis.
- No Tp53 mutations/abnormalities.

- Progressive increase in chromosomal instability from benign to borderline to malignant.

Molecular (High Grade Serous)

- Tp53 mutations- early in evolution-seen in early microscopic tumours, e.g., BRCA1/2. p53 dysfunction found in almost 100% high grade serous using stringent criteria.
- BRCA1/2 abnormalities- germline or somatic mutations or hypermethylation.
- No BRAF and only occasional KRAS mutations.
- High chromosome instability even in small early tumours.

Behaviour and Prognosis (Low Grade Serous)

- Usually advanced at diagnosis.
- Indolent behavior-median survival 4.2 years; 5 year survival approx. 55%; many cases survive longer, e.g., >20 years.
- Often eventually fatal.
- Poor response to chemotherapy.
- Role of hormone therapy- aromatase inhibitors, etc. (ER/PR positive).
- Possible targeted therapies- MEK inhibitors in tumours with RAS mutations.
- Rarely coexist or evolve into high grade serous/undifferentiated carcinoma/ carcinosarcoma.

Behaviour and Prognosis (High Grade Serous)

- Usually advanced at diagnosis.
- Aggressive behavior.
- Median survival 1.7 years.
- 5 year survival rate approx. 25-30%.
- Responds well initially to chemotherapy but then usually recurs.
- Role of PARP inhibitors especially in BRCA abnormalities.

Primary Peritoneal Serous Carcinoma (PPSC)

- Usually high grade.
- Now being diagnosed more frequently.
- Post-chemotherapy cases which probably cannot be diagnosed.
- Use GOG criteria, adopted by WHO, but often has to be diagnosed clinically/ radiologically.

Gog Criteria for PPSC

- Ovaries normal in size or enlarged by a benign process.
- Tumour must be serous in type.
- Microscopy-no tumour in ovary; tumour confined to surface; <5mm invasion into stroma of ovary (arbitrary figure).
- Review slides (if <5 years) and, or report of previous oophorectomy to document absence of tumour.

Ovarian Mucinous Tumours

Mucinous ovarian tumours form a spectrum of diseases along a continuum of differentiation from benign cystadenomas through borderline tumours (MOB) to carcinomas (MOC). They are composed of epithelium showing an intestinal differentiation, and thus the term mucinous is no longer applied to the seromucinous tumours, with mullerian-type epithelium. Mucinous ovarian tumours are usually large and frequently heterogeneous, composed of benign and carcinomatous areas. This implies that their accurate diagnosis requires rigorous and extensive sampling. MOC is uncommon (3-4% of ovarian cancer). The WHO 2014 histological classification has recognized two different types of invasion, first characterized by Riopel et al. in 1999; being expansile or infiltrative. The pattern of invasion in MOC, has important prognostic and therapeutic implications.

The accurate histological diagnosis of mucinous ovarian tumours remains challenging. The two main difficulties are the classification as benign, borderline, or carcinoma and the identification of the invasion pattern, expansile or infiltrative. Another problem with ovarian mucinous tumours is the distinction between a primary and a secondary lesion. A combination of clinical, pathological and immunohistochemical investigations is useful in distinguishing primary mucinous ovarian tumour from metastatic to the ovary.

Mucinous Cystadenoma and Adenofibroma

- *Definition.* Mucinous cystadenoma and adenofibroma are benign neoplasms composed of cysts and glands lined by gastrointestinal or Müllerian type mucinous epithelium lacking architectural complexity or cytologic atypia. They can be ovarian or retroperitoneal. May be associated with mature teratoma or Brenner tumor.
- *Clinical findings & epidemiology.* Symptoms related to an abdominal or pelvic mass. Rarely, patients present with estrogenic or androgenic manifestations, secondary to stromal luteinization. These tumours are seen in patients over a wide age range (range 13–79). Median age 50 years. Benign mucinous neoplasms account for approximately 80% of all primary ovarian mucinous tumours, with mucinous cystadenomas and adenofibromas.
- *Gross appearance.* Mucinous cystadenomas, are usually unilateral (95%) and multilocular with a smooth or bosselated outer surface. Mean size 10 cm, rarely > 30 cm. Cystadenoma is a uni- or multilocular cyst with variably sized smooth walled

locules, filled with dense, viscous, sticky, gelatinous material. No solid areas or papillary excrescences. Adenofibromas are usually smaller, predominantly white and solid with variable amounts of small cysts.

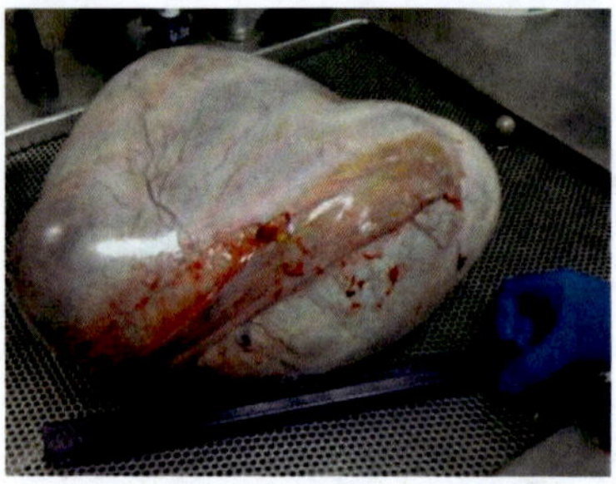

Figure 8. Macroscopic appearance of a mucinous cystadenoma with a smooth outer surface and a size of approximately 20 cm.

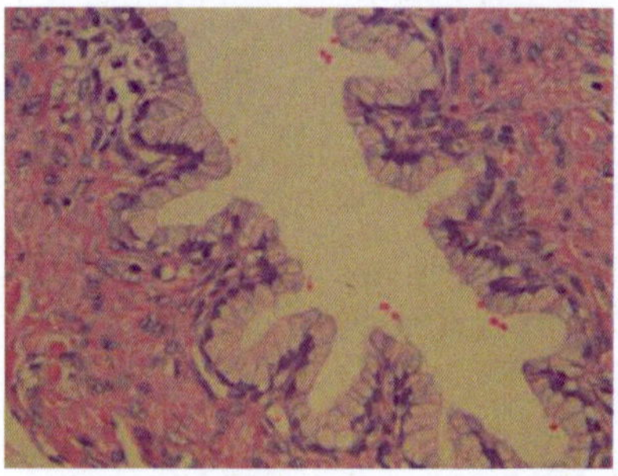

Figure 9. H&E. Histological section of a mucinous cystadenoma/adenofibroma lined by tall columnar cells with abundant mucinous cytoplasm and bland basically based nuclei.

- *Microscopic appearance*. Mucinous cystadenomas are composed of multiple cysts and glands lined by simple non-stratified mucinous epithelium resembling Mullerian, gastric-folveolar-type, or intestinal epithelium containing goblet cells and sometimes neuroendocrine cells or Paneth cells. Adenofibromas have small cysts and glands lined by a single layer of bland mucinous epithelium embedded in a prominent variably cellular fibromatous stroma with or without luteinization. Nuclei are small without cytological atypia, with absent or minimal mitotic activity. A component of dermoid cyst or Brenner tumour may be found. Rarely, mucinous cystadenomas can contain mural nodules, or be associated with clear cell carcinoma, large cell neuroendocrine carcinoma (LNEC), endometrioid carcinoma and sex cord-stromal tumour.
- *Prognosis*. Excellent prognosis. Recurrences may occur after cystectomy or rupture and spillage.

Mucinous Borderline Tumour

- *Definition*. Mucinous borderline tumour (MBT) is a non invasive mucinous neoplasm with complex architecture and gastrointestinal type differentiation. It can be ovarian or retroperitoneal. It may arise from mucinous cystadenoma. Also associated with Brenner tumor and mature cystic teratoma.

- *Clinical findings.* Symptoms are most often related to pelvic mass. MBTs occur over a wide age range, including paediatric patients (mean patient age: 45 years). Second most common subtype of ovarian borderline tumor in Western countries and the most common subtype in Asia
- *Pathogenesis. KRAS* mutations are the most frequent molecular alterations.
- *Gross appearance.* More than 90% of the tumors are unilateral. Mean size: 22 cm; some tumors can measure as large as 50 cm. Cysts are multiloculated with mucinous contents and smooth external surface. Solid areas and necrosis may be present. Solid areas should be preferentially sampled, because these may represent areas of invasion or mural nodules. It is recommended to sample one section per 1cm of tumour for tumours <10cm and two sections per 1cm for tumours =>10cm.
- *Microscopic appearance.* These tumours contain multiple cysts lined by gastrointestinal-type mucinous epithelium with complex architecture with tufting and villus formation. Epithelium resembles low grade dysplasia of the intestine with goblet cells, neuroendocrine cells and occasional Paneth cells. Neoplastic cells have hyperchromasia, crowding, stratification and mitotic activity. They have glands with luminal mucin. May be associated with intraepithelial carcinoma (foci with high grade cytologic atypia) and microinvasion (stromal invasion by single cells or small nests, measuring < 5 mm). A component of benign mucinous cystadenoma is often present. Epithelial proliferation must account for >10% of the epithelial volume for a tumour to qualify as MBT; otherwise, the tumour should be classified as mucinous cystadenoma with focal epithelial proliferation. The presence of focal or patchy marked cytological atypia, often associated with mitotic activity, warrants a diagnosis of intraepithelial carcinoma in these tumours. In the presence of diffuse marked cytological atypia, a diagnosis of mucinous carcinoma (primary or metastatic) should be considered. Some tumours are associated with a Brenner tumour or a mature cystic teratoma. When associated with a teratoma, MBT may have prominent mucin extravasation in the ovarian stroma and the peritoneum. Mural nodules may be present and classified as reactive sarcoma-like, anaplastic carcinoma, or sarcoma. MBT has the same immunohistochemical profile as mucinous carcinoma.
- *Prognosis.* Excellent prognosis; Stage I at diagnosis. Mucinous borderline tumor with intraepithelial carcinoma: 95-100% overall survival rate. Recurrences may occur following cystectomy. Tumors with microinvasion are associated with a recurrence rate of 5%. Anaplastic carcinoma and sarcoma mural nodules are associated with adverse clinical behavior and increased mortality rate; however, anaplastic carcinoma in unruptured Stage I tumors does not necessarily carry an adverse prognosis. A sarcoma-like mural nodule does not have effect on prognosis. MBTs arising in teratomas may be associated with extraovarian disease, including pseudomyxoma peritonei, but they do not seem to be associated with an adverse outcome.

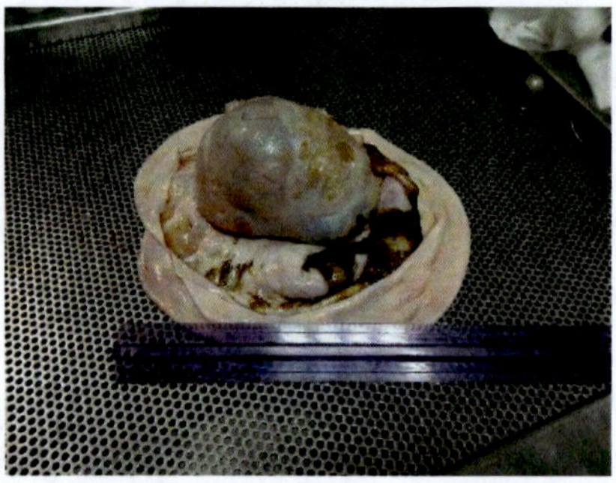

Figure 10. Macroscopic appearance of a MBT developed on the grounds of benign mucinous cystadenoma. A unilocular cystic mass with smooth outer and inner surface and an area of a mural tumour nodule.

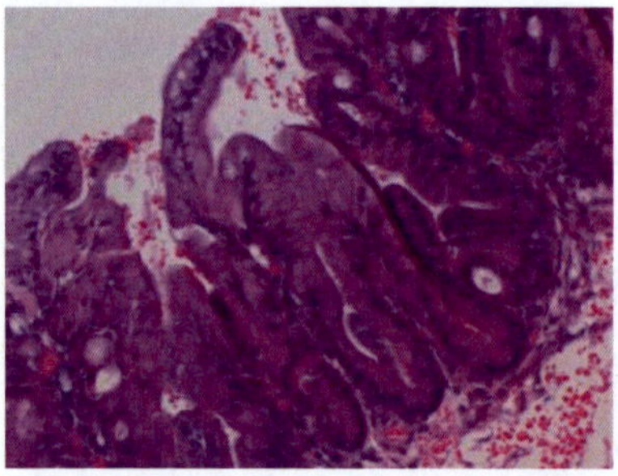

Figure 11. H&E. Histological section of a mucinous borderline tumour. The cyst lining shows architectural complexity with some villous architecture and epithelial stratification.

Mucinous Carcinoma of the Ovary

- *Definition.* Mucinous carcinoma is an invasive mucinous neoplasm composed of gastrointestinal-type cells. It can be ovarian or retroperitoneal. 77% of ovarian mucinous carcinomas are metastases, 23% are ovarian primaries. Of the ovarian primaries, most arise in a benign or borderline tumor; only 5-10% are pure.
- *Clinical findings.* Patients typically present with symptoms related to a pelvic mass. Most tumours are confined to the ovary at presentation. Advanced-stage disease is very rare. The median patient age at presentation is 55 years.
- *Pathogenesis.* Many mucinous carcinomas develop from mucinous borderline tumours, although some may arise from a mature cystic teratoma or a Brenner tumour.
- *Macroscopic appearance.* Primary tumors are usually unilateral, > 10 cm, with smooth capsule, cystic and solid areas and mucoid contents.
- *Microscopic appearance.* There is often a coexistence of benign, borderline and carcinomatous areas, with a continuum of architectural and cytological atypia. Carcinomas are characterized by two different patterns of invasion: expansile/confluent and infiltrative/destructive, each measuring at least 5mm in linear extent. The two patterns may coexist, although the expansile/confluent pattern is more common. The expansile/confluent invasive pattern displays marked glandular crowding, with little or absent intervening stroma, creating a labyrinthine appearance.

The infiltrative/destructive pattern is characterized by irregular glands, nests, and single cells with malignant cytological features, often in a desmoplastic stroma. An infiltrative pattern, in particular in the setting of bilateral ovarian involvement should always raise suspicion for metastatic mucinous carcinoma and prompt evaluation for an extraovarian primary.

- *Grading:*
  - Not standardized, and does not predict prognosis independent of stage.
  - Grade 1-no solid areas.
  - Grade 2-up to 50% solid foci.
  - Grade 3-more than 50% solid foci.
  - Severe nuclear atypia can increase/raise grade I or II carcinomas by one grade.

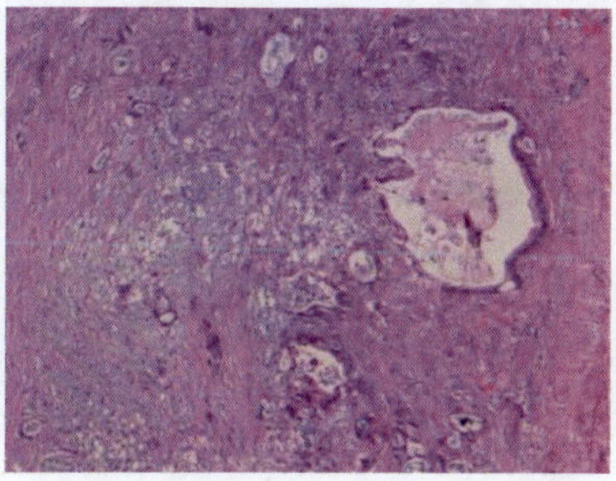

Figure 12. H&E. Histological section of mucinous carcinoma. The tumour exhibits infiltrative/ destructive growth, with irregularly shaped glands arranged haphazardly within desmoplastic stroma.

Ovarian mucinous carcinomas are typically diffusely positive for CK7, and variably positive for CK20, CEA, and CDX2. CA 19-9 is often diffusely positive; CA 125, WT1, Napsin A, vimentin, ER, and PR are usually negative. PAX8, usually focal and weak, is positive in a subset of tumours. P53 may show wild-type or mutation-type staining; p16 is usually negative or focally positive. Diffuse strong positivity for SATB2 can be seen in mucinous tumours associated with mature teratomas.

- *Prognosis.* Distant metastases are rare. Survival: 95% for Stage I vs. 32% for Stages II or greater. Carcinomas with expansile/confluent invasion have a better prognosis than those with infiltrative/destructive one. Recurrences tend to occur within 3 years of diagnosis and have low rates of response to chemotherapy. Most patients with extraovarian disease at presentation die of disease. Anaplastic carcinoma, when found with unruptured Stage I mucinous cystic tumours, may be associated with a favourable prognosis, although data are limited.

Mucinous Carcinoma - Primary or Secondary?

- In most cases, it can be accomplished by pathological examination (gross and microscopic).
- Distribution of disease is important.
- Immunohistochemistry may help but there is a lot of overlap and it's often not paramount.

Features Favouring Metastasis with Mucinous Ovarian Carcinoma

- Bilateral.
- Small tumours.
- Nodular pattern of ovarian involvement.
- Microscopic surface deposits of tumour.
- Marked LVI (especially outside ovary and in hilum).
- Marked variation in growth pattern from one nodule to another.
- Destructive stromal invasion.
- Single cell infiltration and signet ring cells.
- Cells 'floating' in mucin.
- Extraovarian spread.
- NONE PATHOGNOMONIC BUT OFTEN IN COMBINATION.

Endometrioid Cystadenoma and Adenofibroma

- *Definition.* Endometrioid cystadenoma and adenofibroma are benign epithelial tumours exhibiting endometrioid differentiation. Adenofibroma: endometroid and fibroma-like features; may have occasional mitotic figures. There should be no cytologic or architectural atypia. Endometrioid adenofibromas are sometimes associated with endometriosis or an endometriotic cyst.
- *Gross appearance.* Endometrioid cystadenomas are usually unilocular cysts. Endometrioid adenofibromas are solid, with small cysts. They may form a nodule in the wall of an endometriotic cyst.
- *Microscopic appearance.* Endometrioid cystadenomas are cysts lined by endometrioid epithelium without underlying endometrial-type stroma (indicative of endometriosis). Endometrioid adenofibromas are characterized by fibromatous stroma containing cytologically bland, endometrioid glands. Endometrioid cystadenomas may have squamous morules, ciliated or mucinous features.
- *Prognosis.* Benign tumours.

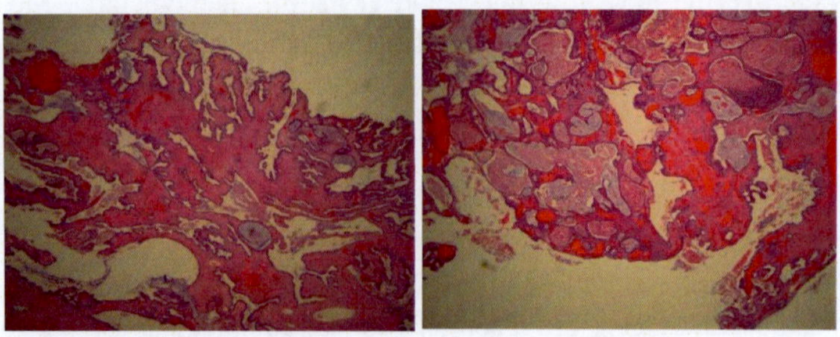

(a) (b)

Figure 13a, b. H&E. Endometrioid cystadenoma/adenofibroma. Endometrial glands are widely spaced within fibromatous stroma.

Endometrioid Borderline Tumour

- *Definition.* Endometrioid borderline tumour is an epithelial tumour composed of crowded endometrioid glands without confluent or destructive invasion.
- *Clinical findings.* Mean age 55 years, range 28-86 years. Patients may present with symptoms related to a pelvic mass, or the tumour may be an incidental finding. 97% present with Stage I disease. 36% associated with endometriosis. Rare tumours. They may coexist with endometrial hyperplasia and/or endometrial endometrioid carcinoma (39%)
- *Gross appearance.* Endometrioid borderline tumours are usually unilateral (3-10% are bilateral), with smooth outer surface. The tumours are often large (mean size: 9cm) and have a solid cut surface, but they may be cystic, with friable haemorrhagic contents.
- *Microscopic appearance.* Endometrioid borderline tumours exhibit two growth patterns: adenofibromatous and intracystic, with prevalence of the former. They may have architectural atypia including non-branching villous papillae, cribriform glands but lacks destructive stromal invasion, glandular confluence or stromal disappearance. The glands in borderline tumours with an adenofibromatous pattern resemble atypical hyperplasia of the endometrium but with a lobular architecture. Squamous metaplasia is common. Microinvasion (<5mm) has been described, but criteria are difficult to apply. More than 5mm of confluent invasion (back-to-back glandular architecture uninterrupted by stroma) or destructive invasion is diagnostic of endometrioid carcinoma.
- *Prognosis.* The prognosis is excellent. Typically, there is no recurrent disease or metastasis on follow-up, even if intraepithelial carcinoma or microinvasion.

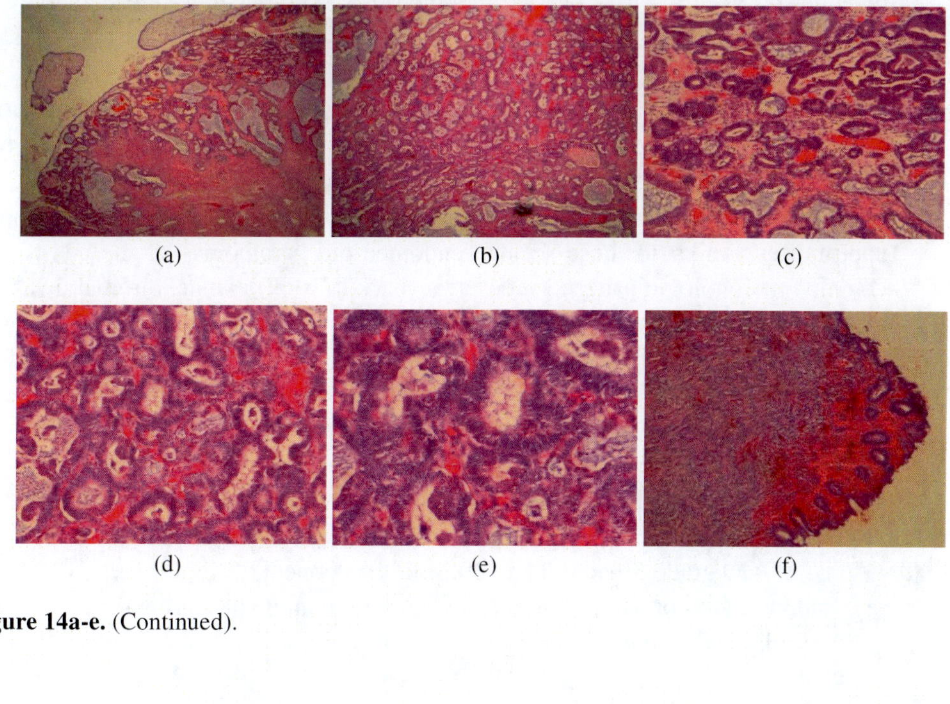

(a) (b) (c)

(d) (e) (f)

Figure 14a-e. (Continued).

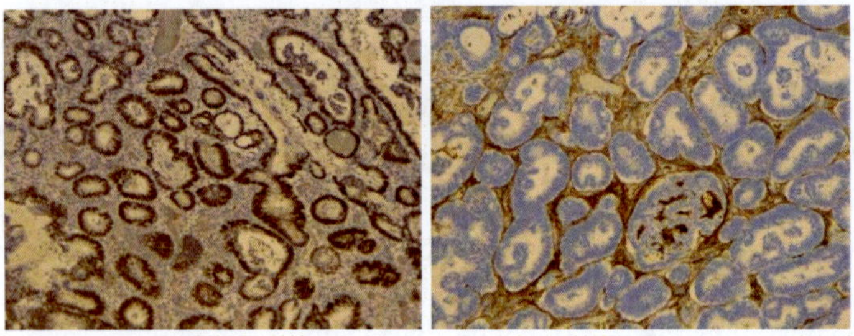

(g) (h)

Figure 14a-e. H&E. Endometrioid borderline tumour. Proliferation of endometrial glands with features resembling atypical hyperplasia (f). H&E. Focus of endometriosis (g-h). Immunostaining for ER ((g), positive) and WT1 (h, negative).

Endometrioid Carcinoma of the Ovary

- *Definition.* Ovarian carcinoma resembling endometrioid carcinoma of the endometrium.

  Seromucinous carcinoma is included as a subtype of endometrioid ovarian carcinoma in the 2020 WHO blue book for female genital tumors.

- *Clinical findings.* Symptoms are related to a pelvic mass, or an incidental finding. There are 10% of primary ovarian carcinomas. Mean patient age is 55 years. Associated with endometriosis/endometriotic cyst (85-90%), endometrioid adenofibroma, synchronous endometrial endometrioid adenocarcinoma or endometrial hyperplasia (15-30%). Risk factors: endometriosis, hormone replacement therapy, first degree family history of breast carcinoma. May occur in the setting of Lynch syndrome.
- *Gross appearance.* Usually unilateral; only 5% bilateral. Cystic with solid component and areas of hemorrhage. With or without polypoid nodule in endometriotic cyst. Mean tumor size: 11 cm (range: 3-22 cm) with a smooth outer surface.
- *Microscopic appearance.* Endometrioid carcinomas show a wide spectrum of appearances similar to those seen in endometrioid carcinomas of the uterus. Most common morphologic pattern is confluent (back to back) glands. Stromal invasion is usually by expansion; rarely, destructive stromal invasion can be observed. Squamous metaplasia (morules or keratin pearls), cytoplasmic mucin, intracytoplasmic vacuoles, oncocytic changes, clear cell changes and cilia and sex cord-like elements (sertoliform) can be observed; none of these morphologic features affect the histologic grade.
  - Histologic grading: same as for endometrial endometrioid adenocarcinoma.
    - FIGO grade 1: less than 5% solid component.
    - FIGO grade 2: 6 - 50% solid component.
    - FIGO grade 3: more than 50% solid component.
  - Endometriosis or adenofibroma may be present in the background.
  - Vascular invasion is rare.

- Might be associated with serous, undifferentiated carcinoma and yolk sac tumor (mixed carcinoma).

Morphologic features in favor of synchronous endometrial and ovarian tumors:

- Both tumors are low grade.
- No myometrial invasion or less than 50% myometrial invasion.
- There is no involvement in any other anatomical sites.
- No lymphovascular involvement in either tumor.
- Background atypical endometrial hyperplasia in the endometrium.
- Unilateral ovarian involvement and unifocal parenchymal distribution of tumor.
- Lack of ovarian capsular, multifocal or hilar involvement.
- Presence of endometriosis or adenofibroma in the ovary.

- *Prognosis.* Stage is the most important prognostic factor. Most tumors are confined to the ovary at diagnosis. Survival rates: > 95% for Stage IA and IB and 51% for Stage III and IV. *CTNNB1* (beta catenin) mutation and low tumor grade are associated with a favorable outcome. Squamous differentiation is associated with CTNNB1 mutation, low tumour grade and favourable outcome. Synchronous endometrioid carcinomas of the endometrium and ovaries are often clonally related but typically have indolent clinical behavior.

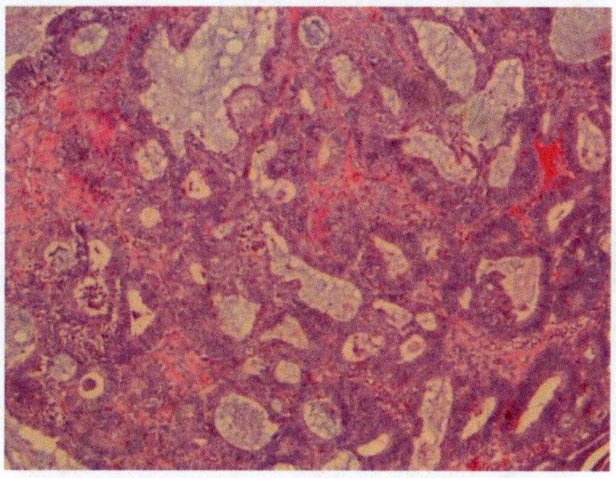

Figure 15. H&E. Endometrioid carcinoma of the ovary.

Clear Cell Adenoma and Cystadenofibroma

- *Definition.* Clear cell adenoma and cystadenofibroma are benign epithelial tumours composed of small glands which are composed of clear or oxyphilic cells within a fibromatous stroma.
- *Clinical findings.* They can be an incidental finding, or patients may present with symptoms of a pelvic mass. The median patient age is early in the sixth decade of life (18-63 years). Association with endometriosis has been reported.
- *Gross appearance.* Unilateral tumours with a smooth and lobulated surface. Reported tumour size ranges from 3.5cm to 26cm. Solid appearance with small cysts.

- *Microscopic appearance.* Clear cell cystadenomas contain small to medium-sized, widely spaced glands in a fibromatous stroma. The constituent cells are bland, flat or low cuboidal, clear, or eosinophilic. Extensive sampling is required to exclude borderline tumours or carcinoma. Papillae, crowded glands, nuclear atypia and stromal desmoplasia, if present, are exclusive of the diagnosis.
- *Prognosis.* Benign tumours.

Clear Cell Borderline Tumour

- *Definition.* A clear cell borderline tumour (CCBT) is an adenofibromatous clear cell tumour with glandular crowding and low grade nuclear atypia, but no stromal invasion. Pure CCBTs account for <1% of all ovarian borderline tumours and in most of the cases are components of clear cell carcinoma.
- *Clinical findings.* Symptoms of a pelvic mass, including an incidental finding. Most of the patients are postmenopausal. Clear cell adenofibroma and CCBT are typically present in combination and are sometimes associated with endometriosis. CCBTs that accompany clear cell carcinoma show genetic changes similar to those of the carcinomatous component, including PIK3CA and ARID1A abnormalities.
- *Gross appearance.* CCBTs are solid or predominantly solid, with small to large cysts with a firm white or tan cut surface. The mean size is 6 cm.
- *Microscopic appearance.* Variably sized glands embedded in a fibromatous stroma, with low cuboidal or flat cells, with enlarged nuclei and clear or eosinophilic cytoplasm. The glands are more irregular and crowded, and less uniform in size, than in adenofibroma. Minimal nuclear stratification is permitted, but densely aggregated glands and papillary or tubulocystic architecture are absent by definition.
- *Prognosis.* No reported recurrences.

Clear Cell Carcinoma of the Ovary

- *Definition.* A malignant epithelial tumor composed of clear, eosinophilic or hobnail cells with tubulocystic, papillary and solid growth. Ovary or any extraovarian site with endometriosis.
- *Clinical features.* The mean patient age is 56 years old. Patients present with symptoms related to a pelvic mass, or the mass may be an incidental finding. CCC is the ovarian carcinoma, most commonly related to paraneoplastic hypercalcaemia and venous thromboembolism.

Increased risk associated with:

- Endometriosis, including endometriotic cysts (50-74%).
- Less frequently, Lynch syndrome and:
  - Mismatch repair (MMR) deficiency in 6-43.75% of cases.
  - Younger patients.

- 10% develop endometriosis associated carcinomas, including clear cell carcinoma.

- Family history of ovarian cancer in a first degree relative.
- Decreased risk associated with:
  - Late menarche (>15 years), early menopause (<40 years), tubal ligation, parity, hysterectomy, smoking, oral contraceptives.
- Expression of the genetic susceptibility locus (HNF1β) via epigenetic mechanisms.

Gross appearance. Usually unilateral and:

- Mean size 13 cm (range 0.8-35 cm).
- Variable appearance on cut surface.
- Mainly cystic, with fleshy nodules protruding into the cyst lumen.
- Solid and cystic (spongy appearance due to small cysts).
- Solid (may be arising from clear cell adenofibroma or borderline clear cell tumor).
- Cyst may contain chocolate brown fluid.
- Pale yellow to brown appearance.
- Necrosis or hemorrhage.
- Ovarian surface involvement in 11% of cases.

- *Microscopic appearance.* Three classic growth patterns (papillary, tubulocystic, solid), frequently admixed, but one pattern may predominate. The tubulocystic pattern exhibits tubules and cysts, lined by a single layer of hobnail or cuboidal cells, sometimes with dense eosinophilic secretions. The papillary pattern comprises simple, non-branching papillae; some hierarchical branching is permitted. Cells are cuboidal and/or hobnail (but not columnar), arranged in a single layer with only minimal stratification. The solid pattern exhibits sheets of polyhedral cells separated by delicate septa. The cytoplasm ranges from clear to eosinophilic. Nuclei are large and monomorphic, with rounded to angulated contours, hyperchromasia, prominent nucleoli and (rarely) intranuclear pseudo-inclusions. Hyaline and psammoma bodies are infrequent.

CCCs are typically positive for PAX8, Napsin A, and HNF 1β, and negative for WT1, ER and PR. WT1, Napsin A and ER together are recommended for distinction from high-grade serous carcinoma and Napsin A and PR for distinction from endometrioid carcinoma.

- *Prognosis.* Stage is the most important prognostic factor. Most CCCs are limited to the ovary (FIGO Stage I) with 72-74% confined to the pelvis (Stage I-II). The 5-year survival rates are 87%, 70% and 24% respectively, for Stages IA/IB, IC/II and III/IV ovarian cancers. A better prognosis than high grade serous carcinoma when confined to the pelvis but a worse prognosis if advanced stage except for some MMR deficient tumors. Grading is not applicable.

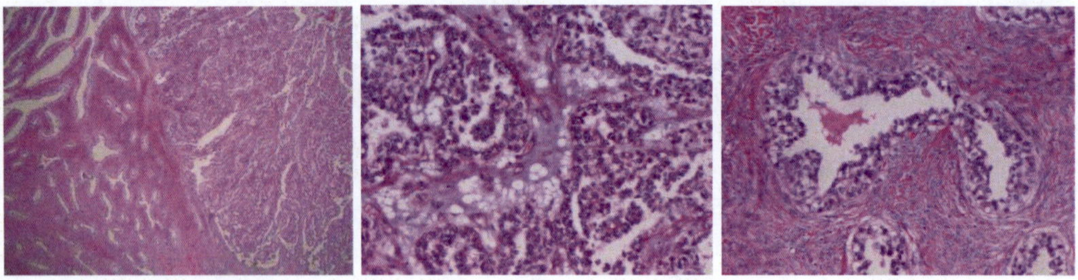

(a) (b) (c)

Figure 16a, b, c. H&E. Clear cell carcinoma of the ovary (clear cell borderline tumour on the left of (a)).

Seromucinous Cystadenoma and Adenofibroma

- *Definition.* Seromucinous cystadenoma is a benign cystic neoplasm composed of glands and cysts lined by an admixture of bland Mullerian-type epithelia. Seromucinous adenofibroma has a prominent fibromatous component. Sometimes associated with endometriosis or an endometriotic cyst.
- *Clinical findings.* Symptoms related to a pelvic mass, or an incidental finding. Mean age 35 years old.
- *Gross appearance.* Adenofibromas are predominantly solid, with a dense fibrous cut surface. They may form a nodule in the wall of an endometriotic cyst. Cystadenomas are usually unilocular, but sometimes there are multilocular.
- *Histopathology.* Adenofibromas are characterized by a prominent fibromatous stroma with glands lined by an admixture of cytologically bland Mullerian-type epithelia in varying proportions, including ciliated, endocervical-type mucinous, and endometrioid (which may have a squamous and/or mucinous differentiation). Mucinous, serous, endometrioid and squamous epithelium. Cystadenomas are composed of cysts lined by a mixture of benign, Mullerian-type epithelia.
- *Prognosis and prediction.* Benign tumours.

Seromucinous Borderline Tumour

- *Definition.* Seromucinous borderline tumour is an architecturally complex papillary neoplasm composed of an admixture of Mullerian-type epithelia, lacking confluent or destructive invasion. They architecturally resemble serous borderline tumors but are much more frequently associated with endometriosis.
- *Clinical findings.* Tumours present over a wide age range (mean age: 34-39 years). Symptoms related to a pelvic mass, or an incidental finding.
- *Epidemiology.* Seromucinous borderline tumours are uncommon ovarian neoplasms. A significant number of patients have associated endometriosis, most commonly an endometriotic cyst (31-35%).

- *Gross appearance.* Seromucinous borderline tumours have a smooth outer surface, with a mean tumour size of 9cm. 30% are bilateral. The tumours comprise a unilocular cyst with friable papillary excrescences in the inner cyst lining.
- *Microscopic appearance.* Seromucinous borderline tumours are composed of papillae exhibiting a hierarchical branching. The epithelium lining the papillae is cytologically bland, stratified and often tufted. It represents an admixture of Mullerian epithelia types in varying proportions, including endometrioid, ciliated, hobnail, clear and eosinophilic cells. Sometimes, mucinous differentiation greatly predominates. Microinvasion has been described. A portion of the cystic lining may exhibit features of an endometriotic cyst.
- *Prognosis.* Excellent.

Seromucinous Carcinoma

Seromucinous carcinoma was included in the previous classification and was defined as a carcinoma composed predominantly of serous and endocervical-type mucinous epithelium, often with foci containing clear cells and areas of endometrioid and squamous differentiation. It has been removed from this classification because this is a poorly reproducible diagnosis and there is significant overlap with other tumour types, especially endometrioid carcinoma. Immunohistochemical and molecular studies have also suggested that most cases represent unusual morphological patterns of endometrioid carcinoma, therefore, seromucinous carcinoma is now considered a subtype of endometrioid carcinoma.

Brenner Tumour

- *Definition.* Tumor composed of transitional/urothelial-like epithelium, typically embedded in fibromatous stroma.

  Benign, borderline and malignant variants are recognized, based on the growth pattern and cytological features of the epithelial cells.

  These tumours occur in the ovary. Extraovarian Brenner tumours have also been reported. Cell of origin of Brenner tumors is controversial; they may arise from Walthard nests, which are nests of metaplastic transitional epithelium in paratubal tissue.
- *Clinical findings.* Brenner tumors are an incidental finding in an ovary removed for other reasons. These are usually unilateral but are occasionally bilateral. Occasionally, Brenner tumours with functioning stoma are associated with endocrine features. Brenner tumours account for approximately 5% of benign ovarian epithelial tumours. Brenner tumors are most common in the fifth and sixth decades but can occur across a wide age range.
- *Gross appearance.* Benign Brenner tumor:
  - Small (usually < 2 cm), circumscribed, fibrous tumor with a firm rubbery cut surface.
  - Calcifications may be present.

One quarter of Brenner tumours are associated with other tumour types, predominantly of the mucinous type.

Histopathology. Benign:

- Smooth contoured nests of bland transitional epithelium within fibromatous stroma.
- Transitional cells have uniform oval nuclei and may have a longitudinal nuclear groove.
- There may be mucinous epithelium at the center of the nests, with microcyst formation.
- Ciliated or nondescript glandular epithelium may be present; a coexistent mucinous cystadenoma is present in 10% of cases.
- Calcification is common.

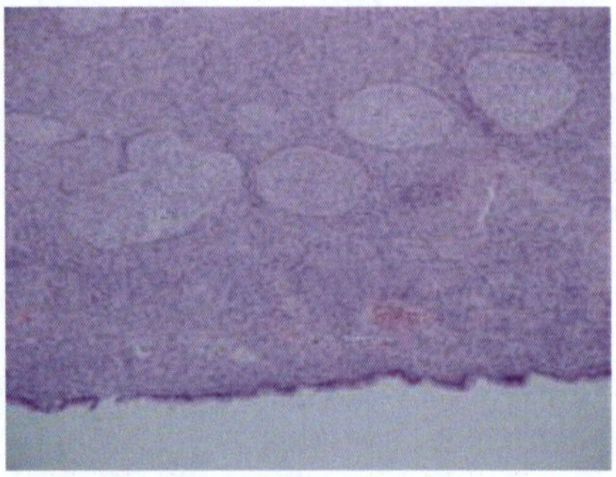

Figure 17. H&E. Mucinous cystadenoma with Brenner tumour.

- *Immunohistochemistry.* Brenner tumours express GATA3, CK7, p63, S100p, AR, uroplakin, and thrombomodulin, but they do not express (or only focally express) CK20. PAX8, ER and PR, which are typically negative.
- *Prognosis.* Benign tumours.

Borderline Brenner Tumour

- *Definition.* A borderline Brenner tumour is a tumour displaying papillary architecture with papillae covered by multilayered transitional epithelium and lacking stromal invasion. Tumours are unilateral and confined to the ovary. There is variable but usually low grade cytological atypia. They are presumed to arise from benign Brenner tumours.
- *Clinical findings.* Pelvic mass. A very uncommon tumour. Patients are usually >50 years old.
- *Gross appearance.* Unlike benign Brenner tumours, borderline Brenner tumours are typically large (usually > 10cm) and cystic. Smooth surface, with fleshy, polypoid masses projecting into cystic cavity(s). Rarely is the tumour is completely solid.
- *Microscopic appearance.* The tumours resemble low-grade papillary urothelial neoplasms of the urothelial tract. Papillary architecture with papillae covered by multilayered transitional epithelium. There is variable cytological atypia, usually low

grade but occasionally moderate or marked cytological atypia may be present. Mucinous or squamous metaplasia is often found. A benign Brenner tumor component is often present.

- *Immunohistochemistry.* Immunohistochemistry is usually positive for p63 and GATA3 and negative for ER, PR and WT1. P53 shows a wild type immunoreactive pattern, and p16 can show loss of staining.
- *Prognosis.* Borderline Brenner tumor has a benign course, although local recurrence has rarely been reported.

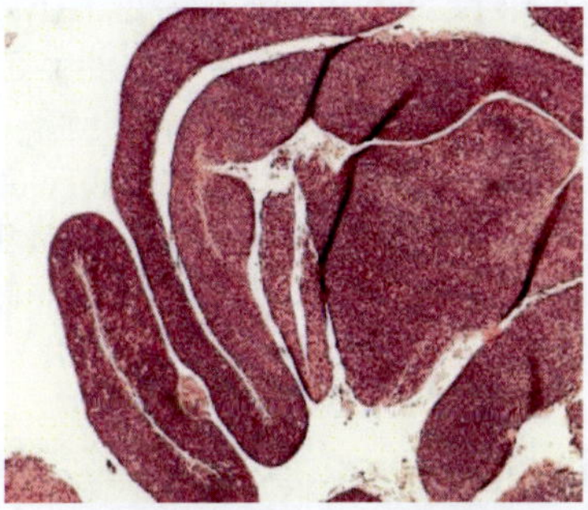

Figure 18. H&E. Borderline Brenner tumour. The tumour shows an endophytic, ribbon-like growth pattern, lined by transitional-type epithelium.

Malignant Brenner Tumour

- *Definition.* Stromal invasion by carcinoma with transitional cell features, associated with a benign or borderline Brenner tumor.
- *Clinical findings.* Patients present with an abdominal mass or pain. Some may have abnormal vaginal bleeding. Tumours are unilateral (>80%) and occasionally bilateral. They account for <5% of all Brenner tumours and occur in women aged >50 years.
- *Pathogenesis.* Malignant Brenner tumours arise from benign and borderline Brenner tumours. PIK3CA mutations and MDM2 amplification have been reported.
- *Gross appearance.* Smooth surface, larger (usually > 10 cm) with fleshy, polypoid masses projecting into cystic cavity(s).

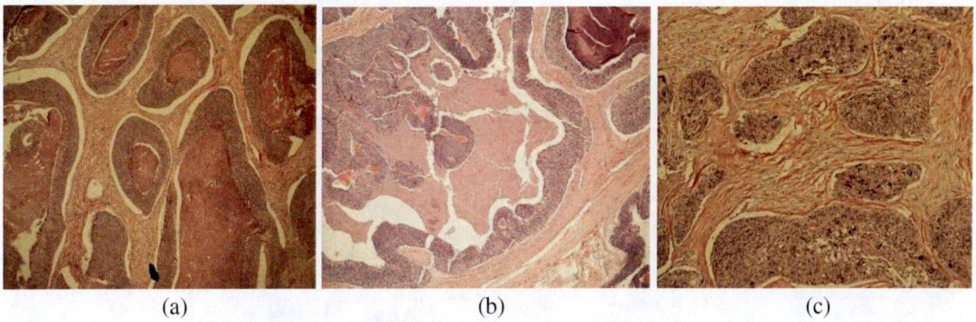

(a) (b) (c)

Figure 19a, b, c. H&E. Malignant Brenner tumour. Confluent sheets of tumour with cystic papillary and solid growth, lined by multilayered epithelium which resembles invasive urothelial carcinoma with areas of squamous differentiation (in (c)).

- *Microscopic appearance.* Stromal invasion by carcinoma with transitional cell features, with irregular nests of cells and single cells in an infiltrative pattern.
  - Squamous or mucinous differentiation may be present.
  - Benign or borderline Brenner tumor component is present.
  - Mucinous glandular elements and (more rarely) mucinous adenocarcinoma coexist within the Brenner component. The absence of a benign or borderline Brenner component should raise the possibility of high-grade serous or endometrioid carcinoma with transitional cell-like differentiation.
- *Immunohistochemistry.* These tumours are usually negative for WT1, negative or weakly positive for ER and PR, and focally positive for p16, showing a wild pattern for TP53. p63 was positive in all Brenner tumours.
- *Prognosis.* Most tumours are confined to the ovary at diagnosis. Patients with Stage I tumours have disease-specific 5-year survival rate of 94.5% and 51.3% in patients with extraovarian spread (Stages II, III, IV).

Mesonephric-Like Adenocarcinoma

- *Definition.* A carcinoma displaying mesonephric differentiation.
- *Clinical findings.* Pelvic or abdominal pain. Most cases are Stage I. The majority of tumours occur in postmenopausal women.
- *Pathogenesis.* The pathogenesis remains unclear. Some tumours are thought to arise from mesonephric remnants. Others may arise from Mullerian carcinomas that exhibit secondary mesonephric differentiation. The latter is supported by the association of mesonephric-like carcinomas with endometriosis, cystadenomas, adenofibromas, borderline tumours and low-grade serous carcinomas.
- *Gross appearance.* The tumours are usually unilateral, with variable size (4-32 cm). The cut surface is solid or mixed solid and cystic.
- *Microscopic appearance.* The histological features are identical to those of mesonephric carcinomas occurring at other sites in the female genital tract, including tubular, glandular (pseudoendometrioid), ductal, papillary and solid patterns. Eosinophilic colloid-like material can be present within the lumen. No association with mesonephric remnants has been described. Associated endometriosis is common.
- *Prognosis*. Unknown.

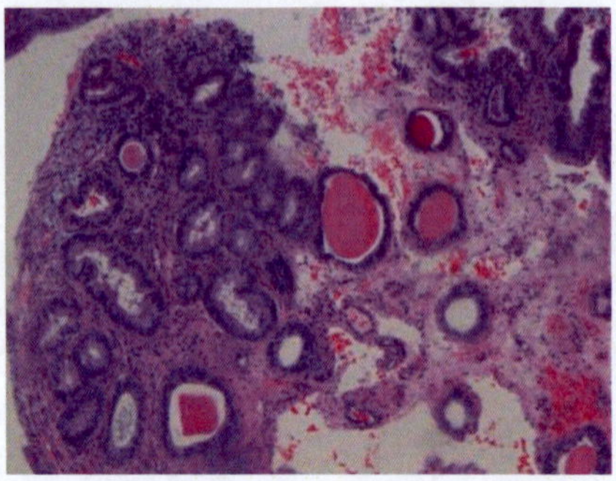

Figure 20. H&E. Mesonephric-like adenocarcinoma.

Undifferentiated and Dedifferentiated Carcinomas of the Ovary

- *Definition.* Undifferentiated carcinoma is a malignant epithelial tumour lacking overt evidence of a specific line of differentiation. Dedifferentiated carcinoma is composed of an undifferentiated carcinoma and a differentiated component.
- *Clinical findings.* Tumours are usually high-stage at presentation. These are rare tumours, representing approximately 0.5% of ovarian carcinomas. Patients are diagnosed at a median age of 53 years (range: 21-82 years).
- *Pathogenesis.* Association with low-grade endometrioid carcinoma suggests progression from endometrioid carcinoma in a subset of tumours.
- *Gross appearance.* The tumours are typically large solid masses with extensive necrosis.
- *Microscopic appearance.* The morphological characteristics are similar to those observed in undifferentiated/dedifferentiated endometrial carcinomas. At least focal sheet-like growth pattern with lack of glandular or papillary differentiation, frequently associated with geographical necrosis. The mitotic activity is high. In dedifferentiated carcinomas, the two components can vary in proportion and the interphase between the two components can be abrupt, imparting a biphasic appearance. The differentiated component can be either endometrioid carcinoma (commonly) or serous carcinoma (rarely).

  Undifferentiated areas show only focal EMA, pankeratin and CK18 staining. PAX8 is either focally positive or completely negative. Tumour cells are usually negative for ER, PR and e-cadherin. Loss of SMARCA4 (BRG1), SMARCA2 (BRM), SMARCB1 (INI1) or ARID1A and DNA mismatch repair abnormalities are common, similar to their endometrial counterparts. p53 usually exhibits wild-type immunoreactivity.
- *Prognosis.* These are highly aggressive neoplasms. Patients, typically present with advanced-stage disease, usually with bulky, pelvic and para-aortic lymph node metastases. The median survival time is 9 months.

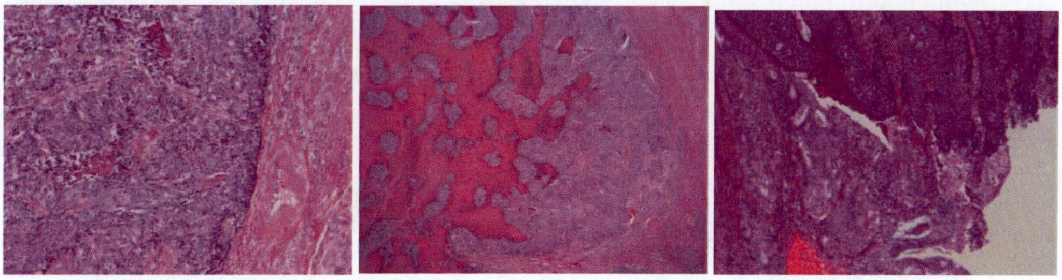

(a) (b) (c)

Figure 21a, b, c. H&E. Ovarian undifferentiated/dedifferentiated carcinoma. (a) The carcinoma consists of sheets of dyscohesive cells that are small to intermediate in size with scant cytoplasm. (b) Extensive geographic necrosis. (c) Dedifferentiated carcinoma is composed of an undifferentiated carcinoma component (upper half) and a differentiated component (lower half). The interphase between the two components is abrupt, imparting a biphasic appearance. The differentiated component is endometrioid carcinoma.

Carcinosarcoma of the Ovary

- *Definition.* Carcinosarcoma is a biphasic neoplasm composed of malignant epithelial and sarcomatous components. They are often high-stage at the time of diagnosis. They account for approximately 2% of all ovarian malignancies. Mostly in postmenopausal, low parity women, with peak incidence in the sixth decade of life.
- *Clinical findings.* Abdominal mass, pain, vaginal bleeding. Risk factors include advanced age, excess estrogen exposure, nulliparity, prior pelvic irradiation, tamoxifen use.
- *Gross appearance.* The tumour is characteristically large (mean size: 14cm) and predominantly solid, with frequent cystic degeneration and extensive haemorrhage and necrosis.
- *Microscopic appearance.* High grade malignant epithelial and sarcomatous elements. The two components are distinct but are typically intermingled with one another. One or the other may predominate. Sarcomatous elements can be homologous (non-specific malignant stroma) or heterologous (malignant elements not normally found, particularly cartilage). The carcinomatous component is most often HGSC, but other histological types may occur.
- *Prognosis.* Very poor prognosis; stage is best predictor and most patients present at an advanced stage. The median survival time is <24 months and the 5-year survival rate is 15-30%, which compares unfavourably with those of HGSC. Tumours with an epithelial component of HGSC may exhibit BRCA1 or BRCA2 mutations, with potential therapeutic impact.

Mixed Carcinoma of the Ovary

- *Definition.* Mixed carcinoma of the ovary is an ovarian carcinoma composed of two or more different histological types.
- *Clinical findings.* Patients usually present with symptoms related to an ovarian mass. Mixed ovarian carcinomas are rare (<1% of ovarian carcinomas). Most mixed carcinomas are composed of histological types that are associated with endometriosis.
- *Gross appearance.* The macroscopic appearance is related to the histological types present.
- *Microscopic appearance.* At least two histological types of any percentage must be clearly recognizable on H&E stained sections. The different histological components should be confirmed by ancillary testing when possible. Mixed carcinomas should be differentiated from pure histological types with ambiguous and/or heterogeneous histomorphology and from collision tumours, which do not share molecular alterations. The most common mixed tumour is endometrioid and clear cell. A combination of Napsin A (expressed in the clear cell component) and PR (expressed in the endometrioid component) helps to discriminate between the two components. Dedifferentiated carcinoma is a special type of mixed carcinoma. Mixed carcinomas with neuroendocrine carcinomas have also been described.
- *Prognosis.* Depends on the histological types present.

References

Histological classification of mucinous ovarian tumors: inter-observer reproducibility, clinical relevance, and role of genetic biomarkers, Catherine Genestie, Aurelie Auguste, Miriam Al Battal, et al. Virchows Archiv, *European Journal of Pathology* (2021) 478:885-891.

Ovarian Epithelial Tumours: Morphologic Types, New Developments and Pathogenesis W Glenn McCluggage, Royal Group of Hospitals, Belfast.

WHO Classification of Tumours Editorial Board. Female Genital Tumours. Lyon (France): *International Agency for Research on Cancer*; 2020. (WHO Classification of tumours series, 5th ed.; vol. 4). Available from: https://tumourclassification.iarc.who.int/.

Chapter 10

Pathology of Non-epithelial Ovarian Tumors

Christos Iavazzo[1,*], MD, PhD
Alexandros Fotiou[1], MD
John Spiliotis[2], MD, PhD
and Agathi Kondi-Pafiti[3], MD, PhD
[1]Department of Gynecologic Oncology, Metaxa Memorial Cancer Hospital, Piraeus, Greece
[2]Department of Surgical Oncology and HIPEC, European Interbalkan Medical Center, Thessaloniki, Greece
[3]Department of Pathology, Aretaieion Hospital, University of Athens, School of Medicine, Athens, Greece

Introduction

The histologic classification of primary ovarian tumors is based on the histogenesis from the various ovarian tissue components. Most ovarian tumors are derived from ovarian surface (coelomic) epithelium. Less common tumors are derived from primitive germ cells, specialized sex cords and gonadal stroma, non specific ovarian mesenchyme or are metastatic mainly from extragenital sites such as breast or gastrointestinal tract, or from genital tract primaries.

The classification of ovarian tumors, based on the current World Health Organization proposed Classification of Ovarian tumors (2003) is presented in Table 1.

For the purpose of this chapter a simplified classification will be provided, omitting the very rare and unclassified ovarian non-epithelial tumors.

According to Scully, most human ovarian tumors can be classified into one of several categories based on presumed histogenesis and direction of differentiation. Separate categories are reserved for neoplasms composed of cells of several origins and many ovarian tumors present similarities with corresponding tumors of the testis, derived from the non-epithelial components of the gonads (Figure 1).

* Corresponding Author's Email: christosiavazzo@hotmail.com.

In: Ovarian Cancer
Editors: Christos Iavazzo, Alexandros Fotiou and John Spiliotis
ISBN: 979-8-88697-633-5

Table 1. Classification of Ovarian tumors (2003)

Derivation	Type of tumor
A. Surface epithelial origin (80-85%)	
	I. Common epithelial tumors; benign, borderline, malignant
	Serous
	Mucinous
	Endometrioid
	Clear cell
	Transitional (Brenner) and Squamous cell (Epidermoid)
	II. Mixed epithelial tumors III. Undifferentiated carcinoma
B. Germ cell origin (10-15%)	
	I. Teratoma
	1. Immature 2. Mature
	Solid
	Cystic (Dermoid)
	3. Monodermal Struma ovarii Carcinoid Neuroectodermal, various forms
	4. Mixed forms
	II. Dysgerminoma
	III. Yolk sac (Endodermal sinus) tumor
	IV. Embryonal carcinoma
	V. Choriocarcinoma
	VI. Polyembryoma
	VII. Tumors composed of germ cells and sex cord-stromal derivatives Gonadoblastoma
C. Sex Cord -Stromal origin (5-10%)	
	I. Granulosa-theca cells
	1. Granulosa cell tumors Adult-Juvenile
	2. Theca cell
	Thecoma-Fibroma-Variants-
	II. Sertoli-Stromal cell tumors, Mixed and Unclassified Forms
	Sertoli Cell tumor Sertoli-Leydig cell tumor
	III. Gynandroblastoma IV. Sex cord tumor with annular tubules
	V. Steroid Cell tumor
	Stromal Luteoma Steroid cell tumor Leydig cell tumor Hilus cell tumor
	VI. Ovarian tumors with functioning stroma
D. Non-specific miscellaneous primary ovarian tumors (<1%)	I. Non specific mesenchymal origin
	I. Fibroma, hemangioma, leiomyoma, lipoma et al. and malignant forms;
	II. Small cell carcinomas, neuroendocrine carcinomas, other forms III. Other primary tumors of uncertain histogenesis
Secondary Neoplasms (5-10%)	I. Extragenital (stomach, GI tract, breast other primeries) II. From genital tract primaries

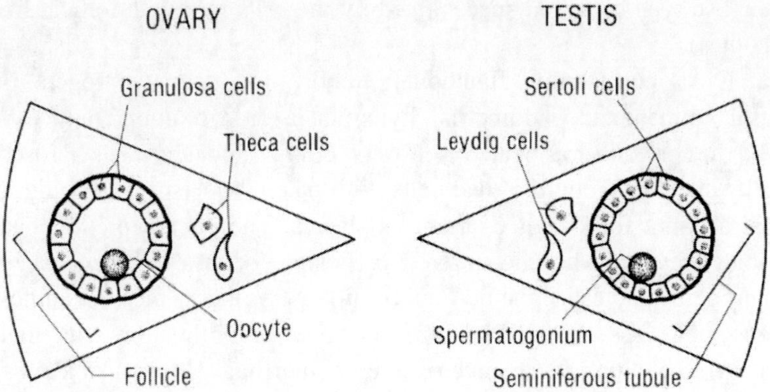

Figure 1. Schematic representation of the main non-epithelial components of the gonads.

In a brief introduction, the main points of the tumors discussed in this chapter are presented. Of special interest for Gynecological Oncology is the group of germ cell tumors, because of their prevalence to the pediatric population and young adults. These tumors are classified according to their origin from the undifferentiated germ cells (dysgerminomas, embryonal carcinomas) or the differentiated germ cells to embryonic (teratomas) or the extra embryonic tissues (yolk sac tumors).

In this group, teratomas are the most common tumors and are further divided into benign cystic teratomas (dermoid cysts), immature, and monodermal teratomas (Struma ovarii composed entirely of thyroid tissue and Carcinoid). Immature teratomas are the most common malignant germ cell tumors and are mostly solid tumors with necrosis and hemorrhage. Histological examination shows various immature tissues are normally observed in embryonal tissues, with the predominance of immature neural tubules or neural elements.

Dysgerminoma is the ovarian counterpart of the testicular seminoma, accounting for 2% of all ovarian malignancies. It is the most common malignant germ cell tumor in the younger population and primarily affects young girls in the second and third decade of life. It is remarkable that this is the most frequently encountered ovarian malignancy in pregnancy, characterized by an excellent prognosis after radiotherapy. Dysgerminomas is usually a solid, ovulated mass with foci of hemorrhage, where microscopically, sheets of monotonous rounded cells with pale cytoplasm and central nuclei are found, divided by septa infiltrated by lymphocytes.

Endodermal sinus tumor (yolk sac carcinoma) is a highly malignant and clinically aggressive neoplasm which is most frequently detected in children and young females. It accounts for 20% of malignant germ cell tumors and is usually fatal within 2 years of diagnosis. Schiller-Duval bodies are characteristic of the tumor.

The group of Sex Cord-Stromal tumors is of special interest, because this is the only group of ovarian tumors hormonally active. The most common types are the granulosa-cell tumors, thecomas, fibromas and the group of Sertoli-Leydig cell tumors.

Granulosa-cell tumors are hormonally active tumors and the most common ovarian neoplasm with estrogenic action. The adult form occurs mainly in postmenopausal women, associated with endometrial hyperplasia and carcinoma, while the juvenile type occurs in the first two decades causing precocious sexual development. Granulosa-cell tumor is usually unilaterally solid and yellowish with microcystic areas or, characterised microscopically by sheets of granulosa type cells and spaces lined by the cells to give a follicle-like appearance (Call-Exner bodies).

Thecoma is a hormonally functional tumor, producing estrogen. It occurs in postmenopausal women and endometrial hyperplasia or carcinoma may develop. It is a unilateral solid tumor with variegated yellow - orange appearance. Microscopically, it is characterized by sheets of round to oval cells with pale cytoplasm containing lipids. Sertoli-Leydig tumors account for 1% of ovarian neoplasms. They occur predominantly in young women although they may be encountered in postmenopausal women as well. They are commonly androgenic and cause the de-feminization of women which is manifested by breast atrophy, amenorrhea, loss of hair and hip fat and even virilization with male-type facial hirsutism. They are solid tumors characterized by hemorrhage. Microscopically, tubules lined by Sertoli-like cells and sheets of Leydig cells are identified.

Of special interest is a small group of ovarian neoplasms with hormonal activity, mostly arising from luteinized ovarian stroma. These lesions comprise a group distinct from the hormone- producing sex cord-stromal tumors.

Rarely are other tumors observed in the ovary. Most are of uncertain histogenesis or resembling common mesenchymal tumors of soft tissues.

About 5-10% of malignant ovarian tumors are secondary. The most common primary site is the breast followed by the large intestine, stomach, and other extra genital and genital tract organs. The term Krukenberg tumor is applied to the uniform enlargement of the ovaries (usually bilaterally) to kidney-shaped tumors. Microscopically, a diffuse infiltration of the ovarian stroma by metastatic signet-ring, mucus containing cells is the hallmark of these tumors. The most common primary site is the stomach followed by other GI tract tumors.

Colon cancers, including primaries from appendix, produce large mucinous neoplasms similar to primary ovarian cystic neoplasms. These group of ovarian secondary tumors are of special interest because many are diagnosed as ovarian primaries and their true nature goes undetected for a long time.

We are going to focus on the most common entities of non epithelial ovarian tumors.

Germ Cell Tumors

Ovarian Teratomas

The term teratoma is derived from the Greek word "teras" which means monster. Teratomas were first described 300 years ago. People believed them to be embryonic structures or aborted embryos and one of the greatest concerns at that time was whether these structures should be baptized or not.

Teratomas account for 10% of all ovarian neoplasms from childhood to old age and they are the most frequent ovarian tumors of childhood accounting for about 25% of all cases. Teratomas represent a complex group of germ-cell tumors of the ovary resembling derivatives of the embryonic layers (ecto-meso-endoderm) or from one of the layers, except mesoderm (monodermal). They usually develop in young women of reproductive age. *Benign or mature cystic* teratomas, also known as *dermoid cysts,* are composed of mature tissues, which can contain elements of all three germ cell layers. Ectodermal elements usually predominate. All tissue elements encountered in benign teratomas represent mature and easily recognised tissues.

Immature teratomas of the ovary are less common and more aggressive germ cell tumors of the ovary. *Monodermal Teratomas* are composed of one type of tissue, although there may be slight traces of other tissue found within the tumor itself. A monodermal teratoma may be malignant or benign and can occur in girls as well as adult women.

Pathogenesis of Teratomas

Cytogenetic techniques support the parthenogenetic theory, which suggests an origin from the primordial germ cells after the first meiotic division. The anatomic distribution of the tumors along lines of migration of the primordial germ cells from the yolk sac to the primitive gonads supports this theory. The absence of cytogenetic abnormalities (including isochromosome 12p {i(12p)} in mature teratomas, suggests that these tumors might be analogous to prepubertal testicular teratomas. Moreover, the Patched/Hedgehog and PI3K/Akt pathways, as well as cyclin D protein are implicated in the pathogenesis. Cycloxygenase-2 is associated with tumor growth and progression in teratomas with squamous cell malignant transformation, as opposed to mature benign teratomas and teratomas associated with adenocarcinomas.

Clinical Findings

Teratomas are often discovered incidentally at routine pelvic examination. They grow slowly and cause minimal symptoms until becoming large enough to present with abdominal enlargement, discomfort, pressure on adjacent organs, and pain. They have been reported to have a right ovary predisposition. However, they are bilateral in 12-20% of cases, and frequently there is more than one in an ovary. Many retrospective studies show that mature teratomas occur most frequently in younger women during their reproductive years (mean age of 35.4 years). The mean size of a mature cystic teratoma was 4-6 cm, in contrast to cases in which malignancy coexisted where 78.7% of tumors were larger than 10 cm. Teratomas may be complicated with torsion (16%), rupture (1-4%), malignant transformation (2%), infection (1%) and autoimmune hemolytic anemia (<1%). Due to the weight of the tumor contents, the infundibulo-pelvic ligament might be stretched. This is the reason why this tumor has greater mobility within the abdomen and may "migrate" from one abdominal area to another, especially if it has a long pedicle. For this reason, they are also prone to torsion, presenting with symptoms of acute abdomen. The leakage of the tumor contents into the peritoneal cavity may cause chemical peritonitis with giant cell granulomas formation caused by keratin and sebum. In these cases, the differential diagnosis includes tuberculosis or peritoneal cancer. Rarely, gliomatosis peritonei after tumor rupture are reported with the characteristic neuroglial elements being disseminated in the peritoneal cavity. In some cases development of sebaceous gland adenoma and development of breast tissue with hyperplasia and secretory activity is reported.

Malignant transformation of mature teratomas occurs in approximately 2% of cases. The frequency of this type of transformation is age- related and is most common in the fifth and sixth decades of life. The malignant changes might involve one, two or three germ layers and are more common in solid rather than cystic teratomas. Squamous cell carcinoma is the most commonly associated malignancy. In such cases, malignant teratomas could present with abdominal distention, bloating or pain. Other rare malignant tumors that may originate from mature teratomas are adenocarcinomas, malignant melanomas, transitional cell carcinomas, thyroid adenocarcinomas and sarcomatous changes.

There is no pathognomonic diagnostic criterion to diagnose immature teratomas, although the presence of a larger, predominantly solid tumor and increased serum α-FP levels may be associated with these tumors. In immature teratomas, tumor grading is based on the amount of immature tissue present. The determination of the amount of undifferentiated neural tissue in immature teratomas is of prognostic importance. A grade 1 tumor is one in which less than one low-power microscopic field (LPF) contains immature neural elements. A grade 2 tumor has one to three LPFs with immature elements. A grade 3 tumor has more than three LPFs with these elements. Immature teratomas are frequently unilateral, associated with ascites, and generally curable if the diagnosis is made at an early stage.

Apart from corpora lutea, the majority of ovarian masses discovered during pregnancy are benign dermoid cysts which account for 20–40% of ovarian neoplasms during this period. Pregnancy complicated by an immature teratoma is rare, with a reported incidence of 0.07%. After the discovery of a teratoma during pregnancy, the obstetrician should weigh the risks of surgery and anesthesia versus the risks of a persistent adnexal mass which include rupture, torsion, as well as preterm labor or obstruction of labor. Hess et al. in a study of 54 patients showed that pregnant women who underwent elective removal of an adnexal mass had less morbidity than those who underwent emergency laparotomy for a symptomatic mass in an emergency setting. So it is recommended that pregnant women with persistent adnexal masses undergo elective extirpation of the mass in the second trimester of pregnancy.

Imaging Studies

A teratoma could be diagnosed by pelvic radiography as the presence of abortive teeth and osseous structures is characteristic. The diagnosis of an ovarian dermoid cyst can often be made with ultrasound. The most characteristic ultrasound finding is a Rokitansky nodule (a densely echogenic tubercle projecting in the cystic lumen). An echogenic mass demonstrating sebaceous material or multiple thin echogenic bands demonstrating hair are other con findings. The gross appearance of teratomas with malignant transformation is similar to the benign teratomas but they tend to present solid consistency. Usually this solid component tends to extend transmurally with direct invasion of the pouch of Douglas, uterus and vagina. It is described that the findings of a solid mass larger than 5 cm in diameter with an irregular border forming an obtuse angle with the inner wall of cyst is suspect for malignant transformation. The CT appearance of a mature teratoma is typically characterized by negative fat attenuation within a cyst with, or without, calcification within the wall. Teeth, and other calcified structures, have been reported in 56% of patients. In uncertain cases, a MRI will increase diagnostic accuracy because of high sensitivity for fat content. Fat shows high signal intensity in T1-weight images, but signal drop on fat-saturated T1-weighted images. Immature teratomas appearance at CT and MRI is characterized by a large irregular solid component containing coarse calcifications and small foci of fat with co 3*Q143ncomitant hemorrhage.

Management

Usually, mature cystic teratomas are characterized by slow growth (1.8 mm per year), and for this reason a non-surgical management of the smaller (<6 cm) lesions is proposed. Radical surgical treatment is not necessary for this type of tumor because conservative surgery usually brings full recovery. Cystectomy with preservation of normal ovarian tissue and close inspection of the contralateral ovary is proposed. Laparoscopic surgery has been used increasingly the last years for the treatment of mature teratomas. However, gynaecologists should keep in mind the possibility of a malignant transformation of a mature teratoma when using laparoscopy to treat such an ovarian mass in order to avoid rupture and possible spillage.

In premenopausal women unilateral oophorectomy and surgical staging may be performed. In postmenopausal women, a total abdominal hysterectomy and bilateral salpingo-oophorectomy is suggested.

The combination of patient's age (above 40 years) with elevated serum SCC antigen level (>2.5 ng/ml) has been considered a useful marker for the diagnosis of malignant transformation. CA 125 does not have specific value as a diagnostic tool. In case of teratomas complicated with malignant change, especially in advanced stage cases, optimal debulking is proposed. Omentectomy does not effect overall survival, whereas lymphadenectomy improves the chances of survival in patients with advanced stages. At present, the optimal adjuvant therapy is not clarified.

For patients with Stage Ia, grade 1 immature teratomas, no adjuvant therapy is required, while teratomas of greater than Stage Ia, grades 2 or 3, adjuvant chemotherapy should be used. Combined concurrent chemo- and radiotherapy is used including platine agents and paclitaxel. 5-fluorouracil/leucovorin infusion has also been used. The use of a combination chemotherapy with bleomycin, etoposide and cisplatin after surgery has dramatically improved the prognosis of women with immature teratomas. In a recent systematic review, it has been shown that postoperative radiotherapy does not have any benefit and might adversely affect survival. It is proposed that radiotherapy should be reserved for patients with localized persistent disease after chemotherapy.

Pathology

Benign mature teratomas are divided into cystic and solid types. Both usually contain mature, well-differentiated adult-type tissues. The cystic type (dermoid cysts) consists mainly of skin and skin appendages, with few heterotopic tissues being present. The solid types arise from totipotential germ cells and may therefore contain elements of heterotopic tissue of any or all three germ layers, although ectodermal structures usually predominate.

Macroscopically, they are rounded tumors, tending to be somewhat flattened after surgical excision. They are usually of moderate size, but rarely grow to great sizes and a case is reported of a teratomas that that weighted 7000 grams.

The external surface of the cystic teratomas is smooth with a whitish wall. Hard areas of bone consistency, may be present within the tumor which is generally semifluid in consistency. Cystic tyeratomas are filled with sebaceous material containing various amounts of hair, usually diffusely attached to the cyst wall or inserted into one or more plaque-like elevations containing a combination of heterotopic tissue such as teeth. This particular area is designated as the dermoid nipple. Within these areas, fully developed cysts and crypts are often present. Occasionally, the cyst wall contents might become inspissated, forming "butter balls" which are yellow, rounded lumps. Benign solid teratomas appear smooth and firm on palpation. Solid areas predominate while cartilage and osseous tissue may be seen.

Beneath the squamous epithelial lining, dermal appendages such as sebaceous glands, hair follicles and sweat glands are found. Other tissues that could be identified are thyroid or breast tissue, respiratory or alimentary tract epithelium, salivary gland, retina, choroid plexus, pancreas, and neural tissue. Rarely, the contents of the cyst become inspissated and aggregated into solid balls, each being separate and not adherent either to the wall of the cyst or to each other (boules de graisse or caviarlike bodies). Foreign body giant cells (single or in clusters) are found in the cyst wall. It should be mentioned that decalcification of the osseous structures, particularly of the dermoid nipple, is often essential for the diagnosis. Benign teratomas may be one component of a combined tumor, in association with epithelial ovarian tumors, such as mucinous cystadenomas and Brenner tumors

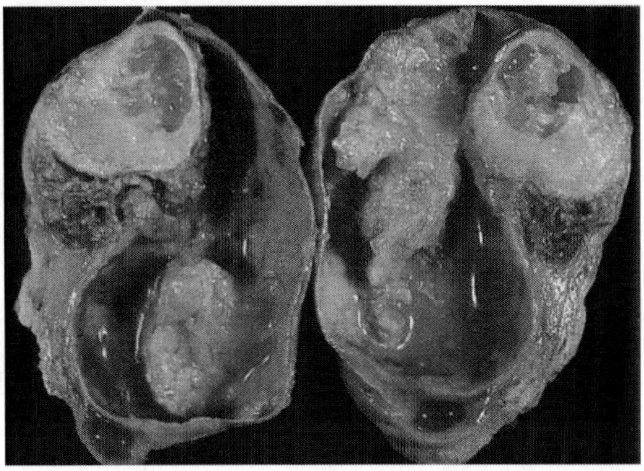

Figure 2. Gross view of a mature cystic teratoma (dermoid cyst), after removal of sebaceous material and hair, with semi-solid areas.

Histologically, the cyst wall is found to be composed of ovarian stroma. The cyst lining consists of squamous epithelial cells, coated with sebum or desquamated keratin.

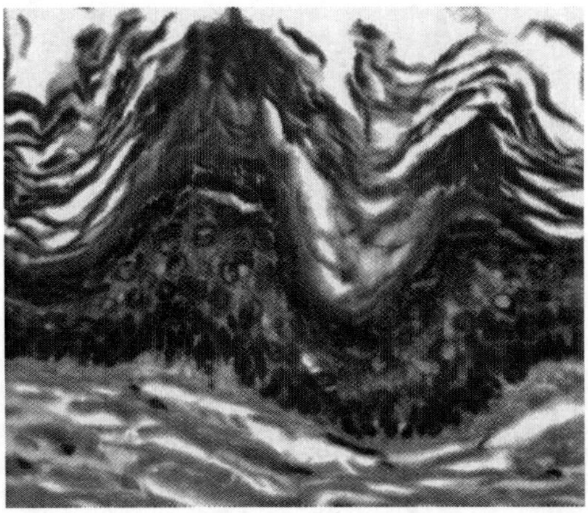

Figure 3. Histological section of a mature cystic teratoma lined by hyperkeratotic squamous cell epithelium (X 120).

Immaturity is characterized by the presence of neural tissue in the form of neuroectodermal rosettes and tubules, and/or less commonly by cellular and mitotically active glia. Tumors with rare foci of immature neural tissue occupying less than one low power field on any histological section are characterized as grade 1 and have at least 95% survival. Those with similar elements occupying more than 1 but less than 4 low power fields in any histological slide are characterized as grade 2 and those with a large amount of immature neural tissue occupying more than 4 low power fields (403) in any slide are characterized as grade 3.

Based on the relative amount of mature and immature neuroepithelial tissues, mitotic activity, and degree of differentiation, the following histologic grading system is proposed:

Grade 0-Mature tissue only
Grade 1-Limited immature neuroepithelial tissue and mitotic activity
Grade 2-Moderate amount of immature tissue and mitotic activity
Grade 3-Large quantities of immature tissue and mitotic activity

Immature teratomas are usually tumors solid or partly microcystic, presenting usually a smooth or lobular exterior surface.

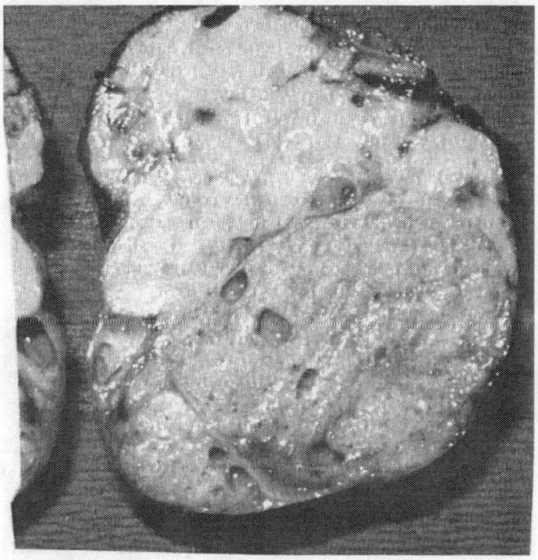

Figure 4. Gross view of an immature solid teratoma composed of whitish cerebroid tissue and small cystic areas.

Malignant teratomas are currently diagnosed only by post-operative pathological examination in most cases. Histologically, squamous cell carcinoma or rarely adenocarcinoma may be found. Sarcomatous lesions are extremely rare.

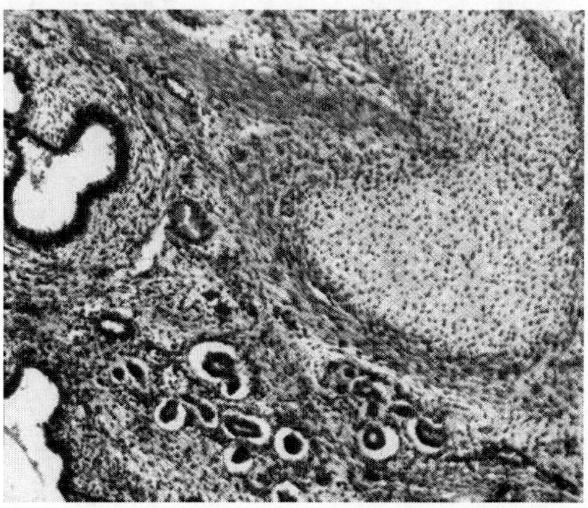

Figure 5. Histological section of an immature teratomas showing immature neural and mesenchymal elements (X120).

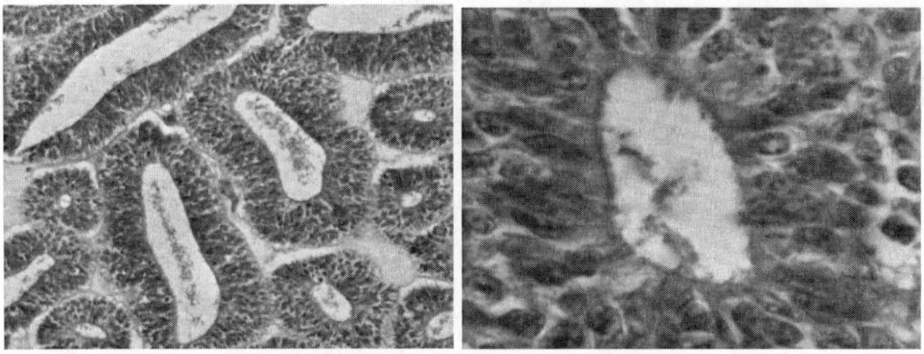

Figure 6. Histological sections of immature teratomas showing primitive nervous elements and tubules (X 250 left, X 400 right).

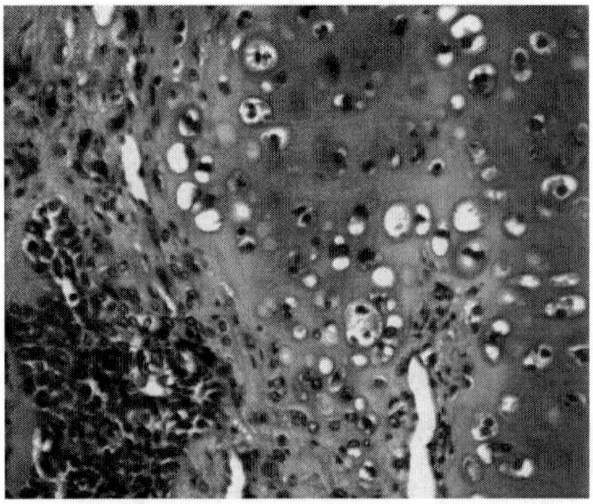

Figure 7. Histological section showing immature chondro-osseous tissues observed in an immature teratomas (X250).

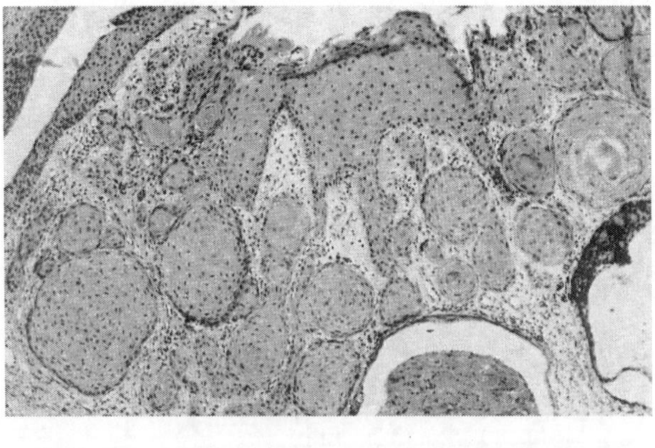

Figure 8. Histological section of a squamous cell carcinoma which infiltrates the wall of a dermoid cyst (X 25).

Prognosis

The prognosis of mature teratomas is excellent, but cases are reported characterized by frequent recurrences.

In immature teratomas the prognosis correlates with the histologic grade of immature neural elements. The quantity of neuroepithelium in immature teratomas correlates with tumor grade and patient survival. Women with Stage Ia grade 1 disease who are surgically treated, and with a complete staging procedure, have a good prognosis High-grade tumors (grades 2 and 3) have overall lower survival of approximately 85%.

In malignant teratomas, the prognosis tends to be poor. Overall, a 5-year survival rate of 52% has been reported by Hirakawa et al. in their series of 28 patients. It seems to be better in cases where the malignancy is an epidermoid carcinoma rather than other types. Prognosis generally depends on the type of the tumor, the extent of spread, and the presence or not of tumor rupture. Optimal cytoreduction has been shown to improve the outcome.

Monodermal Teratomas

World Health Organization Histological Classification of Ovarian Tumors (2003), includes struma ovarii and malignant thyroid tumors arising within struma, in the "thyroid tumor group" under the heading "monodermal teratomas and somatic-type tumors associated with dermoid cysts." Specifically, monodermal teratomas mainly include the thyroid tumor group (struma ovarii – benign or malignant), as well as the carcinoid group (insular, trabecular, mucinous, strumal carcinoid), and neuroectodermal group (ependymoma, primitive neuroectodermal tumor, glioblastoma, multiform, medulloblastoma). Less common groups are the melanocytic tumors, sarcomas, carcinomas, and sebaceous tumor groups.

Struma ovarii is the most common type of monodermal teratomas, accounting for nearly 3% of all ovarian teratomas. Struma ovarii is a neoplasm formed solely of thyroid tissue, however only 20% of such tumors are composed entirely of thyroid tissue and in reality, thyroid tissue overshadows the other teratomatous elements quantitatively (usually over 50%). It was initially described by Bottlin in 1888 and, later, by Pick in 1902 and 1903. Malignancy of struma ovarii is rare. Specifically, malignant transformation of the thyroid tissue in the ovary ranges from 5-10% of all struma ovarii cases. Malignant struma was first described by Wetteland in 1956. Papillary and follicular thyroid carcinomas are the most frequent types of malignancy observed. Metastases from a struma ovarii have also been reported in the literature. *Strumal carcinoid*, a neoplasm apparently unique to the ovary, is composed of both monodermal teratoma (struma) and secondary somatic tumor (carcinoid), and has been misdiagnosed as 'malignant struma ovarii' in the past. *Carcinoid tumor* of the ovary was first described by Stewart in 1939. In the literature, carcinoid tumors are reported in association with gastrointestinal or respiratory type epithelium, mucinous cystadenomas, Brenner tumors and androblastomas. They are observed in untreated teratomas (cystic or solid) in the sixth and seventh decade of life. However, ovarian carcinoids could also be metastatic from gastrointestinal or respiratory tract primaries and this must be considered in the differential diagnosis.

Pathogenesis

The pathogenesis of monodermal teratomas is still controversial. Struma ovarii is composed by mature thyroid tissue growing within ovarian teratomas. Multiple genetic abnormalities have been described in malignancies arising in struma ovarii including alterations in the mitogen-activated protein kinase pathway. So, mutations in BRAF, HRAS, NRAS, PTEN, and RET gene have been described.

Clinical Findings

The peak age incidence of struma ovarii is in the fifth decade, but cases have been reported in older post-menopausal women and rarely in prepubertal girls. Struma ovarii is usually a unilateral tumor that may be greatly enlarged, its diameter ranging from 1 cm to 40 cm and weighting up to 4000 grams. Women may experience acute abdominal pain (12%), but are asymptomatic in almost half of the cases (40%). The typical presentation of struma ovarii is that of a palpable pelvic mass, however, unusual clinical manifestations such as abnormal vaginal bleeding, hyperthyroidism (5%), thyrotoxicosis (15%), ascites (about 35%), and Pseudo-Meigs' syndrome have been reposted. Chronic non-specific thyroiditis and Hashimoto's disease are also described in the literature. Struma ovarii is the most common type of ovarian tumor which is associated with stromal steroid cell formation. Histological findings of malignancy in struma do not necessarily equate with biological malignancy, and the majority of thyroid-type carcinomas do not spread beyond the ovary.

Ovarian carcinoids may reach a large size, up to 20 cm in diameter and the largest reported case weighed 12 kgs. These tumors may produce carcinoid syndrome without liver metastases. In fact, metastases of strumal carcinoid are rather rare, occurring in about 2% of cases. Ovarian carcinoids are often hormonally active, secreting serotonin, bradykinin, and other peptide hormones directly into the systemic circulation and are not inactivated during their pass through the liver. In these cases, episodic cutaneous flushing, diarrhea, and bronchospasm are observed. Cushing's syndrome is another common finding if the tumor arises from Kulschitsky enterochromaffin cells.

Imaging

The most characteristic ultrasound finding is the "struma pearl." This is a smooth round solid ball within a fluid-filled cyst, similar to the round white ball consisting of hair and sebum described in the setting of dermoid ovarian cysts. It could contain areas of cystic degeneration, appearing as hypoechoic spots in the otherwise hyperechoic struma pearl. Doppler could also be used in the diagnosis as these struma pearls are often vascularized areas of ovarian cysts, representing the thyroid tissue components. C/T and MRI appearance might be helpful for diagnosis, as well as in clarifying the extent of the disease or possible lymph node involvement. Struma ovarii usually appears as a multicystic mass with no or moderate cystic wall enhancement. MRI findings are characterized by a multilobulated complex mass with thickened septa, multiple cysts or variable signal intensities and enhancing solid components.

Differential Diagnosis

It includes lesions causing hyperthyroidism and thyroid carcinoma metastatic to the ovary. Differential diagnosis of extra-ovarian spread of struma includes the usual types of thyroid cancer and peritoneal "stromatosis" (struma ovarii with peritoneal dissemination). Ovarian carcinoids must be differentiated from primaries of the gastrointestinal tract.

Management

Work-up for suspected *struma ovarii* includes laboratory assessment of thyroglobulin levels and thyroid function tests. Struma ovarii could be associated with elevated thyroglobulin levels. CA 125 is a non specific marker. In such cases, preoperative referral to a gynecology oncologist for operative management is essential. Fertility sparing surgery (e.g., unilateral cystectomy or oophorectomy) should be considered in women of reproductive age. However, it should be attempted only if there is a unilateral lesion without evidence of capsular invasion or gross metastasis. Any case exhibiting gross metastasis, capsular invasion, or an intra-operative frozen section demonstrating malignant struma ovarii should have complete staging for ovarian cancer with total abdominal hysterectomy, bilateral salpingo-oophorectomy, omentectomy, peritoneal washings and lymph node sampling. The findings of hyperthyroidism usually disappear over several weeks after surgery.

In cases of malignancies arising in the struma ovarii, a combination of gynecologic and endocrine approaches is proposed. Optimal debulking with total abdominal hysterectomy, bilateral salpingo-oophorectomy and even omentectomy to cytoreduce the total mass of intra-abdominal disease is suggested. Adjuvant therapy includes external radiotherapy, chemotherapy, and thyroid suppression. Chemotherapeutic approaches should be tailored more to a metastatic thyroid cancer rather than to ovarian cancer. It is also proposed that women with thyroid cancer arising in the ovary should undergo total thyroidectomy by surgeons to allow for treatment with ^{131}I ablation. To optimize the chances for response to ^{131}I treatment, pretreatment with lithium is also used and a strict low-iodine diet is proposed. Monitoring of thyroglobulin levels can be performed with greater sensitivity in women with or without thyroidectomy. Sequential thyroglobulin levels' monitoring are key to early detection of possible recurrence of malignancy. So, an increase in thyroglobulin levels greater than baseline should lead to further evaluation for recurrent disease. *Carcinoid tumors* should be excised, while in cases of metastases, actinomycin D may be used

Pathology

On gross examination, *struma ovarii* is a solid and sometimes nodular tumor. On section it is a brown or green-brown semi-solid, gelatinous mass and resembles thyroid tissue. Cystic and hemorrhagic areas are common findings.

Histologically, the thyroid tissue is prominent. Many acini appear small and undeveloped, while others are distended with colloid.

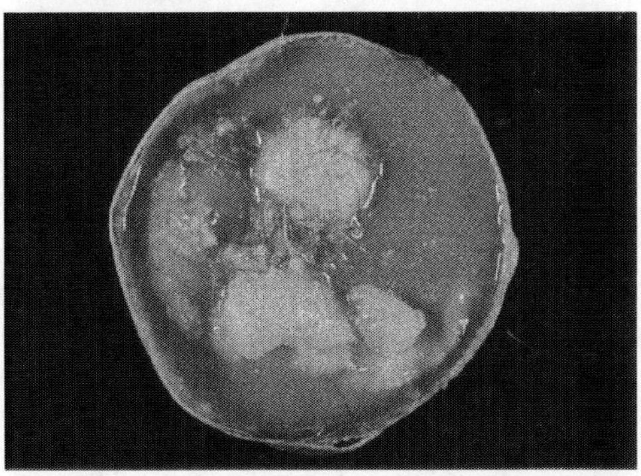

Figure 9. Gross view of a struma ovarii. A gelatinous consistency with nodular areas is prominent. A smooth and intact capsule is observed.

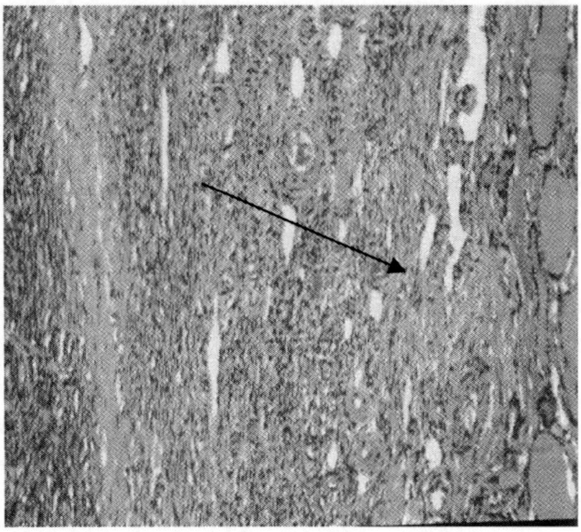

Figure 10. Histological section of a monodermal teratoma showing thyroid follicles (arrow) and ovarian cortex (left) (X120).

Occasionally, the thyroid tissue shows changes associated with hyperactivity, hypoactivity, or have the appearance of an adenomatous nodule or nodular goitre. Sometimes, the cells are arranged in slender cords or trabeculae and should be distinguished from a carcinoid.

Rather unusual findings include solid patterns, prominent microfollicles conveying a pseudotubular appearance, abundant eosinophilic cytoplasm imparting an oxyphilic appearance, and abundant clear cytoplasm. In such atypical cases, a careful search for thyroid follicles, the presence in some cases of birefringent calcium oxalate crystals in the colloid, and immunohistochemical investigation for thyroglobulin or thyroid transcription factor-1 immunoreaction will lead to the diagnosis. Regarding thyroid type carcinoma associated with struma ovarii, papillary carcinoma is the most common type. It is characterised by overlapping, ground glass, irregularly contoured nuclei lining papillary formations with fibrovascular cores. It exhibits nuclear features similar to those of their counterparts in the thyroid gland including grooves, intranuclear cytoplasmic inclusions, and finely granular chromatin. The identification of psammoma bodies in the context of a thyroid-type papillary neoplasm is highly supportive of the diagnosis of malignancy.

Follicular carcinoma is the second most common type of carcinoma to arise in the struma ovarii. The identification of invasion into the surrounding ovarian tissue, vascular invasion, or metastases is evidence of malignancy. The oncocytic variant of follicular carcinoma is similar in appearance to that of Hurthle cell thyroid carcinoma, with cytoplasm abundant, eosinophilic, and granular. Insular carcinoma is infrequent. It is a morphologically distinct type of poorly differentiated thyroid carcinoma of follicular cell origin that forms nests or islands composed of monotonous small cells with rounded nuclei and scant cytoplasm. Although the tumor predominantly has a solid infiltrative growth pattern, microfollicles are frequently encountered, some of which contain colloid. Vascular invasion is common, and variable numbers of mitoses are present.

Carcinoid tumors are solid, firm and yellowish in color.

Histologically solid clumps and strands of polyhedral cells presenting the typical carcinoid morphology are observed. Occasional acinar formations are found lined by cells with granular eosinophilic cytoplasm with fairly well-demarcated cell borders. The nuclei are vesicular with scattered clumping. Argentaffin granules are identified as large, intracytoplasmic, golden brown granules and a positive immunoreaction to chromogranine and synaptoiphysin is observed. The differential diagnosis includes granulosa cell tumors which are immunopositive to inhibin and vimentin and negative to for chromogranine and synaptophysine.

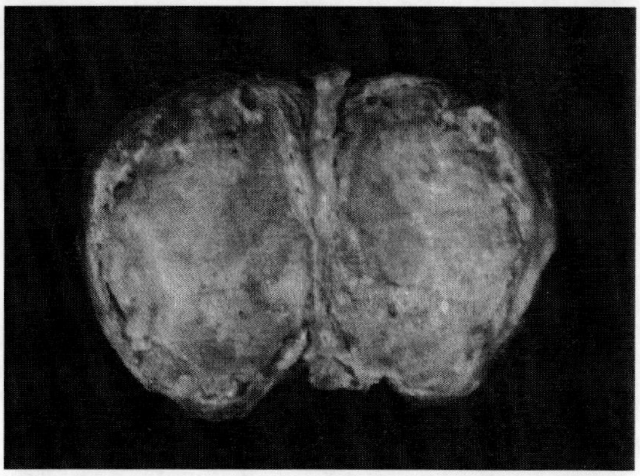

Figure 11. Gross view of a carcinoid tumor, showing a compact tumor with smooth contour.

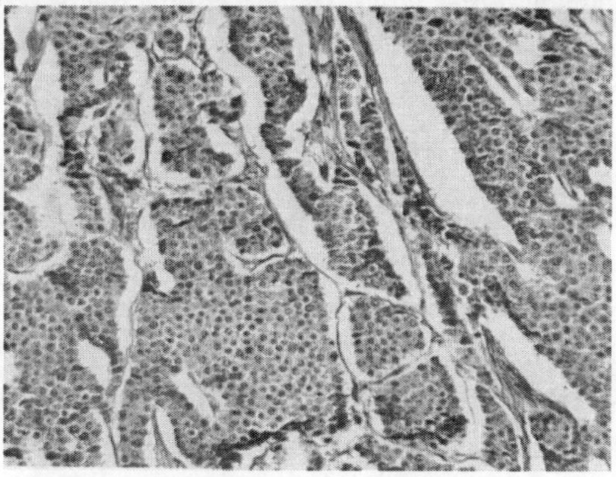

Figure 12. Histological section of an ovarian carcinoid tumor, composed of uniform neoplastic cells arranged in sheets, separated by delicate fibrous septa (X120).

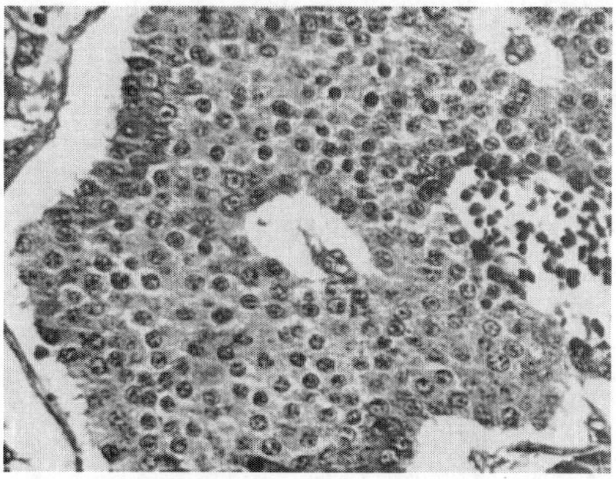

Figure 13. Under higher magnification in this histological section the uniformity of the cells and the nuclei, arranged in islands, is evident (X240).

Thyroid and carcinoid components of ovarian *strumal carcinoid* may be intimately admixed, but it could also be distinct macroscopically and/or histologically. However, even in those cases, there is usually an admixture of these elements at their interface, suggesting that the carcinoid arises from the struma.

Strumal carcinoids present neoplastic neuroendocrine cells invading the struma component and replacing the follicular cells. Glands or cysts lined by goblet cells may also occur, and occasionally the tumor is associated with a mucinous (goblet cell) carcinoid. The carcinoid component may have a trabecular pattern in about one-half of cases, a mixed trabecular and insular pattern, and occasional cases have a pure insular appearance. Immunohistochemically, the thyroidal component of strumal carcinoid expresses thyrormone and the carcinoid element is usually positive for chromogranin and synaptophysin and in some cases for somatostatin, peptide YY and serotonin.

Prognosis

Devaney et al. in a retrospective study report excellent prognosis for struma ovarii tumors. Specifically, in a follow-up period of 3-16 years for 22 patients with struma ovarii and from 2 to 18 years for 8 patients with malignant struma ovarii, all patients were alive except one patient with "proliferative" struma, who succumbed to congestive heart failure. However, in another study, extensive peritoneal adhesions, large size of a struma ovarii (<5 cm, 0%; 5–6 cm, 40%; 7–15 cm, 60%; >15 cm, 75%), and solid histologic architecture, were associated with an increased incidence of recurrence or metastasis in malignant cases. Recurrence rates in women with malignant struma ovarii which are surgically treated without subsequent radioablation reach 50%.

Ovarian Dysgerminoma

Ovarian dysgerminomas, considered the female equivalent of seminomas, is the most common histologic type of malignant germ cell tumor accounting for about 50% of cases. They may occur in a pure form or mixed with other types of germ cell tumors including embryonal carcinoma, yolk sac tumor, choriocarcinoma, and teratoma Most cases arise from dysgenetic gonads of patients with 46, XY pure gonadal dysgenesis (Swyer syndrome). Dysgerminomas were first described on 1931 by Meyer. They usually present in a young age group with a median age of 20 years. Seven per cent of cases occur in the first decade of life and 15-20% of seminomas are diagnosed during pregnancy.

Pathogenesis

Dysgerminomas arise from undifferentiated or neuter germ cells that do not have or have lost the properties to differentiate and are not capable of hormone production. There is an increased tendency (in 30% of patients) to occur in dysgenetic or "dysplastic" ovaries, and frequently develop in association with gonadoblastomas. Mutations of the SRY gene are found in 20% of the patients and the main etiologic factor is considered to be a short arm Y chromosome deletion involving SRY. Other gene mutations such as SF1, SOX9, Wnt4, Dax1, and WT1 involved in testis differentiation are also be implicated. KIT is a growth factor receptor important for normal germ cell migration and development. KIT mutations occur in 27% of cases of dysgerminomas and are associated with advanced stage of tumor presentation and may be used as a prognostic factor in malignant ovarian germ cell tumors. This theory is based on evidence of a detected codon 816 mutation in an aggressive high-stage tumor that was resistant to carboplatin-based chemotherapy. For this reason, KIT is a potential therapeutic target for those dysgerminomas that have the mutation.

Clinical Presentation

Patients with pure gonadal dysgenesis are characterised by the absence of complete pubertal development (incomplete breast development, immature uterus or abnormal menstrual bleeding), even at older ages, caused by the absence of gonadal hormonal secretion from the streak gonads. These patients are phenotypically female with an unambiguously female genital appearance from birth and normal Müllerian structures. They are usually first diagnosed in adolescence with delayed puberty and primary amenorrhea and often present tall stature with minimal breast development (reflecting peripheral aromatization of androgens). The pubic hair distribution, although adult in type, is usually decreased in total quantity. However, cases with precocious puberty are also reported in the current literature, characterized by undifferentiated tumors containing trophoblastic elements associated with high levels of estradiol.

Dysgerminomas are associated with gonadoblastomas in about 50% of cases and may present high HCG levels. Patients with gonadoblastomas are usually phenotypic females with varying degrees of virilization, although some patients are phenotypic males with a variable degree of feminization. Gonadoblastomas have a propensity to give rise to malignant germ cell neoplasms.

Dysgerminomas are unilateral in 90% of cases and present as abdominal masses associated with acute pain in cases of rupture, haemorrhage, or torsion of the mass pedicle. 70% of patients are diagnosed early and present with Stage I disease. However, it should be noted that dysgerminomas disseminate via lymphatics very early.

Rarely, dysgerminoma is diagnosed during pregnancy. The natural course of pregnancy in cases of dysgerminoma is extremely difficult, due to the large size of the tumor, metrotrrhagias, abdominal collection of fluid as well as tubal adhesions, as indicated by various case reports. It is also observed that the abdominal distention is more pronounced than that expected for pregnancy age. In these cases, ultrasound guided fine needle cytology is proposed to achieve the diagnosis. Early diagnosis and excision of the ovarian tumor while it is still intact would offer the best outcome for the mother and fetus.

Dysgerminomas are not hormone-producing tumors; however, they are associated with increased FSH, HCG, CA-125, and LDH levels. Although, LDH levels are found to be elevated, AFP levels are usually normal. Patients with normal gonadal development are expected to have a low FSH level during the prepubertal period, however patients with pure gonadal dysgenesis would have high FSH levels.

Management

Complete gynecological examination is suggested in order to stage the pubertal development according to Tanner's classification and to diagnose a possible pubertal delay. The menstruation of such patients could be controlled by hormone replacement treatment. Genetic counseling of those families is essential. More specifically, a preoperative diagnosis of pure gonadal dysgenesis is important to avoid multiple surgical procedures or delayed diagnosis of the underlying genetic condition. For this reason, karyotype with fluorescence in situ hybridization is proposed in order to identify 46, XY karyotype or various forms of mosaicism. Ultrasound, color Doppler, C/T, as well as MRI are the proposed imaging methods to clarify the condition of the uterus, gonads, and lymph nodes. However, current practice consists of early removal of the two gonads in order to avoid the risk of malignant transformation by laparotomy or laparoscopy in all symptomatic patients.

The first step in the treatment of dysgerminoma is surgery. The surgical management of young patients with Stage IA disease is proposed to be fertility sparing. Routine biopsy of the contra-lateral ovary is unnecessary if it is normal in appearance. Adequate staging should be performed, which includes omental and peritoneal biopsies and sampling of suspicious pelvic and peri-aortic lymph nodes. The staging work-up should also involve an imaging study of the para-aortic lymph nodes and the lungs. In fertility sparing cases, there is always the possibility of pregnancy by oocyte donation if the uterus is present. Several cases of pregnancies after treatment of dysgerminomas with surgery and chemotherapy have been reported.

In Stage IA disease, adjuvant treatment is not recommended. Dysgerminomas are very sensitive to both radiation and chemotherapy. Radiotherapy doses of 2,500 to 3,500 cGy may be curative, even for gross metastatic disease. Radiation should rarely be used as first-line treatment, because of the increased risk of fertility loss. Chemotherapy such as PVB (cisplatin, vinblastine, and bleomycin), PEB (cisplatin, etoposide, and bleomycin), and JEB (carboplatin, etoposide, and bleomycin) are administered to patients with metastases.

Pathology

The dysgenetic gonads are fibrous streaks and the fallopian tubes are slender. Both gonads display fibrous tissue that vaguely resembles ovarian stroma but contains no ovarian follicles. The uterus is usually atrophic and the endometrium show atrophic changes.

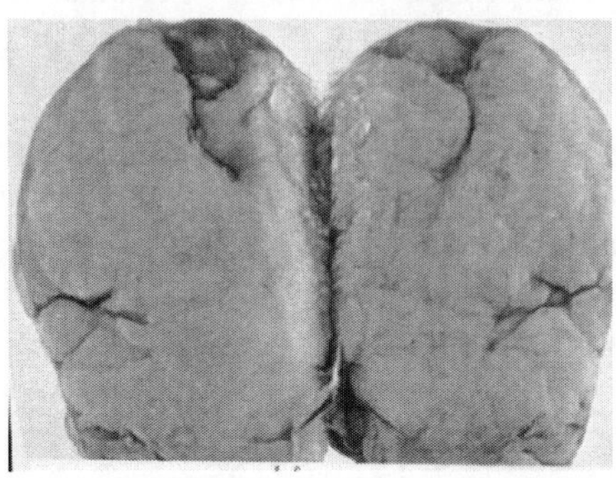

Figure 14. Gross view of a dysgerminoma showing ovoid shape, smooth external surface and lobular cut surface.

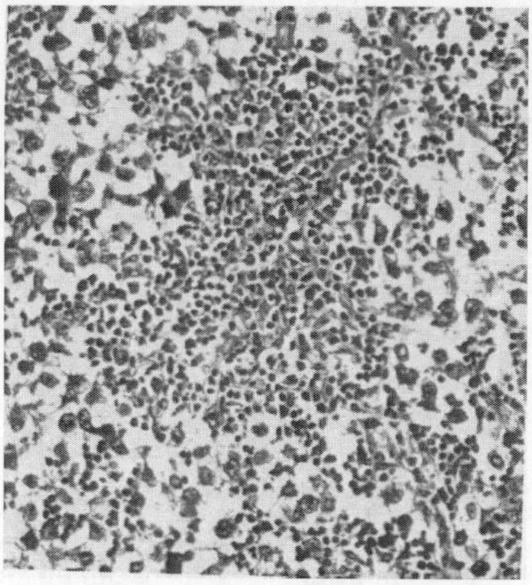

Figure 15. Histological section of dysgerminoma showing a central lymphocytic reaction and the clusters of large neoplastic cells at the periphery (X120).

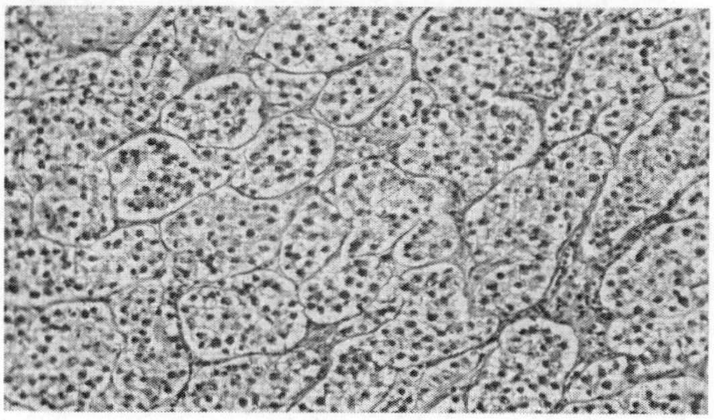

Figure 16. Histological section of a dysgerminoma showing large neoplastic cells in a alveolar pattern divided by delicate fibrous diaphragms (X120).

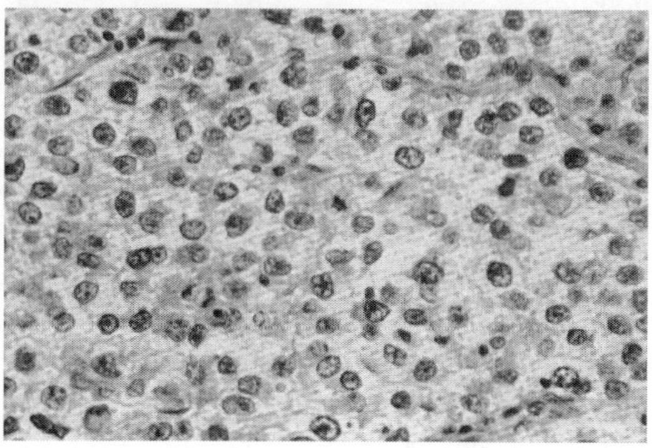

Figure 17. In a larger magnification, large neoplastic cells with round nuclei and prominent nucleoli are observed (X250).

Dysgerminomas vary in size from 3 to 10 cm in diameter and are round to ovoid, usually firm or rubbery tumors, with a smooth external surface. Larger tumors are softer and friable, with an increased tendency to undergo focal necrosis and hemorrhage. Cyst formation is uncommon. The tumor is composed by lobules of grey-pink, moderately firm to soft tissue.

Microscopically, dysgerminomas show a fairly uniform appearance with the presence of large cells with a clear or granular slightly basophilic cytoplasm. The nuclei are round with irregularly clumped chromatin and prominent nucleoli. Mitotic figures are found in moderate numbers. The cells are arranged in clusters, sheets or cords and separated by fibrous connective tissue stroma with marked infiltration by lymphocytes. Focal lymphocytic reaction forming follicles with germinal centers and non specific granulomatous reaction are common findings.

Multinucleated giant cells, similar to the Langhans type and necrotic areas are rarely present. A better prognosis is associated with marked lymphocytic or granulomatous infiltration. In about 5% of cases, syncytiotrophoblastic cells are observed, representing differentiation of germ cells to trophoblasts, secreting b-HCG. Common histochemical findings of dysgerminoma cells are alkaline phosphatase and positive periodic acid Schiff reaction, indicating the presence of intracellular proteoglucans. Immunohistochemically, the tumor cells are positive for PLAP, CD117, and CK, but negative for LCA or CD30. It should also be mentioned that multiple sections from different areas of the tumor are necessary in order to exclude other germ cell patterns.

Differential Diagnosis

It includes diffuse large B cell lymphoma, poorly differentiated carcinoma, embryonal carcinoma and gonadoblastoma. The coexistence of dysgerminoma and gonadoblastoma is seen in about half of the patients and the histologic diagnosis in these cases may be altered by extensive hyalinization and calcification and/or overgrowth of a one element neoplastic element. Immunohistochemistry, as described above is a valuable aid in the differential diagnosis.

Prognosis

With accurate staging, complete resection, and adjuvant chemotherapy, patients should be expected to have excellent survival rates. For Stage IA disease, unilateral gonadectomy alone results in a 5-year disease-free survival rate of greater than 95%. However, early recurrences are mentioned to be very common in other stages (15-25% of cases). The most common sites of recurrence are the peritoneal cavity and the retroperitoneal lymph nodes. Usually, such recurrences are found within the first two years especially in patients whose contra-lateral ovary has been preserved (5-10%). Later recurrences have also been noted. For this reason, careful clinical, radiologic, and serologic follow-up is required. The recurrence rate is higher in sub-optimally staged early disease. Several studies demonstrate the importance of serum tumor markers (AFP and beta-hCG), and the early stage of the disease as predictors of overall survival, whereas the age at the diagnosis has no prognostic significance. Lymph node involvement is proposed to be an independent predictor of poor survival. Fertility sparing operations were found to be significantly associated with the risk of primary treatment failure. However, other studies showed that fertility-sparing surgery is a safe, reasonable treatment option that does not compromise survival. Another prognostic factor is the presence of elements of yolk sac tumor in the metastatic disease. Adjuvant treatment is considered in an effort to reduce the risk of recurrence. Late recurrence may be associated with a poorer prognosis and bleomycin/

etoposide/cisplatin (BEP) chemotherapy may play only a limited role in its management or prevention of late-relapse dysgerminoma.

Yolk Sac Tumor (Endodermal Sinus Tumor, Teilum Tumor)

Most yolk sac tumors (endodermal sinus or Teilum tumors) occur in the ovary and make up the second most common malignant germ cell tumor of the ovary representing approximately 20% of ovarian malignant germ cell neoplasms. It arises from primordial germ cells that occur in young age, usually in the second decade of life (mean age 19 years, ranging from 14 to 45 years), although there have been case reports of yolk sac tumors occurring in infancy and in postmenopausal women. Its relative frequency is higher in Japan (up to 19% of ovarian malignancies) than in North America and Western European countries. Yolk sac tumors present either as a pure form or combined with other germ cell neoplastic elements.

Pathogenesis

Endodermal sinus tumors appear to arise from germ cells misplaced during embryogenesis. During the fourth through the sixth weeks of development, the germ cells migrate through the midline dorsal mesentery, proceeding to the developing gonadal ridge. A remnant of this germinal tissue anywhere along the migration course may become the site of neoplastic growth.

Clinical Findings

Endodermal sinus tumors are unilateral in 99% of cases. The median diameter is 15 cm, ranging from 7 to 28cm. Most patients present with disease confined to the ovary (71% of the cases are Stage 1). The most common finding is abdominal pain occurring in 55% to 80% of the patients. The presence of an abdominal or pelvic mass with abdominal enlargement is another finding. Fever is present in one fourth of the patients. Less frequent findings are ascites or peritonitis secondary to torsion, infection, or rupture of the ovarian tumor. Endocrine manifestations as a direct consequence of hormone secretion are rare findings. The tumor exhibits malignant change in a cell line committed to extra embryonic differentiation, and secretes alpha-fetoprotein. However, preoperative serum AFP levels before initial surgery has no significant correlation with the prognosis. Because of the predilection of this tumor for young patients it may co-exist with pregnancy. No fetal malformations are correlated to the tumor. A total of 10 cases of ovarian yolk sac tumors have been described in postmenopausal patients, associated with endometrial carcinomas. Metastases to the peritoneum, bowel serosa, omentum, liver or lymph nodes occur in 30% of cases. The most common extra-gonadal sites reported are the mediastinum, vagina, brain, and retro-peritoneum.

Imaging Studies

Characteristic features consist of a complex mass of a mixed solid and cystic nature. The tumor may be predominantly solid with areas of hemorrhage and cysts, displaying a heterogeneous appearance. The ultrasound reveals a pelvic mass depicting both echogenic solid and hypo/anechoic cystic components. Concurrent ovarian cystic tyeratomas (occurring in 14% cases), ascites, or urinary obstruction are common findings. CT recognizes the cystic nature because of the multiple internal septations with hemorrhage or protein content and this method could be used for the staging of the tumor. Hemorrhage and necrosis are identified on MRI as high intensity foci on T1-weighted images. Hyper-vascularity in the form of prominent enhancement on post-contrast CT images or signal voids on MRI could also be seen.

Differential Diagnosis

Many benign and malignant lesions are included in the differential diagnosis of a yolk sac tumor, such as teratomas, tubo-ovarian abscess, appendiceal abscess, mesenteric cysts, or gastrointestinal duplication cysts as well as other germ cell and epithelial tumors (dysgerminomas, papillary carcinomas, endometrioid carcinomas). Increased serum alpha-fetoprotein levels are a useful aid to the correct diagnosis.

Management

Total abdominal hysterectomy with bilateral salpingo-oophorectomy, peritoneal cytology, omentectomy and multiple peritoneal biopsies and lymph node dissection is proposed in older patients. Fertility sparing is proposed in younger patients including unilateral salpingo-oophorectomy, peritoneal washing for cytology and careful inspection of the abdominal cavity (biopsies of omentum, peritoneum). With the advent of chemotherapy, the extent of the surgical procedure required has progressively been reduced and become more conservative. Various combinations of chemotherapy have been used i.e., vincristine, actinomycin, cyclophosphamide or cisplatin, vinblastine, bleomycin or bleomycin, etoposide, and platinum. However, BEP given at 21-day intervals is favored for its effectiveness and lower rate of adverse effects. Fifty to 80% of women who underwent fertility sparing surgery and received platinum based chemotherapy subsequently became pregnant. Follow-up is performed by physical examinations, chest and abdominal C/T, as well as serum α-fetoprotein levels every three months during the first year and every 6 months during subsequent years. The role of a second-look laparotomy in the management of patients with endodermal sinus tumors of the ovary is controversial. As demonstrated by Mitchell et al. the routine use of second-look laparotomy after chemotherapy is unnecessary.

Pathology

On gross section, the tumor is multicystic and partially solid, with areas of hemorrhage and necrosis. Cysts of varying sizes are scattered throughout the tissue, giving the tumor a honeycombed appearance.

Microscopically, the tumor presents an epithelial-reticular pattern, with a network of spaces lined by primitive cells. A wide range of histologic patterns may be observed; microcystic, resembling fetal endodermal sinus, solid, alveolar-glandular, poly-vesicular vitelline, with myxomatous stroma, papillary formations, macrocystic, hepatoid, and glandular or primitive endodermal of intestinal type. A mixture of three or four subtypes might have a better prognosis than those composed of one or two subtypes. The majority of cells usually contain vesicular nuclei with moderate nuclear atypia and a low mitotic rate.

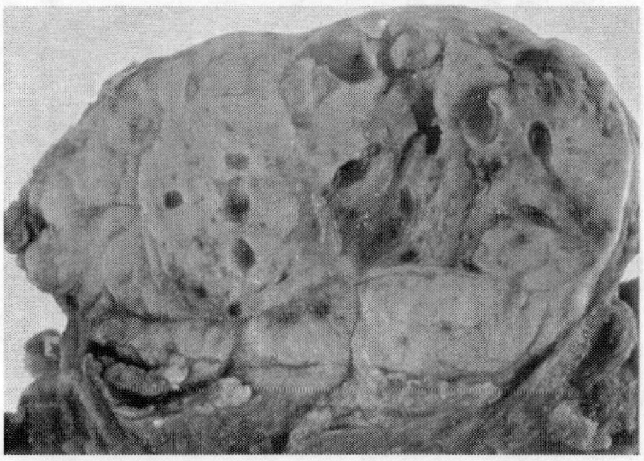

Figure 18. Gross view of a yolk sac tumor, with solid and cystic areas, and a nodular whitish surface.

Numerous Schiller–Duval bodies resembling superficially immature renal glomeruli are also present. Schiller–Duval bodies are characterized as peri-vascular formations consisting of a narrow band of connective tissue with a capillary blood vessel in the center and lined by a layer of cuboidal or low columnar embryonal epithelial-like cells. The surrounding capsular sinusoid space is lined by a single layer of flattened cells with prominent hyper-chromatic nuclei.

Immunohistochemically, endodermal sinus tumors typically express AFP and are consistently positive for cytokeratines, while placental-like alkaline phosphatase is found in 50% of cases. They lack oestrogen and progesterone receptors.

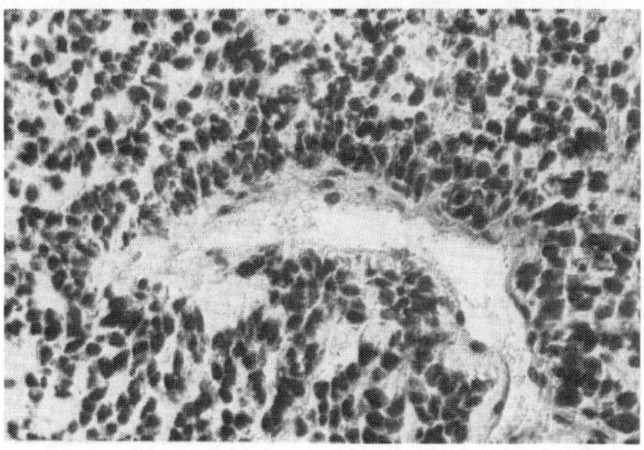

Figure 19. Histological section of yolk sac tumor showing a central capillary surrounded by small undifferentiated tumor cells (X120).

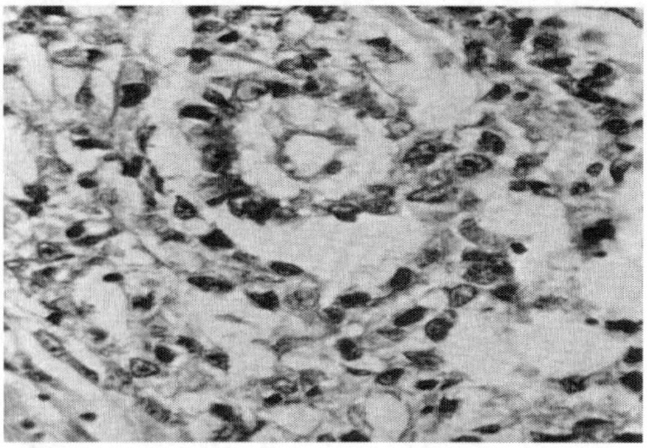

Figure 20. Histological section of a yolk sac tumor showing a Sciller-Duval body Which is glomeruloid formation of neoplastic cells, arranged round a central capillary in a loose stroma (X120).

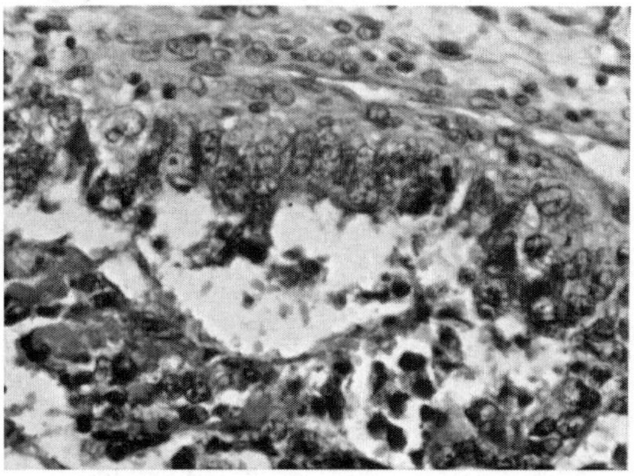

Figure 21. Histological section showing a positive AFP immunohistochemical reaction of the neoplastic cells (X240).

Prognosis

Among all subtypes of germ cell tumors, endodermal sinus tumors are highly malignant and have the worst prognosis. Two different studies showed that age is not a significant prognostic factor, but tumor stage significantly affected survival. In the study of Nawa et al. the 5-year survival rate was 95.2% for patients with Stage I disease, 75% for those with Stage II disease, 30% for those with Stage III disease and 25% for those with Stage IV disease, while in the study of Kawai et al. the 5-year survival rates were 92%, 44%, 29% and 24% for Stage I, II, III and IV, respectively. Surgical treatment alone has a poor prognosis (13% 3-year survival), while in combination with chemotherapy (cisplatin, vinblastine, and bleomycin) there is an 82.5% survival with early stage disease. Early diagnosis and treatment proves an important prognostic factor.

The presence and quantity of ascites before initial surgery and optimal cytoreduction were significant factors in both studies. Patients with residual tumors of 2 cm or less in diameter had a 5-year survival rate of 78% compared to 29.2% in cases where the residual tumor was larger than 2 cm.

Fertility sparing surgery and intrapelvic node dissection seem to have no correlation with the prognosis once effective chemotherapy regimens had been introduced.

Non-gestational Choriocarcinoma

Choriocarcinomas that affect the female genital tract are classified as either gestational or non-gestational in origin. Non-gestational choriocarcinoma arising from a teratoma or from an embryonal nest is an extremely rare germ cell tumor (under 1% of the total number of germ cell tumors). It could be a pure or mixed form, coexisting with other components of germ cell neoplasms such as dysgeminomas, immature teratomas and Teilum tumors. Pure choriocarcinoma is mostly seen in childhood and adolescence. The diagnosis of non-gestational choriocarcinoma may be achieved with certainty only in a woman who is sexually immature, unable to conceive, or has never had sexual intercourse. In women of reproductive age, the presence of other germ cell components is helpful in distinguishing non gestational choriocarcinoma. Less than 45 cases are retrieved in the literature.

Pathogenesis

Non-gestational choriocarcinomas develop from pluripotential germ cells, located in the gonads. It must be noted that various poorly differentiated germ cell tumors may show focal areas of differentiation to choriocarcinoma. Cytogenetic and molecular studies, revealed the impact of oncogenes, tumor suppressor genes and imprinting genes on its pathogenesis. Microsatellite DNA polymorphism analysis using two or three appropriate VNTR loci from the tumor and the patient for identification of paternal sequences establishes the diagnosis.

Clinical Findings

The mean age of patients is 15 years, with a range of 1 to 39 years. Common findings are lower abdominal pain and vaginal bleeding. Moreover, nausea, vomiting, weight loss, and micturition disturbances such as dysuria and increased frequency may be identified. Non-gestational choriocarcinomas are usually unilateral tumors. In pre-pubertal girls, simultaneous enlargement of the contralateral ovary may be observed, caused by the formation of multiple theca-lutein cysts. Precocious puberty may be caused in cases with high hCG levels (50% of cases). Tumor rupture and hemoperitoneum could be found, and more than 90% of patients with extra-uterine gestational choriocarcinoma will present lung metastasis. Brain metastases are reported as well. Increased serial and/or urine hCG levels is another characteristic finding. In a retrospective study, it is reported that the tumor was diagnosed in Stage I in 41%, Stage II in 27%, Stage III in 14%, and Stage IV in 18% of patients.

Imaging

Pelvic ultrasound shows a heterogeneous hyperechoic mass. Abdominal and chest C/T are helpful in the tumor staging. CT reveals a unilateral mass without fat. A large vascularized ovarian pedicle and irregular oversized arterial vessels could be seen at the periphery of the mass during the arterial phase of dynamic CT. Significant contrast material uptake could be observed in the peripheral solid portion of the tumor. On T2-weighted MRI, abnormal vessels and small cystic cavities in the irregular peripheral solid portion could be displayed. High-signal-intensity foci in the solid portion and a large central area with high and intermediate signal intensities could be suggestive of hemorrhage. Significant gadolinium uptake in the solid portion could be suggestive of a highly vascularized tumor.

Differential Diagnosis

Saito et al. was the first to describe the diagnostic criteria for non-gestational choriocarcinoma which include an absence of disease in the uterine cavity, pathological confirmation of disease, exclusion of molar pregnancy and exclusion of co-existence of intrauterine pregnancy. The differential diagnosis includes appendicitis, intussusception, ectopic pregnancy, threatened or incomplete abortion and various types of ovarian malignant tumors.

Management

Treatment with fertility sparing surgery, by ophorectomy/salpingooophorectomy is proposed for Stage I tumors combined subsequent platin-based (BEP-bleomycin, etoposide, cisplatin) or methotrexate-based chemotherapy (MAC-methotrexate, actinomycin D, cyclophosphamide). For stages > I as well as in cases where fertility is not the main consideration, total abdominal hysterectomy and bilateral salpingo-oophorectomy is performed. If the disease is extended, cytoreductive surgery, including pelvic lymphadenectomy, para-aortic lymph node sampling, omentectomy, appendicectomy, and peritoneal biopsies could be performed in order to achieve optimal debulking with no macroscopic residual tumor. Measurement of hCG levels, as well as imaging examinations can be useful in monitoring the patient's response to treatment.

Pathology

One section of the tumor presents as a solid/cystic and friable mass with areas of necrosis and hemorrhage. Microscopically, both vacuolated cytotrophoblasts and multinucleated syncytiotrophoblasts, foci of hemorrhage and necrosis are present. Chorionic villi are absent.

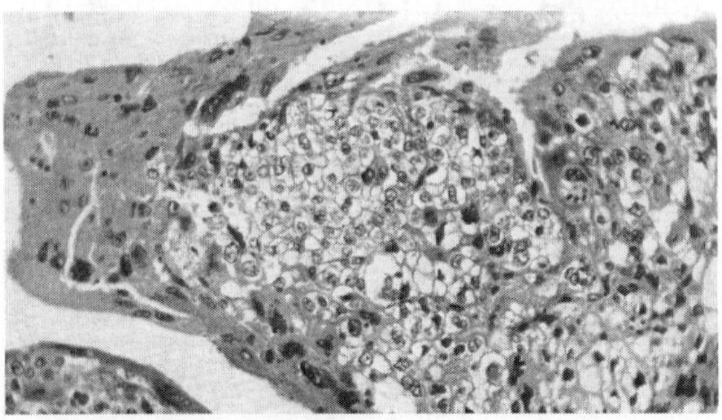

Figure 22. Histological section of a choriocarcinoma showing admixture of trophoblastic and syncytiotrophoblastic cellular elements (X120).

There are no distinctive ultrastructural or immunohistochemical differences between gestational and non-gestational choriocarcinomas. They are highly aggressive malignancies, strongly positive for Ki-67 and show positive immunohistochemical staining with hCG and placental lactogen. Molecular genetic analysis may prove a useful method for identifying the genetic origin of non-gestational choriocarcinomas and usually the presence of paternal human leucocytic antigens or a Y chromosome establishes the origin of the tumor as a gestational choriocarcinoma of paternal origin.

Prognosis

Non-gestational choriocarcinoma carries a worse prognosis than the gestational type. In a recent review at a 6-month follow-up, survival was 86.1% for patients who received adjuvant chemotherapy versus 33.3% for those who received surgical management. Among the chemotherapy group, a 100% survival rate was achieved in patients receiving cisplatin-based chemotherapy and 83.9% in patients receiving methotrexate-based chemotherapy.

Mixed forms of non-gestational choriocarcinomas do not respond well to methotrexate schemes.

Mixed Germ Cell –Sex Cord –Stromal Tumors

Gonadoblastoma

Gonadoblastomas are tumors composed of germ cells and sex cord-stromal elements. They are regarded as benign or as *"in situ"* neoplasms depending on the nature of their components. These tumors consist of aggregates of large, round germ cells, and immature Sertoli/granulosa cells within an ovarian type stroma. If untreated they develop into more aggressive germ cell tumors, such as dysgerminoma. Scully was the first to describe gonadoblastoma as a specific histopathologic entity. Such a neoplasm recapitulates gonadal development and often occurs in indeterminate gonads of individuals with abnormal sexual development. According to his description, gonadoblastomas are composed of primitive germ cells, Sertoli-granulosa type cells and Leydig or theca-lutein type cells of sex cord derivation.

Pathogenesis

Most gonadoblastomas occur in dysgenetic gonads, in patients with a Y chromosome. Approximately 80% of cases occur in phenotypic females, and 20% are in cases with phenotypic male pseudo-hermaphrodism. The tumor is associated with complete androgen insensitivity (46,XY), pure gonadal dysgenesis or Swyer syndrome (46,XY), mixed gonadal dysgenesis (45,X/46,XY), Turner syndrome (45,XO usually with evidence of XY mosaicism), and Frasier syndrome (a rare 46,XY DSD caused by a mutation in the WT1 gene. There is a high incidence of gonadoblastoma in patients with familial XY gonadal dysgenesis. However, it may arise in patients without gonadal dysgenesis. Gonadoblastomas may be found in patients with the androgen insensitivity syndrome or in the ovotestes of a true hermaphrodite with a

46XX, 46XY karyotype. A normal or partially deleted Y chromosome or marker chromosome derived from Y has also been found in 6-9% of patients with Turner syndrome. There is evidence that there is a locus on the Y chromosome termed "gonadoblastoma" locus, which has a normal function in the testis and acts as an oncogene only in the dysgenetic gonads predisposing to gonadoblastoma development. This gene disrupts the normal cell cycle regulation by stimulating protein synthetic activities, accelerating cell proliferation, and promoting carcinogenesis as it has been shown in mice. Specifically, it binds to type B- cyclins, enhances an activated cyclin B-CDK1 kinase activity, and propels a rapid G2/M transition in the cell cycle, while it also counteracts the normal functions of its X-homologue, TSPX. Also mutations of Foxl-2, WT1 and RET genes which are involved in ovary development are implicated to tumorigenesis. Foxl-2 dysregulation could also be found in DSD and DSD associated tumors such as gonadoblastoma and gonadoblastoma-like intratubular undetermined germ cell neoplasia. Although gonadoblastomas are associated with gonad dysgenesis, this is not a prerequisite for its occurrence, and certain cases occurring in pregnancy are reported in the literature. The germ cell element of gonadoblastoma may undergo proliferation, regression or malignancy development especially towards dysgerminoma (50%). Calcification found within a dysgerminoma is highly indicative of a prior gonadoblastoma. In 10% of cases, embryonal carcinoma, yolk sac tumor, immature teratoma, or choriocarcinoma could develop in cases with gonadoblastoma.

Clinical Findings

The external appearance of the patient could vary from a normal sexually developed female to a eunuchoid male. Abnormal genitourinary anatomy could be identified in the neonatal period. Gonadoblastoma is more commonly located in the right gonad, and is bilateral in more than one third of the cases. In some cases poorly developed fallopian tubes and uterus are found. Virilization (e.g., clitoris enlargement, abnormal hirsutism) occurs in approximately 60% of cases. Complete or partial regression of the virilization after tumor excision shows that the steroid hormone production is related to the neoplasm. Hot flushes and other menopausal symptoms have been found after gonad excision suggesting a partially estrogen secretion

Primary amenorrhea or developmental abnormalities of the genitalia are other common findings. Breast development is normal, but secondary sexual characteristics are abnormal, including complete absence of genital and axillary hair growth. A pelvic mass may be palpated during the gynecological examination. Although at the time of diagnosis there is usually no evidence of hormonal activity of the tumor, it seems probable that the tumor once secreted steroid hormones which are responsible for the development of the female secondary sexual characteristics.

Imaging

Gonadoblastomas appear as solid tumors, well circumscribed with heterogenous echo-texture in the lower abdomen on US and CT, while some cases with bloody ascites have also been reported in the literature. Foci of calcification are characteristic of the tumor and lead to the correct X-ray diagnosis.

Differential Diagnosis

It includes mixed germ cell-sex cord-stromal tumor, pure dysgerminoma, and sex cord tumor with annular tubules. Mixed germ cell-sex cord-stromal tumors do not occur in dysgenetic gonads. They lack the discrete nested pattern of gonadoblastoma, and exhibit proliferative activity in the sex cord component, while no regressive changes of hyalinization and calcification are found. Dysgerminomas lack a sex cord component, contain fibrous septa infiltrated by lymphocytes and do not form discrete islands. Sex cord tumors with annular tubules contain hyaline bodies and frequently calcified material, but lack a germ cell component. The sex cord elements are characterized by an antipodal arrangement of the nuclei with prominent nuclear-free zones.

Management

A family history regarding any existence of genital ambiguity, infertility, or amenorrhea is necessary in order to clarify the possible existence of a hereditary factor. A karyotype analysis is proposed in the evaluation of the young females with a pelvic mass and any symptoms of abnormal sexual development. The treatment of choice is bilateral gonadectomy. Prophylactic gonadectomy is recommended at an early age to patients with gonadal dysgenesis who have a Y chromosome in order to avoid development of malignant germ cell tumors.

Pathology

The tumor is usually small ranging from 3 to 5 cm but may reach a great size, acquiring the weight of 3000 grams in a case report. The lesions tend to be larger in cases with a secondary malignant neoplastic component and this component is usually distinctly identifiable. Gonadoblastoma is usually solid with a smooth, glistening external surface. On section it is gritty and grey characterized by fine granularity. Histological examination reveals large, clear germ cells which are scattered throughout, forming well-defined small alveolar aggregates. Occasionally, Call-Exner bodies are found, while granulosa cells, Sertoli or Leydig cells in association with the germ cells are described.

These elements are arranged in three typical patterns within the islands of gonadoblastoma; coronal, follicular, or Call-Exner-like. More specifically, in the coronal pattern, the sex cord elements line the periphery of the nest. In the follicular pattern, they surround individual or collections of germ cells in the way that the follicular epithelium surrounds the ovum of the primary follicle, and in the Call-Exner-like pattern, they surround small round amorphous hyaline eosinophilic bodies present within the cellular nests.

Foci of calcification are also distinct. Various degrees of hyalinization is found in the stroma which is usually dense and fibrous. Immunohistochemically, the immature germ cells of gonadoblastoma are positive for OCT3/4 (octamer-binding transcription factor 3/4), whereas the mature germ cells are negative for this marker but positive for TSPY (testis-specific protein on the Y chromosome).

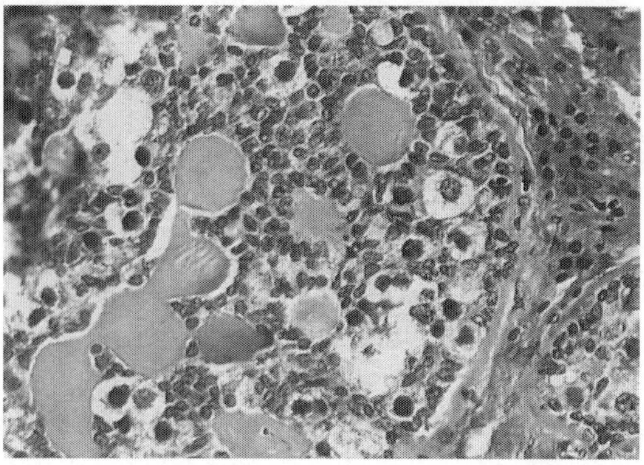

Figure 23. Histological section of gonadoblastoma showing small round spaces with hyaline material surrounded by granulosa –type cells, admixed with large round germ cells (X250).

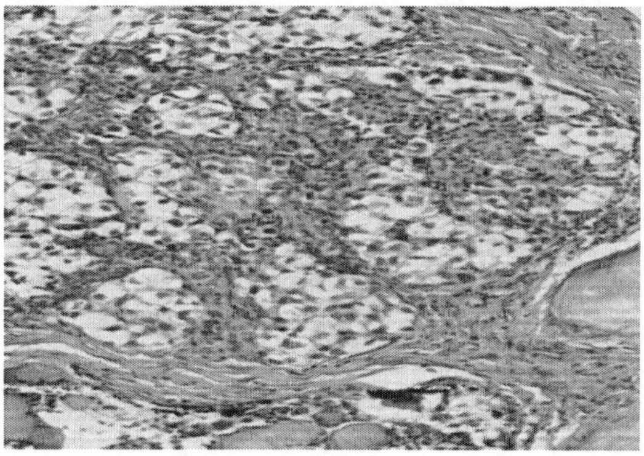

Figure 24. Histological section of gonadoblastoma showing large germ cells, in clusters, stronal-like elements and calcification (bottom) (X120).

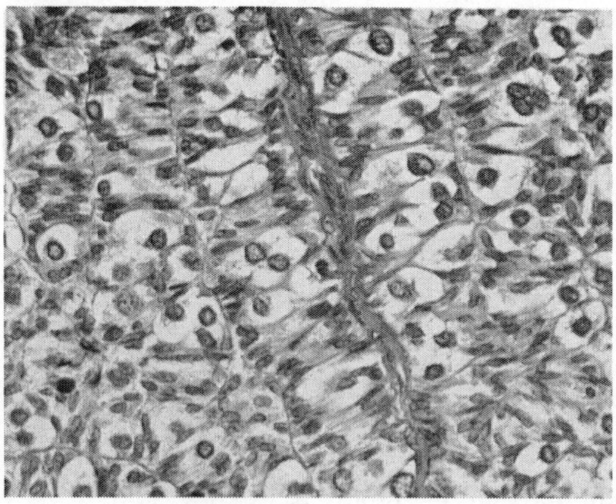

Figure 25. Histological section of gonadoblastoma showing a elongated Sertoli type cells around rounded germ cells (X250).

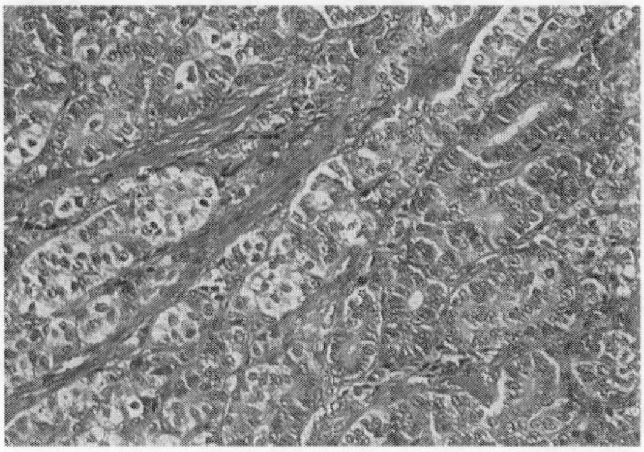

Figure 26. Gonadoblastoma. stromal cells separate clusters of large, rounded cells germ cell-like and tubule lined by Sertoli type cells (right) X (250).

Prognosis

The tumor is mostly clinically benign and the prognosis of patients with pure gonadoblastoma is excellent. In cases presenting ovarian dysgerminoma foci, platinum-based adjuvant chemotherapy offers high cure rates over 90%. The prognosis for gonadoblastoma accompanied by germ cell tumors other than dysgerminoma was very poor in the past, but it has been better nowadays. Combination chemotherapy (BEP) results in significant improvement.

Sex Cord-Stromal Tumors

Granulosa Cell Tumors of the Ovary

Granulosa cell tumors of the ovary (GCT) are the most frequent hormone-secreting ovarian tumors which are included in the sex cord-stromal tumor category. The long natural history of GCT and their tendency to recur years after the initial diagnosis are the most prominent of their characteristics.

Incidence

They represent 2% to 5% of all ovarian tumors. GCTs most commonly present during the perimenopausal or early postmenopausal period, with the peak incidence occurring between the ages of 50-54 years GCTs can be divided on the basis of histopathological features into two subgroups juvenile GCT and adult GCT reflecting the usual age group of presentation. More specifically, the juvenile type is diagnosed in patients less than 30, 20, and 10 years of age in 90%, 80%, and 50% of cases, respectively. However, the adult type can also be found in children, although this is rare. The adult-type is most frequently diagnosed in perimenopausal women, at a mean age that is 10 years younger than that of women diagnosed with epithelial ovarian cancer. The much less common juvenile type also occurs and represents approximately 5% of all GCTs.

Pathogenesis

Little is known about the pathogenesis of ovarian GCTs. Past efforts to understand the molecular pathogenesis of GCTs have been limited. Since pre-ovulatory growth of normal granulosa cells is induced by FSH, alterations in the FSH pathway were proposed to participate in GCTs pathogenesis. However, neither FSH receptors nor associated G-protein mutations have been identified in GCTs. Mutations in the *GNAS* gene, which codes for a stimulatory G protein, have been described in a minority of juvenile GCTs but not in adult type. It is known that GCTs show very little chromosomal instability. Recently, Kobel et al. identified a point mutation 402C-G (C134W) in *FOXL2*, a member of the forkhead-winged helix family of transcription factors, by using whole-transcriptome paired-end RNA sequencing. FOXL2 is a highly conserved transcription factor among species and is expressed as a nuclear protein in the developing eye, pituitary, embryonic and adult ovary, and elsewhere. It is not expressed in developing male gonads and therefore it is considered to be the earliest sexually dimorphic marker of ovarian determination. FOXL2 plays a significant role in the postnatal ovary and follicle maintenance. It suppresses steroid synthesis by suppressing expression of *StAR* gene, which encodes cholesterol transport from the outer to inner mitochondrial membrane. FOXL2 also increases estrogen conversion by inducing the aromatase gene *CYP19A1 in the* granulosa cells from androgens derived from theca cells. Mutations of FOXL2 lead to disorders of ovarian function ranging from premature follicle depletion and ovarian failure to unregulated granulosa cell proliferation leading to GCT formation.

Kalfa et al. recently reported the presence of the *gsp* oncogene in 30% of juvenile GCT cases examined. However, no gsp ongogene evidence has been reported in adult GCTs. The *gsp* oncogene protein product results in the constitutive activation of cAMP-dependent PKA signalling, which leads to abnormal cell proliferation. Regarding the correlated chromosomal abnormalities, these include trisomy 12, monosomy 22, and deletion of chromosome 6, monosomy 22, trisomy 14, as well as deletions in 22q.

Diagnosis

Abdominal swelling, pain, and a palpable mass in the lower abdomen are the presenting symptoms in all patients. All GCTs are hormonally active, producing estradiol. In the juvenile type, 80% to 90% of patients can have signs of isosexual precocious pseudo-, puberty including precocious breast development, increased pubic hair, vaginal bleeding, advanced growth, and bone age. A hormonally active juvenile GCT could also cause menstrual irregularities and rarely virilization in older patients.

The juvenile type was found to be correlated with Potter's syndrome, multiple congenital abnormalities with ambiguous genitalia, Ollier's disease (multiple enchondromatosis), and Maffucci's syndrome (Ollier's disease with hemangioma). If the tumor ruptures, signs of acute abdominal pain and hemoperitoneum may be found. Ovarian torsion can cause more acute onset of pelvic pain. Ascites is present in 10% of patients. GCTs are unilateral in 90-95% of cases. Occasionally, it may be associated with pregnancy. As GCT presents functional activity similar to normal granulosa cells, they may be diagnosed either by the common symptoms caused by any ovarian tumor or by the endometrial pathology due to an estrogenic effect. Symptoms caused by estrogen production can also give rise to different clinical manifestations depending on whether they appear in postmenopausal or young women. Women of reproductive age may have menstrual irregularities or secondary amenorrhea, endometrial polyps and/or hyperplasia. Postmenopausal bleeding could be a common finding. In such a case endometrioid endometrial cancer may be diagnosed and an ovarian tumor (GCT) could be detected in the exploration. Approximately 25% to 50% of GCTs are associated with endometrial hyperplasia, whereas 5% to 13% are associated with an endometrial carcinoma. GCTs are usually large, either solid or entirely cystic tumors measuring up to 40 cm. In the majority of cases the cystic fluid is serous. Tumors are usually round to ovoid and encapsulated with a smooth external surface which may appear lobulated. Its consistency is soft and its color is yellowish, but may be pearl-grey to white. The majority of patients with GCT are diagnosed as having Stage I disease (78-91%). The spread of GCTs is local, by direct extension and intra-peritoneal seeding. The tumors may also spread hematogenously, and patients can develop lung, liver or brain metastases even many years after initial diagnosis. Postmortem examinations have shown that 8% of cases had lymph node metastasis. In general, slow growth with a tendency for late recurrence characterizes the natural history.

Biological markers such as serum estradiol, Inhibin A and B, and AMH may be helpful for diagnosis, though their sensitivity is not always excellent. Inhibin A could be an important tumor marker, particularly in patients with androgenic or hyper-estrogenic symptoms, especially in cases characterized by young age, non increased levels of classic cancer tumor markers, and benign ultrasonographic appearance without any signs of malignancy.

One of the substances secreted by the theca cell component of GCTs is estradiol, and so it may serve as a possible tumor marker. However, estradiol levels are not a reliable marker of disease activity, because fluctuating (instead of very high) levels of estradiol have been found in patients with bulky disease, and patients have varied in their response to treatment. Thus, although estradiol may be helpful in monitoring the course of disease, it is not sensitive enough to serve as a reliable tumor marker in this disease.

Mom et al. evaluated the applicability of serum Inhibin A and B levels for the assessment of GCTs. The sensitivity of Inhibin A testing for the diagnosis of GCTs was 67% with a specificity of 100%, compared to 89% and 100% for Inhibin B, respectively. Serum Inhibin A and B concentrations were elevated in 58% and 85% of patients, respectively, at recurrence, with elevations in Inhibin B concentrations predating recurrences by a median of 11 months (range 8–19 months).

AMH is expressed by granulosa cells of the ovary during the reproductive age and controls the formation of primary follicles by inhibiting excessive follicular recruitment by FSH. Anttonen et al. found AMH gene expression correlated inversely with GCT size, with reduced expression in 87% of tumors of greater than 10 cm in size. This finding may suggest AMH is a less useful marker than the inhibin assay in more advanced disease.

Preoperative imaging diagnosis by using ultrasound, C/T or MRI scanning remains challenging due to the wide variability in morphology. The findings vary widely, including solid masses, tumors with varying degrees of hemorrhagic or fibrotic changes, multilocular cystic lesions, and completely cystic tumors. They are categorized in five morphologic lesions: multilocular cystic, thick-walled unilocular cystic, thin-walled unilocular cystic, homogenously solid, and heterogeneously solid. Evidence of hemorrhage has been reported in 60% to 71.4% of cases. It should be mentioned that they do not have intracystic papillary projections, have less propensity for peritoneal seeding, and are confined to the ovary at the time of diagnosis. Ultrasound often shows increased vascularity by color flow Doppler due to the tumor characteristics Estrogenic effects on the uterus may manifest as uterine enlargement or as endometrial thickening.

Treatment

The treatment of GCTs depends on the age of the patient and the extent of the disease. The role of frozen section should be underlined, however cystectomy is not appropriate. Conventional treatment for GCTs has predominantly been surgical followed by chemotherapy (based on platinum and taxanes) in which recurrent or advanced disease or both has occurred. Treatment in young women who desire reproductive function and where the tumor is grossly confined unilaterally, usually consists of a unilateral salpingo-oophorectomy with a complete staging including an assessment of the contra-lateral ovary. Lymphadenectomy is not an essential part of staging especially in young women. For these patients in whom the uterus is left in situ, an endometrial biopsy or curettage should be performed to clarify the possibility of a coexistent endometrial carcinoma. Minimally invasive surgery (laparoscopy with or without robotic assistance) is appropriate in the occasional patient with a small solid adnexal mass or complex ovarian cyst. For full surgical staging, surgery should include a total abdominal hysterectomy and bilateral salpingo-oophorectomy in postmenopausal women. Colombo et al. suggested that there is a place for conservative surgery without hysterectomy in younger women based on the large retrospective analysis of Zhang et al. in which the results with conservative surgery did not differ from those using a standard surgery with hysterectomy. However, due to the rarity of GCTs, a standard chemotherapeutic regimen has not emerged. Platinum-based therapy including the PAC, VBP, and BEP regimens in selected patients with Stage III/IV disease have been the most successful, with a 5-year survival of 50%. Radiation therapy has also been used with varying success in small studies especially to palliate isolated pelvic recurrences.

Aromatase inhibitors as well as tyrosine- kinase inhibitors (such as Gleevec - imatinib mesylate) have already been used in late tumor recurrence as reported in a number of of case reports. The results are intriguing, but the numbers treated in these studies are too low to allow a conclusion to be drawn. So further confirmation in larger cohort studies is required.

Pathology

Tumors are unilateral, solid with yellow-tan surface and small cystic spaces. Hemorrhage and necrosis may be observed as well. In the hysterectomy specimen, hyperplastic changes of the endometrium, polyps or even endometrial neoplasms may be observed.

Histological examination reveals variations in the appearance of GCTs. The granulosa cell component present as small, cuboidal to polygonal cells, which form cords, strands, or sheets. GCTs have been classified according to certain features of growth of the cells and the stroma into the following type

- Macrofollicular type with the characteristic Call-Exner bodies.
- Microfollicular type formed by islands of fairly uniform granulosa cells.
- Alveolar type, with scanty connective tissue and early stromal yalinization.
- Trabecular or cylindromatous type, with granulosa cells arranged in a trabecular fashion mimicking the pattern of the sex cords.
- Sarcomatoid or diffuse type, with poorly differentiated cells which have lost their epithelial appearance and resemble thecomatous tumors.

Microscopic features that distinguish juvenile GCTs from the adult type are the hyperchromatism of the tumor cells, which generally lack grooves, and the frequent luteinization of both the granulosa and theca cells. Moreover, the follicles are usually immature. Call-Exner bodies, which are pathognomonic of the adult type, are rarely present in the juvenile type. In the differential diagnosis of this tumor, carcinoid and small cell carcinomas should be considered as well as common carcinomas, teratoid tumors, and poorly differentiated mesothelial tumors.

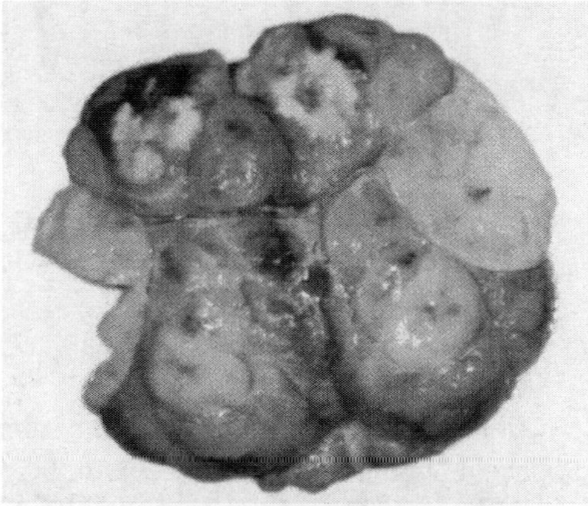

Figure 27. Gross view of a solid granulosa tumor with large yellowish nodules and small cystic spaces.

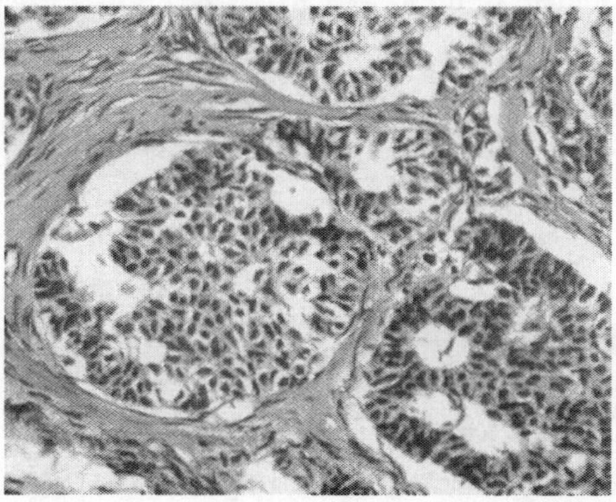

Figure 28. Histological section of a granulosa tumor showing multiple Call-Exner bodies and a follicular pattern of the uniform granulosa cells (X240).

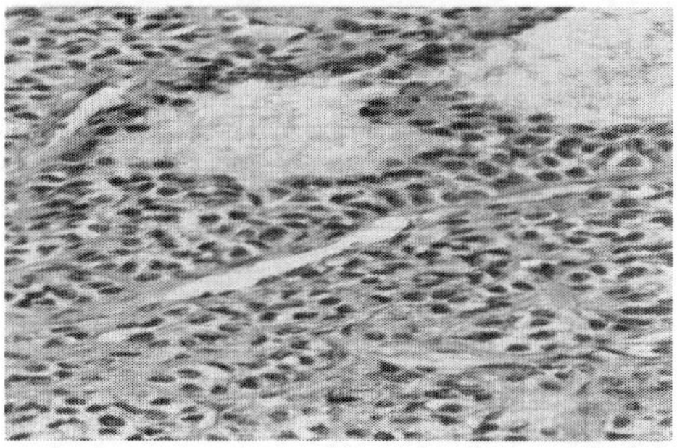

Figure 29. Histological section of a granulosa cell tumor with a macrofollicular pattern of cellular growth (X250).

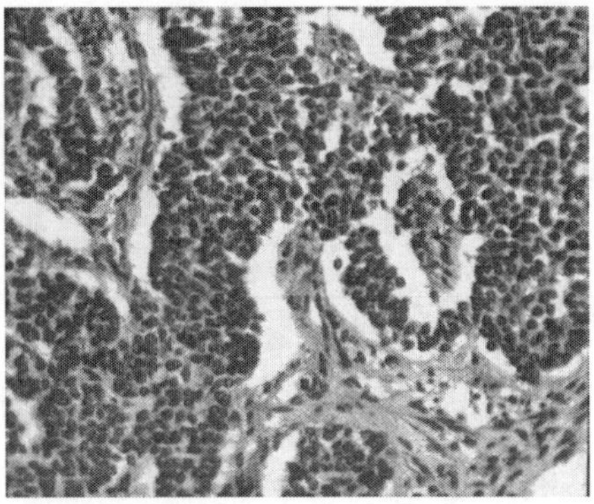

Figure 30. Histological section of a granulosa cell tumor showing atypical cells, absence of Call-Exner bodies and a similarity to a small cell carcinoma (X240).

Immunohistochemistry shows a positive immunoreaction of granulosa tumor cells to inhibin, CD 99,calretinin, vimentin, often a positive to ER, PgR, S100 and smooth muscle actin and a negative immunoreaction to cytokeratin 7, epithelial membrane antigen (EMA), Chromogranine and synaptophysine immunoreaction is negative.

The most characteristic feature which differentiates GCTs from carcinoid is that the granulosa cells, both normal and neoplastic, are devoid of cytoplasmic endocrine granules which are found in the cytoplasm of the neuroendocrine cells.

Prognosis

GCTs are characterized by their slow growth and late recurrence. Auranen et al. in a recent retrospective study of 35 patients showed that there was no difference in tumor size, nuclear atypia, mitotic index, presence of Call-Exner bodies, or Ki-67 staining between nonrecurred and recurred patients. In this study, the only factor associated with risk of recurrence was rupture of the tumor ($P < 0.0001$), and the only factor associated with overall survival was FIGO stage ($P = 0.032$). Most histologic types have the same prognosis, but patients with the more poorly differentiated diffuse or sarcomatoid type tend to do worse. The DNA ploidy of the tumors and Ki-67 expression, markers of cellular proliferation, have also been correlated with survival. Moreover, the disease-free and overall survivals were not statistically different between patients treated or not treated with adjuvant therapy. So, stage is clearly the most important prognostic factor. In a recent retrospective analysis, early-stage disease and age 50 or less were identified as statistically significant predictors of survival. The reported 5-year-survival rate for patients with Stage I disease ranges from 75% to greater than 90%. Recurrence is, however, associated with poor prognosis, with over 80% of patients succumbing to the disease.

In conclusion, GCTs have a low malignancy potential and generally have a good prognosis, but recurrences are very common even after many years post-treatment.

Ovarian Thecoma

Lastra and Collilas were the first to describe ovarian thecomas in 1926. They are also known as theca-cell tumors. They are usually estrogen-producing or hormonally inert tumors. They are tumors of the ovarian stroma and should be differentiated from fibromas. Thecomas are less common than granulosa-cell tumors accounting for 2% of all ovarian tumors. They present mainly in the peri- or postmenopausal period. The median age is 57.5 years. Less than 10% of patients are younger than 30 years of age. However, cases of thecomas which developed in a 30-month-old girl, as well as in a 92-year-old woman are reported in the literature. Thecomas are divided into typical and luteinized subtypes, the latter containing steroid-type cells resembling luteinized theca and luteinized stromal cells. Luteinized thecomas occur in a younger age group than typical thecomas. Fifty per cent of luteinized thecomas are estrogenic, 39% are nonfunctioning, and 11% are androgenic. Typical thecomas are stromal tumors composed of lipid-containing cells resembling those of the theca interna and may have a variable component of fibroblasts.

Pathogenesis

Rather than arising as a de novo tumor, thecomas may represent changes occurring in the background of cortical stromal hyperplasia. However, consistent numerical chromosomal aberrations were recently described. Trisomy 12 or tetrasomy 12 was identified in 71.5% of the cases with chromosomal abnormalities. Thecomas often show trisomy 12 and tetrasomy 12. Moreover, loss of heterozygosity at the *PTCH* gene, unaccompanied by losses at 19p13.3 was also seen in 25% of luteinized thecomas. Further cytogenetic and molecular genetic studies are necessary to understand the pathogenesis of thecomas.

Clinical Findings

The vast majority of thecomas consisting mainly of theca-like cells are benign tumors and asymptomatic except for symptoms of local pressure. Thecomas are rare causes of peripheral precocious puberty. Treatment is surgical and an excellent prognosis is possible for early stage disease. Premenopausal women may present menstrual disorders such as irregular menstruation. Estrogen-producing thecomas change the morphologic characteristics of the uterus to those of a woman of reproductive age and cause varying symptoms related to the enlarged uterus, especially thickened endometrium. They are associated with endocrine symptoms such as endometrial hyperplasia, especially in postmenopausal women may associated with endometrioid endometrial carcinoma. Sixty percent of postmenopausal patients present with uterine bleeding, and more than 20% have endometrial carcinoma. Moreover, six out of 13 cases of thecoma described by Sternberg and Gaskill (1950) were associated with uterine leiomyomas, another type of estrogen-dependent neoplasm.

Nocito et al. (2008) reported that thecomas appeared to be associated with endometrial hyperplasias in 15/50 patients, were an incidental finding in a gynecologic routine examination in 14/50 patients and were found during a cesarean delivery in 1/50 patients. During pregnancy, thecoma is an extremely rare finding. However, luteinized thecoma accounts for 20% of all ovarian tumors in pregnant women. Such patients could present with an estrogen-producing thecoma accompanied by accumulation of ascites in an early phase of pregnancy. The patient should undergo abdominal surgery to remove the tumor with excellent results for the mother and the fetus. Other authors propose treatment only if complications such as torsion or rupture appear.

Thecomas could rarely (in about 2% cases) cause raised circulating serum androgens leading even to acne, enlargement of clitoris, deepening of the voice, muscular development, androgenetic alopecia, frontal balding, and hirsuitism of women. Such symptoms are totally cured after surgical excision of the tumor. Exceptionally progesterone or corticosteroids are produced.

Thecomas are rarely associated with extensive sclerosing peritonitis. In such cases, the ovarian stromal proliferations are typically bilateral, can have an exceedingly high mitotic rate, often incorporate non-neoplastic ovarian structures at their periphery, and are responsive to medical treatment, and so they could lead to complete relief of symptoms and allow preservation of fertility.

Thecoma may also present as Meigs syndrome which is defined as the triad of a compact benign ovarian tumor with ascites and pleural effusion that resolves after resection of the tumor. The ovarian tumor in Meigs syndrome is usually a fibroma, however a thecoma is not a rare finding.

Physical examination usually reveals a unilateral tumor. The tumor size could range from a nonpalpable incidental finding to a large solid tumor with a diameter of 15 to 20 cm.

Ultrasound and CT imaging are used for the diagnosis. Ultrasound shows a solid mass with an intact capsule. Thecomas may manifest as an echogenic mass with distal acoustic attenuation, a well-defined hypo-echoic mass, or an anechoic lesion with through-transmission. Furthermore, secondary features of hyperestrogenism, such as endometrial thickening, could also be seen. CT scan of the abdomen and pelvis reveals a well-defined solid tumor of different size in the adnexal region. MRI scans could reveal thecoma components. Smaller thecomas have homogeneous low signal intensity on both T1- and T2-weighted images, while large thecomas have varying amounts of high-signal-intensity areas, which are caused by edema and cystic degeneration. Theca cells in the normal ovary are highly vascularized, whereas fibrous tissue is known for delayed weak enhancement at dynamic contrast-enhanced imaging. Therefore, the degree of contrast enhancement varies with the amount of fibrous tissue in the thecoma.

Management

The management of thecomas depends mainly on patient's age. An ovarian tumourectomy or unilateral salpingo-oophorectomy is proposed in cases with benign unilateral tumors in patients who desire to retain fertility, while a hysterectomy with bilateral salpingo-oophorectomy is performed in peri- or postmenopausal patients. Special attention is necessary during surgery, as thecomas are usually adherent to adjacent structures or rupture at the time of operation.

Pathology

Thecomas are benign unilateral ovarian tumors, round to oval, and relatively firm in consistency, weighting from a few up to 6000 grams. On section, thecomas present a characteristic whorled pattern resembling fibromas, except that thecomas are characteristically bright yellow in color.

Histologically, they are composed of spindle-shaped cells resembling theca cells of the ovarian follicle. They are formed by interlacing bundles of elongated epithelioid cells. The distinct whorled pattern is characteristic. The cytoplasm contains lipid granules, while small groups of vacuolated cells might be present, filled with fatty material, some of which is crystalloid and doubly refractive. Such cells could be identified with the cholesterol esters. Stromal hyalinization or interstitial edema could occasionally exist. The most characteristic finding of cellular steroid storage is their marked ad frequent luteinization. Special staining with Oil Red "O" shows the presence of lipid intracellularly, while reticulin stains reveal thecomas to be rich in reticulin fibers, a fact that helps in the differential diagnosis from granulosa cell tumors or fibromas. Thecomas are also considerably more likely to stain with inhibin and calretinin. Moreover, thecomas are rather vascular tumors. Furthermore, extensively calcified thecomas appear to occur in younger women. It should be noted that calcified thecomas are benign. Usual the mixed forms with elements resembling granulosa cells observed.

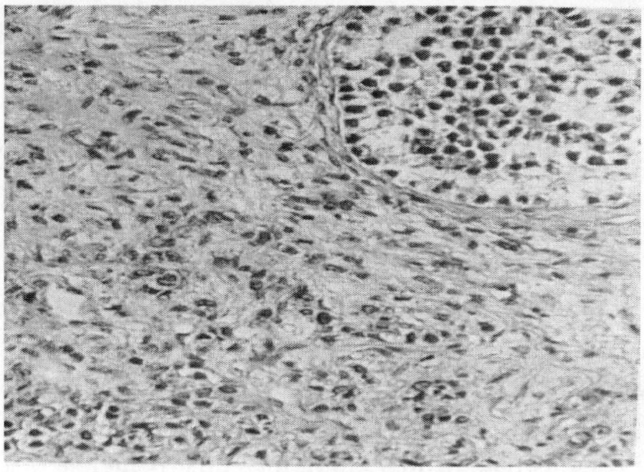

Figure 31. Histological section of thecoma showing an area (upper right) resembling granulosa cell tumor (X250).

Nocito et al. (2008) performed a retrospective study of 50 thecoma cases, studied to establish the most useful diagnostic criteria helpful in characterizing this ovarian stromal tumor. Arteries, veins, lymphatics, and mast cells are normally present in the ovarian medulla and are absent in the cortical area. Thecoma growth appeared to cause atrophy or compression of the ovarian cortical area and contained the above mentioned structures and these findings are significant for diagnosis and supported that this tumor originates in the ovarian medulla. It is proposed that fibroma and thecoma seem to be different neoplasms and should be considered distinct, separate entities because they have different origin, morphology, and potential functionality.

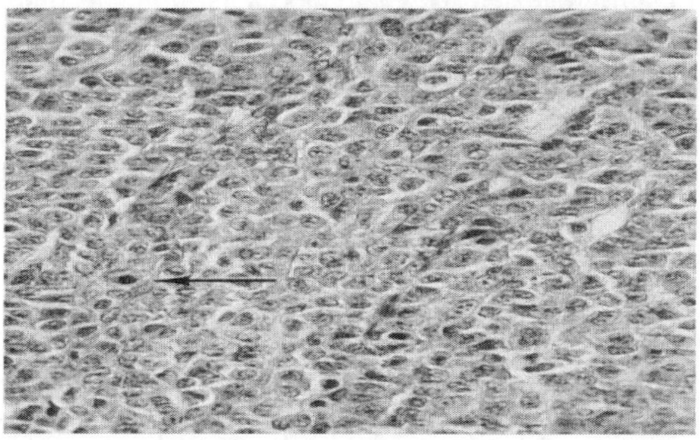

Figure 32. Histological section of a thecoma with mitotic activity (arrow) (X250).

Rare thecomas (2-5%) may show malignant change. In those cases, there is a marked increase in the cellularity of the tumor with cellular pleomorphism and prominent atypical mitoses.

The tumor is usually large and the sectioned surface shows hemorrhage and necrosis. Criteria for identifying malignant thecomas are the diffuse moderate or severe nuclear atypia and a usually high mitotic rate (4 or more MFs/10 HPFs). However, according to Waxman et al. (1979) most of the cases reported in the literature as malignant thecomas were either inadequately documented or misdiagnosed and were better interpreted as fibrosarcomas, stromal sarcomas, or granulosa cell tumors with a diffuse pattern of growth.

The differential diagnosis includes fibroma, granulosa cell tumor, thecomatosis and stromal hyperplasia. Thecomas often secrete clinically significant amounts of steroid hormones, whereas fibromas do not.

Prognosis

The prognosis is excellent. Thecomas are almost always benign and have low malignant potential. However, the prognosis of malignant thecomas is poor. More specifically, Wu et al. (2002) showed in a retrospective study that among eight patients with malignant thecoma, four without postoperative treatment or with non-standard chemotherapy died in the first two years of follow-up, the other four patients received an operation, post-operational radiotherapy and/or chemotherapy, 1 of 4 patients died of irradiation intestinal fistulae 4 years later; two patients were alive without disease more than 10 years, another one for 2 years. So, postoperative systemic chemotherapy or radiotherapy to the patients with malignant thecomas can improve their survival.

Ovarian Fibroma

Fibromas are pure ovarian stromal tumors. They account for 4% of all ovarian neoplasms. They most frequently occur in perimenopausal patients with a median age of 45 years. Rarely (1–1.6%), they present in childhood. They are usually hormonally inert, but may be accompanied by ascites and pleural effusion (Meigs' syndrome). Fibromas include typical fibroma, cellular fibroma and fibrosarcoma.

Pathogenesis

Fibromas arise from undifferentiated mesenchyme which normally furnishes the interstitial fibrous stroma of the ovary. Trisomy 12 or tetrasomy 12 was identified in cases with ovarian fibromas; however, they could be an age-related chromosomal abnormality. Loss of heterozygosity at the human homolog of the Drosophila patched gene (*PTCH*), localized on chromosome 9q22.3, is relatively frequent in cellular fibroma. Trisomy 8 cells were identified in fibrosarcoma cases.

Clinical Findings

They are usually found in peri- or postmenopausal women. In a recent retrospective study, 47.8% of the cases with ovarian typical fibromas were postmenopausal. They are usually unilateral (up to 92%) and nodular tumors. The smaller tumors are usually asymptomatic, while the larger tumors might produce symptoms caused by pressure on neighboring organs. On gynecological examinations, large fibromas are palpable masses that may reach up to the umbilicus area. The main presenting symptom is abdominal pain in 43.5%. Fibromas over 10 cm in diameter are associated with ascites in up to 40% of the cases and Meigs' syndrome in about 1% of the cases. Ascites is generated by a combination of inefficient lymphatic drainage through a small-for-size pedicle and a lack of a real tumor capsule to prevent leakage of lymph in the peritoneal cavity. Hydrothorax is secondary to ascites due to trans-diaphragmatic passage. Fibroma is also identified in women with a hereditary basal cell nevus syndrome, characterized by early-appearing basal cell carcinomas, keratocysts of the jaw, calcification of the dura, and mesenteric cysts (Gorlin syndrome). Torsion followed by acute abdominal findings is an occasional complication. Increased CA 125 is a common finding. Regarding cellular fibromas, they occur in patients with a mean age of 51 years, ranging from 24 to 88 years. It is approximately 10% as common as typical fibroma, and presents as an adnexal mass. There is no steroid hormone activity described or associated endometrial abnormalities causing uterine bleeding.

Fibrosarcoma although rare is the most common type of ovarian sarcoma. It tends to occur in older women (mean age: 58 years) presenting as a large mass.

Imaging

Fibromas can display a wide variety of ultrasound features. It usually appears as a hypoechoic mass with attenuation of the ultrasound beam and internal vascularity with high flow ($RI < 0.4$ or $PI > 1.0$) in Doppler evaluation. The occurrence of edema, cystic degeneration, hemorrhage, and calcification in fibromas will influence the ultrasound features. CT also appears to be non specific. It presents as a well-defined, solid mass with mild heterogeneity. An ovarian fibroma may calcify and/or exhibit cystic degeneration. MRI could show a large, primarily hypointense soft tissue mass with central areas of hyperintensity. It demonstrates low signal on T2 relative to the myometrium due to the predominantly fibrous composition of the mass.

Differential Diagnosis

It includes thecoma, fibromatosis, uterine fibroid and ovarian malignancy. The typical findings of a fibroma are residual primordial follicles at the periphery of the tumor. Both thecomas and fibromas are derived from ovarian stromal cells and it is not uncommon to have both components in a tumor. Tumors bearing a majority of cells with abundant lipid-laden vacuolated cytoplasm or those associated with estrogenic manifestations are classified as thecomas. Fibromatosis of the ovary may resemble a fibroma. It is characterized by small follicular cysts on the cut surface, and microscopically, fibromatosis is less cellular enveloping residual follicles. If follicles, corpora lutea, and corpora albicans are present in a fibroma, they are usually displaced to its periphery. Moreover, fibroma is not characterised by neither lipid-containing cells nor clinically abnormal endocrine functions.

Management

Exploratory laparotomy is performed followed by frozen section. Conservative surgery or total abdominal hysterectomy with bilateral salpingo-oophorectomy could be performed. Minimal-access surgery is an option, especially when the tumor is of moderate or small size. Meigs syndrome usually resolves after resection of the pelvic tumor.

Pathology

Typical fibromas are firm and white on section as shown in the picture.

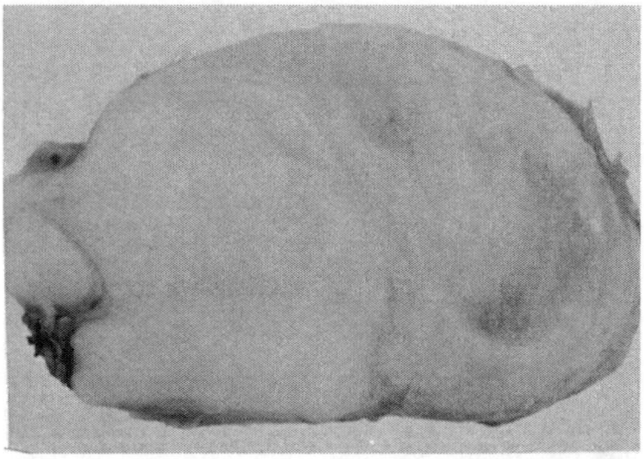

Figure 33. Gross view of a ovarian fibroma, solid, well circumscribed and white.

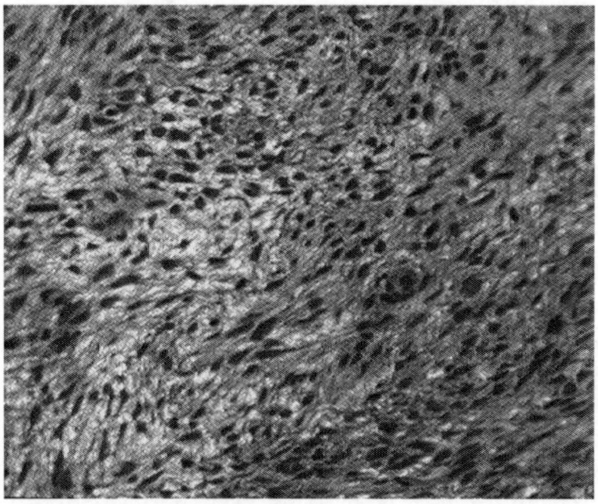

Figure 34. Histological section of a fibroma showing fibloblastic-like cells (X240).

Histologically fibromas consist of oval or round spindle cells resembling fibroblasts within an abundant collage. Mitotic figures are rare. The spindle-shaped cells are usually arranged in intersecting bundles and may occasionally form a storiform pattern. Hyaline plaques could also be found. Focal or extensive intercellular edema can be observed. Calcification is observed in less than 10% of cases. They do not contain stainable lipid. Immunohistochemically, the tumor cells stain for inhibin and calretinin in a minority of cases and are negative for fat stains (Oil Red "O") which are recommended to exclude thecomas.

Cellular fibromas grossly tend to be larger and softer than typical fibromas. They are usually whitish, but some are described as pale yellow or tan. They exhibit increased cellularity compared with typical fibroma, and no more than mild nuclear atypia with the exception that focally moderate nuclear atypia can be found in areas surrounding necrosis. The neoplastic cells often proliferate in an intersecting pattern, and the nuclei are typically elongated and spindle-shaped when sectioned longitudinally. The mitotic rate is 1- 3 mitotic figures/10 HPFs but no significant atypia is observed. Higher mitotic rate and atypia in a cellular fibroma is considered consistent with a neoplasm of low malignant potential, intermediate between typical fibroma and fibrosarcoma. Fibrosarcomas are large, solid tumors with foci of hemorrhage and necrosis. Histologically, they are densely cellular neoplasms composed of spindle-shaped cells exhibiting a herringbone or storiform pattern. The cells have amphi-philic or baseophilic cytoplasm, indistinct borders, and hyperchromatic nuclei with prominent nucleoli. Characteristic features include diffuse moderate-to-marked nuclear pleomorphism and usually > 4 MFs/10 HPFs. They have higher MIB-1 labeling and proliferative index than those of cellular fibroma and also show a gain in trisomy 8 cells that is not detected in the latter. However, they maintain a degree of resemblance to ovarian stromal cells in contrast to undifferentiated ovarian sarcoma.

Prognosis

Typical fibroma is a benign tumor, however, surgical removal of these solid ovarian tumors is recommended because of the low probability of malignancy. Long-term clinical follow-up is recommended in cases with cellular fibroma, as it is characterised by local recurrence or regional spread many years after excision of the primary neoplasm.

Sertoli-Stromal Cell Tumors (Androblastomas)

This group of tumors consist of pure forms or various combinations of Sertoli cells, Leydig cells, cells resembling rete epithelial cells and cells resembling stromal cells-fibroblasts. Some investigators prefer the term "androblastoma" to describe these tumors but in view of the fact that these neoplasms did not originate from male genital "blastema" and do not always produce androgens, the term Sertoli-Stromal tumors is preferable. The most clinically important forms will be presented.

Sertoli-Leydig Cell Tumors

Sertoli-Leydig cell tumor is a member of the sex cord-stromal tumor group. It was first described by Pick in 1905. It shows histological similarity to the embryonic testis. They are very rare tumors accounting for 0.2-0.5% of all ovarian tumors and according to WHO histological classification of ovarian tumors (2003), they are divided in the following categories:

1. Well-differentiated tumors or "tubular adenoma of pick"
2. Tumors of intermediate differentiation or "tubular type of Sertoli-Leydig cell tumor"
   a. tumors with heterologous elements
3. Poorly differentiated (sarcomatoid)
   a. With heterologous elements
4. Retiform type of Sertoli-Leydig cell tumor
   a. With heterologous elements

Pathogenesis

These tumors may result from an aborted differentiation of a primordial follicle and from the ovarian stroma. They represent a mixed mesodermal tumor containing epithelial Mullerian and testicular derivatives. A few cases have been identified in close relatives and so germ-line mutations in the DICER1 gene could be correlated. More specifically, in a recent study, DICER1 mutations in the RNase IIIb domain were found in 30 of 102 non-epithelial ovarian tumors (29%), predominantly in Sertoli-Leydig cell tumors (26 of 43, or 60%), including four tumors with additional germline DICER1 mutations.

Clinical Findings

The median age is 25 years, ranging from 2 to 79 years. Less than 10% of the tumors occur in women older than 50 years, and fewer than 5% occur in pre-pubertal girls. Well-differentiated types present in older ages (average 35 years), while a retiform variant occurs in younger age groups (average 15 years). These tumors usually exhibit as a pelvic or abdominal mass. Patients complain of abdominal swelling or pain. Most tumors are Stage I, unilateral and well circumscribed masses, averaging 10 cm in diameter. More specifically, in a recent study it was shown that the FIGO stage was: 81% IA, 4.8% IC, 4.8% IIB and 2 9.5% IIIC. 23.8% had G1 tumors, 47.6% had G2, and 28.6% had G3 in the same study.

Most tumors are clinically nonfunctional and in the case of tumors that produce hormones masculine or feminine phenotypes may be observed. In cases where there are Leydig cells present, androgens may be produced and this causes relevant clinical manifestations. Virilization develops in only 50% of patients leading to oligo-menorrhea followed by amenorrhea, breast atrophy, acne, hirsutism, temporal balding, deepening of the voice, and enlargement of the clitoris. In some cases patients may experience some form of estrogenic effect, such as endometrial hyperplasia (leading to menorrhagia or menometrorrhagia) or isosexual precocious pseudopuberty. Measurement of plasma androgens may reveal elevated testosterone and androstenedione, with normal or slightly elevated dehydroepiandrosterone sulphate. The serum AFP level may be increased and may be useful as a tumor marker.

Thyroid abnormalities may also coexist with the tumors. An association between Sertoli-Leydig cell tumors and Peutz-Jeghers syndrome has been reported.

Imaging

They generally appear as solid on ultrasound. As they are often richly vascularized, they may have a lower vascular resistive index, and may have peripheral necrosis. Malignant cases present neo-vascularization and distension of preexisting vessels, which result in a low resistance to blood flow. On CT, the tumor appears as a well-defined enhancing solid mass with intratumoral cysts, while it is hypointense with multiple variable-sized cystic areas on MRI. Low signal intensity on T2-weighted imaging depends on the extent of fibrous stroma. Multicystic areas develop as a result of heterologous elements.

Differential Diagnosis

The differential diagnosis includes ovarian papillary serous tumors and yolk sac tumors which present as large unilateral neoplasms with hemorrhage and necrosis. Papillary serous neoplasms demonstrate a positive cytokeratine 7, EMA, CAM5.2 and AE1/AE immunoreaction and yolk sac tumors which also occur in young females typically have an increased serum AFP. Other neoplasms included in the differential diagnosis are undifferentiated carcinoma, carcinoid tumor, struma ovarii, endometrioid carcinoma, or carcinosarcoma. Moreover, Sertoli-Leydig cell tumors should be distinguished from other virilizing tumors, such as adrenal tumors, which often are associated with an elevated urinary level of 17-ketosteroids.

Management

It usually depends on patients' age and tumor stage, degree of differentiation, and presence of heterologous elements in the tumor. Fertility-sparing surgery with a unilateral salpingo-oophorectomy is indicated, as the majority of these tumors are benign or early-stage malignant neoplasms (Stage Ia). De-bulking surgery, including hysterectomy and bilateral salpingo-oophorectomy, tumor resection, and staging procedure may be indicated in postmenopausal patients or those with more advanced disease. Rarely, they are poorly differentiated and aggressive. Chemotherapy is recommended but due to the rarity of these tumors no safe conclusions are reported. Platinum-based schemes have been used such as PAC, VBP, and BEP regimens. It seems that patients with advanced stage or grade 2-3 tumors appear to benefit from postoperative chemotherapy. Radiotherapy has also been used in a limited number of cases.

Pathology

Sertoli-Leydig cell tumors are grossly solid, yellow to brown, usually lobulated with a smooth external surface. Hemorrhage and necrosis frequently are seen in the poorly differentiated tumors. The microscopic examination of the differentiated subtype reveals hollow or solid tubules composed of Sertoli or Leydig cells interspersed with a fibrous stroma. Sertoli cells form tubules and Leydig cells are found in the intervening stroma. Sertoli cells are cytologically bland, and mitotic figures are rare. Leydig cells may contain abundant lipochrome pigment or crystalloids of Reinke.

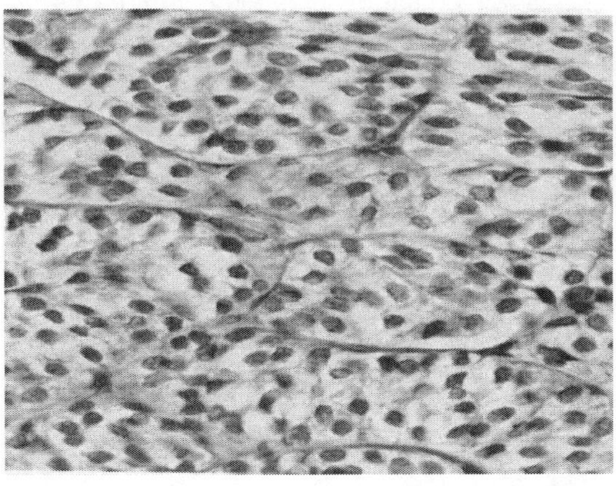

Figure 35. Histological section of a Sertoli cell tumor showing Sertoli cells lining tubules (X400).

The less differentiated histologic subtypes exhibit a less structured appearance characterized by more immature components of the Sertoli and Leydig cells. Cartilage, mucinous epithelium, skeletal muscle, and other heterologous elements are found in 20% to 25% of these tumors. When more heterologous elements exist, the tumors are clinically malignant. Moderate cytologic atypia, brisk mitotic activity, and tumor cell necrosis are indicators of greater malignant potential. To conclude, they are categorized into four subtypes, based on their microscopic characteristics; well differentiated (grade 1), intermediately differentiated (grade 2), poorly differentiated (grade 3) and retiform pattern. Immunohistochemistry is a useful aid in the correct diagnosis. EMA, inhibin, and chromogranin represent the most helpful triad of immunomarkers serving to exclude two common mimics of Sertoli cell tumors (endometrioid carcinoma [inhibin-; EMA+; chromogranin-] and carcinoid tumor [inhibin-; EMA+; chromogranin+]). WT-1, melan A, vimentin and calretinin are helpful in the diagnosis of poorly differentiated type.

Prognosis

Stage and tumor differentiation appear to be important prognostic factors. Young and Scully (1985) in a retrospective study of 207 cases, reported that 18% of the cases were malignant, while only 2.5% had spread beyond the limits of the ovary. The 5-year survival rate ranges from 70% to 90%. Recurrences are uncommon usually in rupture or leakage of the tumor before or during surgery, and if the woman has the very rare retiform or poorly differentiated lesions.

Conclusion

These tumors present a challenge to the gynecologist and pathologist and this mandates the need for a close collaboration, which is necessary for all of the tumors presented in this chapter.

References

Atlas of Tumor Pathology -3rd series, fascicle 23, Scully RE, Young RH Clement PB. *Tumors of the Ovary, Maldeveloped Gonads, Fallopian Tube and Broad Ligament,* Ed, J. Rosai, Armed Forces Institute of Pathology (AFIP), 1998, Washington, USA.

Chen VW, Ruiz B, Killeen JL, Coté TR, Wu XC, Correa CN. Pathology and classification of ovarian tumours. *Cancer.* 2003 May 15;97(10 Suppl):2631-42.

IARC WHO Classification of Tumors No4. *Pathology and genetics tumors of the breast and female genital system.* Tavassoli FA, DeViley P, 2003, IARC, Lyon.

Kurman RJ, Ellenson LH, Ronnett BM *Blaustein's Pathology of the Female Genital Tract*, 6th Ed, Springer New York, 2011.

Roth LM, Talerman A. Recent advances in the pathology and classification of ovarian germ cell tumors. *Int J Gynecol Pathol.* 2006 Oct;25(4):305-20.

Scully RE, Sobin LH, & Serov SF. Histological typing of ovarian tumors World Health Organization - International Histological Classification of Tumors, 2nd Ed, 1999, Springer-Verlag Berlin Heiderberg.

Talerman A, Roth LM. Recent advances in the pathology and classification of gonadal neoplasms composed of germ cells and sex cord derivatives. *Int J Gynecol Pathol.* 2007 Jul;26(3):313-21.

Chapter 11

The Role of Immunohistochemistry in Ovarian Tumors

Christos Valavanis*
Efthymia Souka
and Gabriela-Monica Stanc
Department of Pathology, Molecular Pathology Unit, Metaxa Cancer Hospital of Piraeus, Piraeus, Greece

Introduction

Ovarian cancer is the 6th most common malignancy and the 5th worldwide leading cause of death in women [1]. More than 70% of ovarian cancer cases are diagnosed at an advanced stage with a poor prognosis and the overall 5-year survival rate is around 49% [2].

A wide variety of tumors can be derived from ovarian tissue including mainly epithelial tumors (benign, border-line and malignant), sex cord-stromal tumors, germ cell tumors and mesenchymal tumors [3].

In this chapter we will focus mostly on the epithelial ovarian malignant tumors and in a lesser degree on sex cord-stomal and germ cell tumors of the ovary. We will present the role of immunohistochemistry in identifying them and differentially diagnosing them from other neoplasms.

Epithelial ovarian malignant tumors represent 90% of ovarian cancer cases. They comprise a heterogeneous group of neoplastic diseases with distinct morphologic features, pathogenetic mechanisms, molecular profiles, and clinical courses [3]. Based on pathologic, immunophenotypic and molecular features, epithelial ovarian malignant tumors are classified in five main subtypes: high-grade serous carcinoma (HGSC), low-grade serous carcinoma (LGSC), endometrioid, mucinous and clear cell carcinomas [3-5].

High-grade serous carcinoma is the most common subtype and is frequently related to *BRCA1* and *BRCA2* genetic alterations [6].

Less common types are seromucinous carcinoma, malignant Brenner tumor, mesonephric-like carcinoma, undifferentiated and dedifferentiated carcinomas and carcinosarcoma [3, 4].

The morphologic variation within these groups do not pose major diagnostic difficulties, although problems of differential diagnosis can arise between a primary ovarian

* Corresponding Author's Email: cvalapath@yahoo.com.

In: Ovarian Cancer
Editors: Christos Iavazzo, Alexandros Fotiou and John Spiliotis
ISBN: 979-8-88697-633-5

adenocarcinoma and a metastatic adenocarcinoma of gastrointestinal, mammary or pancreatobiliary origin. There might also be diagnostic difficulties in characterizing an endometrioid carcinoma of the ovary versus a sex cord stromal tumor of Sertoli or granulosa cell origin. Immunohistochemical analysis can also be helpful in identifying the origin of peritoneal disease in cases of intra-abdominal carcinomatosis and in distinguishing it from malignant mesothelioma [7, 8].

The use of immunohistochemical biomarkers has offered valuable assist in these diagnostic difficulties and might provide additional information in prognosis, prediction of therapeutic response and evaluation of post-treatment residual disease. Nevertheless, morphologic evaluation remains the mainstay in histopathological diagnosis.

Immunohistochemical Biomarkers

The majority of malignant epithelial tumors of the ovary are easily identifying based on their morphologic features and only a small number of antibodies are used in order to confirm the diagnosis. The most relevant of these antibodies are presented in the following sections.

Cytokeratin 7 (CK7)

CK7 is an intermediate filament protein expressed in a variety of epithelial cells of different organs. It is a type II basic low molecular weight cytokeratin (LMWCK) with a cytoplasmic and/or membranous expression pattern in ovarian malignant epithelial tumors. It should be evaluated along with other antibodies, because this cytokeratin is also expressed in a plethora of epithelial metastatic tumors of extra-ovarian origin [9-11].

Cytokeratin 20 (CK20)

CK20 is a type I acidic low molecular weight cytokeratin (LMWCK) expressed in primary mucinous ovarian tumors and in various metastatic carcinomas in the ovary of gastrointestinal or pancreatobiliary origin [10-12]. CK20 is also expressed in urothelial carcinoma and Merkel cell carcinoma [13]. The vast majority of primary ovarian non mucinous carcinomas are CK20 negative [14].

Carbohydrate Antigen 125 (CA 125)

CA 125 is a high molecular weight transmembrane glycoprotein expressed in primary non mucinous ovarian epithelial carcinomas and its extracellular domain can be recognized by the monoclonal antibody OC125 [15]. It should be evaluated carefully in the context of a panel of antibodies, taken into account that is also expressed in adenocarcinomas from other organs (breast, lung, colon, pancreas, thyroid) metastatic to the ovaries and in carcinomas of the cervix, endometrium and fallopian tube as well [16-19]. CA 125 also exhibits positive immunoreactivity in mesothelial proliferations and mesothelioma [20].

PAX8

PAX8 belongs to the paired box family of transcription factors that regulate organogenesis and is strongly and diffusely expressed in the nucleus of tumor cells of Müllerian tract origin [21]. PAX8 is also expressed in thyroid, parathyroid, renal and thymic carcinomas. It is very helpful in distinguishing primary malignant epithelial tumors of the ovary from malignant mesotheliomas and metastatic in the ovary, breast, lung and colon adenocarcinomas [22, 23]. It should be noted that focal weak staining is not specific and can be seen in many other tumors. Monoclonal antibodies are preferentially used, because polyclonal antibodies cross-react with PAX5 (B-cell lymphomas) and PAX6 (pancreatic islet cells and some neuroendocrine neoplasms) [24, 25].

Wilms Tumor 1 (WT1)

WT1 is a transcription factor involved in urogenital development with a tumor suppression function [26]. It is strongly expressed in the nucleus of neoplastic cells and positive immunoreactivity can be seen in a broad spectrum of tumors such as Wilms tumor, malignant mesothelioma, desmoplastic malignant melanoma, desmoplastic small round cell tumor, malignant and benign vascular tumors [27-29].

WT1 is normally expressed in the fallopian tube and ovarian surface epithelium and in inclusion cysts of the ovary as well. Malignant ovarian epithelial tumors display strong nuclear immunopositivity, with the highest percentage in serous carcinomas [30].

Other Immunohistochemical Markers

Antibodies useful in distinguishing primary malignant epithelial tumors of the ovary from malignant mesotheliomas are CD15, BerEP4, mCEA, B72.3 (TAG-72) and MOC-31.

CD15 displays positive granular cytoplasmic or membranous immunoreaction in ovarian serous, endometrioid and clear cell adenocarcinomas [8, 31].

Monoclonal antibody BerEP4 exhibits diffuse membranous positivity with high sensitivity in serous adenocarcinomas of the ovary and peritoneum [32].

Monoclonal CEA is positive in ovarian mucinous carcinomas and very rarely in serous adenocarcinomas. Polyclonal CEA is less specific than mCEA and can be positive in mucinous carcinomas and in a relatively higher percentage of ovarian carcinomas compared to mCEA [33].

B72.3 (TAG-72) is a sensitive monoclonal antibody that displays cytoplasmic immunopositivity in ovarian carcinomas [34].

Monoclonal MOC-31 antibody exhibits strong sensitive membranous expression pattern in almost all ovarian carcinomas [35].

All of the above mentioned antibodies are negative in mesotheliomas which show nuclear positivity against WT1 and calretinin and cytoplasmic immunoreaction against cytokeratin 5/6 and mesothelin [35, 36].

Malignant ovarian epithelial tumors can be distingushied from sex-cord stromal tumors by using a panel of antibodies such as inhibin A, calretinin, FOXL2, EMA and Steroidogenic Factor (SF-1) along with the above mentioned ones [37, 38].

Ovarian clear cell carcinoma should be differentiated from yolk sac tumor using antibodies against CK7, Napsin A (cytoplasmic expression in ovarian clear cell carcinoma), SALL4, Glypican-3 and AFP [38-41].

All these antibodies and their staining patterns are more precisely analysed in the next sections in the context of different ovarian cancer pathological entities.

Immunophenotypic Features of Epithelial Ovarian Tumors

Ovarian Serous Carcinomas (OSCs)

Ovarian serous carcinoma is the most common pathologic subtype of ovarian cancer and comprises a group of two distinct neoplastic disease entities, *high-grade serous carcinoma* (HGSC) and *low-grade serous carcinoma* (LGSC) with different histogenesis and clinical outcomes [3].

HGSCs are considered to arise from the surface epithelium or inclusion cysts of the ovary and/or the fimbrial end epithelium of the fallopian tube with putative precursor lesion the serous tubal intraepithelial carcinoma (STIC) [42-44].

On the other hand, LGSCs are thought to have a different histogenesis, arising from preexisting cystadenomas or serous borderline tumors and following a progression course through microinvasions to invasive carcinomas [45].

Immunohistochemical analysis can be useful in cases of small biopsies and in the evaluation of post-therapy specimens, in which ovarian clear cell carcinoma should be differentially diagnosed. Also, in cases of peritoneal carcinomatosis, immunohistochemical procedures should be performed in order to distinguish ovarian serous carcinoma from mesothelioma or other poorly differentiated carcinomas.

Both HGSCs and LGSCs exhibit positive immunoreactivity against CK7, PAX8, WT1, ER (estrogen receptor) and PgR (progesterone receptor) and these biomarkers are enough to establish an ovarian serous carcinoma diagnosis. In addition, 30% to 50% of HGSCs can show three different aberrant expression patterns for p53, strong, diffuse nuclear expression in > 80% of cells correlated with TP53 missense mutation, complete absence of expression implying loss of function mutation and cytoplasmic expression with intensity similar to wild-type immunoreactivity associated with loss of function mutation disrupting the nuclear localization signal domain [46-49]. HGSCs also display cytoplasmic and/or nuclear expression for p16 along with a high Ki-67 cell proliferation index (>75%) [50]. Conversely, LGSCs display patchy or negative expression for p16, low levels of Ki-67 proliferation index and wild-type immunoreactivity for p53 [46, 47].

In the differential diagnosis between mesotheliomas and ovarian serous carcinomas, a panel of various antibodies can be used such as PAX8, Ber-EP4, MOC-31, ER (positive expression in ovarian serous carcinomas) and Calretinin, CK5/6 (both positive in mesotheliomas) [8, 32].

A solid morphologic pattern can pose diagnostic difficulties between an ovarian serous carcinoma and a poorly differentiated endometrioid carcinoma. In such a case WT1, p53 and p16 can be used with diffuse strong staining in serous carcinoma [47-49, 51].

It should be noted that positive p53 immunoreactivity is also helpful in identifying small foci of intraepithelial carcinoma on the ovarian surface or in the fallopian tube epithelium.

Serous carcinoma of the endometrium is WT1 negative or focally weakly positive but p53 positive, thus metastatic serous carcinoma with this staining pattern should be considered of endometrial than ovarian origin [51].

WT1 positivity is also observed in serous borderline tumors and in sex cord-stromal tumors [52-54]. On the other hand, serous borderline and benign tumors show negative immunoreactivity for p53 [46, 52-54].

Ovarian Mucinous Carcinomas (OMCs)

Primary ovarian mucinous tumors are relatively rare, approximately 3% and most of the mucinous carcinomas in the ovary are of metastatic origin, particularly from the gastrointenstinal or pancreatobiliary tract [3, 55].

Ovarian mucinous tumors display a variety of lesions from cystadenoma areas to borderline mucinous tumor regions. Morphologically, there are two major histotypes, the intestinal and the endocervical. Intestinal type is more common than the endocervical. Both types can be encountered as borderline and malignant tumors, with the malignant counterpart of endocervical type, seromucinous carcinoma, is composed of serous and endocervical mucinous epithelium and is frequently associated with endometriosis [3, 55-57].

Immunohistochemistry can be useful in distinguishing primary ovarian mucinous carcinoma of intestinal type from metastatic ones. Antibodies used for this differential diagnosis are mainly CK7 and CK20, along with CDX2, SATB2, PAX8, ER, whereas mucinous ovarian tumors show diffuse immunopositivity for CK7 and focal positive immunoreaction for CK20 [56, 58, 59]. Metastatic mucinous carcinomas from the colon and appendix are negative for CK7 and diffusely positive for CK20 [58] It should be noted that microsatellite unstable (MSI high) right-sided colon adenocarcinomas can show diffuse CK7 positivity and CK20 negativity [60, 61]. The transcription factor CDX2 displays positive nuclear expression in adenocarcinomas from the gastrointestinal tract and is often positive in mucinous ovarian tumors, thus its utility in differential diagnosis between those tumors is limited [62-64]. In addition, PAX8, ER and PgR are positive in primary mucinous tumors of the ovary and can be used, but with caution because of their low sensitivity [65-67]. SATB2 is rarely expressed in ovarian mucinous tumors (5-7%), whereas appendiceal and colonic adenocarcinomas show high diffuse expression (82% in appendiceal and 88% in colorectal) [68, 69].

Differential diagnosis of primary ovarian mucinous tumors from metastatic pancreatobiliary adenocarcinomas is very challenging due to overlapping expression of different immunohistochemical markers. Both tumors have the same expression pattern for CK7 (positive), CK20 (negative) and CDX2 (often positive), on the other hand PAX8, ER and PgR may be helpful due to their positive immunoreaction in ovarian tumors [65-67]. In addition, pancreatic ductal adenocarcinomas show loss of SMAD4/DPC4 nuclear expression in 55% of the cases and positive IMP3 immunoreactivity in 90% ones [70-72], while ovarian mucinous tumors retains SMAD4/DPC4 expression, but are also positive for IMP3 which is an independent factor for ovarian tumor progression [70-72].

Distinction between primary ovarian mucinous tumor and metastatic gastric carcinoma can be made based on the expression of CA125 and PAX8 which are negative in gastric carcinomas and positive in 24% and 35% of ovarian mucinous carcinomas respectively [73].

Endocervical-type mucinous ovarian tumors and seromucinous carcinomas display diffuse immunoreactivity for PAX8, ER and PgR. Seromucinous carcinoma of the ovary should be distinguished from endometrioid ovarian carcinoma with mucinous differentiation. In this case, immunohistochemistry is not useful, the distinction is difficult and can be made based on the morphologic features (back-to-back glands) and expansile than infiltrative pattern of invasion [74-76].

Ovarian Endometrioid Carcinomas (OECs)

Endometrioid carcinomas of the ovary present as unilateral mass in the ovary, are associated with endometriosis and frequently arise from precursor lesions of adenofibroma or borderline tumors [77]. These tumors have a variety of morphologic features with characteristic back-to-back glands expansile rather than infiltrative pattern of invasion [3].

Immunohistochemistry can be helpful in distinguishing primary ovarian endometrioid carcinomas from metastatic colon carcinomas by using CK7, PAX8, ER and PgR markers which are mainly positive in endometrioid carcinomas and negative in colonic ones [78]. Approximately 33% of endometrioid carcinomas display membranous and/or cytoplasmic expression for vimentin [79]. Conversely, CK20 and CDX2 are positive in adenocarcinomas of the colon and negative in endometrioid carcinomas. It should be noted that microsatellite unstable (MSI high) right-sided colon adenocarcinomas can show diffuse CK7 positivity and CK20 negativity [60, 61] and CDX2 can be positive in the squamous morules of endometrioid tumors [80]. Squamous morules of endometrioid tumors also display intense CD10 cytoplasmic expression [81]. Endometrioid ovarian borderline tumors and carcinomas exhibit β-catenin membranous and/or cytoplasmic expression. Nuclear β-catenin expression is associated with *CTNNB1* mutations and favorable prognosis [82].

Sertoliform variants of endometrioid carcinoma can be differentiated from sex cord–stromal tumors by using EMA (positive in endometrioid tumors), inhibin and calretinin (both positive in sex cord stromal tumors) [83].

Differential diagnosis between high-grade endometrioid carcinomas with solid architectural pattern and high-grade serous carcinomas can be made based on the strong diffuse immunoreactivity of WT1, p53 and p16 in HGSCs, while ECs show patchy expression for p16, wild-type expression for p53 and loss of WT1 immunoreactivity [74, 84].

It is worth mentioning that almost 10% of patients with ovarian malignant tumors may present with synchronous endometrial cancer [85] Whether these tumors are metachronous metastatic from the endometrium or ovary to either site, or may be synchronous primaries can not be based on immunohistochemistry but rather on morphologic, clinical, radiologic and to a lesser degree molecular features [85-87]. Features favor the metastatic nature of an ovarian tumor from the endometrium are mainly, absence of ovarian endometriosis lesions, direct tissue invasion of the fallopian tube or ovary, hilar and surface ovarian epithelium involvement, presence of bilateral ovarian tumor masses and deep endometrial tumor invasion of the myometrium with lymphovascular involvement [88, 89]. Clinically, patients with synchronous ovarian and endometrial endometrioid carcinomas are premenopausal women of younger age and frequently characterized by obesity and nulliparity [88].

Ovarian Clear Cell Carcinomas (OCCCs)

Ovarian clear cell carcinomas comprise 10% of ovarian carcinomas, are frequently associated with endometriosis lesions and present mostly as unilateral mass in clinical stage I or II [90]. They have solid, tubular and papillary architectural patterns and are composed by neoplastic cells characterised as hobnail-like cells with clear cytoplasm and distinct nucleoli [3, 90].

Differential diagnosis of CCCs should be made among ECs and HGSCs because both these tumors can show clear cell change, sometimes due to prior therapy. Immunohistochemistry can be useful in distinguishing CCCs from the abovementioned tumors by using antibodies against WT1, ER, Napsin A and hepatocyte nuclear factor-1 beta (HNF1β) [91]. CCCs are negative for WT1 and ER, while HGSCs display positive immunoreactivity for both biomarkers and ECs show positivity for ER [91-93]. In addition, CCCs are strongly immunopositive for Napsin A (80-85%) and HNF1β (80-92%) [94, 95].

Yolk sac tumor might pose a differential diagnostic problem with ovarian clear cell carcinoma, due to morphologic similarities between these tumors. Clear cell carcinomas show positive expression for CK7, EMA, CD15, Napsin A and negative for glypican 3, SALL4 and AFP, whereas Yolk sac tumors display the opposite immunoprofile [96-98].

Clear cell renal cell carcinoma has also morphologic resemblance with clear cell carcinoma of the ovary. Differential diagnosis between these tumors can be made by using a panel of immunohistochemical markers such as CK7, CD10 and RCC. Clear cell renal cell carcinoma is negative for CK7 and positive for CD10 and RCC, whereas clear cell carcinoma of the ovary shows the opposite immunophenotype [99, 100]. Both neoplasms are positive for Pax-8 and HNF-1β [91, 101].

Brenner Tumors - Ovarian Transitional Cell Tumors

Ovarian Brenner tumors are neoplasms composed of transitional/urothelial-like epithelial cells in a fibromatous stroma. They comprise 1% to 2% of ovarian tumors and classified in three variants, benign, borderline and malignant tumors, based on architectural growth patterns, stromal invasion and morphological features of the neoplastic cells [3]. Histogenetically, these tumors may arise from Walthard rests, although the cell of origin is controversial [102]. Malignant Brenner tumor show stromal invasion and in most cases, areas of benign and borderline Brenner tumors can be found within the main tumor [103, 104].

Differential diagnosis between malignant Brenner tumor and metastatic transitional carcinoma of urothelial origin can be problematic. The distinction should be based on that metastatic urothelial carcinomas in the ovary are bilateral multinodular masses and lack a benign Brenner tumor component. Immunohistochemicaly both tumors are positive for GATA3, p63, uroplakin III, thrombomodulin and CK7 [105-107]. Brenner tumors are negative or weakly positive for CK20, while urothelial carcinomas are CK20 positive. Malignant Brenner tumors show loss or weak expression of p53 with mutant staining pattern, while benign and borderline Brenner tumors display loss or weak p53 expression with wildtype staining pattern. On the other hand high-grade metastatic urothelial carcinomas strongly express p53 with a diffuse mutant staining pattern [108, 109].

Distinction should also be made between malignant Brenner tumor and the transitional variant of HGSC. This variant is typically immunopositive for WT1, p53, p16 and ER, while Brenner tumors are negative [110].

Other Ovarian Epithelial Tumors

The immunophenotype of ovarian dedifferentiated and undifferentiated carcinoma are not well characterized. Dedifferentiated carcinoma is defined as the presence of an undifferentiated component in the context of a low-grade endometrioid carcinoma or the end point of the evolutionary process of HGSC, regardless of the percentage present in them. These tumors have a worse prognosis and should be managed accordingly [3, 111]. Ovarian undifferentiated carcinomas may express neuroendocrine biomarkers, but less than 10%. Expression of neuroendocrine markers with a diffuse staining pattern designate the presence of a neuroendocrine carcinoma, primary or metastatic to the ovary [112, 113]. Neuroendocrine carcinomas of small cell type can be of primary ovarian origin or of metastatic origin, more frequently from the lungs. TTF1 expression is not indicative of pulmonary origin of a small cell carcinoma metastatic to the ovary, because TTF1 can also be immunopositive in extrapulmonary small cell carcinomas [114, 115]. Both primary and metastatic neuroendocrine carcinomas show immunopositivity for NSE, CD56, synaptophysin and Chromogranin A. NSE and CD56 are nonspecific and thus their usefulness is limited. CD56 can also be positive in PNETs, rhabdomyosarcomas and sex cord stromal tumors, such as granulosa cell tumor, [116-118].

Another highly malignant neoplasm of neuroendocrine origin that can be found in the ovaries of mainly young women, is the small cell carcinoma of hypercalcemic type. This tumor shows positive diffuse immunoreactivity for EMA and cytokeratins, and focal staining for WT1, CD10, p53, NSE, chromogranin A, CD99 and vimentin [119, 120]. Small cell carcinoma of hypercalcemic type exhibits lack of *SMARCA4* (BRG1) expression, a finding that can be used for diagnosing SCOC-HT immunohistochemically [121, 122]. Absence of inhibin expression, weak staining of calretinin and diffuse positive expression of EMA and CD99 differentiate ovarian small cell carcinoma from juvenile granulosa cell tumor [123].

Immunophenotypic Features of Ovarian Sex Cord-Stromal Tumors (OSCSTs)

Ovarian sex cord-stromal tumors derive from the sex cord stroma or ovarian mesenchyme and comprise 5% to 12% of ovarian tumors [2, 3]. They are classified in mainly five groups: (1) Fibroma-Thecoma and related tumors, (2) Granulosa cell tumors, (3) Sertoli-Leydig cell tumors

(4) Sertoli cell tumors and (5) Leydig cell tumors. Other less common are sex cord tumor with annular tubules and steroid cell tumor [3, 124].

Fibroma – Thecoma and Related Tumors

Diagnosis of benign fibroma-thecoma is based on their morphologic features and rarely needs immunohistochemical staining. Fibromas are positive for FOXL2 and calretinin and rarely for inhibin. In the contrary thecomas are positive for both inhibin and calretinin and for FOXL2 and SMA as well [125-127].

Granulosa Cell Tumors

Granulosa cell tumors are divided in two types, the adult type which is more common and the juvenile type [3, 128].

Adult type granulosa cell tumors are neoplasms of low malignant potential with low mitotic and cell proliferation index, but can spread beyond the ovaries and tend to recur even after many years [129]. They compose of small uniform cells with microfollicular, insular, trabecular and diffuse architectural patterns. They are strongly and diffuse immunopositive for FOXL2, inhibin and calretinin [38]. Inhibin can also stain in a patchy pattern. They also display positive immunoreaction for low molecular weight cytokeratins in a patchy pattern, but are negative for EMA [130, 131]. These tumors frequently show positive immunoreactivity for WT1, SF1, CD99, SMA, CD56, S-100, ER and PgR [132-135].

Differential diagnosis should be made from poorly differentiated carcinomas and carcinoids. Poorly differentiated carcinomas are positive for cytokeratins such as CK7 or CK20 and for EMA, and negative for inhibin FOXL2 and calretinin [37, 38].

Carcinoids display the typical immunoprofile of neuroendocrine differentiation, are positive for cytokeratins and negative for FOXL2, inhibin and calretinin [37, 38].

Juvenile granulosa cell tumors occurs mainly in young persons but can also be found in postmenopausal women. They compose of large cells with atypical nuclei and distinct nucleoli with frequent mitotic figures. They share the same immunoprofile with adult type granulosa cell tumors [3, 128, 130, 131].

Immunohistochemical analysis can assist in differentiating juvenile granulosa cell tumor from ovarian small cell carcinoma of hypercalcemic type. Juvenile granulosa cell tumor displays immunopositivity for FOXL2, inhibin and CD99, whereas ovarian small cell carcinoma shows absence of inhibin and FOXL2 expression, weak staining of calretinin and diffuse positive expression of EMA [123, 125].

Sertoli-Leydig Cell Tumors

Sertoli-Leydig cell tumors occur mainly in young persons and are classified in well differentiated, intermediate and poorly differentiated variants with distinct morphologic features [3, 136]. Immunohistochemically Sertoli cells are positive for cytokeratins, WT1 and CD99 but negative for EMA. Leydig cells are cytokeratins and EMA negative [137-140]. These tumors display patchy staining for inhibin and calretinin and about 50% of them show FOXL2 positive immunoreaction [126]. Detection of DICER1 and FOXL2 mutations along with immunohistochemical analysis may provide a more effective approach for establishing the diagnosis of ovarian Sertoli-Leydig cell tumors. [141, 142].

Heterologous elements can be found in 20% of these tumors, with gastrointestinal epithelium the most common among them, showing positive immunoreactivity for EMA and cytokeratins and negative for inhibin [143]. Rarely hepatoid differentiation can occur in Sertoli-Leydig tumors exhibiting positive immunoreaction for CK8/18, HepPar1 and AFP and negative for inhibin [144, 145].

Differential diagnosis should be made from sertoliform variant of endometrioid carcinoma which displays immunopositivity for cytokeratins and EMA and is negative for inhibin, calretinin and FOXL2 [83, 146].

Sertoli Cell Tumors

Sertoli cell tumors are benign neoplasms that lack Leydig cells and the primitive stroma found in Sertoli-Leydig cell tumors [147]. They are positive for inhibin, calretinin, CD99, vimentin and cytokeratins and negative for EMA [146]. They should be distinguished from sertoliform variant of endometrioid carcinoma which display immunopositivity for cytokeratins and EMA and is negative for inhibin, calretinin and FOXL2 [83, 126, 146].

Leydig Cell Tumors

Leydig cell tumors are benign neoplasms secreting testosterone and compose of polygonal cells with characteristic cytoplasmic hyaline globules known as crystalloids of Reinke. Most of these tumors occur in the hilum of the ovary. Immunohistochemically these tumors are positive for inhibin, melan A, calretinin, and negative for cytokeratins and EMA [38, 123,125, 147, 148]. Insulin-like 3 (INSL3) immunohistochemical analysis can be used to differentiate Leydig cell hyperplasia from Leydig cell tumors. INSL3 is positive in Leydig cell hyperplasia whereas Leydig cell tumors are negative or display decreased expression [149].

Immunophenotypic Features of Ovarian Malignant Germ Cell Tumors (OMGCTs)

Ovarian germ cell tumors are classified in three groups. The first group includes benign cystic teratomas with tissues derived from different lines of differentiation or germ cell layers. The second group comprises monodermal cystic teratomas including struma ovarii, carcinoid tumors and a variety of somatic tumors such as adenocarcinoma, squamous cell carcinoma, melanoma and other malignant non-germ cell tumors arisen in benign cystic teratomas. The third group, on which we will focus in this chapter, comprises malignant GCTs including dysgerminoma, yolk sac tumor, embryonal carcinoma, choriocarcinoma, immature teratoma and mixed GCTs such as gonadoblastoma. These tumors are rare and tend to occur in young women [3, 150, 151].

Dysgerminoma

Dysgerminoma composes of large polygonal cells with well defined cell membrane, clear or eosinophilic cytoplasm, round nuclei and distinct nucleoli. It represents the ovarian analog of testicular seminoma [3, 152]. Immunohistochemically these tumors show diffuse cytoplasmic and membranous immunoreaction for placental alkaline phosphatase (PLAP) and podoplanin (D2-40), membranous immunopositivity for CD117/c-Kit and strong nuclear immunoreaction for pluripotency stem cell transcription factors OCT3/4, SALL4 and NANOG [153-157]. Positive cytoplasmic dot-like immunoreactivity in a patchy pattern can be seen for cytokeratins in some dysgerminoma cases [158]. EMA, CD30, S-100, neuroendocrine and lymphoid biomarkers are negative in dysgerminoma [158]. A small percentage of dysgerminomas (5%) contain areas of syncytiotrophoblastic giant cells that display strong cytoplasmic immunoreaction for β-human chrorionic gonadotropin (hCG) and cytokeratins [159-161]. RNA-binding protein LIN28 is another sensitive biomarker for dysgerminoma with cytoplasmic immunopositivity [162].

Yolk Sac Tumor

Yolk sac tumor is a malignant neoplasm of germ cell tumors and is characterized by different morphological patterns of growth. It arises from undifferentiated and multipotent embryonal carcinoma through differentiation towards yolk sac structures or endodermal somatic tissues [3, 163, 164].

Immunohistochemically, yolk sac tumor shows patchy or diffuse cytoplasmic immunopositivity for AFP and glypican-3, particularly the hepatoid variant of this tumor, although these markers can not differentiate this variant from hepatoid ovarian carcinoma or from metastatic hepatocellular carcinoma [165-168]. Yolk sac tumor displays strong cytoplasmic staining for pancytokeratin AE1/AE3 and for a broad spectrum of cytokeratins, but is negative for EMA, CK7 and CD15 [169, 170] Embryonal carcinoma shows membrane positive staining for CKAE1/AE3 and this pattern of expression can be used to differentiate embryonal carcinoma from yolk sac tumor. Yolk sac tumor is also positive for PLAP among other germ cell tumors [171]. ZBTB16 is a novel highly sensitive (100%) and specific (96%) biomarker for yolk sac tumor [183]. Other markers positive for yolk sac tumor are LIN28, CD117, IMP3 and SALL4. Negative markers are SOX2, D2-40, NANOG, OCT3/4 and CD30 [172-174]. Tissues with endodermal somatic differentiation can be positive for different relevant markers such CDX2 (intestinal), TTF1 (respiratory/foregut) or HepPar1 (hepatoid), but endometrioid glandular differentiation shows negative immunoreaction for ER and PgR [174].

Embryonal Carcinoma

Ovarian embryonal carcinoma is an uncommon malignant neoplasm and rarely occurs as a pure form. It occurs most often as a component of mixed germ cell tumors and immunochemistry can be useful in distinguishing embryonal carcinoma areas from other mixed tumor patterns [3, 175, 176]. As previously mentioned, membrane positive staining for CKAE1/AE3 is characteristic of embryonal carcinoma as opposed to the cytoplasmic staining seen in yolk sac tumor [177]. Embryonal carcinoma shows diffuse strong nuclear immunopositivity for OCT3/4, SALL4 and SOX2 and diffuse strong cytoplasmic staining for CD30 and LIN28 [39, 158, 162, 177]. It may also be patchy positive for AFP and for β-human chrorionic gonadotropin (hCG) in areas with syncytiotrophoblastic giant cells adjacent to tumor cells or isolated in the stroma [178].

Embryonal carcinoma displays negative immunoreaction for EMA, CD117 and podoplanin (D2-40). Diffuse positive immunoreactivity for cytokeratins and CD30 along with negative immunoreactivity for CD117 and D2-40 differentiate embryonal carcinoma from dysgerminoma [179].

Choriocarcinoma

Choriocarcinoma occurs most often as a component of mixed germ cell tumors of the ovary and is composed of syncytiotrophoblastic, cytotrophoblastic and intermediate trophoblastic cells [3, 180-182].

Syncytiotrophoblastic giant cells show cytoplasmic positivity for β-human chrorionic gonadotropin (hCG), pancytokeratin AE1/AE3 and inhibin. [184-186]. Cytotrophoblastic cells are positive for β-catenin [188], whereas intermediate trophoblastic cells are positive for CD10 and pancytokeratin and negative for EMA [184-188]. Intermediate mononucleate trophoblasts are also positive for MUC-4, HLA-G, and Mel-CAM [188]. In addition, transcriptomics and immunohistochemical studies demonstrated that HLA-G might be a predictive biomarker for gestational choriocarcinoma resistance to monochemotherapy [189-191].

Immature Teratomas

Immature teratomas are composed of tissues from the three germ layers along with the presence of immature embryonal structures and immature neuroectodermal tissue [3, 192-194].

Glial tissue is abundant in immature neuroectodermal tissues which are positive for glial fibrillary acidic protein (GFAP) and glial cell line–derived neurotrophic factor receptor α-1 (GFR-α1) [195, 196]. Neuroectodermal elements like neuroepithelial tubules and trabeculae show high cell proliferation index Ki-67 and this staining can be used to differentiate immature teratomas from mature teratomas which show low proliferative activity [196, 197]. Immunohistochemical stainings are not necessary for the diagnosis, which is mainly morphological, however immunohistochemistry can be used to identify immature neuroectodermal elements and immunopositivity for different antibodies such as SALL4, SOX2, Oct4, glypican-3, Fascin, CD99, CDX2 and others has been observed in immature teratoma tissues of different origin [196-200].

Conclusion

In general, the diagnosis of ovarian neoplasms is based mainly on morphological features and immunohistochemistry can assist in confirming the diagnosis, distinguishing the different ovarian histiotypes and differentially diagnosed a metastatic tumor in the ovary from a primary one.

Immunohistochemical data should be interpreted very carefully and always in the context of histological patterns and cytological features. It is also worthy to mention that immunohistochemical procedures should be performed strictly and standardised accordingly to the different antibodies used, taken into account all the necessary preanalytical parameters.

From a prognostic and therapeutic viewpoint, pathologic stage and tumor grade rather than histiotype and immunoprofile are the most important factors to determine the biological behavior of an ovarian neoplasm and make therapeutic decisions, However, this approach may change based on additional information from molecular pathology and precision medicine studies which can lead to novel molecular biomarkers for prognostication and personalized therapy.

References

[1] Momenimovahed, Z., Tiznobaik, A., Taheri, S., and Salehiniya, H. (2019). Ovarian cancer in the world: epidemiology and risk factors. *Int J Womens Health*., Apr 30, 11, 287-299.

[2] *Cancer statistics-Ovarian Cancer*. 2011-2017. https://seer.cancer.gov/statfacts/html/ovary.html.

[3] WHO Classification of Tumors Editorial Board. *WHO classification of tumours: female genital tumours.* vol. 4. 5th edition. Lyon (France): International Agency for Research on Cancer; 2020.

[4] Romero, I., Leskelä, S., Mies, B. P., Velasco, A. P., and Palacios, J. (2020). Morphological and molecular heterogeneity of epithelial ovarian cancer: Therapeutic implications. *EJC Suppl*., Aug 22, 15, 1-15.

[5] Prat, J., D'Angelo, E., and Espinosa, I. (2018). Ovarian carcinomas: at least five different diseases with distinct histological features and molecular genetics. *Hum Pathol*., Oct, 80, 11-27.

[6] Matulonis, U. A., Sood, A. K., Fallowfield, L., Howitt, B. E., Sehouli, J., and Karlan, B. Y. (2016). Ovarian cancer. *Nat Rev Dis Primers*., Aug 25, 2, 16061.

[7] McCluggage, W. G., and Wilkinson, N. (2005). Metastatic neoplasms involving the ovary: a review with an emphasis on morphological and immunohistochemical features. *Histopathology*., Sep, 47(3), 231-47.

[8] Ordóñez, N. G. (1998). Role of immunohistochemistry in distinguishing epithelial peritoneal mesotheliomas from peritoneal and ovarian serous carcinomas. *Am J Surg Pathol*., Oct, 22(10), 1203-14.

[9] Moll, R., Franke, W. W., Schiller, D. L., Geiger, B., and Krepler, R. (1982). The catalog of human cytokeratins: patterns of expression in normal epithelia, tumors and cultured cells. *Cell*., Nov, 31(1), 11-24.

[10] Lagendijk, J. H., Mullink, H., van Diest, P. J., Meijer, G. A., and Meijer, C. J. (1999). Immunohistochemical differentiation between primary adenocarcinomas of the ovary and ovarian metastases of colonic and breast origin. Comparison between a statistical and an intuitive approach. *J Clin Pathol*., Apr, 52(4), 283-90.

[11] Cathro, H. P., and Stoler, M. H. (2002). Expression of cytokeratins 7 and 20 in ovarian neoplasia. *Am J Clin Pathol*., Jun, 117(6), 944-51.

[12] Moll, R., Löwe, A., Laufer, J., and Franke, W. W. (1992). Cytokeratin 20 in human carcinomas. A new histodiagnostic marker detected by monoclonal antibodies. *Am J Pathol*., Feb, 140(2), 427-47.

[13] Miettinen, M. (1995). Keratin 20: immunohistochemical marker for gastrointestinal, urothelial, and Merkel cell carcinomas. *Mod Pathol*., May, 8(4), 384-8.

[14] Tot, T. (2002). Cytokeratins 20 and 7 as biomarkers: usefulness in discriminating primary from metastatic adenocarcinoma. *Eur J Cancer*., Apr, 38(6), 758-63.

[15] Bast, R. C. Jr, Xu, F. J., Yu, Y. H., Barnhill, S., Zhang, Z., and Mills, G. B. (1998). CA 125: the past and the future. *Int J Biol Markers*., Oct-Dec, 13(4), 179-87.

[16] Koelma, I. A., Nap, M., Rodenburg, C. J., and Fleuren, G. J. (1987). The value of tumour marker CA 125 in surgical pathology. *Histopathology*., Mar, 11(3), 287-94. doi: 10.1111/j.1365-2559.

[17] Loy, T. S., Quesenberry, J. T., and Sharp, S. C. (1992). Distribution of CA 125 in adenocarcinomas. An immunohistochemical study of 481 cases. *Am J Clin Pathol*., Aug, 98(2), 175-9.

[18] Keen, C. E., Szakacs, S., Okon, E., Rubin, J. S., and Bryant, B. M. (1999). CA125 and thyroglobulin staining in papillary carcinomas of thyroid and ovarian origin is not completely specific for site of origin. *Histopathology*., Feb, 34(2), 113-7.

[19] Devan, S. M., Pailoor, J., Sthaneshwar, P., and Narayanan, V. (2013). Pattern of tissue expression of CA-125 and HE4 in primary epithelial ovarian tumours and correlation with serum CA-125 levels. *Asian Pac J Cancer Prev*., 14(8), 4545-8.

[20] Friedman, M. T., Gentile, P., Tarectecan, A., and Fuchs, A. (1996). Malignant mesothelioma: immunohistochemistry and DNA ploidy analysis as methods to differentiate mesothelioma from benign reactive mesothelial cell proliferation and adenocarcinoma in pleural and peritoneal effusions. *Arch Pathol Lab Med*., Oct, 120(10), 959-66.

[21] Ordóñez, N. G. (2012). Value of PAX2 immunostaining in tumor diagnosis: a review and update. *Adv Anat Pathol*., Nov, 19(6), 401-9.

[22] Laury, A. R., Perets, R., Piao, H., Krane, J. F., Barletta, J. A., French, C., Chirieac, L. R., Lis, R., Loda, M., Hornick, J. L., Drapkin, R., and Hirsch, M. S. (2011). A comprehensive analysis of PAX8 expression in human epithelial tumors. *Am J Surg Pathol*., Jun, 35(6), 816-26.

[23] Khizer, K., Padda, J., Khedr, A., Tasnim, F., Al-Ewaidat, O. A., Patel, V., Ismail, D., Campos, V. Y. M., and Jean-Charles, G. (2021). Paired-Box Gene 8 (PAX8) and Its Association With Epithelial Carcinomas. *Cureus*., Aug 16, 13(8), e17208.

[24] Toriyama, A., Mori, T., Sekine, S., Yoshida, A., Hino, O., and Tsuta, K. (2014). Utility of PAX8 mouse monoclonal antibody in the diagnosis of thyroid, thymic, pleural and lung tumours: a comparison with polyclonal PAX8 antibody. *Histopathology*., Oct, 65(4), 465-72.

[25] Moretti, L., Medeiros, L. J., Kunkalla, K, Williams, M. D., Singh, R. R., and Vega, F. (2012). N-terminal PAX8 polyclonal antibody shows cross-reactivity with N-terminal region of PAX5 and is responsible for reports of PAX8 positivity in malignant lymphomas. *Mod Pathol*., Feb, 25(2), 231-6.

[26] Lee, S. B., and Haber, D. A. (2001). Wilms tumor and the WT1 gene. *Exp Cell Res*., Mar 10, 264(1), 74-99.

[27] Salvatorelli, L., Parenti, R., Leone, G., Musumeci, G., Vasquez, E., and Magro, G. (2015). Wilms tumor 1 (WT1) protein: Diagnostic utility in pediatric tumors. *Acta Histochem*., May-Jun, 117(4-5), 367-78.

[28] Tandon, R. T., Jimenez-Cortez, Y., Taub, R., and Borczuk, A. C. (2018). Immunohistochemistry in Peritoneal Mesothelioma: A Single-Center Experience of 244 Cases. *Arch Pathol Lab Med*., Feb, 142(2), 236-242.

[29] Lae, M. E., Roche, P. C., Jin, L., Lloyd, R. V., and Nascimento, A. G. (2002). Desmoplastic small round cell tumor: a clinicopathologic, immunohistochemical, and molecular study of 32 tumors. *Am J Surg Pathol*., Jul, 26(7), 823-35.

[30] Shimizu, M., Toki, T., Takagi, Y., Konishi, I., and Fujii, S. (2000). Immunohistochemical detection of the Wilms' tumor gene (WT1) in epithelial ovarian tumors. *Int J GynecolPathol*., Apr, 19(2), 158-63.

[31] Ramalingam, P., Malpica, A., Silva, E. G., Gershenson, D. M., Liu, J. L., and Deavers, M. T. (2004). The use of cytokeratin 7 and EMA in differentiating ovarian yolk sac tumors from endometrioid and clear cell carcinomas. *Am J Surg Pathol*., Nov, 28(11), 1499-505.

[32] Ordóñez, N. G. (2006). Value of immunohistochemistry in distinguishing peritoneal mesothelioma from serous carcinoma of the ovary and peritoneum: a review and update. *Adv Anat Pathol*., Jan, 13(1), 16-25

[33] Neunteufel, W., and Breitenecker, G. (1989). Tissue expression of CA 125 in benign and malignant lesions of ovary and fallopian tube: a comparison with CA 19-9 and CEA. *Gynecol Oncol*., Mar, 32(3), 297-302.

[34] Ponnusamy, M. P., Venkatraman, G., Singh, A. P., Chauhan, S. C., Johansson, S. L., Jain, M., Smith, L., Davis, J. S., Remmenga, S. W., and Batra, S. K. (2007). Expression of TAG-72 in ovarian cancer and its correlation with tumor stage and patient prognosis. *Cancer Lett*., Jun 28, 251(2), 247-57.

[35] Ordóñez, N. G. (2006). The diagnostic utility of immunohistochemistry and electron microscopy in distinguishing between peritoneal mesotheliomas and serous carcinomas: a comparative study. *Mod Pathol.*, Jan, 19(1), 34-48.
[36] Chapel, D. B., Schulte, J. J., Husain, A. N., and Krausz, T. (2020). Application of immunohistochemistry in diagnosis and management of malignant mesothelioma. *Transl Lung Cancer Res.*, Feb, 9(Suppl 1), S3-S27.
[37] Young, R. H. (2018). Ovarian sex cord-stromal tumours and their mimics. *Pathology.*, Jan, 50(1), 5-15.
[38] Rabban, J. T., and Zaloudek, C. J. (2013). A practical approach to immunohistochemical diagnosis of ovarian germ cell tumours and sex cord-stromal tumours. *Histopathology.*, Jan, 62(1), 71-88.
[39] Ulbright, T. M. (2005). Germ cell tumors of the gonads: a selective review emphasizing problems in differential diagnosis, newly appreciated, and controversial issues. *Mod Pathol.*, Feb, 18 Suppl 2, S61-79.
[40] Cao, D., Guo, S., Allan, R. W., Molberg, K. H., and Peng, Y. (2009). SALL4 is a novel sensitive and specific marker of ovarian primitive germ cell tumors and is particularly useful in distinguishing yolk sac tumor from clear cell carcinoma. *Am J Surg Pathol.*, Jun, 33(6), 894-904.
[41] Yamashita, Y., Nagasaka, T., Naiki-Ito, A., Sato, S., Suzuki, S., Toyokuni, S., Ito, M., and Takahashi, S. (2015). Napsin A is a specific marker for ovarian clear cell adenocarcinoma. *Mod Pathol.*, Jan, 28(1), 111-7.
[42] Li, H. X., Lu, Z. H., Shen, K., Cheng, W. J., Malpica, A., Zhang, J., Wei, J. J., Zhang, Z. H., and Liu, J. (2014). Advances in serous tubal intraepithelial carcinoma: correlation with high grade serous carcinoma and ovarian carcinogenesis. *Int J Clin Exp Pathol.*, Feb 15, 7(3), 848-57
[43] Shih, I. M., Wang, Y., and Wang, T. L. (2021). The Origin of Ovarian Cancer Species and Precancerous Landscape. *Am J Pathol.*, Jan, 191(1), 26-39.
[44] Zhang, S., Dolgalev, I., Zhang, T., Ran, H., Levine, D. A., and Neel, B. G. (2019). Both fallopian tube and ovarian surface epithelium are cells-of-origin for high-grade serous ovarian carcinoma. *Nat Commun.*, Nov 26, 10(1), 5367.
[45] Slomovitz, B., Gourley, C., Carey, M. S., Malpica, A., Shih, I. M., Huntsman, D., Fader, A. N., Grisham, R. N., Schlumbrecht, M., Sun, C. C., Ludemann, J., Cooney, G. A., Coleman, R., Sood, A. K., Mahdi, H., Wong, K. K., Covens, A., O'Malley, D. M., Lecuru, F., Cobb, L. P., Caputo, T. A., May, T., Huang, M., Siemon, J., Fernández, M. L., Ray-Coquard, I., and Gershenson, D. M. (2020). Low-grade serous ovarian cancer: State of the science. *Gynecol Oncol.*, Mar, 156(3), 715-725.
[46] O'Neill, C. J., Deavers, M. T., Malpica, A., Foster, H., and McCluggage, W. G. (2005). An immunohistochemical comparison between low-grade and high-grade ovarian serous carcinomas: significantly higher expression of p53, MIB1, BCL2, HER-2/neu, and C-KIT in high-grade neoplasms. *Am J Surg Pathol.*, Aug, 29(8), 1034-41.
[47] Manu, V., Hein, T. A., Boruah, D., and Srinivas, V. (2020). Serous ovarian tumors: Immunohistochemical profiling as an aid to grading and understanding tumorigenesis. *Med J Armed Forces India.*, Jan, 76(1), 30-36.
[48] Köbel, M., Piskorz, A. M., Lee, S., Lui, S., LePage, C., Marass, F., Rosenfeld, N., Mes Masson, A. M., and Brenton, J. D. (2016). Optimized p53 immunohistochemistry is an accurate predictor of *TP53* mutation in ovarian carcinoma. *J Pathol Clin Res.*, Jul 13, 2(4), 247-258.
[49] Köbel, M., Ronnett, B. M., Singh, N., Soslow, R. A., Gilks, C. B., and McCluggage, W. G. (2019). Interpretation of P53 Immunohistochemistry in Endometrial Carcinomas: Toward Increased Reproducibility. *Int J GynecolPathol.*, Jan, 38 Suppl 1(Iss 1 Suppl 1), S123-S131.
[50] Chen, M., Yao, S., Cao, Q., Xia, M., Liu, J., and He, M. (2016). The prognostic value of Ki67 in ovarian high-grade serous carcinoma: an 11-year cohort study of Chinese patients. *Oncotarget.*, Dec 23, 8(64), 107877-107885.
[51] Al-Hussaini, M., Stockman, A., Foster, H., and McCluggage, W. G. (2004). WT-1 assists in distinguishing ovarian from uterine serous carcinoma and in distinguishing between serous and endometrioid ovarian carcinoma. *Histopathology.*, Feb, 44(2), 109-15.

[52] Hashi, A., Yuminamochi, T., Murata, S., Iwamoto, H., Honda, T., and Hoshi, K. (2003). Wilms tumor gene immunoreactivity in primary serous carcinomas of the fallopian tube, ovary, endometrium, and peritoneum. *Int J GynecolPathol.*, Oct, 22(4), 374-7.

[53] Waldstrøm, M., and Grove, A. (2005). Immunohistochemical expression of wilms tumor gene protein in different histologic subtypes of ovarian carcinomas. *Arch Pathol Lab Med.*, Jan, 129(1), 85-8.

[54] Zhao, C., Vinh, T. N., McManus, K., Dabbs, D., Barner, R., and Vang, R. (2009). Identification of the most sensitive and robust immunohistochemical markers in different categories of ovarian sex cord-stromal tumors. *Am J Surg Pathol.*, Mar, 33(3), 354-66.

[55] Cheasley, D., Wakefield, M. J., Ryland, G. L., Allan, P. E., Alsop, K., Amarasinghe, K. C., Ananda, S., Anglesio, M. S., Au-Yeung, G., Böhm, M., Bowtell, D. D. L., Brand, A., Chenevix-Trench, G., Christie, M., Chiew, Y. E., Churchman, M., DeFazio, A., Demeo, R., Dudley, R., Fairweather, N., Fedele, C. G., Fereday, S., Fox, S. B., Gilks, C. B., Gourley, C., Hacker, N. F., Hadley, A. M., Hendley, J., Ho, G. Y., Hughes, S., Hunstman, D. G., Hunter, S. M., Jobling, T. W., Kalli, K. R., Kaufmann, S. H., Kennedy, C. J., Köbel, M., Le Page, C., Li, J., Lupat, R., McNally, O. M., McAlpine, J. N., Mes-Masson, A. M., Mileshkin, L., Provencher, D. M., Pyman, J., Rahimi, K., Rowley, S. M., Salazar, C., Samimi, G., Saunders, H., Semple, T., Sharma, R., Sharpe, A. J., Stephens, A. N., Thio, N., Torres, M. C., Traficante, N., Xing, Z., Zethoven, M., Antill, Y. C., Scott, C. L., Campbell, I. G., and Gorringe, K. L. (2019). The molecular origin and taxonomy of mucinous ovarian carcinoma. *Nat Commun.*, Sep 2, 10(1), 3935.

[56] Lin, X., Lindner, J. L., Silverman, J. F., and Liu, Y. (2008). Intestinal type and endocervical-like ovarian mucinous neoplasms are immunophenotypically distinct entities. *Appl Immunohistochem Mol Morphol.*, Oct, 16(5), 453-8.

[57] Taga, Y., Chigusa, Y., Minamiguchi, S., Kido, A., Horikawa, N., Horie, A., Hamanishi, J., Kondoh, E., Mandai, M., and Yamaguchi, K. (2020). Three cases of seromucinous carcinoma of the ovary arising in endometriotic cysts. *Int Cancer Conf J.*, Sep 21, 10(1), 46-53.

[58] Vang, R., Gown, A. M., Barry, T. S., Wheeler, D. T., Yemelyanova, A., Seidman, J. D., and Ronnett, B. M. (2006). Cytokeratins 7 and 20 in primary and secondary mucinous tumors of the ovary: analysis of coordinate immunohistochemical expression profiles and staining distribution in 179 cases. *Am J Surg Pathol.*, Sep, 30(9), 1130-9.

[59] Vang, R., Gown, A. M., Wu, L. S., Barry, T. S., Wheeler, D. T., Yemelyanova, A., Seidman, J. D., and Ronnett, B. M. (2006). Immunohistochemical expression of CDX2 in primary ovarian mucinous tumors and metastatic mucinous carcinomas involving the ovary: comparison with CK20 and correlation with coordinate expression of CK7. *Mod Pathol.*, Nov, 19(11), 1421-8.

[60] Chapusot, C., Martin, L., Bouvier, A. M., Bonithon-Kopp, C., Ecarnot-Laubriet, A., Rageot, D., Ponnelle, T., Laurent Puig, P., Faivre, J., and Piard, F. (2002). Microsatellite instability and intratumoural heterogeneity in 100 right-sided sporadic colon carcinomas. *Br J Cancer.*, Aug 12, 87(4), 400-4.

[61] Bayrak, R., Yenidünya, S., and Haltas, H. (2011). Cytokeratin 7 and cytokeratin 20 expression in colorectal adenocarcinomas. *Pathol Res Pract.*, Mar 15, 207(3), 156-60.

[62] Werling, R. W., Yaziji, H., Bacchi, C. E., and Gown, A. M. (2003). CDX2, a highly sensitive and specific marker of adenocarcinomas of intestinal origin: an immunohistochemical survey of 476 primary and metastatic carcinomas. *Am J Surg Pathol.*, Mar, 27(3), 303-10.

[63] Groisman, G. M., Meir, A., and Sabo, E. (2004). The value of Cdx2 immunostaining in differentiating primary ovarian carcinomas from colonic carcinomas metastatic to the ovaries. *Int J GynecolPathol.*, Jan, 23(1), 52-7.

[64] Tornillo, L., Moch, H., Diener, P. A., Lugli, A., and Singer, G. (2004). CDX-2 immunostaining in primary and secondary ovarian carcinomas. *J Clin Pathol.*, Jun, 57(6), 641-3.

[65] AtesOzdemir, D., and Usubutun, A. (2016). PAX2, PAX8 and CDX2 Expression in Metastatic Mucinous, Primary Ovarian Mucinous and Seromucinous Tumors and Review of the Literature. *Pathol Oncol Res.*, Jul, 22(3), 593-9.

[66] Sieh, W., Köbel, M., Longacre, T. A., Bowtell, D. D., DeFazio, A., Goodman, M. T., Høgdall, E., Deen, S., Wentzensen, N., Moysich, K. B., Brenton, J. D., Clarke, B. A., Menon, U., Gilks, C. B., Kim, A., Madore, J., Fereday, S., George, J., Galletta, L., Lurie, G., Wilkens, L. R., Carney, M. E.,

Thompson, P. J., Matsuno, R. K., Kjær, S. K., Jensen, A., Høgdall, C., Kalli, K. R., Fridley, B. L., Keeney, G. L., Vierkant, R. A., Cunningham, J. M., Brinton, L. A., Yang, H. P., Sherman, M. E., García-Closas, M., Lissowska, J., Odunsi, K., Morrison, C., Lele, S., Bshara, W., Sucheston, L., Jimenez-Linan, M., Driver, K., Alsop, J., Mack, M., McGuire, V., Rothstein, J. H., Rosen, B. P., Bernardini, M. Q., Mackay, H., Oza, A., Wozniak, E. L., Benjamin, E., Gentry-Maharaj, A., Gayther, S. A., Tinker, A. V., Prentice, L. M., Chow, C., Anglesio, M. S., Johnatty, S. E., Chenevix-Trench, G., Whittemore, A. S., Pharoah, P. D., Goode, E. L., Huntsman, D. G., and Ramus, S. J. (2013). Hormone-receptor expression and ovarian cancer survival: an Ovarian Tumor Tissue Analysis consortium study. *Lancet Oncol.*, Aug, 14(9), 853-62. doi: 10.1016/S1470-2045(13)70253-5.

[67] Tkalia, I. G., Vorobyova, L. I., Svintsitsky, V. S., Nespryadko, S. V., Goncharuk, I. V., Lukyanova, N. Y., and Chekhun, V. F. (2014). Clinical significance of hormonal receptor status of malignant ovarian tumors. *Exp Oncol.*, Jun, 36(2), 125-33.

[68] Schmoeckel, E., Kirchner, T., and Mayr, D. (2018). SATB2 is a supportive marker for the differentiation of a primary mucinous tumor of the ovary and an ovarian metastasis of a low-grade appendiceal mucinous neoplasm (LAMN): A series of seven cases. *Pathol Res Pract.*, Mar, 214(3), 426-430.

[69] Meagher, N. S., Wang, L., Rambau, P. F., Intermaggio, M. P., Huntsman, D. G., Wilkens, L. R., El-Bahrawy, M. A., Ness, R. B., Odunsi, K., Steed, H., Herpel, E., Anglesio, M. S., Zhang, B., Lambie, N., Swerdlow, A. J., Lubiński, J., Vierkant, R. A., Goode, E. L., Menon, U., Toloczko-Grabarek, A., Oszurek, O., Bilic, S., Talhouk, A., García-Closas, M., Wang, Q., Tan, A., Farrell, R., Kennedy, C. J., Jimenez-Linan, M., Sundfeldt, K., Etter, J. L., Menkiszak, J., Goodman, M. T., Klonowski, P., Leung, Y., Winham, S. J., Moysich, K. B., Behrens, S., Kluz, T., Edwards, R. P., Gronwald, J., Modugno, F., Hernandez, B. Y., Chow, C., Kelemen, L. E., Keeney, G. L., Carney, M. E., Natanzon, Y., Robertson, G., Sharma, R., Gayther, S. A., Alsop, J., Luk, H., Karpinskyj, C., Campbell, I., Sinn, P., Gentry-Maharaj, A., Coulson, P., Chang-Claude, J., Shah, M., Widschwendter, M., Tang, K., Schoemaker, M. J., Koziak, J. M., Cook, L. S., Brenton, J. D., Daley, F., Kristjansdottir, B., Mateoiu, C., Larson, M. C., Harnett, P. R., Jung, A., DeFazio, A., Gorringe, K. L., Pharoah, P. D. P., Minoo, P., Stewart, C., Bathe, O. F., Gui, X., Cohen, P., Ramus, S. J., and Köbel, M. (2019). A combination of the immunohistochemical markers CK7 and SATB2 is highly sensitive and specific for distinguishing primary ovarian mucinous tumors from colorectal and appendiceal metastases. *Mod Pathol.*, Dec, 32(12), 1834-1846.

[70] Ji, H., Isacson, C., Seidman, J. D., Kurman, R. J., and Ronnett, B. M. (2002). Cytokeratins 7 and 20, Dpc4, and MUC5AC in the distinction of metastatic mucinous carcinomas in the ovary from primary ovarian mucinous tumors: Dpc4 assists in identifying metastatic pancreatic carcinomas. *Int J GynecolPathol.*, Oct, 21(4), 391-400.

[71] Burdelski, C., Jakani-Karimi, N., Jacobsen, F., Möller-Koop, C., Minner, S., Simon, R., Sauter, G., Steurer, S., Clauditz, T. S., and Wilczak, W. (2018). IMP3 overexpression occurs in various important cancer types and is linked to aggressive tumor features: A tissue microarray study on 8,877 human cancers and normal tissues. *Oncol Rep.*, Jan, 39(1), 3-12.

[72] Zhu, Q., Qu, Y., Zhang, Q., Lu, L., Weng, W., Zhang, H., Zhang, L., Ning, Y., and Wang, Y. (2017). IMP3 is upregulated in primary ovarian mucinous carcinoma and promotes tumor progression. *Am J Transl Res.*, Jul 15, 9(7), 3387-3398.

[73] McCluggage, W. G. (2012). Immunohistochemistry in the distinction between primary and metastatic ovarian mucinous neoplasms. *J Clin Pathol.*, Jul, 65(7), 596-600.

[74] Tabrizi, A. D., Kalloger, S. E., Köbel, M., Cipollone, J., Roskelley, C. D., Mehl, E., and Gilks, C. B. (2010). Primary ovarian mucinous carcinoma of intestinal type: significance of pattern of invasion and immunohistochemical expression profile in a series of 31 cases. *Int J GynecolPathol.*, Mar, 29(2), 99-107.

[75] Taylor, J., and McCluggage, W. G. (2015). Ovarian seromucinous carcinoma: report of a series of a newly categorized and uncommon neoplasm. *Am J Surg Pathol.*, Jul, 39(7), 983-92.

[76] Shappell, H. W., Riopel, M. A., Smith Sehdev, A. E., Ronnett, B. M., and Kurman, R. J. (2002). Diagnostic criteria and behavior of ovarian seromucinous (endocervical-type mucinous and mixed cell-

type) tumors: atypical proliferative (borderline) tumors, intraepithelial, microinvasive, and invasive carcinomas. *Am J Surg Pathol.*, Dec, 26(12), 1529-41.

[77] Terada, T. (2012). Endometrioid adenocarcinoma of the ovary arising in atypical endometriosis. *Int J Clin Exp Pathol.*, 5(9), 924-7.

[78] Assem, H., Rambau, P. F., Lee, S., Ogilvie, T., Sienko, A., Kelemen, L. E., and Köbel, M. (2018). High-grade Endometrioid Carcinoma of the Ovary: A Clinicopathologic Study of 30 Cases. *Am J Surg Pathol.*, Apr, 42(4), 534-544.

[79] Köbel, M., Rahimi, K., Rambau, P. F., Naugler, C., Le Page, C., Meunier, L., de Ladurantaye, M., Lee, S., Leung, S., Goode, E. L., Ramus, S. J., Carlson, J. W., Li, X., Ewanowich, C. A., Kelemen, L. E., Vanderhyden, B., Provencher, D., Huntsman, D., Lee, C. H., Gilks, C. B., and Mes Masson, A. M. (2016). An Immunohistochemical Algorithm for Ovarian Carcinoma Typing. *Int J GynecolPathol.*, Sep, 35(5), 430-41.

[80] Houghton, O., Connolly, L. E., and McCluggage, W. G. (2008). Morules in endometrioid proliferations of the uterus and ovary consistently express the intestinal transcription factor CDX2. *Histopathology.*, Aug, 53(2), 156-65.

[81] Chiarelli, S., Buriticá, C., Litta, P., Ciani, S., Guarch, R., and Nogales, F. F. (2006). An immunohistochemical study of morules in endometrioid lesions of the female genital tract: CD10 is a characteristic marker of morular metaplasia. *Clin Cancer Res.*, Jul 15, 12(14 Pt 1), 4251-6.

[82] Zyla, R. E., Olkhov-Mitsel, E., Amemiya, Y., Bassiouny, D., Seth, A., Djordjevic, B., Nofech-Mozes, S., and Parra-Herran, C. (2021). CTNNB1 Mutations and Aberrant β-Catenin Expression in Ovarian Endometrioid Carcinoma: Correlation With Patient Outcome. *Am J Surg Pathol.*, Jan, 45(1), 68-76.

[83] Misir, A., and Sur, M. (2007). Sertoliform endometrioid carcinoma of the ovary: a potential diagnostic pitfall. *Arch Pathol Lab Med.*, Jun, 131(6), 979-81.

[84] Lim, D., Murali, R., Murray, M. P., Veras, E., Park, K. J., and Soslow, R. A. (2016). Morphological and Immunohistochemical Reevaluation of Tumors Initially Diagnosed as Ovarian Endometrioid Carcinoma With Emphasis on High-grade Tumors. *Am J Surg Pathol.*, Mar, 40(3), 302-12.

[85] Yoneoka, Y., Yoshida, H., Ishikawa, M., Shimizu, H., Uehara, T., Murakami, T., and Kato, T. (2019). Prognostic factors of synchronous endometrial and ovarian endometrioid carcinoma. *J Gynecol Oncol.* Jan, 30(1), e7.

[86] Ishikawa, M., Nakayama, K., Nakamura, K., Ono, R., Yamashita, H., Ishibashi, T., Minamoto, T., Iida, K., Razia, S., Ishikawa, N., and Kyo, S. (2019). High frequency of POLE mutations in synchronous endometrial and ovarian carcinoma. *Hum Pathol.*, Mar, 85, 92-100.

[87] Reijnen, C., Küsters-Vandevelde, H. V. N., Ligtenberg, M. J. L., Bulten, J., Oosterwegel, M., Snijders, M. P. L. M., Sweegers, S., de Hullu, J. A., Vos, M. C., van der Wurff, A. A. M., van Altena, A. M., Eijkelenboom, A., and Pijnenborg, J. M. A. (2020). Molecular profiling identifies synchronous endometrial and ovarian cancers as metastatic endometrial cancer with favorable clinical outcome. *Int J Cancer.*, Jul 15, 147(2), 478-489.

[88] Heitz, F., Amant, F., Fotopoulou, C., Battista, M. J., Wimberger, P., Traut, A., Fisseler-Eckhoff, A., Harter, P., Vandenput, I., Sehouli, J., Schmidt, M., Kimmig, R., du Bois, R., and du Bois, A. (2014). Synchronous ovarian and endometrial cancer--an international multicenter case-control study. *Int J Gynecol Cancer.*, Jan, 24(1), 54-60.

[89] Stewart, C. J. R., Crum, C. P., McCluggage, W. G., Park, K. J., Rutgers, J. K., Oliva, E., Malpica, A., Parkash, V., Matias-Guiu, X., and Ronnett, B. M. (2019). Guidelines to Aid in the Distinction of Endometrial and Endocervical Carcinomas, and the Distinction of Independent Primary Carcinomas of the Endometrium and Adnexa From Metastatic Spread Between These and Other Sites. *Int J GynecolPathol.*, Jan, 38 Suppl 1(Iss 1 Suppl 1), S75-S92.

[90] Iida, Y., Okamoto, A., Hollis, R. L., Gourley, C., and Herrington, C. S. (2021). Clear cell carcinoma of the ovary: a clinical and molecular perspective. *Int J Gynecol Cancer.*, Apr, 31(4), 605-616.

[91] Köbel, M., Kalloger, S. E., Carrick, J., Huntsman, D., Asad, H., Oliva, E., Ewanowich, C. A., Soslow, R. A., and Gilks, C. B. (2009). A limited panel of immunomarkers can reliably distinguish between clear cell and high-grade serous carcinoma of the ovary. *Am J Surg Pathol.*, Jan, 33(1), 14-21.

[92] Fadare, O., and Parkash, V. (2019). Pathology of Endometrioid and Clear Cell Carcinoma of the Ovary. *Surg Pathol Clin.*, Jun, 12(2), 529-564.

[93] Lim, D., Ip, P. P., Cheung, A. N., Kiyokawa, T., and Oliva, E. (2015). Immunohistochemical Comparison of Ovarian and Uterine Endometrioid Carcinoma, Endometrioid Carcinoma With Clear Cell Change, and Clear Cell Carcinoma. *Am J Surg Pathol*., Aug, 39(8), 1061-9.

[94] Skirnisdottir, I., Bjersand, K., Akerud, H., and Seidal, T. (2013). Napsin A as a marker of clear cell ovarian carcinoma. *BMC Cancer*., Nov 5, 13, 524.

[95] Li, Q., Zeng, X., Cheng, X., Zhang, J., Ji, J., Wang, J., Xiong, K., Qi, Q., and Huang, W. (2015). Diagnostic value of dual detection of hepatocyte nuclear factor 1 beta (HNF-1β) and napsin A for diagnosing ovarian clear cell carcinoma. *Int J Clin Exp Pathol*., Jul 1, 8(7), 8305-10.

[96] Esheba, G. E., Pate, L. L., and Longacre, T. A. (2008). Oncofetal protein glypican-3 distinguishes yolk sac tumor from clear cell carcinoma of the ovary. *Am J Surg Pathol*., Apr, 32(4), 600-7.

[97] Cao, D., Guo, S., Allan, R. W., Molberg, K. H., and Peng, Y. (2009). SALL4 is a novel sensitive and specific marker of ovarian primitive germ cell tumors and is particularly useful in distinguishing yolk sac tumor from clear cell carcinoma. *Am J Surg Pathol*., Jun, 33(6), 894-904.

[98] Ramalingam, P., Malpica, A., Silva, E. G., Gershenson, D. M., Liu, J. L., and Deavers, M. T. (2004). The use of cytokeratin 7 and EMA in differentiating ovarian yolk sac tumors from endometrioid and clear cell carcinomas. *Am J Surg Pathol*., Nov, 28(11), 1499-505.

[99] Cameron, R. I., Ashe, P., O'Rourke, D. M., Foster, H., and McCluggage, W. G. (2003). A panel of immunohistochemical stains assists in the distinction between ovarian and renal clear cell carcinoma. *Int J Gynecol Pathol*., Jul, 22(3), 272-6.

[100] Zhou, M., Roma, A., and Magi-Galluzzi, C. (2005). The usefulness of immunohistochemical markers in the differential diagnosis of renal neoplasms. *Clin Lab Med*., Jun, 25(2), 247-57.

[101] Kato, N., and Motoyama, T. (2009). Hepatocyte nuclear factor-1beta (HNF-1beta) in human urogenital organs: its expression and role in embryogenesis and tumorigenesis. *Histol Histopathol*., Nov, 24(11), 1479-86.

[102] Kuhn, E., Ayhan, A., Shih IeM, Seidman, J. D., and Kurman, R. J. (2014). The pathogenesis of atypical proliferative Brenner tumor: an immunohistochemical and molecular genetic analysis. *Mod Pathol*., Feb, 27(2), 231-7.

[103] Zheng, R., and Heller, D. S. (2019). Borderline Brenner Tumor: A Review of the Literature. *Arch Pathol Lab Med*., Oct, 143(10), 1278-1280.

[104] Zhang, Y., Staley, S. A., Tucker, K., and Clark, L. H. (2019). Malignant Brenner tumor of the ovary: Case series and review of treatment strategies. *Gynecol Oncol Rep*., Feb 12, 28, 29-32.

[105] Ordóñez, N. G., and Mackay, B. (2000). Brenner tumor of the ovary: a comparative immunohistochemical and ultrastructural study with transitional cell carcinoma of the bladder. *Ultrastruct Pathol*., May-Jun, 24(3), 157-67.

[106] Ogawa, K., Johansson, S. L., and Cohen, S. M. (1999). Immunohistochemical analysis of uroplakins, urothelial specific proteins, in ovarian Brenner tumors, normal tissues, and benign and neoplastic lesions of the female genital tract. *Am J Pathol*., Oct, 155(4), 1047-50.

[107] Liao, X. Y., Xue, W. C., Shen, D. H., Ngan, H. Y., Siu, M. K., and Cheung, A. N. (2007). p63 expression in ovarian tumours: a marker for Brenner tumours but not transitional cell carcinomas. *Histopathology*. Oct, 51(4), 477-83.

[108] Cuatrecasas, M., Catasus, L., Palacios, J., and Prat, J. (2009). Transitional cell tumors of the ovary: a comparative clinicopathologic, immunohistochemical, and molecular genetic analysis of Brenner tumors and transitional cell carcinomas. *Am J Surg Pathol*., Apr, 33(4), 556-67.

[109] Prat, J. (1999). Ovarian tumors of borderline malignancy (tumors of low malignant potential): a critical appraisal. *Adv Anat Pathol*., Sep, 6(5), 247-74.

[110] Magrill, J., Karnezis, A. N., Tessier-Cloutier, B., Talhouk, A., Kommoss, S., Cochrane, D., Chow, C., Cheng, A., Soslow, R., Hauptmann, S., du Bois, A., Pfisterer, J., Gilks, C. B., Huntsman, D. G., and Kommoss, F. (2019). Tubo-Ovarian Transitional Cell Carcinoma and High-grade Serous Carcinoma Show Subtly Different Immunohistochemistry Profiles. *Int J Gynecol Pathol*., Nov, 38(6), 552-561.

[111] Tafe, L. J., Garg, K., Chew, I., Tornos, C., and Soslow, R. A. (2010). Endometrial and ovarian carcinomas with undifferentiated components: clinically aggressive and frequently underrecognized neoplasms. *Mod Pathol*., Jun, 23(6), 781-9.

[112] Yasuda, M., Kajiwara, H., Osamura, Y. R., Hirasawa, T., Muramatsu, T., Murakami, M., Takagi, M., Tadokoro, M., Kobayashi, Y., Inayama, Y., Miyagi, E., and Nakatani, Y. (2006). Ovarian carcinomas with neuroendocrine differentiation: Review of five cases referring to immunohistochemical characterization. *J Obstet Gynaecol Res.*, Aug, 32(4), 387-95.

[113] Veras, E., Deavers, M. T., Silva, E. G., and Malpica, A. (2007). Ovarian nonsmall cell neuroendocrine carcinoma: a clinicopathologic and immunohistochemical study of 11 cases. *Am J Surg Pathol.*, May, 31(5), 774-82.

[114] Volante, M., Birocco, N., Gatti, G., Duregon, E., Lorizzo, K., Fazio, N., Scagliotti, G. V., and Papotti, M. (2014). Extrapulmonary neuroendocrine small and large cell carcinomas: a review of controversial diagnostic and therapeutic issues. *Hum Pathol.*, Apr, 45(4), 665-73.

[115] van der Heijden, H. F., and Heijdra, Y. F. (2005). Extrapulmonary small cell carcinoma. *South Med J.*, Mar, 98(3), 345-9.

[116] McCluggage, W. G., McKenna, M., and McBride, H. A. (2007). CD56 is a sensitive and diagnostically useful immunohistochemical marker of ovarian sex cord-stromal tumors. *Int J Gynecol Pathol.*, Jul, 26(3), 322-7.

[117] Ohishi, Y., Kaku, T., Oya, M., Kobayashi, H., Wake, N., and Tsuneyoshi, M. (2007). CD56 expression in ovarian granulosa cell tumors, and its diagnostic utility and pitfalls. *Gynecol Oncol.*, Oct, 107(1), 30-8.

[118] Mechtersheimer, G., Staudter, M., and Möller, P. (1991). Expression of the natural killer cell-associated antigens CD56 and CD57 in human neural and striated muscle cells and in their tumors. *Cancer Res.*, Feb 15, 51(4), 1300-7.

[119] McCluggage, W. G., Oliva, E., Connolly, L. E., McBride, H. A., and Young, R. H. (2004). An immunohistochemical analysis of ovarian small cell carcinoma of hypercalcemic type. *Int J Gynecol Pathol.*, Oct, 23(4), 330-6.

[120] Young, R. H., Oliva, E., and Scully, R. E. (1994). Small cell carcinoma of the ovary, hypercalcemic type. A clinicopathological analysis of 150 cases. *Am J Surg Pathol.*, Nov, 18(11), 1102-16.

[121] Jelinic, P., Schlappe, B. A., Conlon, N., Tseng, J., Olvera, N., Dao, F., Mueller, J. J., Hussein, Y., Soslow, R. A., and Levine, D. A. (2016). Concomitant loss of SMARCA2 and SMARCA4 expression in small cell carcinoma of the ovary, hypercalcemic type. *Mod Pathol.*, Jan, 29(1), 60-6.

[122] Genestie, C., Blanc-Durand, F., Auguste, A., Pautier, P., Dunant, A., Scoazec, J. Y., Gouy, S., Morice, P., Bentivegna, E., Maulard, A., LeFormal, A., Devouassoux-Shisheboran, M., and Leary, A. (2020). Clinical utility of SMARCA4 testing by immunohistochemistry in rare ovarian tumours. *Br J Cancer.*, Feb, 122(4), 564-568.

[123] Riopel, M. A., Perlman, E. J., Seidman, J. D., Kurman, R. J., and Sherman, M. E. (1998). Inhibin and epithelial membrane antigen immunohistochemistry assist in the diagnosis of sex cord-stromal tumors and provide clues to the histogenesis of hypercalcemic small cell carcinomas. *Int J Gynecol Pathol.*, Jan, 17(1), 46-53.

[124] Hanley, K. Z., and Mosunjac, M. B. (2019). Practical Review of Ovarian Sex Cord-Stromal Tumors. *Surg Pathol Clin.*, Jun, 12(2), 587-620.

[125] Movahedi-Lankarani, S., and Kurman, R. J. (2002). Calretinin, a more sensitive but less specific marker than alpha-inhibin for ovarian sex cord-stromal neoplasms: an immunohistochemical study of 215 cases. *Am J Surg Pathol.*, Nov, 26(11), 1477-83.

[126] Al-Agha, O. M., Huwait, H. F., Chow, C., Yang, W., Senz, J., Kalloger, S. E., Huntsman, D. G., Young, R. H., and Gilks, C. B. (2011). FOXL2 is a sensitive and specific marker for sex cord-stromal tumors of the ovary. *Am J Surg Pathol.*, Apr, 35(4), 484-94.

[127] Tiltman, A. J., and Haffajee, Z. (1999). Sclerosing stromal tumors, thecomas, and fibromas of the ovary: an immunohistochemical profile. *Int J Gynecol Pathol.*, Jul, 18(3), 254-8.

[128] Levin, G., Zigron, R., Haj-Yahya, R., Matan, L. S., and Rottenstreich, A. (2018). Granulosa cell tumor of ovary: A systematic review of recent evidence. *Eur J Obstet Gynecol Reprod Biol.*, Jun, 225, 57-61.

[129] Färkkilä, A., Haltia, U. M., Tapper, J., McConechy, M. K., Huntsman, D. G., and Heikinheimo, M. (2017). Pathogenesis and treatment of adult-type granulosa cell tumor of the ovary. *Ann Med.*, Aug, 49(5), 435-447.

[130] Costa, M. J., DeRose, P. B., Roth, L. M., Brescia, R. J., Zaloudek, C. J., and Cohen, C. (1994). Immunohistochemical phenotype of ovarian granulosa cell tumors: absence of epithelial membrane antigen has diagnostic value. *Hum Pathol.*, Jan, 25(1), 60-6.

[131] Gitsch, G., Kohlberger, P., Steiner, A., Neumeister, B., and Breitenecker, G. (1992). Expression of cytokeratins in granulosa cell tumors and ovarian carcinomas. *Arch Gynecol Obstet.*, 251(4), 193-7.

[132] Otis, C. N., Powell, J. L., Barbuto, D., and Carcangiu, M. L. (1992). Intermediate filamentous proteins in adult granulosa cell tumors. An immunohistochemical study of 25 cases. *Am J Surg Pathol.*, Oct, 16(10), 962-8.

[133] Cathro, H. P., and Stoler, M. H. (2005). The utility of calretinin, inhibin, and WT1 immunohistochemical staining in the differential diagnosis of ovarian tumors. *Hum Pathol.*, Feb, 36(2), 195-201.

[134] Gordon, M. D., Corless, C., Renshaw, A. A., and Beckstead, J. (1998). CD99, keratin, and vimentin staining of sex cord-stromal tumors, normal ovary, and testis. *Mod Pathol.*, Aug, 11(8), 769-73.

[135] Farinola, M. A., Gown, A. M., Judson, K., Ronnett, B. M., Barry, T. S., Movahedi-Lankarani, S., and Vang, R. (2007). Estrogen receptor alpha and progesterone receptor expression in ovarian adult granulosa cell tumors and Sertoli-Leydig cell tumors. *Int J Gynecol Pathol.*, Oct, 26(4), 375-82.

[136] Wang, G., Zhang, R., Li, C., and Chen, A. (2021). Characteristics and outcomes analysis of ovarian Sertoli-Leydig cell tumors (SLCTs): analysis of 15 patients. *J Ovarian Res.*, Nov 4, 14(1), 150.

[137] Mooney, E. E., Nogales, F. F., Bergeron, C., and Tavassoli, F. A. (2002). Retiform Sertoli-Leydig cell tumours: clinical, morphological and immunohistochemical findings. *Histopathology.*, Aug, 41(2), 110-7.

[138] Deavers, M. T., Malpica, A., Liu, J., Broaddus, R., and Silva, E. G. (2003). Ovarian sex cord-stromal tumors: an immunohistochemical study including a comparison of calretinin and inhibin. *Mod Pathol.*, Jun, 16(6), 584-90.

[139] Matias-Guiu, X., Pons, C., and Prat, J. (1998). Müllerian inhibiting substance, alpha-inhibin, and CD99 expression in sex cord-stromal tumors and endometrioid ovarian carcinomas resembling sex cord-stromal tumors. *Hum Pathol.*, Aug, 29(8), 840-5.

[140] Choi, Y. L., Kim, H. S., and Ahn, G. (2000). Immunoexpression of inhibin alpha subunit, inhibin/activin betaA subunit and CD99 in ovarian tumors. *Arch Pathol Lab Med.*, Apr, 124(4), 563-9.

[141] Zhang, X., Shen, D., and Wang, Y. (2018). Detection of the DICER1 hotspot mutation alongside immunohistochemical analysis may provide a better diagnostic measure for ovarian Sertoli-Leydig cell tumors. *Pathol Res Pract.*, Sep, 214(9), 1370-1375.

[142] Karnezis, A. N., Wang, Y., Keul, J., Tessier-Cloutier, B., Magrill, J., Kommoss, S., Senz, J., Yang, W., Proctor, L., Schmidt, D., Clement, P. B., Gilks, C. B., Huntsman, D. G., and Kommoss, F. (2019). DICER1 and FOXL2 Mutation Status Correlates With Clinicopathologic Features in Ovarian Sertoli-Leydig Cell Tumors. *Am J Surg Pathol.*, May, 43(5), 628-638.

[143] Aguirr, P., Scully, R. E., and DeLellis, R. A. (1986). Ovarian heterologous Sertoli-Leydig cell tumors with gastrointestinal-type epithelium. An immunohistochemical analysis. *Arch Pathol Lab Med.*, Jun, 110(6), 528-33

[144] Mooney, E. E., Nogales, F. F., and Tavassoli, F. A. (1999). Hepatocytic differentiation in retiform Sertoli-Leydig cell tumors: distinguishing a heterologous element from Leydig cells. *Hum Pathol.*, Jun, 30(6), 611-7.

[145] Tetu, B., Ordóñez, N. G., and Silva, E. G. (1986). Sertoli-Leydig cell tumor of the ovary with alpha-fetoprotein production. *Arch Pathol Lab Med.*, Jan, 110(1), 65-8.

[146] Guerrieri, C., Frånlund, B., Malmström, H., and Boeryd, B. (1998). Ovarian endometrioid carcinomas simulating sex cord-stromal tumors: a study using inhibin and cytokeratin 7. *Int J Gynecol Pathol.*, Jul, 17(3), 266-71.

[147] Oliva, E., Alvarez, T., and Young, R. H. (2005). Sertoli cell tumors of the ovary: a clinicopathologic and immunohistochemical study of 54 cases. *Am J Surg Pathol.*, Feb, 29(2), 143-56.

[148] Busam, K. J., Iversen, K., Coplan, K. A., Old, L. J., Stockert, E., Chen, Y. T., McGregor, D., and Jungbluth, A. (1998). Immunoreactivity for A103, an antibody to melan-A (Mart-1), in adrenocortical and other steroid tumors. *Am J Surg Pathol.*, Jan, 22(1), 57-63. Stewart, C. J., Nandini, C. L., and

Richmond, J. A. (2000). Value of A103 (melan-A) immunostaining in the differential diagnosis of ovarian sex cord stromal tumours. *J Clin Pathol.*, Mar, 53(3), 206-11.

[149] Lakis, N. S., Lombardo, K. A., Mangray, S., Netto, G. J., Salles, D., and Matoso, A. (2019). INSL3 Expression in Leydig Cell Hyperplasia and Leydig Cell Tumors. *Appl Immunohistochem Mol Morphol.*, Mar, 27(3), 203-209.

[150] Euscher, E. D. (2019). Germ Cell Tumors of the Female Genital Tract. *Surg Pathol Clin.*, Jun, 12(2), 621-649.

[151] Safdar, N. S., Stall, J. N., and Young, R. H. (2021). Malignant Mixed Germ Cell Tumors of the Ovary: An Analysis of 100 Cases Emphasizing the Frequency and Interrelationships of Their Tumor Types. *Am J Surg Pathol.*, Jun 1, 45(6), 727-741.

[152] Husaini, A. L., Soudy, H., El Din, H., Darwish, A., Ahmed, M., Eltigani, A., A L Mubarak, M., Sabaa, A. A., Edesa, W., A L-Tweigeri, T., and Al-Badawi, I. A. (2012). Pure dysgerminoma of the ovary: a single institutional experience of 65 patients. *Med Oncol.*, Dec, 29(4), 2944-8.

[153] Lifschitz-Mercer, B., Walt, H., Kushnir, I., Jacob, N., Diener, P. A., Moll, R., and Czernobilsky, B. (1995). Differentiation potential of ovarian dysgerminoma: an immunohistochemical study of 15 cases. *Hum Pathol.*, Jan, 26(1), 62-6.

[154] Sever, M., Jones, T. D., Roth, L. M., Karim, F. W., Zheng, W., Michael, H., Hattab, E. M., Emerson, R. E., Baldridge, L. A., and Cheng, L. (2005). Expression of CD117 (c-kit) receptor in dysgerminoma of the ovary: diagnostic and therapeutic implications. *Mod Pathol.*, Nov, 18(11), 1411-6.

[155] Hoei-Hansen, C. E., Kraggerud, S. M., Abeler, V. M., Kaern, J., Rajpert-De Meyts, E., and Lothe, R. A. (2007). Ovarian dysgerminomas are characterised by frequent KIT mutations and abundant expression of pluripotency markers. *Mol Cancer.*, Feb 2, 6, 12.

[156] Trinh, D. T., Shibata, K., Hirosawa, T., Umezu, T., Mizuno, M., Kajiyama, H., and Kikkawa, F. (2012). Diagnostic utility of CD117, CD133, SALL4, OCT4, TCL1 and glypican-3 in malignant germ cell tumors of the ovary. *J Obstet Gynaecol Res.*, May, 38(5), 841-8.

[157] Cossu-Rocca, P., Jones, T. D., Roth, L. M., Eble, J. N., Zheng, W., Karim, F. W., and Cheng, L. (2006). Cytokeratin and CD30 expression in dysgerminoma. *Hum Pathol.*, Aug, 37(8), 1015-21

[158] Iczkowski, K. A., Butler, S. L., Shanks, J. H., Hossain, D., Schall, A., Meiers, I., Zhou, M., Torkko, K. C., Kim, S. J., and MacLennan, G. T. (2008). Trials of new germ cell immunohistochemical stains in 93 extragonadal and metastatic germ cell tumors. *Hum Pathol.*, Feb, 39(2), 275-81. Zaloudek, C. J., Tavassoli, F. A., and Norris, H. J. (1981). Dysgerminoma with syncytiotrophoblastic giant cells. A histologically and clinically distinctive subtype of dysgerminoma. *Am J Surg Pathol.*, Jun, 5(4), 361-7.

[159] Kapp, D. S., Kohorn, E. I., Merino, M. J., and LiVolsi, V. A. (1985). Pure dysgerminoma of the ovary with elevated serum human chorionic gonadotropin: diagnostic and therapeutic considerations. *Gynecol Oncol.*, Feb, 20(2), 234-44.

[160] Mullin, T. J., and Lankerani, M. R. (1986). Ovarian dysgerminoma: immunocytochemical localization of human chorionic gonadotropin in the germinoma cell cytoplasm. *Obstet Gynecol.*, Sep, 68(3 Suppl), 80S-83S.

[161] Xue, D., Peng, Y., Wang, F., Allan, R. W., and Cao, D. (2011). RNA-binding protein LIN28 is a sensitive marker of ovarian primitive germ cell tumours. *Histopathology.*, Sep, 59(3), 452-9.

[162] Wang, Y., Yang, J., Yu, M., Cao, D., Zhang, Y., Zong, X., and Shen, K. (2018). Ovarian yolk sac tumor in postmenopausal females: A case series and a literature review. *Medicine* (*Baltimore*)., Aug, 97(33), e11838.

[163] Cicin, I., Saip, P., Guney, N., Eralp, Y., Ayan, I., Kebudi, R., and Topuz, E. (2009). Yolk sac tumours of the ovary: evaluation of clinicopathological features and prognostic factors. *Eur J Obstet Gynecol Reprod Biol.*, Oct, 146(2), 210-4.

[164] Chaudhary, R. K., Kher, A., Bobhate, S. K., and Grover, S. (1989). Alpha-fetoprotein in germ cell tumors. An immunohistochemical study. *Indian J Pathol Microbiol.*, Jul, 32(3), 167-73.

[165] Zynger, D. L., McCallum, J. C., Luan, C., Chou, P. M., and Yang, X. J. (2010). Glypican 3 has a higher sensitivity than alpha-fetoprotein for testicular and ovarian yolk sac tumour: immunohistochemical investigation with analysis of histological growth patterns. *Histopathology.*, May, 56(6), 750-7.

[166] Devouassoux-Shisheboran, M., Schammel, D. P., and Tavassoli, F. A. (1999). Ovarian hepatoid yolk sac tumours: morphological, immunohistochemical and ultrastructural features. *Histopathology*., May, 34(5), 462-9.

[167] Pitman, M. B., Triratanachat, S., Young, R. H., and Oliva, E. (2004). Hepatocyte paraffin 1 antibody does not distinguish primary ovarian tumors with hepatoid differentiation from metastatic hepatocellular carcinoma. *Int J Gynecol Pathol*., Jan, 23(1), 58-64.

[168] Niehans, G. A., Manivel, J. C., Copland, G. T., Scheithauer, B. W., and Wick, M. R. (1988). Immunohistochemistry of germ cell and trophoblastic neoplasms. *Cancer*., Sep 15, 62(6), 1113-23.

[169] Ramalingam, P., Malpica, A., Silva, E. G., Gershenson, D. M., Liu, J. L., and Deavers, M. T. (2004). The use of cytokeratin 7 and EMA in differentiating ovarian yolk sac tumors from endometrioid and clear cell carcinomas. *Am J Surg Pathol*., Nov, 28(11), 1499-505.

[170] Reiswich, V., Gorbokon, N., Luebke, A. M., Burandt, E., Menz, A., Kluth, M., Hube-Magg, C., Wittmer, C., Weidemann, S., Fraune, C., Möller, K., Lebok, P., Sauter, G., Simon, R., Uhlig, R., Wilczak, W., Jacobsen, F., Minner, S., Krech, R., Bernreuther, C., Marx, A., Steurer, S., Clauditz, T., and Krech, T. (2021). Pattern of placental alkaline phosphatase (PLAP) expression in human tumors: a tissue microarray study on 12,381 tumors. *J Pathol Clin Res*., Nov, 7(6), 577-589.

[171] Cao, D., Guo, S., Allan, R. W., Molberg, K. H., and Peng, Y. (2009). SALL4 is a novel sensitive and specific marker of ovarian primitive germ cell tumors and is particularly useful in distinguishing yolk sac tumor from clear cell carcinoma. *Am J Surg Pathol*., Jun, 33(6), 894-904.

[172] Nogales, F. F., Quiñonez, E., López-Marín, L., Dulcey, I., and Preda, O. (2014). A diagnostic immunohistochemical panel for yolk sac (primitive endodermal) tumours based on an immunohistochemical comparison with the human yolk sac. *Histopathology*., Jul, 65(1), 51-9.

[173] Chang, M. C., Vargas, S. O., Hornick, J. L., Hirsch, M. S., Crum, C. P., and Nucci, M. R. (2009). Embryonic stem cell transcription factors and D2-40 (podoplanin) as diagnostic immunohistochemical markers in ovarian germ cell tumors. *Int J Gynecol Pathol*., Jul, 28(4), 347-55.

[174] Nogales, F. F., Preda, O., and Nicolae, A. (2012). Yolk sac tumours revisited. A review of their many faces and names. *Histopathology*., Jun, 60(7), 1023-33.

[175] Hulewicz, G., Golfier, F., Chatte, G., Vitrey, D., Martel, I., Raudrant, D., and Trillet-Lenoir, V. (1996). Carcinome embryonnaire pur de l'ovaire. Revue de la littérature à propos d'un cas [Pure embryonal carcinoma of the ovary. A review of the literature apropos of a case]. *Bull Cancer*., Sep, 83(9), 718-24.

[176] Wang, Y., Zhou, F., Qian, Z., Qing, J., Zhao, M., and Huang, L. (2014). Mixed ovarian germ cell tumor composed of immature teratoma, yolk sac tumor and embryonal carcinoma. *J Coll Physicians Surg Pak*., Nov, 24 Suppl 3, S198-200.

[177] Cheng, L., Zhang, S., Talerman, A., and Roth, L. M. (2010). Morphologic, immunohistochemical, and fluorescence *in situ* hybridization study of ovarian embryonal carcinoma with comparison to solid variant of yolk sac tumor and immature teratoma. *Hum Pathol*., May, 41(5), 716-23.

[178] Furumoto, M. (1981). Cellular localization of AFP, hCG and its free subunits, and SP1 in embryonal carcinoma of the testis and ovary. *Pathol Res Pract*., Dec, 173(1-2), 12-21.

[179] Lau, S. K., Weiss, L. M., and Chu, P. G. (2007). D2-40 immunohistochemistry in the differential diagnosis of seminoma and embryonal carcinoma: a comparative immunohistochemical study with KIT (CD117) and CD30. *Mod Pathol*., Mar, 20(3), 320-5.

[180] Liu, X., Zhang, X., Pang, Y., Ma, Y., Zhang, X., and Liu, P. (2020). Clinicopathological factors and prognosis analysis of 39 cases of non-gestational ovarian choriocarcinoma. *Arch Gynecol Obstet*., Apr, 301(4), 901-912.

[181] Nishida, T., Oda, T., Sugiyama, T., Kataoka, A., Honda, S., and Yakushiji, M. (1998). Ovarian mixed germ cell tumor comprising polyembryoma and choriocarcinoma. *Eur J Obstet Gynecol Reprod Biol*., May, 78(1), 95-7.

[182] Adow, M. T., Gebresilasie, S. F., and Abebe, N. A. (2021). Primary Ovarian Choriocarcinoma: Rare Entity. *Case Rep Obstet Gynecol*., Sep 24, 2021, 4545375.

[183] Xiao, G. Q., Li, F., Unger, P. D., Katerji, H., Yang, Q., McMahon, L., and Burstein, D. E. (2016). ZBTB16: a novel sensitive and specific biomarker for yolk sac tumor. *Mod Pathol*., Jun, 29(6), 591-8.

[184] Daya, D., and Sabet, L. (1991). The use of cytokeratin as a sensitive and reliable marker for trophoblastic tissue. *Am J Clin Pathol*., Feb, 95(2), 137-41.

[185] Shih, I. M., and Kurman, R. J. (1999). Immunohistochemical localization of inhibin-alpha in the placenta and gestational trophoblastic lesions. *Int J Gynecol Pathol.*, Apr, 18(2), 144-50.

[186] Pelkey, T. J., Frierson, H. F., Jr. Mills, S. E., and Stoler, M. H. (1999). Detection of the alpha-subunit of inhibin in trophoblastic neoplasia. *Hum Pathol.*, Jan, 30(1), 26-31.

[187] Ino, K., Suzuki, T., Uehara, C., Nagasaka, T., Okamoto, T., Kikkawa, F., and Mizutani, S. (2000). The expression and localization of neutral endopeptidase 24.11/CD10 in human gestational trophoblastic diseases. *Lab Invest.*, Nov, 80(11), 1729-38.

[188] Mao, T. L., Kurman, R. J., Huang, C. C., Lin, M. C., and Shih, IeM. (2007). Immunohistochemistry of choriocarcinoma: an aid in differential diagnosis and in elucidating pathogenesis. *Am J Surg Pathol.*, Nov, 31(11), 1726-32.

[189] Bolze, P. A., Lopez, J., Allias, F., Hajri, T., Patrier, S., Devouassoux-Shisheboran, M., Massardier, J., You, B., Golfier, F., and Mallet, F. (2020). Transcriptomic and immunohistochemical approaches identify HLA-G as a predictive biomarker of gestational choriocarcinoma resistance to monochemotherapy. *Gynecol Oncol.*, Sep, 158(3), 785-793.

[190] Polakova, K., Bandzuchova, E., Tirpakova, J., Kuba, D., and Russ, G. (2007). Modulation of HLA-G expression. *Neoplasma.*, 54(6), 455-62.

[191] Akhter, A., Das, V., Naik, S., Faridi, R. M., Pandey, A., and Agrawal, S. (2012). Upregulation of HLA-G in JEG-3 cells by dexamethasone and hydrocortisone. *Arch Gynecol Obstet.*, Jan, 285(1), 7-14

[192] Nogales, F. F., Ruiz Avila, I., Concha, A., and del Moral, E. (1993). Immature endodermal teratoma of the ovary: embryologic correlations and immunohistochemistry. *Hum Pathol.*, Apr, 24(4), 364-70.

[193] Shinkai, T., Masumoto, K., Chiba, F., Shirane, K., Tanaka, Y., Aiyoshi, T., Sasaki, T., Ono, K., Gotoh, C., Urita, Y., Takayasu, H., Suzuki, R., and Sakashita, S. (2020). Pediatric ovarian immature teratoma: Histological grading and clinical characteristics. *J Pediatr Surg.*, Apr, 55(4), 707-710.

[194] Alwazzan, A. B., Popowich, S., Dean, E., Robinson, C., Lotocki, R., and Altman, A. D. (2015). Pure Immature Teratoma of the Ovary in Adults: Thirty-Year Experience of a Single Tertiary Care Center. *Int J Gynecol Cancer.*, Nov, 25(9), 1616-22.

[195] Bing, Z., Pasha, T. L., Lal, P., and Tomaszewski, J. E. (2008). Expression of glial cell line-derived neurotropic factor receptor alpha-1 in immature teratomas. *Am J Clin Pathol.*, Dec, 130(6), 892-6.

[196] Vance, R. P., Geisinger, K. R., Randall, M. B., and Marshall, R. B. (1988). Immature neural elements in immature teratomas. An immunohistochemical and ultrastructural study. *Am J Clin Pathol.*, Oct, 90(4), 397-411.

[197] Hiroshima, K., Toyozaki, T., Iyoda, A., Yusa, T., Fujisawa, T., and Ohwada, H. (2001). Apoptosis and proliferative activity in mature and immature teratomas of the mediastinum. *Cancer.*, Oct 1, 92(7), 1798-806.

[198] Phi, J. H., Park, S. H., Paek, S. H., Kim, S. K., Lee, Y. J., Park, C. K., Cho, B. K., Lee, D. H., and Wang, K. C. (2007). Expression of Sox2 in mature and immature teratomas of central nervous system. *Mod Pathol.*, Jul, 20(7), 742-8.

[199] Umehara, R., Kurata, A., Takanashi, M., Hashimoto, H., Fujita, K., Nagao, T., and Kuroda, M. (2019). Fascin as a Useful Marker for Identifying Neural Components in Immature Teratomas of Human Ovary and Those Derived From Murine Embryonic Stem Cells. *Int J Gynecol Pathol.*, Jul, 38(4), 377-385.

[200] Abiko, K., Mandai, M., Hamanishi, J., Matsumura, N., Baba, T., Horiuchi, A., Mikami, Y., Yoshioka, S., Wakasa, T., Shiozawa, T., and Konishi, I. (2010). Oct4 expression in immature teratoma of the ovary: relevance to histologic grade and degree of differentiation. *Am J Surg Pathol.*, Dec, 34(12), 1842-8.

Chapter 12

Molecular Pathology of Epithelial Ovarian Tumors

Christos Valavanis*, **MD**
Efthymia Souka, MD
and Gabriela-Monica Stanc, MD
Department of Pathology, Molecular Pathology Unit, Metaxa Cancer Hospital, Piraeus, Greece

Introduction

Ovarian cancer affects approximately 300,000 women globally every year leading to 185,000 deaths at the same time. It is a very heterogeneous disease entity with several histiotypes of different cell origin, presented with distinct histopathological and molecular features, and different therapeutic outcomes. It is nearly always detected at an advanced clinical stage with high recurrence rates and poor benefit from several treatment approaches [1, 2]. According to histogenesis and morphological features, ovarian cancer is classified into three main categories, ovarian epithelial tumors, sex cord-stromal tumors and germ cell tumors. Ovarian epithelial tumors are the most common, comprise 90% of all ovarian neoplasms and are subdivided into five main subtypes with different prevalence as follows: high-grade serous carcinoma (HGSC – 70%), low-grade serous carcinoma (LGSC – 5%), endometrioid (EC – 10%), mucinous (MC – 3%) and clear cell carcinomas (CCC – 10%) [3-5]. Less common types are seromucinous carcinoma, malignant Brenner tumor, mesonephric-like carcinoma, undifferentiated and dedifferentiated carcinomas and carcinosarcoma [4-6]. Each histiotype arises through different pathogenetic mechanism and is characterized by specific molecular alterations that dysregulate signal transduction pathways that can be exploited for the design of tailored therapeutics. In this chapter we will focus on the pathogenetic mechanisms involved in the ovarian epithelial tumor histogenesis, the molecular events happened, and the putative molecular targets for prognosis and precision treatment modalities.

---

* Corresponding Author's Email: cvalapath@yahoo.com.

In: Ovarian Cancer
Editors: Christos Iavazzo, Alexandros Fotiou and John Spiliotis
ISBN: 979-8-88697-633-5

Pathogenetic Mechanisms of Epithelial Ovarian Tumors

According to the traditional concept of ovarian carcinogenesis, the primary site of origin is the ovarian surface epithelium which undergoes Müllerian or non-Müllerian metaplasia and progressively leads to neoplastic malignant transformation [7]. Traditional theories hypothesized that ovarian carcinogenesis is due to malignant transformation of endometriosis lesions or to repetitive incessant ovulations through inflamed ovarian tissue damage and subsequent sex-hormone exposure [7-10].

Recent pathological observations have revealed the presence of dysplastic lesions in the fimbria of fallopian tubes in sporadic high-grade serous carcinomas, designated as STIC (Serous Tubal Intraepithelial Carcinoma), but not in the ovarian surface epithelia [11-14].

In addition, advances in molecular genomic studies have shown the presence of mutations in the *BRCA1* and *BRCA2* tumor suppressor genes and common genomic alterations in STIC and serous carcinoma, such as gene mutations in *p53, p16, CCNE1, BRD4*and *RSF1* and centrosome copy number abnormalities, suggesting a clonal histogenetic relationship [15-18]. A clonal histogenetic relationship has also be found among endometriosis, precursor ovarian lesions and endometrioid and clear cell carcinomas based on molecular alterations of *ARID1A, KRAS* and *MET* genes [19-22].

Based on the findings it is now well established that ovarian cancer is not a single disease entity and the cells of origin are extra-ovarian Müllerian epithelia that seeded the ovary as inclusion cysts and then are promoted to malignant transformation under the influence of ovarian microenvironment [23-27].

Combined clinical, morphological, molecular and genetic studies have led to the acceptance of a dualistic model of ovarian carcinogenesis that divides ovarian epithelial carcinomas into two categories, designated as type I and type II. Type I tumors arise from precursor lesions in the ovary while type II neoplasms develop from the tubal and/or surface ovarian epithelium. Type I ovarian epithelial tumors include low-grade serous carcinoma, endometrioid carcinoma, mucinous carcinoma, clear cell carcinoma and malignant Brenner tumor. Type II comprises high-grade serous carcinoma, carcinosarcoma and undifferentiated carcinoma [6, 27-29].

Type I ovarian epithelial tumors have an indolent biological behavior and arise from precursor lesions in the ovary such as cystadenoma or adenofibroma through atypical proliferative lesions or borderline tumors towards malignant transformation and eventually invasive neoplasms. Molecularly, they are characterized by genomic stability, somatic gene mutations with distinctive molecular profile for each histiotype and absence of p53 mutations [30-33].

Type II ovarian epithelial tumors have a more aggressive biological behavior and originate from tubal fimbrium epithelia through dysplastic lesions, serous in situ carcinoma and finally towards invasive carcinomas. They are characterized by genomic instability, p53 mutations and dysfunction of tumor suppressor genes *BRCA1* and *BRCA2* due to mutational events or gene promoter hypermethylation [30-33].

In the following sections we are going to present the molecular genomic alterations that can be found in the different histiotypes of ovarian epithelial tumors and the possible clinical implications that may have in prognosis and therapeutic modalities.

Molecular Features of Epithelial Ovarian Tumors

High-grade Serous Ovarian Carcinomas (HGSCs)

High-grade serous carcinomas (HGSCs) represent the most aggressive and chemoresistant epithelial ovarian tumors with a high incidence of mortality around 70-80%worldwide [34, 35].

These neoplasms are more frequently diagnosed in advanced clinical stage and in postmenopausal women. Predisposition factors towards these neoplasms are mainly the menopausal hormonal therapy and the hereditary breast and ovarian cancer (HBOC) syndrome characterized mostly by germline *BRCA1/2* alterations [36] and less frequently (approximately 2%)by germline alterations in other Homologous Recombination Repair genes such as *BRIP1, ATM, RAD51C* and *RAD51D* [37-39].

Genome-wide and genetic studies have shown that these tumors are characterized by somatic *TP53* mutations mainly in the DNA binding domain in high frequency (>95%) [40, 41] and altered Homologous Recombination Repair (HRR) pathway leading to genomic instability and aneuploidy with recurrent high copy number structural alterations (CNAs). CNAs comprise oncogene amplifications such as *CCNE1* (20%), *MECOM, EMSY* and *MYC* and deletions/breaks of tumor suppressor genes such as *PTEN, RB1, RAD51B* and *NF1* [42-45]. In addition, recurrent mutations have been found in genes such as*NF1* (4%-6%), *RB1* (2%-6%)and *PTEN* (<1%) that along with structural alterations/deletions can lead to overall gene inactivation in relatively high frequency such as 20%, 17% and 7% respectively [46, 47].

HGSCs display alterations in BRCA1/2 genes that are involved in the repair of DNA double-strand breaks through homologous recombination (HR). Almost 15% of HGSCs have *BRCA1/2* germline mutations, 5% somatic mutations and 11% show *BRCA1* epigenetic silencing through promoter hypermethylation of CpG islands [46, 48]. Besides, mutations in other homologous recombination repair related genes have been observed in HGSCs conferring an HRR deficient phenotype in 50% of the cases and leading to high genomic instability [49]. These HRR-related genes include Fanconi anemia genes (*PALB2, FANCA, FANCI, FANCL, FANCC), RAD* family genes (*RAD50, RAD51, RAD51B, RAD51C, RAD54L),* MRN complex genes *[Mre11-Rad50-Nbs1(Nibrin)]* and DNA damage response (DDR) genes (*ATM, ATR, CHEK1, CHEK2)* [50-52].

Based on the HRR pathway status, HGSCs are divided into two morphologically distinct histiotype categories. HRR- proficient tumors display papillary, micropapillary and slit-like spaces morphological patterns with worse progression free survival, while HRR- deficient tumors show SET-like morphology (solid, endometrioid and transitional patterns) and improved progression free survival due to therapeutic response to platinum and poly-ADP-ribose polymerase (PARP) inhibitors [53-55]. HRR-proficient tumors are more likely to be resistant to these therapeutic modalities and are characterized by molecular alterations unrelated and mutually exclusive to *BRCA1/2* pathway such as *CCNE1* gene amplification [56-58].

As mentioned above, HRR deficiency (HRD) can occur due to germline or somatic mutations and epigenetic modifications of HRR genes. In addition, other molecular events can disrupt the physiological function of HRR pathway such as *RAD51* down regulation through *PTEN* inactivation, decreased expression of *BRCA1* through *CDK12* inactivation or *EMSY* gene amplification leading to *BRCA1* deficiency [44, 59-64].

According to NCCN guidelines HRD status should be tested in order to get information for the optimization of PARP inhibitor HGSCs treatment. Most of the HRD assays evaluate the presence of germline or somatic HRR genes mutations and/or assess tumor genomic instability by analyzing the percentage of genomic loss of heterozygocity, telomeric allelic imbalance and genome-wide structural alterations (HRD mutation signatures) [65-68]. PARP is an enzyme involved in the repair of single strand DNA breaks (SSBs) through excision repair and the error-prone Polθ/PARP1-mediated nonhomologous end joining repair pathway [69]. PARP inhibition in HRD ovarian tumors acts through synthetic lethality induction and leads eventually to tumor cell death [70]. It should be noted that primary resistance to PARP inhibition can be encountered in ovarian tumors with functional HRR particularly in the presence of CCNE1 amplification. In addition, acquired resistance or decreased sensitivity to PARPi therapy can occur through BRCA/HRR genes functional restoration by secondary mutations [71, 72]. In this setting a functional assay can be used by assessing the HRD status at RNA or protein levels [73, 74].

Other putative prognostic and therapy predictive biomarkers in HGSCs include tumor subtyping based on transcriptional profiling which divides HGSCs in four categories (differentiated, immunoreactive, mesenchymal and proliferative), the former(differentiated and immunoreactive) with favorable clinical behavior and prognosis and the latter (mesenchymal and proliferative) with aggressive clinical course and worse prognosis [75-77]. Additionally, hypermethylation of *TAP1* promoter region in 6p21.3 chromosomal locus confers unfavorable prognosis, while the presence of increased CD8+ tumor infiltrating T lymphocytes is associated with favorable one [78-80]. Studies on PD-L1 and LAG3 expression and potential use of immunotherapy in ovarian HGSCs showed modest therapeutic results and controversial prognosis [81-83].

Other deregulated pathways in HGSCs are the *PIK3CA/AKT* and *NOTCH* pathways which can be targeted by using PIK3CA or AKT inhibitors [84-86]. *HER2* overexpression/amplification can also be found in ovarian HGSCs in 2%-4% of the cases with no significant impact on progression free survival, albeit a finding that can be exploited for anti-HER2 therapy [87, 88].

Low-grade Serous Ovarian Carcinomas (LGSCs)

Low-grade serous carcinomas (LGSCs) are more commonly found in younger women with a median age of 55 years, are less aggressive with better clinical course and prognosis than HGSCs and constitute approximately 5% of epithelial ovarian tumors [89]. LSGCs originate from benign or borderline serous tumors and display papillary architectural pattern with low-grade nuclear atypia and distinct nucleoli. More aggressive clinical course is associated with borderline serous tumors showing micropapillary histological pattern, microinvasions and bilateral ovarian presence [90].

Low-grade serous carcinomas (LGSCs) are characterized by genomic stability with low mutation rates and less copy number aberrations than HGSCs. Copy number aberrations like gene deletions or amplifications can be found in approximately 86% of LGSCs most commonly the chromosomal loss of 1p36.33, 9p and homozygous deletions of the *CDKN2A/2B* locus [91, 92].

In 80% of the LGSCs cases, activated mutations of the mitogen-activated protein kinase (MAPK) signal transduction pathway are detected, involving upstream regulators like *KRAS* (25-54%), *BRAF* (8-33%), *NRAS* (8-26%) and *ERBB2* (5-6%) [93-95]. *KRAS* mutations are associated with aggressive clinical behavior and worse prognosis whereas *BRAF* mutations are found in early stage tumors [92, 93, 97-99]. LGSCs are usually chemoresistant tumors in advanced clinical stage, a problem that can be overcome by using MEK inhibitors that target the mutated MAPK pathway molecular regulators [96, 100]. Other recurrent driver mutations involved in the pathogenesis of LGSCs have been identified in *PIK3CA*, *FFAR1*, *USP9X* (11%) and *EIF1AX* (15%) [92]. *USPX9* and *EIF1AX*are downstream effectors of MAPK pathway and linked to the mTOR pathway, thus inhibitors of mTOR pathway can be used for molecularly targeted therapies in chemotherapy resistant recurrent tumors [97, 100].

Driver mutations in *KRAS* and *BRAF* genes are early events in LGSCs development and can be found in 85% of benign cystadenomas and serous borderline tumors [101]. Morphological correlations with molecular features have demonstrated that serous borderline tumors with classic morphology are characterized more frequently with *BRAF* mutations, whereas *KRAS* and *BRAF* wild-type tumors display micropapillary histological pattern [102]. Progression and transformation of serous borderline ovarian tumors and/or LGSCs into HGSCs is a rare event, albeit has been occasionally observed [103-105]. This observation is further established based on the presence of *KRAS*, *BRAF* or *NRAS* mutations in p53 wild-type HGSCs of mixed low to intermediate grade histology [106], which leads to further subtyping of p53 wild type HGSCs into LGSC-like (40%) and usual HGSC-like (60%) subtypes [107]. LGSC-like neoplasms display mixed low to intermediate grade morphological patterns and/or presence of *KRAS*, *BRAF* or *NRAS* mutations (60%), with micropapillary histomorphology in 60% of the cases [107]. The category of usual HGSC-like neoplasms show high-grade morphology similar to conventional p53-mutated HGSCs with aberrant p53 immunohistochemical expression (64%), *MDM2* amplification (14%), *ARID1B* loss-of-function by gene fusion or mutations (14%) and *RAD21* loss-of -function by gene fusion (14%) [107, 108]. Approximately 25% of usual HGSC-like tumors show micropapillary histomorphology [107].

Endometrioid Ovarian Carcinomas (EOCs)

Endometrioid ovarian carcinomas represent 10% of epithelial ovarian tumors, are associated with favorable prognosis and are encountered in the age range of 40-70 years [109]. They originate mainly from endometriosis lesions and less frequently from benign or borderline endometrioid ovarian neoplasms, such as adenofibromas [9, 10, 110]. Risk factors for EOCs are endometriosis, hereditary breast and ovarian cancer syndrome, Lynch syndrome, late menopause and post-menopausal hormone therapy [111, 112].

Endometriosis-associated EOCs are characterized by shared mutations in *PIK3CA*, *ARID1A* and *KRAS* genes, whereas borderline endometrioid tumors have *CTNNB1* mutations in 90% of the cases [113-115]. The most mutated genes found in EOCs are *ARID1A* (30-35%), a component of the SW1/SNF chromatin remodelling complex and *CTNNB1* (25-60%) involved in the β-catenin signal transduction pathway [114-117]. Other less common genomic alterations are mutations in *PIK3CA* (15-40%), *PTEN* (20-30%) with frequent loss of heterozygocity (45-75%), *KRAS* (10-30%), *TP53* (10-25%), *POLE* (3-10%) [118, 119], as well as mismatch repair deficiency (MMR, 10-20%) with somatic or germline predisposition MMR genes (MLH1, MSH2, MSH6, PMS2) mutations in Lynch syndrome associated cases [120, 121].

Synchronous organ-confined endometrial and ovarian endometrioid carcinomas can be found in 25% of cases demonstrating clonal relationship and have a favorable clinical course

[122-124]. Seromucinous carcinomas (mixed serous and endocervical-type mucinous carcinomas) are considered by the current WHO classification a subtype of endometrioid carcinomas due to their histogical and molecular features overlapping [125, 126]. Benign seromucinous tumors are frequently related to endometriosis lesions [127, 128] and borderline seromucinous tumors have been demonstrated to have *ARID1A* and *KRAS* genomic aberrations [126, 129].

Based on their molecular features, EOCs are divided in four molecular subcategories: 1. Hypermutated with microsatellite instability due to MMR deficiency (10-20%), 2. Ultramutated with *POLE* mutations (3-10%), *TP53* mutated (10-25%) and with no specific molecular signatures (60-70%) [130-132]. Hypermutated and ultramutated EOCs show high mutational burden, a finding that might be exploited for immunotherapeutic interventions.

POLE-mutated EOCs and MMR-deficient ovarian endometrioid tumors due to somatic or germline MMR genes mutations have favorable clinical course and prognosis [132]. MMR germline mutations are found in the Lynch syndrome (hereditary nonpolyposis colorectal cancer syndrome - HNPCC) and predispose to endometriosis-associated endometrioid tumors [120, 133]. *TP53* mutated EOCs have high genomic complexity with unfavorable prognosis, whereas *CTNNB1*-mutated demonstrate low genomic complexity with good prognosis, unlike their uterine endometrial endometrioid *CTNNB*1-mutated tumors which show worse clinical course [117, 134, 135].

The genomic aberrations found in different genes in EOCs might be used as candidates for targeted therapeutic interventions, such as targeting mutated *ARID1A* with HDAC inhibitors or targeting dysregulated MAPK or PI3K pathways with MEK or PIK3AC inhibitors respectively [136, 137].

Mucinous Ovarian Carcinomas (MOCs)

Mucinous ovarian carcinomas are rare tumors accounting for 2-3% of epithelial ovarian carcinomas with relatively high prevalence in women below 40 years of age [138]. Their histology resemble gastrointestinal tumors and originate mainly from mucinous benign or borderline tumors, with a small percentage originating from mature cystic teratomas or Brenner tumors with gastrointestinal pattern component [4]. Their prognosis is excellent in early clinical stages, albeit in advanced stages they display chemoresistance with poor clinical outcome [139, 140].

Molecularly, MOCs are characterized by *KRAS* mutations (66%), *CDKN2A* inactivation (76%) and *HER2/neu* gene amplification (20%) [141]. *HER2* gene amplification is mutually exclusive with KRAS mutations and is found in most of the cases with mutated *TP53* [64%) [141, 142]. Benign mucinous tumors give rise to MOCs through a progression tumor evolution model starting with *KRAS* or *CDKN2A* mutation, whereas mucinous borderline tumors have both *KRAS* and *CDKN2A* mutations along with extra genomic copy number aberrations [143, 144]. More genomic copy number aberrations, mainly chromosomal locus 9p13.3 amplification and *TP53* mutations are added at the final evolutionary steps of MOCs progressive carcinogenesis [144]. Other less frequently mutated genes in MOCs are *PIK3CA/PTEN*, *BRAF*, *CTNNB1/APC* (regulators of the β-catenin/Wnt signal transduction pathway), *RNF43* and *ARID1A* (8-12%) [141]. MOCs with no *KRAS* or *HER2* gene alterations are considered to be tumors arising from mature cystic teratomas [145]. MOCs with high genomic complexity and mutational burden are associated with high nuclear grade, tumor progression and unfavorable prognosis [141].

MAPK and HER2 targeted therapeutic approaches along with other inhibitors such as HDAC inhibitor for *ARID1A* can be used for more effective tailored treatment of MOCs [146].

Clear Cell Ovarian Carcinomas (CCOCs)

Clear cell ovarian carcinomas constitute approximately 5% of epithelial ovarian tumors with relatively high prevalence in young women of East Asian origin [147]. They arise from endometriosis lesions and/or clear cell benign (adenofibroma) or borderline tumors, pathologic entities with *PIK3CA*and *ARID1A* precursor mutations [148]. Endometriosis and late menopause are the main risk factors associated with the appearance of CCOCs.

CCOCs are characterized by genomic aberrations that involve *PIK3CA* activating mutations (40-50%), *ARID1A* loss of function mutations (50-75%), *MET* gene amplifications, mutations in *ARID1B* (10%), *KRAS* (15%), *PPP2R1A* (15%), *TERT* promoter (15%), *SMARCA4*, *PTEN* (1-5%), *PIK3CA, PIK3R1, AKT2, TP53 (5-20%)* and *ZNF217*transcription factor overexpression which is associated with poor outcome [148-150]. Genes involved in antioxidant cell machinery such as *GPX3* (glutathione peroxidase 3), *GLRX3* (glutaredoxin) and *SOD3* (superoxide dismutase) have been demonstrated to be highly expressed in CCOCs resulting in tumor chemoresistance [151]. Additionally, HER2 gene amplification (15%) and Mismatch Repair genes deficiency (2-3%) have also been identified [152], the germline mutations of the latter may predispose in developing CCOCs [152, 153]. Abnormal p53 expression (7%) has also been reported and is associated with adverse prognosis [154]. Druggable targets might be molecules involved in PIK3/AKT/mTOR pathway and loss of function of *ARID1A*genethrough inhibition of EZH2 transcription factor [155].

Small Cell Ovarian Carcinomas (SCOCs)

Small cell ovarian carcinomas are extremely rare neoplasms accounting for less than 1% of epithelial ovarian tumors with unknown cell origin and poorly understood pathogenesis [156]. Based on morphological features, SCOCs are classified into two types: 1. Hypercalcemic type (SCOC-HT) characterized by chemoresistance and 2. Pulmonary type (SCOC-PT) characterized by chemosensitivity [157]. They are highly malignant neoplasms with poor clinical outcome.

Hypercalcemic type SCOCs affect young women with mean age of 22 years and are characterized by somatic or germline *SMARCA4 (BRG1)* mutations (90%), a component of the SW1/SNF complex of chromatin remodelling, leading to gene loss of function [158]. The lack of *SMARCA4* expression can be used for diagnosing SCOC-HT immunohistochemically [159]. Loss of function of *SMARCA4*leads to EZH2 transcription factor upregulation and overexpression which might be used as a druggable target for SCOC-HT tailored treatment [160, 161].

Pulmonary type SCOCs affect women with mean age of 51 years with poor prognosis, albeit chemosensitive and radiosensitive. There is no data on molecular characterization and pathogenetic mechanisms for pulmonary type SCOCs due to its rarity [162].

Brenner Ovarian Tumors

Brenner tumors of the ovary are uncommon neoplasms accounting for 5% of epithelial ovarian tumors and mostly are benign neoplasms, albeit borderline and malignant Brenner tumors occur as well [163]. Malignant Brenner tumors are very rare accounting for less of 5% of all Brenner tumors [164]. Histogenetically they arise from the ovarian surface epithelium or the paratubal

Walthard cell nests and the tuboperitoneal junction epithelium of the fallopian tube via transitional cell metaplasia via androgenic stimulation (AR and AKR1C3 expression) [165]. They are frequently associated with mucinous tumors and are characterized by *MYC* gene amplification and to a lesser extent *KRAS* and *HRAS* gene mutations, genomic alterations that are mutually exclusive [166]. The pathogenesis of these tumors is not well understood, transformation of benign to borderline tumors is related to *CDKN2A* loss of function due to promoter hypermethylation and homozygous deletions resulting in p16 suppressed expression and to *KRAS* and *PIK3CA* gene mutations in 30% of borderline tumors [165].

Progression to malignant Brenner tumors is associated with *MDM2* and *CCND1* gene amplification leading to cyclin D1 nuclear overexpression and lack of *TP53* and *TERT* mutations unlike urothelial carcinomas despite their histomorphologic similarities [167, 168, 170].

Malignant Brenner tumors display *CDKN2A/2B* loss and oncogenic *FGFR1/3* genomic aberrations in 55% of cases and recurrent *FGFR3 S249C* or *FGFR3-TACC3* fusion in 45% of cases [169]. *FGFR3*mutated tumors are associated with benign or borderline Brenner tumor precursor components. Malignant Brenner tumors with *PIK3CA* mutations are frequently enriched with *FGFR3* alterations, while *FGFR3* wild-type tumors are associated with*MDM2* amplification [169, 170]. Therefore, FGFR pathway could be an ideal target candidate for tailored malignant Brenner tumor treatment.

Mesonephric-like Ovarian Carcinomas (MLOCs)

Mesonephric-like ovarian carcinomas are presumed to either originate from normal or hyperplastic mesonephric remnants or Müllerian tumors with mesonephric differentiation [171]. They have morphologic and immunophenotypic resemblance to cervical mesonephric adenocarcinomas and are characterized by recurrent *KRAS* gene activating mutations (89%) and chromosomal gains in 1q (89%), 10 (43%) and 12 chromosomes [172]. They also have *PIK3CA* activating mutations demonstrating a biological relationship with carcinomas of Müllerian origin, but no mutations in *ARID1A* or *TP53* [173, 174]. They also exhibit PTEN (23%) and CTNNB1 (14%) mutations [174]. As a component of serous borderline tumors or low-grade serous carcinomas, both neoplasms share *KRAS* or NRAS activating mutations implying a clonal relationship and suggesting that some mesonephric-like carcinomas have a Müllerian origin with mesonephric differentiation [175, 176].

Dedifferentiated and Undifferentiated Ovarian Carcinomas and Carcinosarcomas

Dedifferentiated ovarian carcinomas constitute a group of ovarian tumors morphologically characterized by both undifferentiated and differentiated components. They have been demonstrated to have inactivating genomic alterations in SWI/SNF chromatin remodeling complex genes, such as *SMARCA4*/BRG1, *INI1*, *ARID1*And *ARI1B* and MMR genes deficiency as well [177].

Carcinosarcomas are aggressive neoplasms with biphasic histomorphology characterized by carcinomatous and sarcomatous components [178]. They are considered to have epithelial origin due to the concordant molecular profiles in both components, mostly *TP53* mutations/deletions [178]. Recent whole-exome next generation sequencing studies have shown multiple genomic alterations in different genes/pathways including*HER2/neu*, *EGFR*, *PI3K/AKT/mTOR*, *MAPK*, genes related to histones (H2A and H2B) and chromatin structure (*MBD3* deletions, a member of the nucleosome remodeling deacetylase complex) and genes related to cell-cycle regulation [179-181]. Genomic alterations in histone genes suggest a putative role in epithelial-mesenchymal transition and sarcomatous transformation of precursor carcinomatous components of these tumors [181]. In addition, gene amplification of *MYC* (78%) and *ZNF217* (87%) have been shown to occur in both components, whereas *MYC* amplification is observed in a lesser degree in sarcomatous component [182]. Most carcinosarcomas have molecular patterns of genomic aberrations similar to those found in serous carcinomas, an observation compatible with the current hypothesis that carcinosarcomas are in fact metaplastic carcinomas [183, 184].

References

[1] Brett M. Reid, Jennifer B. Permuth, Thomas A. Sellers. Epidemiology of ovarian cancer: a review. *Cancer Biol. Med.* 2017 Feb;14(1):9-32.

[2] Torre LA, Trabert B, DeSantis CE, Miller KD, Samimi G, Runowicz CD, Gaudet MM, Jemal A, Siegel RL. Ovarian cancer statistics, 2018. *CA Cancer J Clin.* 2018 Jul;68(4):284-296.

[3] McCluggage WG. Morphological subtypes of ovarian carcinoma: a review with emphasis on new developments and pathogenesis. *Pathology.* 2011 Aug;43(5):420-32.

[4] WHO Classification of Tumors Editorial Board. *WHO classification of tumours: female genital tumours.* vol. 4. 5th edition. Lyon (France): International Agency for Research on Cancer; 2020.

[5] Romero I, Leskelä S, Mies BP, Velasco AP, Palacios J. Morphological and molecular heterogeneity of epithelial ovarian cancer: Therapeutic implications. *EJC Suppl.* 2020 Aug 22;15:1-15.

[6] Prat J, D'Angelo E, Espinosa I. Ovarian carcinomas: at least five different diseases with distinct histological features and molecular genetics. *Hum Pathol.* 2018 Oct;80:11-27.

[7] Kurman RJ, Shih IeM. The Dualistic Model of Ovarian Carcinogenesis: Revisited, Revised, and Expanded. *Am J Pathol.* 2016 Apr;186(4):733-47.

[8] Fathalla MF. Incessant ovulation--a factor in ovarian neoplasia? *Lancet.* 1971 Jul 17;2(7716):163.

[9] Heidemann LN, Hartwell D, Heidemann CH, Jochumsen KM. The relation between endometriosis and ovarian cancer - a review. *Acta Obstet Gynecol Scand.* 2014 Jan;93(1):20-31.

[10] Králíčková M, Laganà AS, Ghezzi F, Vetvicka V. Endometriosis and risk of ovarian cancer: what do we know? *Arch Gynecol Obstet.* 2020 Jan;301(1):1-10.

[11] Zhang W, Wei L, Li L, Yang B, Kong B, Yao G, Zheng W. Ovarian serous carcinogenesis from tubal secretory cells. *Histol Histopathol.* 2015 Nov;30(11):1295-302.

[12] Hatina J, Boesch M, Sopper S, Kripnerova M, Wolf D, Reimer D, Marth C, Zeimet AG. Ovarian Cancer Stem Cell Heterogeneity. *Adv Exp Med Biol.* 2019;1139:201-221.

[13] Shih IM, Wang Y, Wang TL. The Origin of Ovarian Cancer Species and Precancerous Landscape. *Am J Pathol.* 2021 Jan;191(1):26-39.

[14] Li HX, Lu ZH, Shen K, Cheng WJ, Malpica A, Zhang J, Wei JJ, Zhang ZH, Liu J. Advances in serous tubal intraepithelial carcinoma: correlation with high grade serous carcinoma and ovarian carcinogenesis. *Int J Clin Exp Pathol.* 2014 Feb 15;7(3):848-57.

[15] Kuhn E, Wang TL, Doberstein K, Bahadirli-Talbott A, Ayhan A, Sehdev AS, Drapkin R, Kurman RJ, Shih IeM. CCNE1 amplification and centrosome number abnormality in serous tubal intraepithelial carcinoma: further evidence supporting its role as a precursor of ovarian high-grade serous carcinoma. *Mod Pathol.* 2016 Oct;29(10):1254-61.

[16] Soong TR, Howitt BE, Horowitz N, Nucci MR, Crum CP. The fallopian tube, "precursor escape" and narrowing the knowledge gap to the origins of high-grade serous carcinoma. *Gynecol Oncol.* 2019 Feb;152(2):426-433.

[17] Rhyasen GW, Yao Y, Zhang J, Dulak A, Castriotta L, Jacques K, Zhao W, Gharahdaghi F, Hattersley MM, Lyne PD, Clark E, Zinda M, Fawell SE, Mills GB, Chen H. BRD4 amplification facilitates an oncogenic gene expression program in high-grade serous ovarian cancer and confers sensitivity to BET inhibitors. *PLoS One.* 2018 Jul 23;13(7):e0200826.

[18] Sehdev AS, Kurman RJ, Kuhn E, Shih IeM. Serous tubal intraepithelial carcinoma upregulates markers associated with high-grade serous carcinomas including Rsf-1 (HBXAP), cyclin E and fatty acid synthase. *Mod Pathol.* 2010 Jun;23(6):844-55.

[19] Ayhan A, Mao TL, Seckin T, Wu CH, Guan B, Ogawa H, Futagami M, Mizukami H, Yokoyama Y, Kurman RJ, Shih IeM. Loss of ARID1A expression is an early molecular event in tumor progression from ovarian endometriotic cyst to clear cell and endometrioid carcinoma. *Int J Gynecol Cancer.* 2012 Oct;22(8):1310-5.

[20] Bulun SE, Wan Y, Matei D. Epithelial Mutations in Endometriosis: Link to Ovarian Cancer. *Endocrinology*. 2019 Mar 1;160(3):626-638.

[21] Bulun SE, Yilmaz BD, Sison C, Miyazaki K, Bernardi L, Liu S, Kohlmeier A, Yin P, Milad M, Wei J. *Endometriosis. Endocr Rev.* 2019 Aug 1;40(4):1048-1079.

[22] Ruderman R, Pavone ME. Ovarian cancer in endometriosis: an update on the clinical and molecular aspects. *Minerva Ginecol.* 2017 Jun;69(3):286-294.

[23] Kroeger PT Jr, Drapkin R. Pathogenesis and heterogeneity of ovarian cancer. *Curr Opin Obstet Gynecol.* 2017 Feb;29(1):26-34.

[24] Zhang S, Dolgalev I, Zhang T, Ran H, Levine DA, Neel BG. Both fallopian tube and ovarian surface epithelium are cells-of-origin for high-grade serous ovarian carcinoma. *Nat Commun.* 2019 Nov 26;10(1):5367.

[25] Klotz DM, Wimberger P. Cells of origin of ovarian cancer: ovarian surface epithelium or fallopian tube? *Arch Gynecol Obstet.* 2017 Dec;296(6):1055-1062.

[26] Banet N, Kurman RJ. Two types of ovarian cortical inclusion cysts: proposed origin and possible role in ovarian serous carcinogenesis. *Int J Gynecol Pathol.* 2015 Jan;34(1):3-8.

[27] Kurman RJ, Shih IeM. Molecular pathogenesis and extraovarian origin of epithelial ovarian cancer--shifting the paradigm. *Hum Pathol.* 2011 Jul;42(7):918-31.

[28] Koshiyama M, Matsumura N, Konishi I. Recent concepts of ovarian carcinogenesis: type I and type II. *Biomed Res Int.* 2014;2014:934261. doi: 10.1155/2014/934261.

[29] Devouassoux-Shisheboran M, Genestie C, Ray-Coquard I. La classification histo-moléculaire des cancers épithéliaux ovariens en 2 types est-elle pertinente ? [Dualistic classification of epithelial ovarian cancer: Is it clinically relevant?]. *Bull Cancer.* 2016 Mar;103(3):252-8.

[30] Ramalingam P. Morphologic, Immunophenotypic, and Molecular Features of Epithelial Ovarian Cancer. *Oncology* (Williston Park). 2016 Feb;30(2):166-76.

[31] Rojas V, Hirshfield KM, Ganesan S, Rodriguez-Rodriguez L. Molecular Characterization of Epithelial Ovarian Cancer: Implications for Diagnosis and Treatment. *Int J Mol Sci.* 2016 Dec 15;17(12):2113.

[32] Prahm KP, Karlsen MA, Høgdall E, Scheller NM, Lundvall L, Nedergaard L, Christensen IJ, Høgdall C. The prognostic value of dividing epithelial ovarian cancer into type I and type II tumors based on pathologic characteristics. *Gynecol Oncol.* 2015 Feb;136(2):205-11.

[33] Bergamini A, Candiani M, Taccagni G, Rabaiotti E, Viganò R, De Marzi P, Ferrari D, Mangili G. Different Patterns of Disease Spread between Advanced-Stage Type I and II Epithelial Ovarian Cancer. *Gynecol Obstet Invest.* 2016;81(1):10-4.

[34] Lisio MA, Fu L, Goyeneche A, Gao ZH, Telleria C. High-Grade Serous Ovarian Cancer: Basic Sciences, Clinical and Therapeutic Standpoints. *Int J Mol Sci.* 2019 Feb 22;20(4):952.

[35] Westfall D, Roma AA, Silva EG. High-grade serous carcinoma of the ovary. *Ann Diagn Pathol.* 2009 Aug;13(4):285-90.

[36] Petrucelli N, Daly MB, Pal T. *BRCA1*- and *BRCA2*-Associated Hereditary Breast and Ovarian Cancer. 1998 Sep 4 [updated 2016 Dec 15]. In: Adam MP, Ardinger HH, Pagon RA, Wallace SE, Bean LJH, Gripp KW, Mirzaa GM, Amemiya A, editors. *GeneReviews®* [Internet]. Seattle (WA): University of Washington, Seattle; 1993–2021.

[37] Suszynska M, Ratajska M, Kozlowski P. BRIP1, RAD51C, and RAD51D mutations are associated with high susceptibility to ovarian cancer: mutation prevalence and precise risk estimates based on a pooled analysis of ~30,000 cases. *J Ovarian Res.* 2020 May 2;13(1):50.

[38] Minion LE, Dolinsky JS, Chase DM, Dunlop CL, Chao EC, Monk BJ. Hereditary predisposition to ovarian cancer, looking beyond BRCA1/BRCA2. *Gynecol Oncol.* 2015 Apr;137(1):86-92.

[39] Chandrasekaran D, Sobocan M, Blyuss O, Miller RE, Evans O, Crusz SM, Mills-Baldock T, Sun L, Hammond RFL, Gaba F, Jenkins LA, Ahmed M, Kumar A, Jeyarajah A, Lawrence AC, Brockbank E, Phadnis S, Quigley M, El Khouly F, Wuntakal R, Faruqi A, Trevisan G, Casey L, Burghel GJ, Schlecht H, Bulman M, Smith P, Bowers NL, Legood R, Lockley M, Wallace A, Singh N, Evans DG, Manchanda R. Implementation of Multigene Germline and Parallel Somatic Genetic Testing in Epithelial Ovarian Cancer: SIGNPOST Study. *Cancers* (Basel). 2021 Aug 27;13(17):4344.

[40] Wojnarowicz PM, Oros KK, Quinn MC, Arcand SL, Gambaro K, Madore J, Birch AH, de Ladurantaye M, Rahimi K, Provencher DM, Mes-Masson AM, Greenwood CM, Tonin PN. The genomic landscape of TP53 and p53 annotated high grade ovarian serous carcinomas from a defined founder population associated with patient outcome. *PLoS One.* 2012;7(9):e45484.

[41] Vang R, Levine DA, Soslow RA, Zaloudek C, Shih IeM, Kurman RJ. Molecular Alterations of TP53 are a Defining Feature of Ovarian High-Grade Serous Carcinoma: A Rereview of Cases Lacking TP53 Mutations in The Cancer Genome Atlas Ovarian Study. *Int J Gynecol Pathol.* 2016 Jan;35(1):48-55.

[42] Mittempergher L. Genomic Characterization of High-Grade Serous Ovarian Cancer: Dissecting Its Molecular Heterogeneity as a Road Towards Effective Therapeutic Strategies. *Curr Oncol Rep.* 2016 Jul;18(7):44.

[43] Otsuka I. Mechanisms of High-Grade Serous Carcinogenesis in the Fallopian Tube and Ovary: Current Hypotheses, Etiologic Factors, and Molecular Alterations. *Int J Mol Sci.* 2021 Apr 23;22(9):4409.

[44] Brown LA, Irving J, Parker R, Kim H, Press JZ, Longacre TA, Chia S, Magliocco A, Makretsov N, Gilks B, Pollack J, Huntsman D. Amplification of EMSY, a novel oncogene on 11q13, in high grade ovarian surface epithelial carcinomas. *Gynecol Oncol.* 2006 Feb;100(2):264-70.

[45] Weberpals JI, Pugh TJ, Marco-Casanova P, Goss GD, Andrews Wright N, Rath P, Torchia J, Fortuna A, Jones GN, Roudier MP, Bernard L, Lo B, Torti D, Leon A, Marsh K, Hodgson D, Duciaume M, Howat WJ, Lukashchuk N, Lazic SE, Whelan D, Sekhon HS. Tumor genomic, transcriptomic, and immune profiling characterizes differential response to first-line platinum chemotherapy in high grade serous ovarian cancer. *Cancer Med.* 2021 May;10(9):3045-3058.

[46] Cancer Genome Atlas Research Network. Integrated genomic analyses of ovarian carcinoma. Nature. 2011 Jun 29;474(7353):609-15. doi: 10.1038/nature10166. Erratum in: *Nature.* 2012 Oct 11;490(7419):298.

[47] Ballabio S, Craparotta I, Paracchini L, Mannarino L, Corso S, Pezzotta MG, Vescio M, Fruscio R, Romualdi C, Dainese E, Ceppi L, Calura E, Pileggi S, Siravegna G, Pattini L, Martini P, Delle Marchette M, Mangioni C, Ardizzoia A, Pellegrino A, Landoni F, D'Incalci M, Beltrame L, Marchini S. Multisite analysis of high-grade serous epithelial ovarian cancers identifies genomic regions of focal and recurrent copy number alteration in 3q26.2 and 8q24.3. *Int J Cancer.* 2019 Nov 15;145(10):2670-2681.

[48] Moschetta M, George A, Kaye SB, Banerjee S. BRCA somatic mutations and epigenetic BRCA modifications in serous ovarian cancer. *Ann Oncol.* 2016 Aug;27(8):1449-55.

[49] Pennington KP, Walsh T, Harrell MI, Lee MK, Pennil CC, Rendi MH, Thornton A, Norquist BM, Casadei S, Nord AS, Agnew KJ, Pritchard CC, Scroggins S, Garcia RL, King MC, Swisher EM. Germline and somatic mutations in homologous recombination genes predict platinum response and survival in ovarian, fallopian tube, and peritoneal carcinomas. *Clin Cancer Res.* 2014 Feb 1;20(3):764-75.

[50] Takaya H, Nakai H, Takamatsu S, Mandai M, Matsumura N. Homologous recombination deficiency status-based classification of high-grade serous ovarian carcinoma. *Sci Rep.* 2020 Feb 17;10(1):2757. doi: 10.1038/s41598-020-59671-3.

[51] Pietragalla A, Arcieri M, Marchetti C, Scambia G, Fagotti A. Ovarian cancer predisposition beyond BRCA1 and BRCA2 genes. *Int J Gynecol Cancer.* 2020 Nov;30(11):1803-1810.

[52] Berkel C, Cacan E. Involvement of ATMIN-DYNLL1-MRN axis in the progression and aggressiveness of serous ovarian cancer. *Biochem Biophys Res Commun.* 2021 Sep 17;570:74-81.

[53] Soslow RA, Han G, Park KJ, Garg K, Olvera N, Spriggs DR, Kauff ND, Levine DA. Morphologic patterns associated with BRCA1 and BRCA2 genotype in ovarian carcinoma. *Mod Pathol.* 2012 Apr;25(4):625-36.

[54] Ritterhouse LL, Nowak JA, Strickland KC, Garcia EP, Jia Y, Lindeman NI, Macconaill LE, Konstantinopoulos PA, Matulonis UA, Liu J, Berkowitz RS, Nucci MR, Crum CP, Sholl LM, Howitt BE. Morphologic correlates of molecular alterations in extrauterine Müllerian carcinomas. *Mod Pathol.* 2016 Aug;29(8):893-903.

[55] Banerjee SN, Lord CJ. First-line PARP inhibition in ovarian cancer - standard of care for all? *Nat Rev Clin Oncol.* 2020 Mar;17(3):136-137.

[56] Jiang X, Li X, Li W, Bai H, Zhang Z. PARP inhibitors in ovarian cancer: Sensitivity prediction and resistance mechanisms. *J Cell Mol Med.* 2019 Apr;23(4):2303-2313.

[57] Wang L, Wang Q, Xu Y, Cui M, Han L. Advances in the Treatment of Ovarian Cancer Using PARP Inhibitors and the Underlying Mechanism of Resistance. *Curr Drug Targets.* 2020;21(2):167-178.

[58] Patch AM, Christie EL, Etemadmoghadam D, Garsed DW, George J, Fereday S, Nones K, Cowin P, Alsop K, Bailey PJ, Kassahn KS, Newell F, Quinn MC, Kazakoff S, Quek K, Wilhelm-Benartzi C, Curry E, Leong HS; Australian Ovarian Cancer Study Group, Hamilton A, Mileshkin L, Au-Yeung G, Kennedy C, Hung J, Chiew YE, Harnett P, Friedlander M, Quinn M, Pyman J, Cordner S, O'Brien P, Leditschke J, Young G, Strachan K, Waring P, Azar W, Mitchell C, Traficante N, Hendley J, Thorne H, Shackleton M, Miller DK, Arnau GM, Tothill RW, Holloway TP, Semple T, Harliwong I, Nourse C, Nourbakhsh E, Manning S, Idrisoglu S, Bruxner TJ, Christ AN, Poudel B, Holmes O, Anderson M, Leonard C, Lonie A, Hall N, Wood S, Taylor DF, Xu Q, Fink JL, Waddell N, Drapkin R, Stronach E, Gabra H, Brown R, Jewell A, Nagaraj SH, Markham E, Wilson PJ, Ellul J, McNally O, Doyle MA, Vedururu R, Stewart C, Lengyel E, Pearson JV, Waddell N, deFazio A, Grimmond SM, Bowtell DD. Whole-genome characterization of chemoresistant ovarian cancer. *Nature.* 2015 May 28;521(7553): 489-94.

[59] Popova T, Manié E, Boeva V, Battistella A, Goundiam O, Smith NK, Mueller CR, Raynal V, Mariani O, Sastre-Garau X, Stern MH. Ovarian Cancers Harboring Inactivating Mutations in CDK12 Display a Distinct Genomic Instability Pattern Characterized by Large Tandem Duplications. *Cancer Res.* 2016 Apr 1;76(7):1882-91.

[60] McCormick A, Earp E, Leeson C, Dixon M, O'Donnell R, Kaufmann A, Edmondson RJ. Phosphatase and Tensin Homolog Is a Potential Target for Ovarian Cancer Sensitization to Cytotoxic Agents. *Int J Gynecol Cancer.* 2016 May;26(4):632-9.

[61] Kawahara N, Ogawa K, Nagayasu M, Kimura M, Sasaki Y, Kobayashi H. Candidate synthetic lethality partners to PARP inhibitors in the treatment of ovarian clear cell cancer. *Biomed Rep.* 2017 Nov;7(5):391-399.

[62] Mendes-Pereira AM, Martin SA, Brough R, McCarthy A, Taylor JR, Kim JS, Waldman T, Lord CJ, Ashworth A. Synthetic lethal targeting of PTEN mutant cells with PARP inhibitors. *EMBO Mol Med.* 2009 Sep;1(6-7):315-22.

[63] Hollis RL, Churchman M, Michie CO, Rye T, Knight L, McCavigan A, Perren T, Williams ARW, McCluggage WG, Kaplan RS, Jayson GC, Oza A, Harkin DP, Herrington CS, Kennedy R, Gourley C. High EMSY expression defines a BRCA-like subgroup of high-grade serous ovarian carcinoma with prolonged survival and hypersensitivity to platinum. *Cancer.* 2019 Aug 15;125(16):2772-2781.

[64] Bajrami I, Frankum JR, Konde A, Miller RE, Rehman FL, Brough R, Campbell J, Sims D, Rafiq R, Hooper S, Chen L, Kozarewa I, Assiotis I, Fenwick K, Natrajan R, Lord CJ, Ashworth A. Genome-wide profiling of genetic synthetic lethality identifies CDK12 as a novel determinant of PARP1/2 inhibitor sensitivity. *Cancer Res.* 2014 Jan 1;74(1):287-97.

[65] Miller RE, Leary A, Scott CL, Serra V, Lord CJ, Bowtell D, Chang DK, Garsed DW, Jonkers J, Ledermann JA, Nik-Zainal S, Ray-Coquard I, Shah SP, Matias-Guiu X, Swisher EM, Yates LR. ESMO recommendations on predictive biomarker testing for homologous recombination deficiency and PARP inhibitor benefit in ovarian cancer. *Ann Oncol.* 2020 Dec;31(12):1606-1622.

[66] Sztupinszki Z, Diossy M, Borcsok J, Prosz A, Cornelius N, Kjeldsen MK, Mirza MR, Szallasi Z. Comparative Assessment of Diagnostic Homologous Recombination Deficiency-Associated Mutational Signatures in Ovarian Cancer. *Clin Cancer Res.* 2021 Oct 15;27(20):5681-5687.

[67] Stover EH, Fuh K, Konstantinopoulos PA, Matulonis UA, Liu JF. Clinical assays for assessment of homologous recombination DNA repair deficiency. *Gynecol Oncol.* 2020 Dec;159(3):887-898.

[68] Davies H, Glodzik D, Morganella S, Yates LR, Staaf J, Zou X, Ramakrishna M, Martin S, Boyault S, Sieuwerts AM, Simpson PT, King TA, Raine K, Eyfjord JE, Kong G, Borg Å, Birney E, Stunnenberg HG, van de Vijver MJ, Børresen-Dale AL, Martens JW, Span PN, Lakhani SR, Vincent-Salomon A, Sotiriou C, Tutt A, Thompson AM, Van Laere S, Richardson AL, Viari A, Campbell PJ, Stratton MR, Nik-Zainal S. HRDetect is a predictor of BRCA1 and BRCA2 deficiency based on mutational signatures. *Nat Med.* 2017 Apr;23(4):517-525.

[69] Ceccaldi R, Liu JC, Amunugama R, Hajdu I, Primack B, Petalcorin MI, O'Connor KW, Konstantinopoulos PA, Elledge SJ, Boulton SJ, Yusufzai T, D'Andrea AD. Homologous-recombination-deficient tumours are dependent on Polθ-mediated repair. *Nature.* 2015 Feb 12;518(7538):258-62.

[70] D'Andrea AD. Mechanisms of PARP inhibitor sensitivity and resistance. *DNA Repair* (Amst). 2018 Nov;71:172-176.

[71] Weigelt B, Comino-Méndez I, de Bruijn I, Tian L, Meisel JL, García-Murillas I, Fribbens C, Cutts R, Martelotto LG, Ng CKY, Lim RS, Selenica P, Piscuoglio S, Aghajanian C, Norton L, Murali R, Hyman DM, Borsu L, Arcila ME, Konner J, Reis-Filho JS, Greenberg RA, Robson ME, Turner NC. Diverse *BRCA1* and *BRCA2* Reversion Mutations in Circulating Cell-Free DNA of Therapy-Resistant Breast or Ovarian Cancer. *Clin Cancer Res.* 2017 Nov 1;23(21):6708-6720.

[72] Norquist B, Wurz KA, Pennil CC, Garcia R, Gross J, Sakai W, Karlan BY, Taniguchi T, Swisher EM. Secondary somatic mutations restoring BRCA1/2 predict chemotherapy resistance in hereditary ovarian carcinomas. *J Clin Oncol.* 2011 Aug 1;29(22):3008-15.

[73] Sheta R, Bachvarova M, Plante M, Renaud MC, Sebastianelli A, Gregoire J, Navarro JM, Perez RB, Masson JY, Bachvarov D. Development of a 3D functional assay and identification of biomarkers, predictive for response of high-grade serous ovarian cancer (HGSOC) patients to poly-ADP ribose polymerase inhibitors (PARPis): targeted therapy. *J Transl Med.* 2020 Nov 19;18(1):439.

[74] Fuh K, Mullen M, Blachut B, Stover E, Konstantinopoulos P, Liu J, Matulonis U, Khabele D, Mosammaparast N, Vindigni A. Homologous recombination deficiency real-time clinical assays, ready or not? *Gynecol Oncol.* 2020 Dec;159(3):877-886.

[75] Konecny GE, Wang C, Hamidi H, Winterhoff B, Kalli KR, Dering J, Ginther C, Chen HW, Dowdy S, Cliby W, Gostout B, Podratz KC, Keeney G, Wang HJ, Hartmann LC, Slamon DJ, Goode EL. Prognostic and therapeutic relevance of molecular subtypes in high-grade serous ovarian cancer. *J Natl Cancer Inst.* 2014 Sep 30;106(10):dju249.

[76] Cook DP, Vanderhyden BC. Ovarian cancer and the evolution of subtype classifications using transcriptional profiling†. *Biol Reprod.* 2019 Sep 1;101(3):645-658.

[77] Mota A, S Oltra S, Moreno-Bueno G. Insight updating of the molecular hallmarks in ovarian carcinoma. *EJC Suppl.* 2020 Aug 22;15:16-26.

[78] Wang C, Cicek MS, Charbonneau B, Kalli KR, Armasu SM, Larson MC, Konecny GE, Winterhoff B, Fan JB, Bibikova M, Chien J, Shridhar V, Block MS, Hartmann LC, Visscher DW, Cunningham JM, Knutson KL, Fridley BL, Goode EL. Tumor hypomethylation at 6p21.3 associates with longer time to recurrence of high-grade serous epithelial ovarian cancer. *Cancer Res.* 2014 Jun 1;74(11):3084-91.

[79] Bodelon C, Killian JK, Sampson JN, Anderson WF, Matsuno R, Brinton LA, Lissowska J, Anglesio MS, Bowtell DDL, Doherty JA, Ramus SJ, Talhouk A, Sherman ME, Wentzensen N. Molecular Classification of Epithelial Ovarian Cancer Based on Methylation Profiling: Evidence for Survival Heterogeneity. *Clin Cancer Res.* 2019 Oct 1;25(19):5937-5946.

[80] Li J, Wang J, Chen R, Bai Y, Lu X. The prognostic value of tumor-infiltrating T lymphocytes in ovarian cancer. *Oncotarget.* 2017 Feb 28;8(9):15621-15631.

[81] Wang L. Prognostic effect of programmed death-ligand 1 (PD-L1) in ovarian cancer: a systematic review, meta-analysis and bioinformatics study. *J Ovarian Res.* 2019 Apr 30;12(1):37.

[82] Darb-Esfahani S, Kunze CA, Kulbe H, Sehouli J, Wienert S, Lindner J, Budczies J, Bockmayr M, Dietel M, Denkert C, Braicu I, Jöhrens K. Prognostic impact of programmed cell death-1 (PD-1) and PD-ligand 1 (PD-L1) expression in cancer cells and tumor-infiltrating lymphocytes in ovarian high grade serous carcinoma. *Oncotarget.* 2016 Jan 12;7(2):1486-99.

[83] Whitehair R, Peres LC, Mills AM. Expression of the Immune Checkpoints LAG-3 and PD-L1 in High-grade Serous Ovarian Carcinoma: Relationship to Tumor-associated Lymphocytes and Germline BRCA Status. *Int J Gynecol Pathol.* 2020 Nov;39(6):558-566.

[84] Huang CC, Cheng SH, Wu CH, Li WY, Wang JS, Kung ML, Chu TH, Huang ST, Feng CT, Huang SC, Tai MH. Delta-like 1 homologue promotes tumorigenesis and epithelial-mesenchymal transition of ovarian high-grade serous carcinoma through activation of Notch signaling. *Oncogene.* 2019 Apr;38(17):3201-3215.

[85] Lisio MA, Fu L, Goyeneche A, Gao ZH, Telleria C. High-Grade Serous Ovarian Cancer: Basic Sciences, Clinical and Therapeutic Standpoints. *Int J Mol Sci.* 2019 Feb 22;20(4):952.

[86] Chen S, Cavazza E, Barlier C, Salleron J, Filhine-Tresarrieu P, Gavoilles C, Merlin JL, Harlé A. Beside P53 and PTEN: Identification of molecular alterations of the RAS/MAPK and PI3K/AKT signaling pathways in high-grade serous ovarian carcinomas to determine potential novel therapeutic targets. *Oncol Lett.* 2016 Nov;12(5):3264-3272.

[87] Pfisterer J, Du Bois A, Bentz EK, Kommoss F, Harter P, Huober J, Schmalfeldt B, Burchardi N, Arnold N, Hilpert F. Prognostic value of human epidermal growth factor receptor 2 (Her-2)/neu in patients with advanced ovarian cancer treated with platinum/paclitaxel as first-line chemotherapy: a retrospective evaluation of the AGO-OVAR 3 Trial by the AGO OVAR Germany. *Int J Gynecol Cancer.* 2009 Jan;19(1):109-15.

[88] Ersoy E, Cao QJ, Otis CN. HER2 Protein Overexpression and Gene Amplification in Tubo-Ovarian High-grade Serous Carcinomas. *Int J Gynecol Pathol.* 2021 Jul 28.

[89] Slomovitz B, Gourley C, Carey MS, Malpica A, Shih IM, Huntsman D, Fader AN, Grisham RN, Schlumbrecht M, Sun CC, Ludemann J, Cooney GA, Coleman R, Sood AK, Mahdi H, Wong KK, Covens A, O'Malley DM, Lecuru F, Cobb LP, Caputo TA, May T, Huang M, Siemon J, Fernández ML, Ray-Coquard I, Gershenson DM. Low-grade serous ovarian cancer: State of the science. *Gynecol Oncol.* 2020 Mar;156(3):715-725.

[90] Longacre TA, McKenney JK, Tazelaar HD, Kempson RL, Hendrickson MR. Ovarian serous tumors of low malignant potential (borderline tumors): outcome-based study of 276 patients with long-term (> or =5-year) follow-up. *Am J Surg Pathol.* 2005 Jun;29(6):707-23.

[91] Van Nieuwenhuysen E, Busschaert P, Laenen A, Moerman P, Han SN, Neven P, Lambrechts D, Vergote I. Loss of 1p36.33 Frequent in Low-Grade Serous Ovarian Cancer. *Neoplasia.* 2019 Jun;21(6):582-590.

[92] Hunter SM, Anglesio MS, Ryland GL, Sharma R, Chiew YE, Rowley SM, Doyle MA, Li J, Gilks CB, Moss P, Allan PE, Stephens AN, Huntsman DG, deFazio A, Bowtell DD; Australian Ovarian Cancer Study Group, Gorringe KL, Campbell IG. Molecular profiling of low grade serous ovarian tumours identifies novel candidate driver genes. *Oncotarget.* 2015 Nov 10;6(35):37663-77.

[93] Romero I, Leskelä S, Mies BP, Velasco AP, Palacios J. Morphological and molecular heterogeneity of epithelial ovarian cancer: Therapeutic implications. *EJC Suppl.* 2020 Aug 22;15:1-15.

[94] Anglesio MS, Arnold JM, George J, Tinker AV, Tothill R, Waddell N, Simms L, Locandro B, Fereday S, Traficante N, Russell P, Sharma R, Birrer MJ; AOCS Study Group, deFazio A, Chenevix-Trench G, Bowtell DD. Mutation of ERBB2 provides a novel alternative mechanism for the ubiquitous activation of RAS-MAPK in ovarian serous low malignant potential tumors. *Mol Cancer Res.* 2008 Nov;6(11):1678-90.

[95] Kaldawy A, Segev Y, Lavie O, Auslender R, Sopik V, Narod SA. Low-grade serous ovarian cancer: A review. *Gynecol Oncol.* 2016 Nov;143(2):433-438.

[96] Mert I, Chhina J, Allo G, Dai J, Seward S, Carey MS, Llaurado M, Giri S, Rattan R, Munkarah AR. Synergistic effect of MEK inhibitor and metformin combination in low grade serous ovarian cancer. *Gynecol Oncol.* 2017 Aug;146(2):319-326.

[97] Wong KK, Tsang YT, Deavers MT, Mok SC, Zu Z, Sun C, Malpica A, Wolf JK, Lu KH, Gershenson DM. BRAF mutation is rare in advanced-stage low-grade ovarian serous carcinomas. *Am J Pathol.* 2010 Oct;177(4):1611-7.

[98] Tsang YT, Deavers MT, Sun CC, Kwan SY, Kuo E, Malpica A, Mok SC, Gershenson DM, Wong KK. KRAS (but not BRAF) mutations in ovarian serous borderline tumour are associated with recurrent low-grade serous carcinoma. *J Pathol.* 2013 Dec;231(4):449-56.

[99] Grisham RN, Iyer G, Garg K, Delair D, Hyman DM, Zhou Q, Iasonos A, Berger MF, Dao F, Spriggs DR, Levine DA, Aghajanian C, Solit DB. BRAF mutation is associated with early stage disease and improved outcome in patients with low-grade serous ovarian cancer. *Cancer.* 2013 Feb 1;119(3):548-554.

[100] Farley J, Brady WE, Vathipadiekal V, Lankes HA, Coleman R, Morgan MA, Mannel R, Yamada SD, Mutch D, Rodgers WH, Birrer M, Gershenson DM. Selumetinib in women with recurrent low-grade serous carcinoma of the ovary or peritoneum: an open-label, single-arm, phase 2 study. *Lancet Oncol.* 2013 Feb;14(2):134-40.

[101] Ho CL, Kurman RJ, Dehari R, Wang TL, Shih IeM. Mutations of BRAF and KRAS precede the development of ovarian serous borderline tumors. *Cancer Res.* 2004 Oct 1;64(19):6915-8.

[102] Chui MH, Xing D, Zeppernick F, Wang ZQ, Hannibal CG, Frederiksen K, Kjaer SK, Cope L, Kurman RJ, Shih IM, Wang TL, Vang R. Clinicopathologic and Molecular Features of Paired Cases of Metachronous Ovarian Serous Borderline Tumor and Subsequent Serous Carcinoma. *Am J Surg Pathol.* 2019 Nov;43(11):1462-1472.

[103] Garg K, Park KJ, Soslow RA. Low-grade serous neoplasms of the ovary with transformation to high-grade carcinomas: a report of 3 cases. *Int J Gynecol Pathol.* 2012 Sep;31(5):423-8.

[104] Dehari R, Kurman RJ, Logani S, Shih IeM. The development of high-grade serous carcinoma from atypical proliferative (borderline) serous tumors and low-grade micropapillary serous carcinoma: a morphologic and molecular genetic analysis. *Am J Surg Pathol.* 2007 Jul;31(7):1007-12.

[105] Quddus MR, Rashid LB, Hansen K, Sung CJ, Lawrence WD. High-grade serous carcinoma arising in a low-grade serous carcinoma and micropapillary serous borderline tumour of the ovary in a 23-year-old woman. *Histopathology.* 2009 May;54(6):771-3.

[106] Zarei S, Wang Y, Jenkins SM, Voss JS, Kerr SE, Bell DA. Clinicopathologic, Immunohistochemical, and Molecular Characteristics of Ovarian Serous Carcinoma With Mixed Morphologic Features of High-grade and Low-grade Serous Carcinoma. *Am J Surg Pathol.* 2020 Mar;44(3):316-328.

[107] Chui MH, Momeni Boroujeni A, Mandelker D, Ladanyi M, Soslow RA. Characterization of TP53-wildtype tubo-ovarian high-grade serous carcinomas: rare exceptions to the binary classification of ovarian serous carcinoma. *Mod Pathol.* 2021 Feb;34(2):490-501.

[108] Ayhan A, Kurman RJ, Yemelyanova A, Vang R, Logani S, Seidman JD, Shih IeM. Defining the cut point between low-grade and high-grade ovarian serous carcinomas: a clinicopathologic and molecular genetic analysis. *Am J Surg Pathol.* 2009 Aug;33(8):1220-4.

[109] Nasioudis D, Latif NA, Simpkins F, Cory L, Giuntoli RL 2nd, Haggerty AF, Morgan MA, Ko EM. Adjuvant chemotherapy for early stage endometrioid ovarian carcinoma: An analysis of the National Cancer Data Base. *Gynecol Oncol.* 2020 Feb;156(2):315-319.

[110] Terada T. Endometrioid adenocarcinoma of the ovary arising in atypical endometriosis. *Int J Clin Exp Pathol.* 2012;5(9):924-7.

[111] Helder-Woolderink JM, Blok EA, Vasen HF, Hollema H, Mourits MJ, De Bock GH. Ovarian cancer in Lynch syndrome; a systematic review. *Eur J Cancer.* 2016 Mar;55:65-73.

[112] La Vecchia C. Ovarian cancer: epidemiology and risk factors. *Eur J Cancer Prev.* 2017 Jan;26(1):55-62.

[113] Wiegand KC, Shah SP, Al-Agha OM, Zhao Y, Tse K, Zeng T, Senz J, McConechy MK, Anglesio MS, Kalloger SE, Yang W, Heravi-Moussavi A, Giuliany R, Chow C, Fee J, Zayed A, Prentice L, Melnyk N, Turashvili G, Delaney AD, Madore J, Yip S, McPherson AW, Ha G, Bell L, Fereday S, Tam A, Galletta L, Tonin PN, Provencher D, Miller D, Jones SJ, Moore RA, Morin GB, Oloumi A, Boyd N, Aparicio SA, Shih IeM, Mes-Masson AM, Bowtell DD, Hirst M, Gilks B, Marra MA, Huntsman DG. ARID1A mutations in endometriosis-associated ovarian carcinomas. *N Engl J Med.* 2010 Oct 14;363(16):1532-43.

[114] Samartzis EP, Noske A, Dedes KJ, Fink D, Imesch P. ARID1A mutations and PI3K/AKT pathway alterations in endometriosis and endometriosis-associated ovarian carcinomas. *Int J Mol Sci.* 2013 Sep 12;14(9):18824-49.

[115] Oliva E, Sarrió D, Brachtel EF, Sánchez-Estévez C, Soslow RA, Moreno-Bueno G, Palacios J. High frequency of beta-catenin mutations in borderline endometrioid tumours of the ovary. *J Pathol.* 2006 Apr;208(5):708-13.

[116] Kim S, Jeong S. Mutation Hotspots in the β-Catenin Gene: Lessons from the Human Cancer Genome Databases. *Mol Cells.* 2019 Jan 31;42(1):8-16.

[117] Zyla RE, Olkhov-Mitsel E, Amemiya Y, Bassiouny D, Seth A, Djordjevic B, Nofech-Mozes S, Parra-Herran C. CTNNB1 Mutations and Aberrant β-Catenin Expression in Ovarian Endometrioid Carcinoma: Correlation With Patient Outcome. *Am J Surg Pathol.* 2021 Jan;45(1):68-76.

[118] Cybulska P, Paula ADC, Tseng J, Leitao MM Jr, Bashashati A, Huntsman DG, Nazeran TM, Aghajanian C, Abu-Rustum NR, DeLair DF, Shah SP, Weigelt B. Molecular profiling and molecular classification of endometrioid ovarian carcinomas. *Gynecol Oncol.* 2019 Sep;154(3):516-523.

[119] Leskela S, Romero I, Rosa-Rosa JM, Caniego-Casas T, Cristobal E, Pérez-Mies B, Gutierrez-Pecharroman A, Santón A, Ojeda B, López-Reig R, Palacios-Berraquero ML, Andrada E, Montes S, Pastor F, Gomez MC, López-Guerrero JA, Poveda A, Palacios J. Molecular Heterogeneity of Endometrioid Ovarian Carcinoma: An Analysis of 166 Cases Using the Endometrial Cancer Subrogate Molecular Classification. *Am J Surg Pathol.* 2020 Jul;44(7):982-990.

[120] Leskela S, Romero I, Cristobal E, Pérez-Mies B, Rosa-Rosa JM, Gutierrez-Pecharroman A, Caniego-Casas T, Santón A, Ojeda B, López-Reig R, Palacios-Berraquero ML, García Á, Ibarra J, Hakim S, Guarch R, López-Guerrero JA, Poveda A, Palacios J. Mismatch Repair Deficiency in Ovarian Carcinoma: Frequency, Causes, and Consequences. *Am J Surg Pathol.* 2020 May;44(5):649-656.

[121] Bennett JA, Pesci A, Morales-Oyarvide V, Da Silva A, Nardi V, Oliva E. Incidence of Mismatch Repair Protein Deficiency and Associated Clinicopathologic Features in a Cohort of 104 Ovarian Endometrioid Carcinomas. *Am J Surg Pathol.* 2019 Feb;43(2):235-243.

[122] Anglesio MS, Wang YK, Maassen M, Horlings HM, Bashashati A, Senz J, Mackenzie R, Grewal DS, Li-Chang H, Karnezis AN, Sheffield BS, McConechy MK, Kommoss F, Taran FA, Staebler A, Shah SP, Wallwiener D, Brucker S, Gilks CB, Kommoss S, Huntsman DG. Synchronous Endometrial and Ovarian Carcinomas: Evidence of Clonality. *J Natl Cancer Inst.* 2016 Feb 1;108(6):djv428.

[123] Schultheis AM, Ng CK, De Filippo MR, Piscuoglio S, Macedo GS, Gatius S, Perez Mies B, Soslow RA, Lim RS, Viale A, Huberman KH, Palacios JC, Reis-Filho JS, Matias-Guiu X, Weigelt B. Massively Parallel Sequencing-Based Clonality Analysis of Synchronous Endometrioid Endometrial and Ovarian Carcinomas. *J Natl Cancer Inst.* 2016 Feb 1;108(6):djv427.

[124] Gilks CB, Kommoss F. Synchronous tumours of the female reproductive tract. *Pathology.* 2018 Feb;50(2):214-221.

[125] Kurman RJ, Shih IeM. Seromucinous Tumors of the Ovary. What's in a Name? *Int J Gynecol Pathol.* 2016 Jan;35(1):78-81.

[126] Wu CH, Mao TL, Vang R, Ayhan A, Wang TL, Kurman RJ, Shih IeM. Endocervical-type mucinous borderline tumors are related to endometrioid tumors based on mutation and loss of expression of ARID1A. *Int J Gynecol Pathol.* 2012 Jul;31(4):297-303.

[127] Ben-Mussa A, McCluggage WG. Ovarian seromucinous cystadenomas and adenofibromas: first report of a case series. *Histopathology.* 2021 Feb;78(3):445-452.

[128] Watkins, Jaclyn C. M.D., M.S.; Young, Robert H. M.D. Müllerian Mucinous Cystadenomas of the Ovary: A Report of 25 Cases of an Unheralded Benign Ovarian Neoplasm Often Associated With Endometriosis and a Brief Consideration of Neoplasms Arising From the Latter, *International Journal of Gynecological Pathology:* January 2022 - Volume 41 - Issue 1 - p 68-75.

[129] Kim KR, Choi J, Hwang JE, Baik YA, Shim JY, Kim YM, Robboy SJ. Endocervical-like (Müllerian) mucinous borderline tumours of the ovary are frequently associated with the KRAS mutation. *Histopathology.* 2010 Oct;57(4):587-96.

[130] Parra-Herran C, Lerner-Ellis J, Xu B, Khalouei S, Bassiouny D, Cesari M, Ismiil N, Nofech-Mozes S. Molecular-based classification algorithm for endometrial carcinoma categorizes ovarian endometrioid carcinoma into prognostically significant groups. *Mod Pathol.* 2017 Dec;30(12):1748-1759.

[131] Bosse T, Nout RA, McAlpine JN, McConechy MK, Britton H, Hussein YR, Gonzalez C, Ganesan R, Steele JC, Harrison BT, Oliva E, Vidal A, Matias-Guiu X, Abu-Rustum NR, Levine DA, Gilks CB, Soslow RA. Molecular Classification of Grade 3 Endometrioid Endometrial Cancers Identifies Distinct Prognostic Subgroups. *Am J Surg Pathol.* 2018 May;42(5):561-568.

[132] Hollis RL, Thomson JP, Stanley B, Churchman M, Meynert AM, Rye T, Bartos C, Iida Y, Croy I, Mackean M, Nussey F, Okamoto A, Semple CA, Gourley C, Herrington CS. Molecular stratification of endometrioid ovarian carcinoma predicts clinical outcome. *Nat Commun.* 2020 Oct 5;11(1):4995.

[133] Chui MH, Ryan P, Radigan J, Ferguson SE, Pollett A, Aronson M, Semotiuk K, Holter S, Sy K, Kwon JS, Soma A, Singh N, Gallinger S, Shaw P, Arseneau J, Foulkes WD, Gilks CB, Clarke BA. The histomorphology of Lynch syndrome-associated ovarian carcinomas: toward a subtype-specific screening strategy. *Am J Surg Pathol.* 2014 Sep;38(9):1173-81.

[134] Wang L, Rambau PF, Kelemen LE, Anglesio MS, Leung S, Talhouk A, Köbel M. Nuclear β-catenin and CDX2 expression in ovarian endometrioid carcinoma identify patients with favourable outcome. *Histopathology.* 2019 Feb;74(3):452-462.

[135] Cheasley D, Nigam A, Zethoven M, Hunter S, Etemadmoghadam D, Semple T, Allan P, Carey MS, Fernandez ML, Dawson A, Köbel M, Huntsman DG, Le Page C, Mes-Masson AM, Provencher D, Hacker N, Gao Y, Bowtell D, deFazio A, Gorringe KL, Campbell IG. Genomic analysis of low-grade serous ovarian carcinoma to identify key drivers and therapeutic vulnerabilities. *J Pathol.* 2021 Jan;253(1):41-54.

[136] Fukumoto T, Park PH, Wu S, Fatkhutdinov N, Karakashev S, Nacarelli T, Kossenkov AV, Speicher DW, Jean S, Zhang L, Wang TL, Shih IM, Conejo-Garcia JR, Bitler BG, Zhang R. Repurposing Pan-HDAC Inhibitors for ARID1A-Mutated Ovarian Cancer. *Cell Rep.* 2018 Mar 27;22(13):3393-3400.

[137] Lee JM, Minasian L, Kohn EC. New strategies in ovarian cancer treatment. *Cancer.* 2019 Dec 15;125 Suppl 24(Suppl 24):4623-4629.

[138] Babaier A, Ghatage P. Mucinous Cancer of the Ovary: Overview and Current Status. *Diagnostics* (Basel). 2020 Jan 19;10(1):52.

[139] Gouy S, Saidani M, Maulard A, Bach-Hamba S, Bentivegna E, Leary A, Pautier P, Devouassoux-Shisheboran M, Genestie C, Morice P. Characteristics and Prognosis of Stage I Ovarian Mucinous Tumors According to Expansile or Infiltrative Type. *Int J Gynecol Cancer.* 2018 Mar;28(3):493-499.

[140] Hada T, Miyamoto M, Ishibashi H, Matsuura H, Sakamoto T, Kakimoto S, Iwahashi H, Tsuda H, Takano M. Survival and biomarker analysis for ovarian mucinous carcinoma according to invasive patterns: retrospective analysis and review literature. *J Ovarian Res.* 2021 Feb 14;14(1):33.

[141] Cheasley D, Wakefield MJ, Ryland GL, Allan PE, Alsop K, Amarasinghe KC, Ananda S, Anglesio MS, Au-Yeung G, Böhm M, Bowtell DDL, Brand A, Chenevix-Trench G, Christie M, Chiew YE, Churchman M, DeFazio A, Demeo R, Dudley R, Fairweather N, Fedele CG, Fereday S, Fox SB, Gilks CB, Gourley C, Hacker NF, Hadley AM, Hendley J, Ho GY, Hughes S, Hunstman DG, Hunter SM, Jobling TW, Kalli KR, Kaufmann SH, Kennedy CJ, Köbel M, Le Page C, Li J, Lupat R, McNally OM, McAlpine JN, Mes-Masson AM, Mileshkin L, Provencher DM, Pyman J, Rahimi K, Rowley SM, Salazar C, Samimi G, Saunders H, Semple T, Sharma R, Sharpe AJ, Stephens AN, Thio N, Torres MC, Traficante N, Xing Z, Zethoven M, Antill YC, Scott CL, Campbell IG, Gorringe KL. The molecular origin and taxonomy of mucinous ovarian carcinoma. *Nat Commun.* 2019 Sep 2;10(1):3935.

[142] Anglesio MS, Kommoss S, Tolcher MC, Clarke B, Galletta L, Porter H, Damaraju S, Fereday S, Winterhoff BJ, Kalloger SE, Senz J, Yang W, Steed H, Allo G, Ferguson S, Shaw P, Teoman A, Garcia JJ, Schoolmeester JK, Bakkum-Gamez J, Tinker AV, Bowtell DD, Huntsman DG, Gilks CB, McAlpine JN. Molecular characterization of mucinous ovarian tumours supports a stratified treatment approach with HER2 targeting in 19% of carcinomas. *J Pathol.* 2013 Jan;229(1):111-20.

[143] Hunter SM, Gorringe KL, Christie M, Rowley SM, Bowtell DD; Australian Ovarian Cancer Study Group, Campbell IG. Pre-invasive ovarian mucinous tumors are characterized by CDKN2A and RAS pathway aberrations. *Clin Cancer Res.* 2012 Oct 1;18(19):5267-77.

[144] Mackenzie R, Kommoss S, Winterhoff BJ, Kipp BR, Garcia JJ, Voss J, Halling K, Karnezis A, Senz J, Yang W, Prigge ES, Reuschenbach M, Doeberitz MV, Gilks BC, Huntsman DG, Bakkum-Gamez J, McAlpine JN, Anglesio MS. Targeted deep sequencing of mucinous ovarian tumors reveals multiple overlapping RAS-pathway activating mutations in borderline and cancerous neoplasms. *BMC Cancer.* 2015 May 19;15:415.

[145] Bouri S, Simon P, D'Haene N, Catteau X, Noël JC. P53 and PIK3CA Mutations in KRAS/HER2 Negative Ovarian Intestinal-Type Mucinous Carcinoma Associated with Mature Teratoma. *Case Rep Obstet Gynecol.* 2020 Jul 22;2020:8863610.

[146] Gorringe KL, Cheasley D, Wakefield MJ, Ryland GL, Allan PE, Alsop K, Amarasinghe KC, Ananda S, Bowtell DDL, Christie M, Chiew YE, Churchman M, DeFazio A, Fereday S, Gilks CB, Gourley C, Hadley AM, Hendley J, Hunter SM, Kaufmann SH, Kennedy CJ, Köbel M, Le Page C, Li J, Lupat R, McNally OM, McAlpine JN, Pyman J, Rowley SM, Salazar C, Saunders H, Semple T, Stephens AN, Thio N, Torres MC, Traficante N, Zethoven M, Antill YC, Campbell IG, Scott CL. Therapeutic options for mucinous ovarian carcinoma. *Gynecol Oncol.* 2020 Mar;156(3):552-560.

[147] Liu H, Xu Y, Ji J, Dong R, Qiu H, Dai X. Prognosis of ovarian clear cell cancer compared with other epithelial cancer types: A population-based analysis. *Oncol Lett.* 2020 Mar;19(3):1947-1957. doi: 10.3892/ol.2020.11252.

[148] Iida Y, Okamoto A, Hollis RL, Gourley C, Herrington CS. Clear cell carcinoma of the ovary: a clinical and molecular perspective. *Int J Gynecol Cancer.* 2021 Apr;31(4):605-616.

[149] Huang HN, Lin MC, Huang WC, Chiang YC, Kuo KT. Loss of ARID1A expression and its relationship with PI3K-Akt pathway alterations and ZNF217 amplification in ovarian clear cell carcinoma. *Mod Pathol.* 2014 Jul;27(7):983-90.

[150] Friedlander ML, Russell K, Millis S, Gatalica Z, Bender R, Voss A. Molecular Profiling of Clear Cell Ovarian Cancers: Identifying Potential Treatment Targets for Clinical Trials. *Int J Gynecol Cancer.* 2016 May;26(4):648-54.

[151] Takano M, Tsuda H, Sugiyama T. Clear cell carcinoma of the ovary: is there a role of histology-specific treatment? *J Exp Clin Cancer Res.* 2012 Jun 1;31(1):53.

[152] Bennett JA, Morales-Oyarvide V, Campbell S, Longacre TA, Oliva E. Mismatch Repair Protein Expression in Clear Cell Carcinoma of the Ovary: Incidence and Morphologic Associations in 109 Cases. *Am J Surg Pathol.* 2016 May;40(5):656-63.

[153] Tan DS, Iravani M, McCluggage WG, Lambros MB, Milanezi F, Mackay A, Gourley C, Geyer FC, Vatcheva R, Millar J, Thomas K, Natrajan R, Savage K, Fenwick K, Williams A, Jameson C, El-Bahrawy M, Gore ME, Gabra H, Kaye SB, Ashworth A, Reis-Filho JS. Genomic analysis reveals the molecular heterogeneity of ovarian clear cell carcinomas. *Clin Cancer Res.* 2011 Mar 15;17(6):1521-34.

[154] Parra-Herran C, Bassiouny D, Lerner-Ellis J, Olkhov-Mitsel E, Ismiil N, Hogen L, Vicus D, Nofech-Mozes S. p53, Mismatch Repair Protein, and POLE Abnormalities in Ovarian Clear Cell Carcinoma: An Outcome-based Clinicopathologic Analysis. *Am J Surg Pathol.* 2019 Dec;43(12):1591-1599.

[155] Bitler BG, Aird KM, Garipov A, Li H, Amatangelo M, Kossenkov AV, Schultz DC, Liu Q, Shih IeM, Conejo-Garcia JR, Speicher DW, Zhang R. Synthetic lethality by targeting EZH2 methyltransferase activity in ARID1A-mutated cancers. *Nat Med.* 2015 Mar;21(3):231-8.

[156] Oneda E, Zorzi F, Gorio A, Quaglia F, Abeni C, Rota L, Zaniboni A. Differential Diagnosis of Small Cell Carcinoma of the Ovary or Ovarian Metastases of Small Cell Carcinoma of the Lung: A Case Report and Review of the Literature. *Case Rep Oncol.* 2020 Jul 10;13(2):822-828.

[157] Münstedt K, Estel R, Dreyer T, Kurata A, Benz A. Small Cell Ovarian Carcinomas - Characterisation of Two Rare Tumor Entities. *Geburtshilfe Frauenheilkd.* 2013 Jul;73(7):698-704.

[158] Auguste A, Blanc-Durand F, Deloger M, Le Formal A, Bareja R, Wilkes DC, Richon C, Brunn B, Caron O, Devouassoux-Shisheboran M, Gouy S, Morice P, Bentivegna E, Sboner A, Elemento O, Rubin MA, Pautier P, Genestie C, Cyrta J, Leary A. Small Cell Carcinoma of the Ovary, Hypercalcemic Type (SCCOHT) beyond *SMARCA4* Mutations: A Comprehensive Genomic Analysis. *Cells.* 2020 Jun 19;9(6):1496.

[159] Genestie C, Blanc-Durand F, Auguste A, Pautier P, Dunant A, Scoazec JY, Gouy S, Morice P, Bentivegna E, Maulard A, LeFormal A, Devouassoux-Shisheboran M, Leary A. Clinical utility of SMARCA4 testing by immunohistochemistry in rare ovarian tumours. *Br J Cancer.* 2020 Feb;122(4):564-568.

[160] Wang Y, Chen SY, Karnezis AN, Colborne S, Santos ND, Lang JD, Hendricks WP, Orlando KA, Yap D, Kommoss F, Bally MB, Morin GB, Trent JM, Weissman BE, Huntsman DG. The histone methyltransferase EZH2 is a therapeutic target in small cell carcinoma of the ovary, hypercalcaemic type. *J Pathol.* 2017 Jul;242(3):371-383.

[161] Tischkowitz M, Huang S, Banerjee S, Hague J, Hendricks WPD, Huntsman DG, Lang JD, Orlando KA, Oza AM, Pautier P, Ray-Coquard I, Trent JM, Witcher M, Witkowski L, McCluggage WG, Levine

DA, Foulkes WD, Weissman BE. Small-Cell Carcinoma of the Ovary, Hypercalcemic Type-Genetics, New Treatment Targets, and Current Management Guidelines. *Clin Cancer Res.* 2020 Aug 1;26(15):3908-3917.

[162] Kalampokas E, Sharma V, Gagliardi T, Payne F, Gurumurthy M. Primary small cell ovarian cancer of pulmonary type: A case report. *Gynecol Oncol Rep.* 2018 Feb 8;24:10-13.

[163] Zheng R, Heller DS. Borderline Brenner Tumor: A Review of the Literature. *Arch Pathol Lab Med.* 2019 Oct;143(10):1278-1280.

[164] Zhang Y, Staley SA, Tucker K, Clark LH. Malignant Brenner tumor of the ovary: Case series and review of treatment strategies. *Gynecol Oncol Rep.* 2019 Feb 12;28:29-32.

[165] Kuhn E, Ayhan A, Shih IeM, Seidman JD, Kurman RJ. The pathogenesis of atypical proliferative Brenner tumor: an immunohistochemical and molecular genetic analysis. *Mod Pathol.* 2014 Feb;27(2):231-7.

[166] afe LJ, Muller KE, Ananda G, Mitchell T, Spotlow V, Patterson SE, Tsongalis GJ, Mockus SM. Molecular Genetic Analysis of Ovarian Brenner Tumors and Associated Mucinous Epithelial Neoplasms: High Variant Concordance and Identification of Mutually Exclusive RAS Driver Mutations and MYC Amplification. *Am J Pathol.* 2016 Mar;186(3):671-7.

[167] Cuatrecasas M, Catasus L, Palacios J, Prat J. Transitional cell tumors of the ovary: a comparative clinicopathologic, immunohistochemical, and molecular genetic analysis of Brenner tumors and transitional cell carcinomas. *Am J Surg Pathol.* 2009 Apr;33(4):556-67.

[168] Khani F, Diolombi ML, Khattar P, Huang W, Fallon JT, Epstein JI, Zhong M. Benign and Malignant Brenner Tumors Show an Absence of TERT Promoter Mutations That Are Commonly Present in Urothelial Carcinoma. *Am J Surg Pathol.* 2016 Sep;40(9):1291-5.

[169] Lin DI, Killian JK, Venstrom JM, Ramkissoon SH, Ross JS, Elvin JA. Recurrent urothelial carcinoma-like FGFR3 genomic alterations in malignant Brenner tumors of the ovary. *Mod Pathol.* 2021 May;34(5):983-993.

[170] Pfarr N, Darb-Esfahani S, Leichsenring J, Taube E, Boxberg M, Braicu I, Jesinghaus M, Penzel R, Endris V, Noske A, Weichert W, Schirmacher P, Denkert C, Stenzinger A. Mutational profiles of Brenner tumors show distinctive features uncoupling urothelial carcinomas and ovarian carcinoma with transitional cell histology. *Genes Chromosomes Cancer.* 2017 Oct;56(10):758-766.

[171] Lin DI, Shah N, Tse JY, Killian JK, Hemmerich A, Edgerly C, Haberberger J, Severson EA, Huang RSP, Ramkissoon SH, Vergilio JA, Ross JS, Elvin JA. Molecular profiling of mesonephric and mesonephric-like carcinomas of cervical, endometrial and ovarian origin. *Gynecol Oncol Rep.* 2020 Sep 26;34:100652.

[172] Mirkovic J, McFarland M, Garcia E, Sholl LM, Lindeman N, MacConaill L, Dong F, Hirsch M, Nucci MR, Quick CM, Crum CP, McCluggage WG, Howitt BE. Targeted Genomic Profiling Reveals Recurrent KRAS Mutations in Mesonephric-like Adenocarcinomas of the Female Genital Tract. *Am J Surg Pathol.* 2018 Feb;42(2):227-233.

[173] Pors J, Segura S, Chiu DS, Almadani N, Ren H, Fix DJ, Howitt BE, Kolin D, McCluggage WG, Mirkovic J, Gilks B, Park KJ, Hoang L. Clinicopathologic Characteristics of Mesonephric Adenocarcinomas and Mesonephric-like Adenocarcinomas in the Gynecologic Tract: A Multi-institutional Study. *Am J Surg Pathol.* 2021 Apr 1;45(4):498-506.

[174] da Silva EM, Fix DJ, Sebastiao APM, Selenica P, Ferrando L, Kim SH, Stylianou A, Da Cruz Paula A, Pareja F, Smith ES, Zehir A, Konner JA, Cadoo K, Reis-Filho JS, Abu-Rustum NR, Mueller JJ, Weigelt B, Park KJ. Mesonephric and mesonephric-like carcinomas of the female genital tract: molecular characterization including cases with mixed histology and matched metastases. *Mod Pathol.* 2021 Aug;34(8):1570-1587.

[175] McCluggage WG, Vosmikova H, Laco J. Ovarian Combined Low-grade Serous and Mesonephric-like Adenocarcinoma: Further Evidence for A Mullerian Origin of Mesonephric-like Adenocarcinoma. *Int J Gynecol Pathol.* 2020 Jan;39(1):84-92.

[176] Chapel DB, Joseph NM, Krausz T, Lastra RR. An Ovarian Adenocarcinoma With Combined Low-grade Serous and Mesonephric Morphologies Suggests a Müllerian Origin for Some Mesonephric Carcinomas. *Int J Gynecol Pathol.* 2018 Sep;37(5):448-459.

[177] Coatham M, Li X, Karnezis AN, Hoang LN, Tessier-Cloutier B, Meng B, Soslow RA, Blake Gilks C, Huntsman DG, Stewart CJ, Postovit LM, Köbel M, Lee CH. Concurrent ARID1A and ARID1B inactivation in endometrial and ovarian dedifferentiated carcinomas. *Mod Pathol.* 2016 Dec;29(12):1586-1593.

[178] Jin Z, Ogata S, Tamura G, Katayama Y, Fukase M, Yajima M, Motoyama T. Carcinosarcomas (malignant mullerian mixed tumors) of the uterus and ovary: a genetic study with special reference to histogenesis. *Int J Gynecol Pathol.* 2003 Oct;22(4):368-73.

[179] Rottmann D, Snir OL, Wu X, Wong S, Hui P, Santin AD, Buza N. HER2 testing of gynecologic carcinosarcomas: tumor stratification for potential targeted therapy. *Mod Pathol.* 2020 Jan;33(1):118-127.

[180] Brunetti M, Agostini A, Staurseth J, Davidson B, Heim S, Micci F. Molecular characterization of carcinosarcomas arising in the uterus and ovaries. *Oncotarget.* 2019 Jun 4;10(38):3614-3624.

[181] Zhao S, Bellone S, Lopez S, Thakral D, Schwab C, English DP, Black J, Cocco E, Choi J, Zammataro L, Predolini F, Bonazzoli E, Bi M, Buza N, Hui P, Wong S, Abu-Khalaf M, Ravaggi A, Bignotti E, Bandiera E, Romani C, Todeschini P, Tassi R, Zanotti L, Odicino F, Pecorelli S, Donzelli C, Ardighieri L, Facchetti F, Falchetti M, Silasi DA, Ratner E, Azodi M, Schwartz PE, Mane S, Angioli R, Terranova C, Quick CM, Edraki B, Bilgüvar K, Lee M, Choi M, Stiegler AL, Boggon TJ, Schlessinger J, Lifton RP, Santin AD. Mutational landscape of uterine and ovarian carcinosarcomas implicates histone genes in epithelial-mesenchymal transition. *Proc Natl Acad Sci USA*. 2016 Oct 25;113(43):12238-12243.

[182] Schipf A, Mayr D, Kirchner T, Diebold J. Molecular genetic aberrations of ovarian and uterine carcinosarcomas--a CGH and FISH study. *Virchows Arch.* 2008 Mar;452(3):259-68.

[183] Wessman S, Fuentes BB, Törngren T, Kvist A, Kokaraki G, Menkens H, Hjerpe E, Hugo Y, Petta TB, Borg Å, Carlson JW. Precision Oncology of High-Grade Ovarian Cancer Defined through Targeted Sequencing. *Cancers* (Basel). 2021 Oct 19;13(20):5240.

[184] Berton-Rigaud D, Devouassoux-Shisheboran M, Ledermann JA, Leitao MM, Powell MA, Poveda A, Beale P, Glasspool RM, Creutzberg CL, Harter P, Kim JW, Reed NS, Ray-Coquard I. Gynecologic Cancer InterGroup (GCIG) consensus review for uterine and ovarian carcinosarcoma. *Int J Gynecol Cancer.* 2014 Nov;24(9 Suppl 3):S55-60.

Chapter 13

An Approach to Borderline Ovarian Tumors

Maria Luisa Fais[1], MD
Giorgio Candotti[2], MD
Giulia Carboni[1], MD
Giuseppe Deo[1], MD
Giuseppina Fais[1], MD
Valerio Mais[1], MD, PhD
Stefano Angioni[1], MD, PhD
and Michele Peiretti[1,*], MD, PhD
[1]Department of Surgical Sciences, Division of Gynecology and Obstetrics, University of Cagliari, Italy
[2]Obstetrics and Gynecology Unit, IRCCS San Raffaele Scientific Institute, Milan, Italy

Introduction

Since the early 1970s, the International Federation of Gynecology and Obstetrics (FIGO) and the WHO have recognized an independent group of ovarian epithelial tumors with low malignant potential (Acs, 2005). In 2003, the WHO classification introduced the term "borderline ovarian tumors" (BOTs) (Tavassoli & Devilee, 2003), a subgroup of epithelial ovarian neoplasms characterized by nuclear atypia and modestly increased mitotic activity but, without an infiltrative growth pattern or stromal invasion, unlike ovarian cancer.

The specific criteria for histological diagnosis, the different subtype, the biological behavior of the disease, the controversies about therapeutic indications, particularly in the younger, make the diagnosis and treatment of BOT difficult.

This chapter discusses the current recommendations and the existing literature data on the clinical management of borderline ovarian tumor, highlighting the surgical approach including fertility sparing treatment.

* Corresponding Author's Email: michelepeiretti@hotmail.com.

In: Ovarian Cancer
Editors: Christos Iavazzo, Alexandros Fotiou and John Spiliotis
ISBN: 979-8-88697-633-5

Epidemiology

Borderline ovarian tumors represent 10-20% of all ovarian epithelial tumors (Lenhard, Mitterer, Kumper, & al., 2009), with an incidence of 1.8-4.8 out of 100,000 (Skirnisdottir, Garmo, Wilander, & Holmberg, 2008). The median age of diagnosis is 45 years, but 34% of patients are under 40 years old (Skirnisdottir, Garmo, Wilander, & Holmberg, 2008). Survival, all stages combined, is 95% at 5 years and 90% at 10 years; a 5-year survival for Stages I, II, III, IV is 99.7% (95% CI: 96.2 – 100%), 99.6% (95% CI: 92.6 – 100%), 95.3% (95% CI: 91.8 – 97.4%) and 77.1% (95% CI: 58.0 – 88.3%), respectively (Bourdel, Huchon, Abdel Wahab, & al., 2021). In a systematic review of 6,362 patients of BOTs, it was reported that 78.9% of cases were diagnosed at Stage I (Du Bois, Ewald-Riegler, Du Bois, & Harter, 2009). Extended disease spread within the pelvic or beyond (Stage II – III) was rare, disease beyond the abdomen (Stage IV) represented an exception (Acs, 2005).

An epidemiological association between individual risk of borderline ovarian tumor and family history of BOT or different cancers (pancreatic, lung, bone and leukemia) was described in literature (Bourdel, Huchon, Abdel Wahab, & al., 2021). In a systematic review and pooled analysis, an increased risk of BOT was reported among women with a history of pelvic inflammatory disease (PID). Furthermore, these risks increased with the number of PID episodes. This association was biologically plausible and could be explained by the hypothesis that inflammation, characterized by the production of free radicals, cytokines, prostaglandins, and growth factors with the potential for genetic and epigenetic changes to the DNA, resulted in an increased risk of malignant transformation (Rasmussen, Kjaer, Albieri, Bandera, & et al., 2017).

In the last few years, several studies have shown a link between fertility drugs and BOTs. One of the largest studies looking at incidence of BOTs compared 7,544 infertile women who underwent in vitro fertilization (IVF) with 14,095 women in the non-IVF infertility group. The rate of BOTs in women undergoing IVF was higher with an HR of 2.46 (95% CI 1.20–5.04) (Stewart, Holman, Finn, Preen, & Hart, 2013). Another study compared the incidence of BOTs in a cohort of >19,000 women undergoing IVF with 6,000 women with subfertility who did not undergo IVF and with the general population, with a mean follow-up of 14.7 years. The incidence of BOTs was higher in the IVF cohort when compared with the general population (SIR 1.76, 95% CI 1.16–2.56) as well as compared with the subfertility group (HR 4.23, 95% CI 1.25–14.33) (van Leeuwen, Klip, Mooij, & et. al., 2011). The largest systematic review evaluating the risk of borderline ovarian tumors following the use of fertility drugs identified three case-control and three cohort studies. Three studies reported a 2–3–fold increased risk for BOTs with fertility drug use. However, it is not possible to perform a meta-analysis giving an overall relative risk due to the extreme heterogeneity among studies. Nonetheless, when individual drug use was evaluated, there was no significant increased risk for borderline ovarian tumors with clomiphene citrate (CC) alone, CC and gonadotropins, or gonadotropins alone. While several studies have shown a small increase in the absolute risk of BOTs after fertility treatments, according to the American Society for Reproductive Medicine (ASRM)/ There was insufficient consistent evidence that a particular fertility drug increased the risk of disease and currently there was insufficient evidence to recommend against the use of fertility medications to avoid BOTs (ASRM, Fertility Drugs and Cancer: A Guideline, 2016).

Biopathology

BOTs are neoplasms of epithelial origin characterized by up-regulated cellular proliferation and the presence of slight nuclear atypia but without destructive stromal invasion. Six histologic subtypes of BOT are distinguished based on the epithelial cell type, comprising serous (50%) and mucinous (45%), and less common subtypes including endometrioid, clear cell, seromucinous, and borderline Brenner tumor (Silverberg, et al., 2004). There were three histologic characteristics correlated with biological behavior of the disease: peritoneal implants, classified into "invasive" and "non-invasive"; microinvasion of the tumor; and a micropapillary pattern of serous BOT.

Peritoneal Implants

Approximately one third of serous BOT are associated with peritoneal implants, a serous epithelial proliferations confined to the peritoneal surface without infiltration of the underlying subperitoneal fat, unlike invasive peritoneal implants characteristics of LGSC (Low-Grade Serous Cancer) (Hauptmann, Friedrich, Redline, & Avril, 2017). In a meta-analysis of 97 studies including 4,129 patients with serous borderline tumor, Seidman et al. reported an overall survival rate of virtually 100% for Stage I and 95.3% for advanced stage with non-invasive implants, whereas survival for tumors associated with invasive peritoneal disease was reduced to 66% and the presence of a micropapillary variant of serous BOT was a strong predictor for concurrent invasive peritoneal disease. (Seidman & Kurman, 2000). These results confirm the importance of the pathologist differentiation between "non-invasive" and "invasive" peritoneal implant in terms of clinical management, to optimise histological analysis as well as minimise interobserver variability, for which a pathologist is required (Morice, et al., 2012).

Micropapillary Pattern of Serous BOT

The micropapillary pattern comprising 5–15% of serous BOTs, characterized by the lack of hierarchically branching papillae, showing either elongate filiform "micropapillae" (≥ 5:1 length to width ratio) or cribriform epithelium lining the cyst walls or large caliber fibrovascular papillae, with at least one area of continuous micropapillary or cribriform growth > 5 mm in one dimension (Hauptmann, Friedrich, Redline, & Avril, 2017). The clinical relevance of the micropapillary pattern results in the association with a poorer prognosis than do lesions without this histological feature, so that this histological variant of serous BOTs is described by Kurman as an intermediate entity in the progression from serous BOT to LGSC (Kurman & Shih, The Origin and Pathogenesis of Epithelial Ovarian Cancer: A Proposed Unifying Theory., 2012). Gene expression analysis performed in conventional serous BOT (n = 17), micropapillary variant (n = 9), and LGSC (n = 11) support this view, demonstrating differential gene expression patterns between serous BOT and its micropapillary variant, but no differences in gene expression between micropapillary variant and LGSC (May, et al., 2012). Interesting, the serous BOT with micropapillary patterns without implants (Stage I) or with non-invasive implants (Stage II–III) have the same prognosis as do serous BOT without micropapillary variants (Kurman, Seidman, & Shih, Serous Borderline Tumours of the Ovary., 2005). Therefore, the poorer prognosis in the cases of serous BOTs with micropapillary patterns could perhaps be linked to the increased rate of invasive peritoneal implants and not to the presence of micropapillary patterns themselves. As reported, a micropapillary pattern alone is no independent prognostic factor but is often associated with invasive peritoneal disease, therefore the micropapillary pattern is a feature of a high-risk group likely to develop an invasive recurrence (Morice, et al., 2012) and associated with shorter disease-free survival (DFS) and overall survival (OS).

Microinvasion in Serous BOT

The WHO 2014 classification refined the term "microinvasion" in serous BOT as isolated rounded eosinophilic cells or cell clusters stroma rich in fibroblasts and cannot exceed 5 mm in the largest linear dimension. The microinvasive foci are characterized by cells with morphologic evidence of apoptosis and lower expression of WT1 and Ki67 index, suggesting terminal differentiation and/or senescence of this cells (Maniar, Wang, Visvanathan, Shih Ie, & Kurman, 2014). At the moment, microinvasion in serous BOT is not consistently associated with an adverse prognostic effect. However, in a review by Morice et al. about serous BOT with microinvasion (n=133), 20 patients had recurrence (15%), including 35% (seven of 20) with invasive disease at recurrence. Rate of disease-related death was 6% (eight of 133) (Morice, et al., 2012). In accordance with some studies, this data shown that stromal microinvasion is a prognostic factor for serous BOT, but further investigations are needed to establish whether microinvasion is a prognostic factor *independent* of peritoneal implants or micropapillary patterns.

Diagnosis

Incidental finding upon clinical examination or imaging techniques in asymptomatic women allows the physician to make a diagnosis of adnexal mass. Sometimes the patients experience symptoms such as abdominal discomfort or abdominal pain in the presence of grow dimension of lesion. Acute symptoms, such as a pain secondary to rupture or torsion, are unusual.

Ultrasonography is the first-line of imaging for the diagnosis of adnexal mass (Kaijser, Vandecaveye, Deroose, & et al., 2014). A subjective assessment by expert ultrasound examiners is sufficient for the establishment of the borderline nature of the ovary lesion and for to narrow the diagnosis to a specific histological subtype. Recently, the ESGO/ISUOG/IOTA/ESGE Consensus Statement on pre-operative diagnosis of ovarian tumors reported the typical findings of the main subtype of BOT (Timmerman, Planchamp, Bourne, Landolfo, & et al., 2021). The most common features of ultrasound images of the different subtypes of BOT are summarized in Table 1. Other imaging techniques, such as magnetic resonance imaging (MRI) or Computed Tomography (CT) scan may provide additional information but are not routinely necessary in preoperative evaluation. For lesions indeterminate on ultrasound, an MRI increases the specificity of the imaging evaluation, thus decreasing benign resections. CT is useful in the diagnosis and treatment planning of advanced disease (Bourdel, Huchon, Abdel

Wahab, & al., 2021). The assessment of the invasiveness of peritoneal implants of imaging BOT is not actually defined. No recommendation can be made on imaging prediction of the possibility of conservative BOT treatment (Abdel Wahab, Rousset, Bolze, & Thomassin-Naggara, 2020). A CT scan may be useful in excluding peritoneal carcinomatosis in the cases where there is doubt between a borderline and an invasive tumor (Bourdel, Huchon, Abdel Wahab, & al., 2021).

Table 1. The most common features of ultrasound images of the different subtypes of BOT

Subtype	Laterality	Appearance	Features	Color score
Borderline serous	Uni (73%) Bi(27%)	Unilocular-solid (55%) or multilocular-solid (30%); cystic fluid anechoic (47%) or low-level	>3 irregular papillations (81%) with internal blood flow and anechoic spaces; no shadowing	2/3
Borderline mucinous (intestinal type) (30–50%)	Uni	Multilocular (80%) or unilocular (15%); very large tumor (median diameter 195 mm)	Multiple small loculi, often 'honeycomb nodule'; nopapillations; cystic fluid low-level 2	2/3
Borderline mucinous (endocervical type)	Uni	Unilocular-solid; sometimes multilocular-solid; median diameter 37 mm	Papillations (60%); cystic fluid low-level or ground-glass	2/3
Borderline seromucinous	Uni	Contain endometrioid-, indifferent- and squamous-type epithelium	Frequently associated with endometriosis	/

Regarding markers tumor, according to ESGO/ISUOG/IOTA/ESGE Consensus Statement, CA125 is the best available biomarker identified to date. However, false-positive results may be derived from several conditions, such as endometriosis, pelvic inflammatory disease, menstruation, uterine fibroids or benign cysts. In the past year, multiple studies have highlighted the role of HE4 as a potential complement to CA125, especially in differentiating benign cysts and inflammatory lesions in younger women. The 2018 INCA (Institute National du Cancer) Guidelines recommend the dosage of CA125 and HE4 serum levels in the pre-operative assessment of patients with adnexal masses. The CA19.9 assay may be proposed when a mucinous BOT is suspected on imaging. (Lavoue, Huchon, Akladios, Alfonsi, & et al., 2019).

Staging and Risk Assessment

The standard surgical approach to BOTs is based on total abdominal hysterectomy and bilateral salpingo-oophorectomy (BSO) with a surgical staging procedure that includes peritoneal washing, peritoneal biopsies (pelvic peritoneum, paracolic gutters, diaphragm), omentectomy, and resection of macroscopically suspicious lesions. According to the ESMO-ESGO Consensus Conference, the standard approach is open surgery. The rationale for this choice is based on ensuring adequate exposure and macroscopic exploration of the abdominal cavity and reducing the risk of primary tumor rupture during its dissection and/or removal (Colombo et al., 2019). However, the laparoscopic approach in the early stage seems to be safe, and it is commonly accepted in clinical practice. The development of laparoscopic techniques with the use of Endo-Bag gives less risk of spillage and fewer port-site metastases. In the CNGOF Guidelines, if no risk of tumor rupture is possible, laparoscopy with a protected extraction is recommended over laparotomy (Bourdel, Huchon, Abdel Wahab, et al., 2021). Systematic lymphadenectomy is not recommended, even in advanced-stage BOTs. (Bourdel, Huchon, Abdel Wahab, & al., 2021). Systematic lymphadenectomy is not recommended, even in advanced-stage BOTs (Lesieur, Kane, Duvillard, & et al., 2011). Several studies have reported no effect of node involvement in terms of overall survival (OS) in patients with BOTs. (Morice, et al., 2012).

In cases without completed staging during the first surgery the role of surgical restaging is still controversial. It is known that the omission of staging has an impact on recurrence rate (du Bois, Ewald-Riegler, de Gregorio, & et al., 2013). On the other hand, in literature, similar oncological outcomes for both upstaged and non-upstaged patients with early disease are reported and the benefit on OS of complete surgical staging in macroscopically Stage I BOTs remains unproven (Zapardiel, Rosenberg, Peiretti, Zanagnolo, & et al., 2010). The indication for restaging surgery should be evaluated individually and it should be discussed at a multidisciplinary meeting according to the current evidence, surgical restaging should only be considered (I) for serous BOT with micropapillary patterns that correlate with a higher risk of extraovarian microscopic implants; (II) for mucinous BOT in cases where the appendix was not visualized or where an initial cystectomy has been performed, imposing a unilateral salpingo-oophorectomy; and (III) in cases with incomplete visual exploration of the abdomino-pelvic peritoneum during the first surgery. A laparoscopic approach is recommended. The procedure should include peritoneal washing, complete exploration of the abdominal cavity with peritoneal biopsies, omentectomy, and exploration of the appendix with an appendectomy in case of a pathological macroscopic appearance. In cases of mucinous BOTs, restaging surgery should also include unilateral salpingo-oophorectomy for mucinous BOTs initially treated by cystectomy. For endometrioid BOTs, in the absence of a strategy to maintain fertility, a hysterectomy is recommended (Colombo, et al., 2019) - (Bourdel, Huchon, Abdel Wahab, & al., 2021).

Indications of adjuvant platinum-based chemotherapy remain rare in BOTs and are limited to patients with invasive peritoneal implants or with nodal spread (Leary, Petrella, Pautier, Duvillard, & et al., 2014).

Primary Treatment of Early Stage

When early stage BOTs are suspected on preoperative imaging in a menopausal woman or in those who have fulfilled their reproductive wishes, bilateral salpingo-oophorectomy, peritoneal surgical staging and peritoneal washing are recommended. Conversely, there is no evidence supporting the need of systematic hysterectomy and lymphadenectomy (Bourdel, Huchon, Abdel Wahab, & al., 2021).

Considering the good prognosis of BOTs, fertility-sparing surgery (FSS) - defined as the preservation of the uterus and at least part of one ovary - should be considered for young women who desire to preserve the potential to conceive. In cases of early stage serous BOT with non-invasive implants, unilateral salpingo-oophorectomy (USO) or cystectomy with complete surgical staging may be offered. A meta-analysis and a large multicenter series demonstrated that ultraconservative surgery (cystectomy) increases the risk of recurrence (Darai, Fauvet, Uzan, Gouy, & et al., 2013); (Trillsch, Mahner, Woelber, & et al., 2014). The recurrence rate of USO and cystectomy are 12% and 25%, respectively (Vasconcelos & de Sousa Mendes, 2015). Nonetheless, the ESGO-ESMO Guidelines reported that an adnexectomy not should be preferred over a cystectomy because the latter is associated with a higher fertility rate (Colombo, et al., 2019).

If there is bilateral ovarian involvement and complete resection can be achieved, unilateral or bilateral ovarian cystectomy may be considered. Recent phase III trial demonstrated that the bilateral cystectomy compared with a unilateral adnexectomy and contralateral cystectomy in bilateral serous BOTs increased the fertility rate without increasing the recurrence rate (Palomba, Falbo, Del Negro, Rocca, & et al., 2010).

The preservation of the maximum volume of a healthy ovary should be considered in the context of FSS in early-stage disease, and cystectomy is considered an acceptable approach to optimize fertility preservation in serous BOT. In the patients treated conservatively, the risk of an invasive recurrence is very low and is estimated at 0.5%.

In surgical management, the contralateral normal-appearing ovary should be carefully inspected but a biopsy is not required since it may cause unnecessary damage to the ovarian reserve and the peritoneal adhesions, that is associated with a 20–30% reduction of pregnancy rate (ASRM, Pathogenesis, Consequences and Control of Peritoneal Adhesions in Gynecologic Surgery., 2007). When possible, the uterus should be preserved, in perspective of heterologous fertilization (Luke, Brown, Missmer, Spector, & et al., 2016).

The impact of the histological subtype in surgical management is still debated. Mucinous BOT tend to recur as invasive ovarian carcinoma is more frequent than the serous subtype after conservative treatment (Koskas, Uzan, Gouy, Pautier, & al., 2011). Therefore, the mere excision of the tumor is not feasible and USO is required (Tropé, Kaern, & Davidson, 2012). An appendectomy for the mucinous subtype is also strongly recommended. In the absence of a treatment strategy aimed at maintaining fertility in endometrioid BOT, hysterectomy is considered as a part of the initial surgery. Previous studies reported a correlation between endometrioid BOT with concomitant disorders of the endometrium and occasionally even synchronous endometrioid adenocarcinoma of the uterus, especially in younger and nulliparous patients (Bell & Kurman, 2000). For this reason, a different research group highlights the importance of uterine curettage as part of the diagnostic workup to exclude endometrial pathology in cases of this subtype with envisaged fertility preservation (Reichenbach, Schmoeckel, Mahner, & Trillsch, 2021). However, in the perspective of fertility preservation, it should be recalled that the curettage of the endometrium is one of the more important iatrogenic causes of intrauterine adhesions that may affect pregnancy rate (Santamaria, Isaacson, & Simòn, 2018). To date, the main international guidelines and treatment recommendations do not specifically address the importance of excluding an extraovarian disease in cases of endometrioid BOT when a fertility conserving approach is envisaged.

Fertility Sparing Surgery: Clinical Evaluation and Obstetrical Outcomes

The clinical follow up should be more intensive and a considerable proportion of women require additional surgeries for recurrence of the disease. Therefore, conservative management should always be carefully balanced and it should not be considered if the woman has already fulfilled her reproductive wishes or if future pregnancies are implausible, such as in women older than 40 years old and in those with infertility and concomitant compromised ovarian reserve which are present prior to surgery. An oncofertility counselling is mandatory in all young women with a diagnosis of BOT, if possible before the intervention and then amended after it. Obviously, if BOT is an unexpected finding, only post-surgical counselling can be done. Complete clinical history focusing on menstrual cycles characteristics, parity and eventual history of infertility, transvaginal ultrasound to evaluate the antral follicle count (AFC) and anti-müllerian hormone (AMH) assessments is essential for collected data about fertility statement. Ideally, this evaluation should precede surgery but important insights could emerge also after the intervention and may guide future decisions. Of particular relevance is the monitoring of the ovarian reserve over time after the intervention. Importantly, this information should be collected at least six months after surgery since the re-equilibrium of the ovarian function needs time (Mangili, Somigliana, Giorgione, Martinelli, & et al., 2016).

This setting of patients are also worthy of fertility preservation considerations, because ovarian reserve may be directly injured by surgery and post-surgical peritoneal adhesions may develop and interfere with natural conception. Preserving gametes is an option in women who may be infertile after the end of the treatments and the oocytes cryopreservation following controlled ovarian hyper-stimulation (COH) represent the standard technique. The oocytes cryopreservation after *in vitro* maturation (IVM) of oocytes collected without hormonal stimulation is still experimental but very promising; the ovarian cortex freezing is not recommended in cases of an ovarian tumor, because of the risk of disease spread. Therefore, in adult women, the COH represent the first choice. However, constitutive estrogen and progesterone receptors expression has previously been reported for BOT, particularly in the serous subtype (Høgdall, Christensen, Høgdall, Blaakaer, & et al., 2007), and even if not supported by clear data, a detrimental effect of COH on BOT growth is plausible and COH should not be offered when BOT is still present. Contrary, data about the feasibility and safety of COH in women with previously diagnosed BOT is scanty but reassuring. In a review of literature on this specific issue, a total of 126 cases of BOT subsequently underwent COH to treat infertility are analyzed. Specifically, 104 of them were previously operated on for early stage disease while the remaining 22 were operated on for advanced stages. The pooled estimate of pregnancy was 80% and the rate of recurrences was 23% (45/126). One case of progression to an invasive carcinoma was documented but no deaths were observed (Attar, Berkman, Topuz, Baysal, & et al., 2004).

A neglected but important issue here is the possibility to consider natural pregnancy. If the woman has a partner and she is interested in having a pregnancy, she should be encouraged to have regular intercourse starting as soon as possible (Mangili, Somigliana, Giorgione, Martinelli, & et al., 2016). In cases of a history of infertility, Assisted Reproductive Techniques (ARTs) should be immediately considered. There is actually no consensus on the best timing for conception seeking. Some authors suggested waiting 1–2 years after the initial treatment of BOT mainly because the risk of recurrence after conservative treatment is higher in the first two years (Fauvet, Poncelet, Boccara, Descamps, & et al., 2005). Other authors suggested immediate pregnancy seeking after the diagnosis (Mangili, Somigliana, Giorgione, Martinelli, & et al., 2016). Adequate counselling regarding the risk of potential recurrence in pregnancy is essential, because a sonographic follow-up is complicated. Other imaging techniques are limited by pregnancy and abdominal surgery in pregnancy is feasible but risky.

Regarding the obstetrical outcomes after conservative surgical treatment, the date reported in literature are encouraging. In a review article about fertility outcome after BOTs management which reviewed120 articles, a pregnancy rate (PR) of 54% in the early stage was reported and 34% in advanced stage disease (Darai, Fauvet, Uzan, Gouy, & et al., 2013). In a large series of patients treated conservatively for BOTs considering only patients with childbearing desire and excluding patients with a previous history of infertility, a 84% PR (Delle Marchette, Ceppi, Andreano, Bonazzi, & et al., 2019) was reported. In a recent study conducted on 85 (n. 74, Stage I; n. 3, Stage II; n. 8, Stage III),patients with BOT treated conservatively a PR among childbearing-desiring women was 73% and live birth rate was 67% (Candotti, Peiretti, Mangili, Bergamini, & et al., 2020). Not negligible, the maternal desire and the younger age of diagnosis are the most important factors affecting PR after surgery.

Primary Treatment of Advanced Stage

Advanced stage BOTs are defined by a FIGO stage ≥ II. Radical surgery represents the standard treatment. There is no proven benefit of systematic lymph node dissection in Stage II/III of serous BOT (Colombo, et al., 2019). In patients with a desire to fall pregnant, conservative treatment with uterine and all or part of the ovary preservation may be proposed after a multidisciplinary meeting (Bourdel, Huchon, Abdel Wahab, & al., 2021). Literature does not provide sufficient data to conclude that a hysterectomy should be routinely performed in Stage II or III serous BOT, therefore the FSS can be assessed in selected cases. Data concerning conservative treatment in the presence of peritoneal implants are rare. In a recent study conducted in 65 patients with advanced serous BOT (n. 18, Stage II; n. 47, Stage III), 38 (58%) patients recurred: 8 (21%) under the form of invasive disease. Three of the patients who had a reoccurrence died. The authors reported that 5- and 10-years OS rate in patients treated with a conservative approach were 100% and 92%, respectively and the 5- and 10-years DFS rates were 42% and 25%, respectively. A multivariate analysis shown that the use of conservative treatment impacts DFS, but no OS. In this context, the recurrence rate is higher (Gouy, et al., 2021), but the risk of lethal outcomes is rare if a complete resection of implants is achieved. However, conservative management in Stage II/III BOT should be assessed with caution, due to the limitation in terms of number of cases with invasive implants reported in literature.

Regarding the necessity of chemotherapy in advanced BOT, to date the 2019 ESMO-ESGO Guidelines and 2020 CNGOF Guidelines reported no benefit in adding adjuvant treatment to upfront surgery, even in the case of invasive implants (Colombo, et al., 2019).

Treatment of Recurrent Disease

In cases of recurrence, in a woman of childbearing age, a second conservative surgery can be proposed after informing the patient of the risk of additional recurrences. In the absence of an invasive tumor at the time of BOT recurrence, chemotherapy is not indicated. In cases of an ovary with peritoneal infiltration, chemotherapy should be discussed by a multidisciplinary team.

Conclusion

- The standard surgical approach of borderline ovarian tumor (BOT) is based on total abdominal hysterectomy and bilateral salpingo-oophorectomy with a peritoneal surgical staging, including peritoneal washing, peritoneal biopsies (pelvic peritoneum, paracolic gutters, diaphragm), omentectomy and resection of macroscopically suspicious lesions;
- The laparoscopic approach in early stage BOTs seems to be safe and it is commonly accepted in clinical practices;
- An oncofertility counselling is mandatory in all young women with a suspicious/diagnosis of BOT;
- Fertility sparing surgery with unilateral salpingo-oophorectomy or cystectomy may be an oncological safe option for young patients in childbearing age with early stage disease;
- Conservative treatment can be proposed in younger patients that wish to preserve the potential to conceive with advanced stage of BOTs exclusively in selected cases and previous adequate counselling;
- The obstetrical outcomes after conservative surgical treatment in young patients with BOT are encouraging.

References

Abdel Wahab, C., Rousset, P., Bolze, P. A., & Thomassin-Naggara, I. (2020). Borderline ovarian tumours: CNGOF GuidelinesforClinical Practice - Imaging. *Gynecol Obstet Fertil Senol, 48*(3), 260-276.

Acs, G. (2005). Serous and mucinous borderline (low malignant potential) tumors of the ovary. *Am. J. Clin. Pathol. 123 (Suppl.)*, S13-S57.

Anglesio, M. S., Kommos, S., Tolcher, M. C., Clarke, B., & al., e. (2013). Molecular characterization ofmucinous ovarian tumours supports a stratified treatment approach with HER2 targeting in 19% of carcinomas. *J Pathol, 229*(1), 111–120.

ASRM. (2007). Pathogenesis, consequences and control of peritoneal adhesions in gynecologic surgery. *Fert Steril, 88*, 21-26.

ASRM. (2016). Fertility drugs and cancer: a guideline. *Fertility and Sterility, 106*(7), 1617-1626.

Attar, E., Berkman, S., Topuz, S., Baysal, B., & et al. (2004). Evolutive peritoneal disease after conservative management and the use of infertility drugs in a patients with stage IIIC bordrline micro-papillary serous carcinoma (MPSC) of the ovary: case report. *Hum Reprod, 19*, 1472-1475.

Bell, K. A., & Kurman, R. J. (2000). A clinicopathological analysisof atypical proliferative (borderline) tumors and well-differentiated endometrioid adenocarcinomas of the ovary. *Am J Surg Pathol., 24*, 1465-1479.

Bourdel, N., Huchon, C., Abdel Wahab, C., & al., e. (2021). Borderline ovarian tumors: Guidelines from French national college of obstetricians and gynecologists. *Eur. J. Obst. Gynecol. and Reproduct. Biol., 256*, 492-501.

Candotti, G., Peiretti, M., Mangili, G., Bergamini, A., & et al. (2020). What women want: fertility sparing surgery in borderline ovarian tumours patients and pregnancy outcome. *Europ J Surg Oncol, 46*, 888-892.

Colombo, N., Sessa, C., du Bois, A., Ledermann, J., McCluggage, W., & et al. (2019). ESMO-ESGO consensus conference recommendations on ovarian cancer: pathology and molecular biology, early and advanced stages, borderline tumours and recurrent disease. *Gynecol Cancer, 29*, 728-760.

Darai, E., Fauvet, R., Uzan, C., Gouy, S., & et al. (2013). Fertility and borderline ovarian tumor: a systematic review of conservative management, risk of recurrence and alternative options. *Hum Reprod Update, 19*, 151-166.

Delle Marchette, M., Ceppi, L., Andreano, A., Bonazzi, C., & et al. (2019). Oncologic and fertility impact of surgical approach for borderline ovarian tumours treated with fertility sparing surgery. *Eur J Cancer, 111*, 61-68.

Du Bois, A., Ewald-Riegler, N., Du Bois, O., & Harter, P. (2009). Borderline tumors of the ovary - a systematic review. *Geburtsh Frauenheilk, 69*, 807-833.

Fauvet, R., Poncelet, C., Boccara, J., Descamps, P., & et al. (2005). Fertility after conservative treatment for borderline ovarian tumors: a French multicenter study. *Fertil Steril*, 284-290.

Gouy, S., Maria, S., Faron, M., Maulard, A., Pautier, P., & et al. (2021). Results after conservative surgery of stage II/III serous borderline ovarian tumors. *Ann Surg Oncol, 28*, 3597-3604.

Hauptmann, S., Friedrich, K., Redline, R., & Avril, S. (2017). Ovarian bordeline tumors in the 2014 WHO classification: evolving concepts and diagnostic criteria. *Virchows Arch., 470*, 125-142.

Høgdall, E., Christensen, L., Høgdall, C., Blaakaer, J., & et al. (2007). Prognostic value of estrogen recertor and progesterone receptor tumor expression in Danish ovarian cancer patients: from the 'MALOVA' ovariancancer study. *Oncol Rep, 18*, 1051-1059.

Kaijser, J., Vandecaveye, V., Deroose, C. M., & et al. (2014). Imaging techniques for the pre-surgical diagnosis of adnexal tumours. *Best pract Res Clin Obstet Gynaecol., 28*, 683-685.

Koskas, M., Uzan, C., Gouy, S., Pautier, P., & al., e. (2011). Fertility determinants after conservative surgery for muconous borderline tumours of the ovary (excluding peritoneal pseudomixoma). *Hum Reprod., 26*, 808-814.

Kurman, R. J., & Shih, I. M. (2012). The origin and pathogenesis of epithelial ovarian cancer: a proposed unifying theory. *Am J Surg Pathol., 34*(3), 433-443.

Kurman, R. J., Carcangiu, M. L., Herrington, C. S., & Young, R. H. (2014). *WHO classification of tumours of female reproductive organs.* Lyon: IARC.

Kurman, R. J., Seidman, J. D., & Shih, I. M. (2005). Serous borderline tumoursof the ovary. *Histopathology, 10*, 310-315.

Lavoue, V., Huchon, V., Akladios, C., Alfonsi, P., & et al. (2019). Management of epithelial cancer of the ovary, falloppian tube, and primary peritoneum. Short text of the French Clinical Practice Guidelines issued by FRANCOGYN, CNGOF, SFOG, and GINECO-ARCAGY, and endorsed by INCa. *Obstet Gynecol Reprod Biol., 236*, 214-223.

Leary, A., Petrella, M., Pautier, P., Duvillard, P., & et al. (2014). Adjuvant platinum-based chemotherapy for borderline serous ovarian tumours with invasive implants. *Gynecol Oncol, 132*, 23-27.

Lenhard, M. S., Mitterer, S., Kumper, C., & al., e. (2009). Long-term follow up after ovarian borderline tumor: relapse and survival in a large patient cohort. *Eur. J. Obstet. Gynecol. Reprod. Biol., 145*(2), 189-194.

Luke, B., Brown, M., Missmer, S., Spector, L., & et al. (2016). Assisted reproductive technology use and outcomes among women with a historyof cancer. *Hum Reprod, 31*, 183-189.

Mangili, G., Somigliana, E., Giorgione, V., Martinelli, F., & et al. (2016). Fertility preservation in women with borderline ovarian tumours. *Cancer Treatment Reviews, 49*, 13-24.

Maniar, K. P., Wang, Y., Visvanathan, K., Shih Ie, M., & Kurman, R. J. (2014). Evaluation of microinvasion and lymph node involvement in ovarian serous borderline/atypical proliferative serous tumors: a morphological and immunohistochemical analysis of 37 cases. *Am J Surg Pathol., 38*(6), 743-755.

May, T., Virtanen, C., Sharma, M., Milea, A., Begley, H., Rosen, B., & et al. (2012). Low malignant potential tumors with micropapillary features are molecularly similar to low-grade serous carcinoma of the ovary. *Gynecol Oncol., 117*(1), 9-17.

Morice, P., Uzan, C., Fauvet, R., Gouy, S., Duvillard, P., & Darai, E. (2012). Borderline ovarian tumour: pathological diagnostic dilemma and risk factors for invasive or lethal recurrence. *Lancet Oncol., 13*, 103-115.

Palomba, S., Falbo, A., Del Negro, S., Rocca, M., & et al. (2010). Ultra-conservative fertility-sparing strategy for bilateral borderline ovarian tumours:an 11-years ollow up. *Hum Reprod, 25*, 1966-1972.

Palomba, S., Zupi, E., Russo, T., Falbo, A., & et al. (2007). Comparison of two fertility-sparing approachesfor bilateral borderline ovarian tumours:a randomized controlled study. *Hum Reprod., 22*, 578-585.

Rasmussen, C. B., Kjaer, K., Albieri, V., Bandera, E. V., & et al. (2017). Pelvic inflammatory disease and the risk of ovarian cancer and borderline ovarian tumors: a pooled analysis of 13 case-control studies. *Am J Epidemiol., 185*(1), 8-20.

Reichenbach, J., Schmoeckel, E., Mahner, S., & Trillsch, F. (2021). Diagnostic workup for endometrioid borderline ovarian tumors (eBOT) requires histopathological evaluation of the uterus. *J Ovarian Res, 14*(89), 1-7.

Santamaria, X., Isaacson, K., & Simòn, C. (2018). Asherman's Syndrome: it may not be all our fault. *Hum Reprod, 33*(8), 1374-1380.

Seidman, J. D., & Kurman, R. J. (2000). Ovarian serous borderline tumours: a critical review of the literature with emphasis on prognostic indicators. *Hum Pathol, 31*(5), 539-557.

Silverberg, S., Bell, D. A., Kurman, R. J., Seidman, J. D., Prat, J., & Ronnett, B. M. (2004). Borderline ovarian tumors: key points and workshop summary. *Hum Pathol, 35*(8), 910-917.

Skirnisdottir, I., Garmo, H., Wilander, E., & Holmberg, L. (2008). Borderline ovarian tumors in Sweden 1960-2005: trends in incidence and age at diagnosis compared to ovarian cancer. *Int. J. Cancer, 123*(8), 1897-1901.

Stewart, L. M., Holman, C. D., Finn, J. C., Preen, D. B., & Hart, R. (2013). In vitro fertilization is associated with an increased risk of borderline ovarian tumours. *Gynecol. Oncol., 129*, 372-6.

Tavassoli, F. A., & Devilee, P. (2003). Pathology and genetics of tumours of the breast and female genital organs. *IARC* Press.

Timmerman, D., Planchamp, F., Bourne, T., Landolfo, C., & et al. (2021). ESGO/ISUOG/IOTA/ESGE Consensus Statement on pre-operative diagnosis of ovarian tumors. *Int J Gynecol Cancer*, 1-22.

Trillsch, F., Mahner, S., Woelber, L., & et al. (2014). Age-dependent differences in borderline ovarian tumours (BOT) regarding clinical characteristics and outcomes: results from a sub-analysis of the AGO ROBOT study. *Ann Oncol, 25*, 1320-1327.

Tropé, C., Kaern, J., & Davidson, B. (2012). Borderline ovarian tumpurs. *Best Pract Res Clin Obstet Gynaecol., 24*, 325-336.

Uzan, C., Kane, A., Rey, A., Gouy, S., & et al. (2010). Outcomes after conservative treatment of advanced-stage serous borderline tumours of the ovary. *Ann Oncol, 21*, 55-60.

van Leeuwen, F. E., Klip, H., Mooij, T. M., & et. al. (2011). Risk of borderline and invasive ovarian tumours after ovarian stimulation for in vitro fertilization in a large Dutch cohort. *26*, 3456-65.

Vang, R., Gown, A. M., Barry, T. S., Wheeler, D. T., Yemelyanova, A., & et al. (2006). Cytokeratins 7 and 20 in primary and secondary mucinous tumors of the ovary: analysis of coordinate. *Am J Surg Pathol, 30*(9), 1130–1139.

Vang, R., Gown, A. M., Wu, L. S., Barry, T. S., Wheeler, D. T., & et. al. (2006). Immunohistochemical expression of CDX2 in primary ovarian mucinous tumors and metastatic mucinous carcinomas involving the ovary: comparison with CK20 and correlation with coordinate expression of CK7. *Mod Pathol, 19*(11), 1421–1428.

Vasconcelos, I., & de Sousa Mendes, M. (2015). Conservative surgery in ovarian borderline tumours: a meta-analysis with emphasis on recurrence risk. *Eur J Cancer, 51*, 620-631.

Weinstein, D., & Polishuk, W. (1975). The role of wedge resection of the ovary as a causefor mechanical sterility. *Surg Gynecol Obstet, 141*, 417-418.

Chapter 14

Prophylactic Salpingo-Oophorectomy in High-Risk Patients

Paul I. Stanciu*, MD, PhD and Sabina Mistry, MD

Gynaecological Oncology Department, West Hertfordshire Hospitals, NHS Trust, UK

Introduction

Advances in cancer research in the past decade have established that there is a genetic background predisposing women to develop breast, ovarian, uterine and peritoneal cancers. [1-3] The main gene mutations associated with these malignancies are germline mutations of the BRCA1 and BRCA2 genes, which account for almost 20% of the high-grade serous carcinomas (HGSC) of the ovary [1]. Women with these mutations have a higher risk of developing ovarian cancer (44% and 17%, respectively for BRCA 1 and BRCA 2 carriers) compared to the 1% to 5% baseline risk of the general population [2].

Management options for these high-risk patients include ovarian screening and prophylactic surgery. Currently there is no universal screening strategy for ovarian cancer, [4] but Risk-Reducing Salpingo-Oophorectomy (RRSO) has been proven in several studies to reduce the risk of developing ovarian or fallopian tube cancer in this subset of patients by up to 80% [5-7]. Furthermore, RRSO reduces the overall mortality rates up to 60% and is strongly recommended for the prevention of ovarian cancer in BRCA 1/2 mutation carriers [5, 8)].

For BRCA1 carriers, RRSO is recommended before the age of 40 and for BRCA 2 carriers RRSO is recommended before the age of 45 or in any case when their family is complete [9]. Nevertheless, this prophylactic surgery cannot be recommended in the general population as removal of the ovaries in pre-menopausal women is known to increase the risk of osteoporosis, coronary artery disease, stroke and overall mortality [10]. Even with this strategy, the risk for development of subsequent peritoneal carcinomas remains between 1% and 4.3% [5, 11].

The incidence of occult HGSC in the distal fallopian tube at the time of prophylactic surgery for BRCA 1/2 carriers varies from 5% to 15% [12, 13] and the incidence of Serous Tubal Intraepithelial Carcinoma (STIC) varies from 0.6% to 7%. [14].

* Corresponding Author's Email: paulstanciu.md@gmail.com.

In: Ovarian Cancer
Editors: Christos Iavazzo, Alexandros Fotiou and John Spiliotis
ISBN: 979-8-88697-633-5

STICs and p53 Signatures

Increased evidence in recent literature points out that the precursor of many ovarian and peritoneal HGSCs is represented by a STIC lesion which largely arises in the distal part of the fallopian tube [15, 16]. A diverse spectrum of fallopian tube lesions have been described. These can range from distinctive p53 signature with normal tubal epithelium (Figure 1) and a low proliferation Ki-67 index (Figure 2) to aberrant p53 staining patterns (Figure 3) [17]. Serous tubal intraepithelial lesions (STIL) present cytological atypia but fall short of the criteria necessary to diagnose STIC [18].

P53 immunohistochemistry is one of the most useful markers for STICs and a predictor for the TP53 mutation. More than 90% of STICs have p53 signatures and share identical TP53 mutations with invasive ovarian or peritoneal cancers suggesting that STICs are the site of origin for HGSCs [19]. Germline TP53 mutations constitute the initial event in the development of HGSCs [20, 21] and is suggested that they are playing a significant role in the oncogenesis of several other human cancers [22].

Kuhn et al., [23] demonstrated that TP53 mutations were detectable in 27 out of 29 pairs of STICs and concurrent HGSCs, showing a clonal relationship between the two entities.

In a recent study conducted at the Royal Marsden Hospital in London [24], the incidence of STICs at the time of RRSO was found to be 2.33%. All STIC lesions found in this study presented p53 signatures and 28.57% of these patients developed peritoneal HGSC.

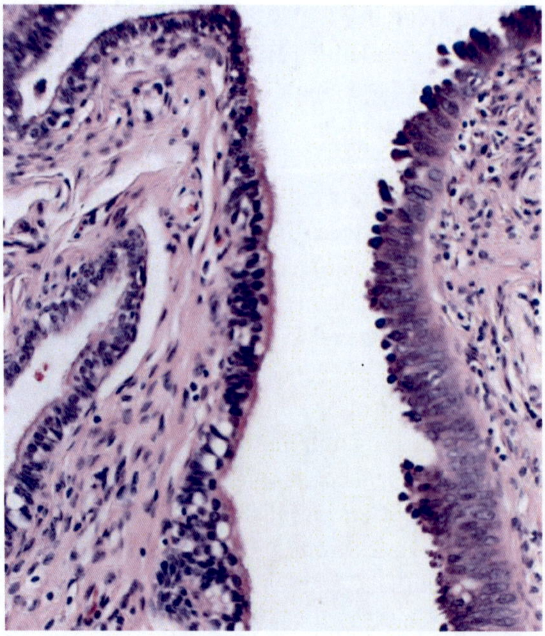

Figure 1. Fallopian tube (x20 magnification). Normal tubal epithelium on the left and STIC present on the right.

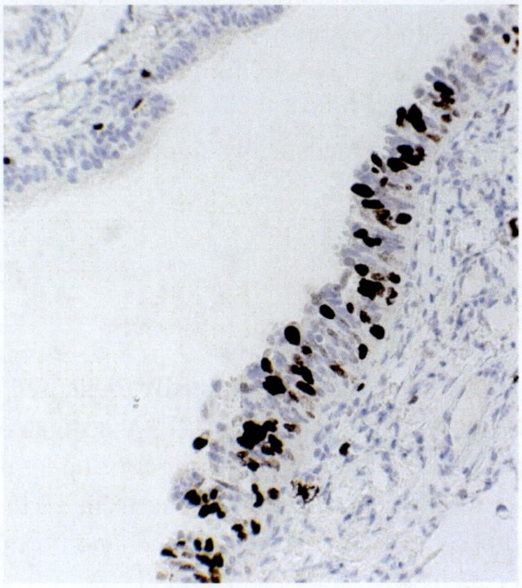

Figure 2. Ki67 (x20 magnification). Occasional nuclei are positive in the normal tubal epithelium (left). STIC (right) demonstrates increased nuclear staining.

Breast Cancer (BC) and Ovarian Cancer (OC) Risk

Multiple studies have proven the efficacy of RRSO in the reduction of both breast and ovarian cancer risk for patients with BRCA mutations.

Domcheck et al., [8] showed that RRSO not only significantly reduces BC-specific and OC-specific mortality, but also decreases the overall mortality in BRCA1 mutation carriers (HR = 0.42; 0.22-0.81) and in BRCA2 mutation carriers (HR = 0.10; 0.01-0.77). The author concluded that prophylactic removal of the tubes and ovaries in patients with no prior BC reduces the risk of developing BC by 37% for BRCA 1 carriers and by 64% for BRCA 2 carriers.

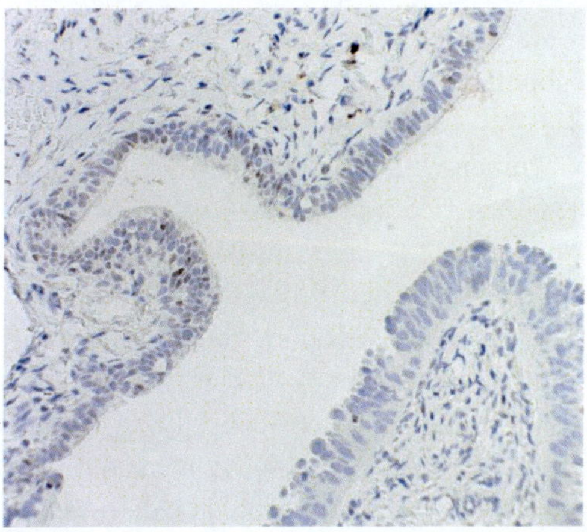

Figure 3. P53 (x20 magnification). Normal tubal epithelium (left) shows patchy, variable intensity nuclear staining and is interpreted as normal. STIC (right) demonstrates complete absence (null) staining and is interpreted as abnormal.

Xiao Li et al., [25] in a recently published meta-analysis reported a 45% reduction of BC risk and a 65% reduction in all-cause mortality for BRCA 1/2 mutation carriers who underwent RRSO.

Kauff et al., [26] also showed a statistically significant reduction in BC risk after RRSO for BRCA 2 mutation carriers.

Peritoneal Cancer Risk

In BRCA carriers, primary peritoneal cancer is usually diagnosed at an advanced stage many years after prophylactic surgery. Iavazzo et al., [27] investigated 1830 BRCA carriers that underwent RRSO and estimated their lifetime risk of developing primary peritoneal cancer at 1.53%. The author found a long-time interval ranging from 12 to 84 months from the initial prophylactic surgery to presentation of peritoneal cancer and for this reason, he proposed long term follow-up for these patients.

The presence of STICs and potential peritoneal seeding of premalignant cells during or before RRSO was regarded by some authors as a possible mechanism that could explain the origin of peritoneal cancer after the prophylactic removal of tubes and ovaries [28].

Two thirds of the patients that developed peritoneal cancer in the RMH study [24] had STICs and p53 signatures at the time of prophylactic surgery and taking into consideration the delayed presentation, the authors concluded that long term follow up could be advocated for all BRCA carriers with STICs and p53 signatures found at the time of RRSO.

Interestingly, the appendix was also suggested by other authors as a potential source of peritoneal cancer in BRCA carriers and appendectomy was advised at the time of prophylactic salpingo-oophorectomy but the evidence to date is scarce to justify this additional procedure [29].

Uterine Cancer Risk

BRCA mutation carriers are also at increased risk of developing serous endometrial cancer compared to the general population and several authors have reported this risk to be higher for BRCA 1 carriers [30-32].

After following 4456 women with BRCA 1 and BRCA 2 mutations for a mean interval of 5.7 years, Segev et al., [31] reported a higher risk of endometrial cancer in BRCA1 patients compared to BRCA 2 patients (13 cases in BRCA1 compared to 4 cases in BRCA2, standardized incidence ratio,1.91; 95% CI, 1.06–3.19; P = .03).

In a recently published prospective cohort study, Saule et al., [30] also found a higher incidence of serous endometrial cancer in BRCA 1/2 carriers than in the control population (standardized incidence ratio = 32.2, 95% confidence interval = 11.5 to 116.4, P < .001). They estimated a 3% lifetime risk of developing BRCA mediated serous endometrial cancer and acknowledged that prophylactic hysterectomy could be discussed at the time of RRSO.

Shu et al., [32] proposed that the endometrium might be susceptible to similar BRCA-mediated carcinogenesis as the fallopian tube. All the serous or serous-like endometrial tumors they found in their series had myometrial invasion and developed at least 7 years apart from the initial prophylactic surgery. They estimated that the 25-year risk for serous or serous-like uterine cancer after RRSO for BRCA 1 carriers ranges from 2.6% to 4.7% and that 21.2 to 37.9 hysterectomies are required in order to prevent one serous endometrial cancer. These figures, combined with low morbidity rates and acceptable costs, could potentially favour adding a hysterectomy at the time of prophylactic salpingo-oophorectomy for BRCA 1 carriers. [32] Furthermore, it was demonstrated that by adding a hysterectomy to a prophylactic salpingo-oophorectomy in a 40-year-old BRCA1 mutation carrier model, it resulted in a mean gain of 4.9 additional months of life and was cost-effective [33].

Conclusion

Prophylactic salpingo-oophorectomy in high-risk patients significantly decreased the incidence of ovarian and fallopian tube cancers, but patients with STICs and p53 signatures need long-term follow up as they have a higher risk of developing primary peritoneal carcinomas. The role of concomitant hysterectomy remains controversial in BRCA mutation carriers. However, it is known that BRCA1 carriers are at higher risk of developing serous endometrial carcinoma even after RRSO and therefore a concomitant hysterectomy could be discussed at the time of the procedure.

References

[1] George A, Kaye S, Banerjee S. Delivering widespread BRCA testing and PARP inhibition to patients with ovarian cancer. *Nat. Rev. Clin. Oncol.* 2017 May;14(5):284-296.

[2] Kuchenbaecker K B, Hopper J L, Barnes D R, Phillips K A, Mooij T M, Roos-Blom M J, Jervis S, van Leeuwen F E, Milne R L, Andrieu N, Goldgar D E, Terry M B, Rookus M A, Easton D F, Antoniou A C; BRCA1 and BRCA2 Cohort Consortium, McGuffog L, Evans D G, Barrowdale D, Frost D, Adlard J, Ong K R, Izatt L, Tischkowitz M, Eeles R, Davidson R, Hodgson S, Ellis S, Nogues C, Lasset C, Stoppa-Lyonnet D, Fricker J P, Faivre L, Berthet P, Hooning M J, van der Kolk L E, Kets C M, Adank M A, John E M, Chung W K, Andrulis I L, Southey M, Daly M B, Buys S S, Osorio A, Engel C, Kast K, Schmutzler R K, Caldes T, Jakubowska A, Simard J, Friedlander M L, McLachlan S A, Machackova E, Foretova L, Tan Y Y, Singer C F, Olah E, Gerdes A M, Arver B, Olsson H. Risks of breast, ovarian, and contralateral breast cancer for BRCA1 and BRCA2 mutation carriers. *JAMA* 2017;317:2402–16.

[3] Sekine M., Enomoto T. (2017) Hereditary Ovarian Cancer. In: Katabuchi H. (eds) Frontiers in Ovarian Cancer Science. *Comprehensive Gynecology and Obstetrics.* Springer, Singapore.

[4] Jacobs I J, Menon U, Ryan A, Gentry-Maharaj A, Burnell M, Kalsi J K, Amso N N, Apostolidou S, Benjamin E, Cruickshank D, Crump D N, Davies S K, Dawnay A, Dobbs S, Fletcher G, Ford J, Godfrey K, Gunu R, Habib M, Hallett R, Herod J, Jenkins H, Karpinskyj C, Leeson S, Lewis S J, Liston W R, Lopes A, Mould T, Murdoch J, Oram D, Rabideau D J, Reynolds K, Scott I, Seif M W, Sharma A, Singh N, Taylor J, Warburton F, Widschwendter M, Williamson K, Woolas R, Fallowfield L, McGuire A J, Campbell S, Parmar M, Skates S J. Ovarian cancer screening and mortality in the UK Collaborative Trial of Ovarian Cancer Screening (UKCTOCS): a randomised controlled trial. *Lancet.* 2016 Mar 5;387(10022):945-956.

[5] Rebbeck T R, Kauff N D, Domchek S M. Meta-analysis of risk reduction estimates associated with risk-reducing salpingo-oophorectomy in BRCA1 or BRCA2 mutation carriers. *J. Natl. Cancer Inst.* 2009;101:80–87.

[6] Finch A, Beiner M, Lubinski J, Lynch H T, Moller P, Rosen B, Murphy J, Ghadirian P, Friedman E, Foulkes W D, Kim-Sing C, Wagner T, Tung N, Couch F, Stoppa-Lyonnet D, Ainsworth P, Daly M,

Pasini B, Gershoni-Baruch R, Eng C, Olopade O I, McLennan J, Karlan B, Weitzel J, Sun P, Narod S A; Hereditary Ovarian Cancer Clinical Study Group. Salpingo-oophorectomy and the Risk of Ovarian, Fallopian Tube, and Peritoneal Cancers in Women With a BRCA1 or BRCA2 Mutation. *JAMA*. 2006;296(2):185–192.

[7] Finch A P, Lubinski J, Møller P, Singer C F, Karlan B, Senter L, Rosen B, Maehle L, Ghadirian P, Cybulski C, Huzarski T, Eisen A, Foulkes W D, Kim-Sing C, Ainsworth P, Tung N, Lynch H T, Neuhausen S, Metcalfe K A, Thompson I, Murphy J, Sun P, Narod S A. Impact of oophorectomy on cancer incidence and mortality in women with a BRCA1 or BRCA2 mutation. *Journal of Clinical* Oncology 2014;32(15):1547–53.

[8] Domchek S M, Friebel T M, Singer C F, Evans D G, Lynch H T, Isaacs C, Garber J E, Neuhausen S L, Matloff E, Eeles R, Pichert G, Van t'veer L, Tung N, Weitzel J N, Couch F J, Rubinstein W S, Ganz P A, Daly M B, Olopade O I, Tomlinson G, Schildkraut J, Blum J L, Rebbeck T R. Association of risk-reducing surgery in BRCA1 or BRCA2 mutation carriers with cancer risk and mortality. *JAMA*. 2010;304(9):967–75.

[9] Hartmann L C, Lindor N M. The role of risk-reducing surgery in hereditary breast and ovarian cancer. *N. Engl. J. Med.* 2016;374:454–68.

[10] Parker W H, Broder M S, Chang E, Feskanich D, Farquhar C, Liu Z, Shoupe D, Berek JS, Hankinson S, Manson J E. Ovarian conservation at the time of hysterectomy and long-term health outcomes in the nurses' health study. *Obstet. Gynecol.* 2009;113(5):1027–37.

[11] Rebbeck T R, Lynch H T, Neuhausen S L, Narod S A, Van't Veer L, Garber J E, Evans G, Isaacs C, Daly M B, Matloff E, Olopade O I, Weber B L; Prevention and Observation of Surgical End Points Study Group. Prophylactic oophorectomy in carriers of BRCA1 or BRCA2 mutations. *N. Engl. J. Med.* 2002;346:1616–1622.

[12] Leeper K, Garcia R, Swisher E, Goff B, Greer B, Paley P. Pathologic findings in prophylactic oophorectomy specimens in high-risk women. *Gynecol. Oncol.* 2002;87(1):52–6.

[13] Lu K H, Garber J E, Cramer D W, Welch W R, Niloff J, Schrag D, Berkowitz R S, Muto M G. Occult ovarian tumors in women with BRCA1 or BRCA2 mutations undergoing prophylactic oophorectomy. *J. Clin. Oncol.* 2000;18(14):2728–32.

[14] Wethington S L, Park K J, Soslow R A, Kauff N D, Brown C L, Dao F, Otegbeye E, Sonoda Y, Abu-Rustum N R, Barakat R R, Levine D A, Gardner G J. Clinical outcome of isolated serous tubal intraepithelial carcinomas (STIC), *Int. J. Gynecol. Cancer* 23(2013):1603–1611.

[15] Tang S, Onuma K, Deb P, Wang E, Lytwyn A, Sur M, Daya D. Frequency of serous tubal intraepithelial carcinoma in various gynecologic malignancies: a study of 300 consecutive cases. *Int. J. Gynecol. Pathol.* 2012;31:103–110.

[16] Li H X, Lu Z H, Shen K, Cheng W J, Malpica A, Zhang J, Wei J J, Zhang Z H, Liu J. Advances in serous tubal intraepithelial carcinoma: correlation with high grade serous carcinoma and ovarian carcinogenesis. *International Journal of Clinical and Experimental Pathology*. 2014;7(3):848-857.

[17] Lee Y, Miron A, Drapkin R, Nucci M R, Medeiros F, Saleemuddin A, Garber J, Birch C, Mou H, Gordon R W, Cramer D W, McKeon F D, Crum C P. A candidate precursor to serous carcinoma that originates in the distal fallopian tube. *J. Pathol.* 2007;211:26–35.

[18] Carcangiu M L, Radice P, Manoukian S, Spatti G, Gobbo M, Pensotti V, Crucianelli R, Pasini B. Atypical epithelial proliferation in fallopian tubes in prophylactic salpingo-oophorectomy specimens from BRCA1 and BRCA2 germline mutation carriers. *Int. J. Gynecol. Pathol.* 2004;23:35–40.

[19] Kurman R J, Shih I M. Molecular pathogenesis and extraovarian origin of epithelial ovarian cancer--shifting the paradigm. *Hum. Pathol.* 2011;42(7):918–31.

[20] Ahmed A A, Etemadmoghadam D, Temple J, Lynch A G, Riad M, Sharma R, Stewart C, Fereday S, Caldas C, Defazio A, Bowtell D, Brenton J D. Driver mutations in TP53 are ubiquitous in high grade serous carcinoma of the ovary. *J. Pathol.* 2010;221:49–56.

[21] Bowtell D D. The genesis and evolution of high-grade serous ovarian cancer. *Nat. Rev. Cancer.* 2010;10:803–808.

[22] Goh A M, Coffill C R, Lane D P. The role of mutant p53 in human cancer. *J. Pathol.* 2011;223:116–126.

[23] Kuhn E, Kurman R J, Vang R, Sehdev A S, Han G, Soslow R, Wang T L, Shih Ie M. TP53 mutations in serous tubal intraepithelial carcinoma and concurrent pelvic high-grade serous carcinoma--evidence supporting the clonal relationship of the two lesions. *J. Pathol.* 2012;226:421–426.

[24] Stanciu P I, Ind T E J, Barton D P J, Butler J B, Vroobel K M, Attygalle A D, Nobbenhuis M A E. Development of Peritoneal Carcinoma in women diagnosed with Serous Tubal Intraepithelial Carcinoma (STIC) following Risk-Reducing Salpingo-Oophorectomy (RRSO). *J. Ovarian Res.* 2019 May 25;12(1):50.

[25] Li X, You R, Wang X, Liu C, Xu Z, Zhou J, Yu B, Xu T, Cai H, Zou Q. Effectiveness of Prophylactic Surgeries in BRCA1 or BRCA2 Mutation Carriers: A Meta-analysis and Systematic Review. *Clin. Cancer Res.* August 1.2016;(22)(15):3971-3981.

[26] Ka Kauff N D, Domchek S M, Friebel T M, Robson M E, Lee J, Garber J E, Isaacs C, Evans D G, Lynch H, Eeles RA, Neuhausen SL, Daly MB, Matloff E, Blum JL, Sabbatini P, Barakat RR, Hudis C, Norton L, Offit K, Rebbeck TR. Risk-Reducing Salpingo-Oophorectomy for the Prevention of BRCA1 and BRCA2 Associated Breast and Gynecologic Cancer: A Multi-Center, Prospective Study. *Journal of Clinical Oncology.* 2008;26(8):1331–1337.

[27] Iavazzo C, Gkegkes ID, Vrachnis N. Primary peritoneal cancer in BRCA carriers after prophylactic bilateral salpingo-oophorectomy. *J. Turk. Ger. Gynecol. Assoc.* 2016;17(2):73-6.

[28] Chene G, Dauplat J, Radosevic-Robin N, Cayre A, Penault-Llorca F. Tu-be or not tu-be: that is the question… about serous ovarian carcinogenesis. *Crit. Rev. Oncol. Hematol.* 2013;88:134–43.

[29] Sitzmann J V, Wiebke E A. Risk-Reducing Appendectomy and the Elimination of BRCA1 -Associated Intraperitoneal Cancer. *JAMA Surg.* 2013;148:285–91.

[30] Saule C, Mouret-Fourme E, Briaux A. Risk of serous endometrial carcinoma in women with pathogenic BRCA1/2 variant after risk-reducing salpingo-oophorectomy. *J. Natl. Cancer Inst.* 2018;110:2017–2019.

[31] Segev Y, Iqbal J, Lubinski J, Gronwald J, Lynch H T, Moller P, Ghadirian P, Rosen B, Tung N, Kim-Sing C, Foulkes WD, Neuhausen SL, Senter L, Singer CF, Karlan B, Ping S, Narod SA; Hereditary Breast Cancer Study Group. The incidence of endometrial cancer in women with BRCA1 and BRCA2 mutations. *Gynecol. Oncol.* 2013;130(1):127–131.

[32] Shu C A, Pike M C, Jotwani A R, Friebel T M, Soslow R A, Levine D A, Nathanson K L, Konner J A, Arnold A G, Bogomolniy F, Dao F, Olvera N, Bancroft E K, Goldfrank D J, Stadler Z K, Robson M E, Brown C L, Leitao M M Jr, Abu-Rustum N R, Aghajanian C A, Blum J L, Neuhausen S L, Garber J E, Daly M B, Isaacs C, Eeles R A, Ganz P A, Barakat R R, Offit K, Domchek S M, Rebbeck T R, Kauff N D. Uterine Cancer After Risk-Reducing Salpingo-oophorectomy Without Hysterectomy in Women With BRCA Mutations. *JAMA Oncol.* 2016;2(11):1434-1440.

[33] Havrilesky L J, Moss H A, Chino J, Myers E R, Kauff N D. Mortality reduction and cost-effectiveness of performing hysterectomy at the time of risk-reducing salpingo-oophorectomy for prophylaxis against serous/serous-like uterine cancers in BRCA1 mutation carriers. *Gynecol. Oncol.* 2017 Jun;145(3):549-554.

Chapter 15

The Management of Early-Stage Epithelial Ovarian Cancer

Virginia García Pineda, MD, PhD
Violeta Romero, MD, PhD
and Ignacio Zapardiel*, MD, PhD
Gynecologic Oncology Unit, La Paz University Hospital, Madrid, Spain

Introduction

It was predicted that in 2018, there would be approximately 22, 240 new cases of ovarian cancer diagnosed and 14, 070 ovarian cancer deaths in the United States (USA). Incidence peak inpostmenopausal women at the average age of 65 years old at the time of diagnosis (USA) [1].

Epithelial ovarian cancer is staged according to the latest classification of International Federation of Gynaecology and Obstetrics (Cancer Report 2018) [2]. In most cases, patients with initial cancer have few symptoms and its development time does not differ from those diagnosed at advanced stages. Most cases are diagnosed in an advanced stage, especially when onset is acute and requires urgent medical attention, while only 25% of cases are diagnosed in early-stages (I or II) [3, 4].

The most frequent type of histology in ovarian cancer is epithelial, accounting for 90% of all cases where high epithelial serous carcinoma implies at least a 70% epithelial histological subtype.

Concerning surgical staging in EOC, it has a dual purpose: first of all, making an accurate approach to the real stage of the tumor since some occult disease in imaging tests might be found during the surgical staging. Last but not least, there is evidence that adequate surgical staging improves overall and disease-free survival [5].

Current guidelines establish standardized quality criteria for the best management of the disease. Over 90% of the procedures in gynaecologic oncology must be performed by a trained surgeon or for those who are accredited as a gynaecologic oncologist in accredited centers for the management of this disease. But this is not the only requirement.. Participation in clinical trials specifically targeted to gynaecological oncology patients has to be an essential element

---

* Corresponding Author's Email: ignaciozapardiel@alumni.harvard.edu.

In: Ovarian Cancer
Editors: Christos Iavazzo, Alexandros Fotiou and John Spiliotis
ISBN: 979-8-88697-633-5

in our daily practice since investigations are a basic requirement, necessary in improving the outcome of patients.

The best treatment for patients is guided by individualized case discussion and decision making in a multidisciplinary tumor board. Decisions that are taken among the different specialists improves management before, during and after the surgery as well as enabling comprehensive resolution in cases of postoperative complications.

As previously said, all recommendations done by ESGO are targeted for advanced stages but there is a systematic review published that suggests this also could be applied for those in early stages and it might be exported to early-stage ovarian cancer [6].

Management of Early Ovarian Cancer

Surgical Staging

The concept of surgical staging of early-stage ovarian carcinoma was developed when there was a better understanding of the natural course of the disease, which was gained in the 1970s and 1980s when the incidence of occult intraperitoneal and retroperitoneal disease was defined in literature [7] (Table 1). Since these tumors have an early and aggressive spread pattern, occult metastasis can be seen even in cases where the tumor is apparently confined to the ovaries. After standardized surgical staging, there is a 30% overall reported rate of upstaging to at least FIGO Stage IIIa in literature [8]. Ayhan et al., reported a 31.4% upstaging rate after surgical staging where the most common occult metastasis was the lymphatic involvement (41.5%) [9] (Table 1). There is a proof from retrospective and randomized clinical trials that the extent of staging is significantly related to the prognosis of early-stage ovarian carcinoma as it defines a real early-stage or advanced-stage disease and therefore, an appropriate adjuvant treatment.

According to recent European consensus guidelines, the standard surgical approach in early-stage ovarian cancer is based on: complete exploration of the abdomino-pelvic peritoneal cavity with careful examination of all peritoneal surfaces, taking washings of peritoneal cavity, peritoneal biopsies (pelvic peritoneum, paracolic gutters and diaphragm); omentectomy (at least infracolic omentectomy); pelvic and paraaortic lymphadenectomy; total complete hysterectomy and bilateral salpingo-oophorectomy. An appendectomy can be omitted even in mucinous tumors if its appearance is normal [10-12] (Figure 1).

The standard approach is open surgery as it confers better macroscopic examination of the abdominal cavity and can reduce the risk of rupture of primary ovarian tumors. However, in recent years, the laparoscopic approach has gained an important role in surgical staging of early-stage ovarian cancer. The most relevant European guidelines recommend midline laparotomy as a first choice but consider laparoscopic surgical management in expertise hands able to perform an adequate surgical staging without tumor spillage and for restaging surgery in cases when the initial ovarian tumor has been removed and there is no risk of rupture of the ovarian lesion [12].

On the other hand, compared with laparotomy, minimally-invasive surgery is associated with fewer complications and shorter recovery period, and has been adopted in early-stage endometrial cancer. Nevertheless, its incorporation to surgical management remains controversial due to the absence of randomized trials comparing oncological results and demonstrating equivalent outcome in both approaches. Moreover, a recent Cochrane Library systematic review concluded that there was no high-quality scientific evidence available to establish the safety of laparoscopic staging in Stage I ovarian cancer [13]. A recent prospective observational study of Melamed et al. which included a total of 4,798 patients, matched patients who underwent laparoscopic staging with similar patients who underwent laparotomic staging comparing survival among matched cohorts. According to their results, planned laparoscopic staging was not associated with time to death after adjustment for receipt of adjuvant chemotherapy, histological type and grade, and pathologic stage (Hazard Ratio 0.82, 95% CI 0.57-1.16). Moreover, planned laparoscopic staging was associated with a slightly higher median lymph node count (14 versus 12, $p = 0.005$) [14]. Another retrospective case-control study of Gallota et al., evaluated the oncologic outcomes of patients with early-stage ovarian cancer including 60 patients who underwent laparoscopic management and 120 patients who underwent open surgery. They concluded that operative time ($p = 0.01$), estimated blood loss ($p = 0.032$), and median hospital stay ($p = 0.001$) were higher in patients submitted to laparotomic versus laparoscopic staging. Four-year progression-free survival (PFS) and overall survival (OS) rates with a median follow-up of 38 months were 89% and 92% in the laparoscopic group, respectively, and 81% and 91% in the laparotomic group, without any statistically significant difference between the groups [15]. In addition, it has been shown that the laparoscopic approach also significantly reduces the time to receive adjuvant chemotherapy and postoperative complications [16, 17].

Therefore, the recent evidence of literature suggests that in the surgical treatment of FIGO Stage I ovarian cancer, laparoscopy is associated with an equivalent oncologic outcome compared with a conventional abdominal approach and can be a safe option in expert hands.

Concerning the role of pelvic and paraaortic lymph node dissection in surgical staging of early-stage ovarian cancer, its therapeutic value is still controversial. Nodal status in early-stage is the most important prognostic factor as when lymph nodal metastases are reported, there is an increased risk of recurrence and death. The risk of occult pelvic and/or para-aortic lymph node metastases in apparent early-stage ovarian cancer ranges from 6.1 to 29.6%, with a mean incidence of 14.2%

EOC metastasizes early and mainly through two routes: direct peritoneal spread into the abdominal cavity and lymphatic spread. Nowadays there is a concept indicating that the histological subtypes of high-grade serous EOC and low-grade EOC are not differentially graded neoplasms of the same type, but rather two distinct tumor types with different pathogenesis. Their different biological behavior explains why not all serous epithelial ovarian tumors respond equally to standard chemotherapy based on carboplatin and paclitaxel and do not present the same pattern of lymph node involvement.

It is now known from recent scientific evidence that the rate of positive nodes in low-grade epithelial ovarian cancer (LGEOC) differs greatly from high-grade subtypes. The results of a multicenter study of Heitz et al., whose aim was to evaluate the rate of lymph node metastases in patients with different tumor stages and histological subtypes, undergoing systematic pelvic and paraaortic lymphadenectomy, showed that low-grade endometrioid and mucinous carcinoma tumors did not present lymph nodes metastases in early stage. Conversely, 20% of low-grade serous carcinoma presented nodal involvement. The authors concluded that the risk of LN metastases in patients with EOC is dependent on stage and histological subtype. Reoperation for systematic lymph node staging only should be discussed individually and with caution given the low risk of nodal involvement in these patients [18]. A multicenter retrospective study of Minig et al. included 163 cases of low-grade epithelial ovarian cancer in early stage in whom pelvic and paraaortic lymphadenectomy were performed with a minimum of 10 lymph nodes retrieved at each level. The rate of lymph node metastases in serous, endometrioid and mucinous ovarian cancer subtypes was 10,7%, 1.5% and 0%, respectively. The overall nodal involvement in ovarian cancer was 4.3%. After surgery, the rate of upstaging was 2.4% of patients. This results in low-grade subtypes raising the question of the potential benefits of lymphadenectomies as part of the staging in these cases. Therefore, large prospective studies are warranted to evaluate the oncologic safety of omitting systematic lymphadenectomy in apparent Stage I non serous low-grade epithelial carcinoma [19].

Table 1. Occult metastasis in apparent early-stage EOC

	Cytology	Omentum	Peritoneum	Diaphragm	Lymphatic involvement
Piver et al. 1978	18.8%	7.1%	9.8%	7.6%	10.9%
Ayhan et al. 2007	35.8%	11.3%	3.8%	0%	41.5%
Hengeveld et al. 2019	15.8%	4.4%	7.7%	2.6%	7.8%

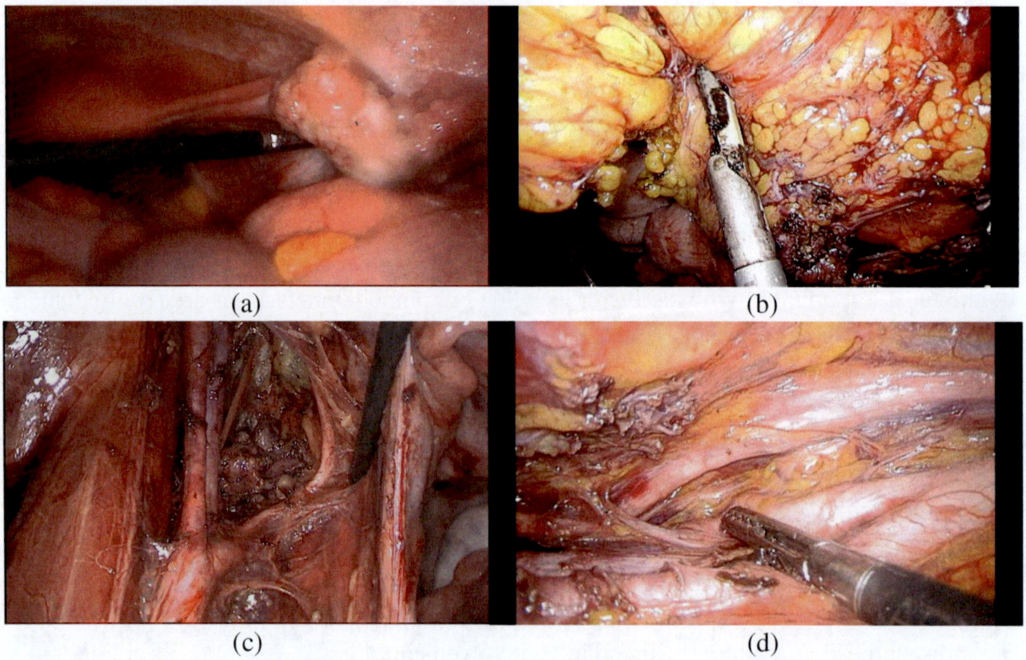

Figure 1. Surgical staging by laparoscopy. (a) Hysterectomy and bilateral salpingo-oophorectomy. (b) infracolic omentectomy. (c) Pelvic Lymphadenectomy (left side). (d) Extraperitoneal para-aortic lymphadenectomy.

The therapeutic role of pelvic and paraaortic lymphadenectomy in surgical staging of early-stage epithelial ovarian cancer is still controversial. A recent retrospective multicenter study of Bizarri et al., evaluated overall survival (OS) and disease-free survival (DFS) in patients with LGEOC early-stage which underwent different types of nodal staging (comprehensive lymphadenectomy, lymph node sampling and no lymphadenectomy). The 5-year-DSF was 79.7% vs. 76.5% vs. 68.3% ($p = 0.006$), and 5-year overall survival (OS) was 92.3% vs. 94.5%

vs. 89.8% ($p = 0.165$) in women who received comprehensive lymphadenectomy vs. lymph node sampling vs. no lymphadenectomy, respectively. Lymphadenectomy represented an independent factor for DFS improvement, HR 0.52 (95% CI 0.37-0.73) ($p < 0.001$) [20]. Nowadays, a lymphadenectomy is part of surgical staging in early-stage ovarian cancer and is recommended in the main guidelines when it influences the decision for adjuvant treatment, however, prospective studies are needed to assess the therapeutic value of lymphadenectomy in early-stage ovarian cancer.

Chemotherapy

Chemotherapy in early-stage ovarian cancer has been largely discussed. Chemotherapy scheme has traditionally been adjuvant after a comprehensive surgical staging.

The most important studies about adjuvant chemotherapy were published at the beginning of the 2000s.. In 2004, Laurie Elit et al., published a meta-analysis that included 13 randomized controlled trials between 1965 and 2004 in patients with FIGO stage I EOC. Trials results were statistically significant with the needfulness of platinum-based chemotherapy in early-stage EOC since it showed an improvement in 5-year-overall survival (absolute survival difference of 8%) and reduced risk of relapse (RR 0.70) [21].

In 2015, a Cochrane Database review of adjuvant chemotherapy in ovarian cancer reported a comprehensive description of the different high-risk subtypes in order to describe subgroups of patients who benefit from receiving adjuvant treatment. Most of the patients were classified as Stage I (>95%) and the main results showed better overall survival (OS) in the chemotherapy group (HR 0.71 among 1.008 women included in 3 studies with high level of evidence) and better progression-free survival (PFS). Results were consistent after a 10-year follow-up (HR 0.72 and 0.67 for OS and PFS respectively). Even though adjuvant treatment was effective in improving overall survival, authors recommended individualized chemotherapy treatment in subgroups of low-risk ovarian cancer since the benefits and possible adverse effects were not well-defined [22].

Nowadays, it is known that some specific characteristics implies a subsequent poorer prognosis such as high-tumor grade (G3), FIGO stage IC (ascites presence) or FIGO stage II and clear cell histology (at any stage). These high-risk subtypes are candidates for adjuvant treatment since their 5-year disease-free-survival rates showed worse outcomes (in some series as low as 75%) when compared with low-risk features [23].

Those women with no-clear-cells ovarian cancer histology in its early-stage (IA or IB) with low-grade tumor, had an excellent 5-year overall survival after complete surgery in 90% of the cases. This low-risk subset of patients did not show a clear benefit from chemotherapy among reported literature and therefore they were not candidates for chemotherapy. Nevertheless, the role of adjuvant chemotherapy in moderate grade tumors (G2) is controversial [24].

Immunotherapy has been a promising new line of treatment for ovarian cancer. It could be a possibility in those patients with incomplete debulking surgery and failure of first-line schemes of chemotherapy. Meanwhile, further studies are requested on the subject.

One of the most important studies in the last years was the ICON7 trial. This multicenter and randomized trial included 1,528 patients with high-risk early-stage ovarian cancer (FIGO Stage I-IIa, Grade 3 or clear cell histology) and in cases of advanced disease. Standard chemotherapy platinum-based scheme was compared to the same regimen plus bevacizumab in terms of progression-free survival. Although this study showed a benefit for those women in an advanced stage with an incomplete cytoreduction, it did not demonstrate benefit in patients with early-stage, including those with high-risk features [25].

Concerning the role of immunotherapy, several studies have been published recently although they mostly involved advanced-stage ovarian cancer. The SOLO1 phase III clinical trial, which evaluated the use of olaparib for advanced-stage ovarian cancer, showed an improvement in overall and progression-free survival of BRCA-mutated patients who responded to first-line chemotherapy. Patients were randomized to receive olaparib or placebo. Olaparib-group had a 70% lower risk of death or progression when compared to the placebo-group (Kaplan-Meier HR 0.30, $p < 0.001$) [26].

Ray-Coquard et al. published the results of a Phase III trial in advanced ovarian cancer which had the innovative feature of including a group platinum-taxane chemotherapy and another group with the same chemotherapy plus bevacizumab. Another novel aspect in this clinical trial was that patients were included in the study regardless of BRCA mutation status. Results were consistent with SOLO1 results, the use of olaparib showed a benefit in progression-free survival, mainly in BRCA-mutated patients (Hazard Ratio 0.33 [95% CI, 0.25 to 0.45]) versus non-BRCA-mutated patients (Hazard Ratio 0.43 [CI 95%, 0.28 to 0.66]) [27].

Meanwhile, the use of olaparib is justified in advanced-stages although there is lack of studies for its use in early stages. The use of olaparib could be interesting in its early-stages due to the special clinical features of the patients.

Nowadays, new fields of investigation are ongoing. The role of the so-called cancer stem cells (CSC) has been largely discussed especially in other localizations such as in breast and colorectal cancers. The involvement of this tumoral cells subpopulation has been investigated in cases of cancer recurrence and in patients with platinum-based chemotherapy resistance. CSCs originate from adult tissue resident stem cells and it is observed that they are able to respond to chemotherapy or radiotherapy by developing adaptations to them. The investigation of plasticity pathways of CSCs is a recent area of study since it might provide new targeted inmuno-based treatment in the future for those patients with recurrences and/or traditional chemotherapy schemes failures [28].

Conclusion

- Most ovarian carcinomas are diagnosed in advanced stages. Only approximately 25% are diagnosed at an early stage.
- Surgical resection and comprehensive staging are the cornerstone of treatment.
- Nodal staging with pelvic and paraaortic lymphadenectomy is not proposed for expansile-mucinous EOC.
- Reoperation for systematic lymph node staging only in LG-EOC should be discussed individually with caution given the low risk of nodal involvement in these patients.
- Laparoscopic approach is safe and accurate for early-stage ovarian cancer in expert hands.
- Chemotherapy is not needed in all cases. Certain subtypes imply a higher relapse risk and poorer prognosis (G3, clear cell carcinoma, IC or superior stages) and these are candidates for adjuvant treatment.

References

[1] Torre, L,Trabert, B, Siegel, R. Ovarian cancer statistics, 2018. *CA Cancer J. Clin.*, 2018 Jul;68(4):284-296.

[2] Bhatla, N. and Denny, L. (2018), FIGO Cancer Report 2018. *Int. J. Gynecol. Obstet.*, 143: 2-3.

[3] Olson SH, Mignone L, Nakraseive C, Caputo TA, Barakat RR, Harlap S. Symptoms of ovarian cancer. *Obstet. Gynecol.* 2001 Aug;98(2):212-7.

[4] Goff BA, Mandel L, Muntz HG, Melancon CH. Ovarian carcinoma diagnosis. *Cancer.* 2000 Nov 15;89(10):2068-75.

[5] Le T, Adolph A, Krepart GV, Lotocki R, Heywood MS. The benefits of comprehensive surgical staging in the management of early-stage epithelial ovarian carcinoma. *Gynecol. Oncol.* 2002 May;85(2):351-5.

[6] Bonte AS, Luyckx A, Wyckmans L, Trinh XB, van Dam PA. Quality indicators for the management of endometrial, cervical and ovarian cancer. *Eur. J. Surg. Oncol.* 2019 Apr;45(4):528-537.

[7] Piver, M, Barlow, J, Lele, S. Incidence of subclinical metastasis in stage I and II ovarian carcinoma. *Obstet. Gynecol.*, 1978 Jul;52(1):100-4.

[8] Hengeveld, EM, Zusterzeel, PLM, Lajer, H, Høgdall, CK, Rosendahl, M. The value of surgical staging in patients with apparent early-stage epithelial ovarian carcinoma. *Gynecol. Oncol.*, 2019; 154:308-313.

[9] Ayhan, A, Gultekin, M, Celik, NY, Dursun, P, Taskiran, C, Aksan, G, & Yuce, K. Occult metastasis in early ovarian cancers: risk factors and associated prognosis. *Am. J. Obstet. Gynecol.* 2007;196:81.e1-81.e6.

[10] Colombo N, Sessa C, du Bois A, Ledermann J, McCluggage WG, McNeish I. ESMO-ESGO Consensus Conference recommendations on ovarian cancer:pathology and molecular biology, early and advanced stages, borderline tumors and recurrent disease. *Ann. Oncol.* 2019;30(5):672-705.

[11] van de Vorst, R, Hoogendam, J, van der Aa, M, Witteveen, P, Zweemer, R, Gerestein, C. The attributive value of comprehensive surgical staging in clinically early-stage epithelial ovarian carcinoma: A systematic review and meta-analysis. *Gynecol. Oncol.* 2021;161(3):876-883.

[12] Querleu, D, Planchamp, F, Chiva, L, Fotopoulou, C, Barton, D, Cibula, D, Aletti, G, Carinelli, S, Creutzberg, C, Davidson, B, Harter, P, Lundvall, L, Marth, C, Morice, P, Rafii, A, Ray-Coquard, I, Rockall, A, Sessa, C, van der Zee, A, Vergote, I. and duBois, A. European Society of Gynaecological Oncology (ESGO) Guidelines for Ovarian Cancer Surgery. *Int. J. Gynecol. Cancer.* 2017;27(7):1534-1542.

[13] Falcetta, FS, Lawrie, TA, Medeiros, LR, da Rosa, MI, Edelweiss, MI, Stein, AT, Zelmanowicz, A, Moraes, AB, Zanini, RR., Rosa, DD., & Platt, J. Laparoscopy versus laparotomy for FIGO stage I ovarian cancer. *Database Syst. Rev.* 2016;10(10):CD005344.

[14] Rauh-Hain, JA, Melamed, A, Wright, A, Gockley, A, Clemmer, JT, Schorge, JO, del Carmen, MG., & Keating, NL. Laparoscopic Staging for Apparent Stage I Epithelial Ovarian Cancer: Analysis of the National Cancer DataBase. *Am. J. Obstet. Gynecol.* 2017;216(1):50.e1-50.e12.

[15] Gallotta, V, Petrillo, M, Conte, C, Vizzielli, G, Fagotti, A, Ferrandina, G, Fanfani, F, Costantini, B, Carbone, V, & Scambia, G. Laparoscopic Versus Laparotomic Surgical Staging for Early-Stage Ovarian Cancer: A Case-Control Study. *J. Minim. Invasive Gynecol.* 2016;23:769-774.

[16] Bogani, G, Cromi, A, Serati, M, Di Naro, E, Casarin, J, Pinelli, C Laparoscopic and open abdominal staging for early-stage ovarian cancer: our experience, systematic review, and meta-analysis of comparative studies. *Int. J. Gynecol. Cancer.* 2014;24(7):1241-9.

[17] Bogani, G, Borghi, C, Maggiore, U, Ditto, A, Signorelli, M,Martinelli, F. Minimally Invasive Surgical Staging in Early-stage Ovarian Carcinoma: A Systematic Review and Meta-analysis. *J. Minim. Invasive Gynecol.* 2017;24(4):552-562.

[18] Heitz, F, Harter, P, Ataseven, B, Heikaus, S, Schneider, S, Prader, S. Stage- and Histologic Subtype-Dependent Frequency of Lymph Node Metastases in Patients with Epithelial Ovarian Cancer Undergoing Systematic Pelvic and Paraaortic Lymphadenectomy. *Ann. Surg. Oncol.* 2018;25:2053-2059.

[19] Minig, L, Heitz, F, Cibula, D, Bakkum-Gamez, J, Germanova, A, Dowdy, S. Patterns of Lymph Node Metastases in Apparent Stage I Low-Grade Epithelial Ovarian Cancer: A Multicenter Study. *Ann. Surg. Oncol.* 2017;24:2720-2726.

[20] Bizzarri, N, du Bois, A, Fruscio, R, De Felice, F, De Iaco, P, Casarin, J, Vizza, E, Chiantera, V, Corrado, G, Cianci, S, Magni, S, Ferrari, D, Giuliani, D, Harter, P, Ataseven, B, Bommert, M, Perrone, AM, Scambia, G, & Fagotti, A. Is there any therapeutic role of pelvic and para-aortic lymphadenectomy in apparent early stage epithelial ovarian cancer? *Gynecol. Oncol.* 2021;160: 56-63.

[21] Elit, L, Chambers, A, Fyles, A, Covens, A, Carey, M, Fung, MF. Systematic review of adjuvant care for women with Stage I ovarian carcinoma. *Cancer.* 2004;101(9):1926-35.

[22] Lawrie, TA, Winter-Roach, BA, Heus, P, Kitchener, HC. Adjuvant (post-surgery) chemotherapy for early-stage epithelial ovarian cancer. *Cochrane Database Syst. Rev.* 2015;(12):CD004706.

[23] Li, S, Zhu, Z. Chemotherapy is not necessary for early-stage serous and endometrioid ovarian cancer after undergoing comprehensive staging surgery. *J. Ovarian Res.* 2020;9;13(1):91.

[24] Chan, JK, Tian, C, Monk, BJ, Herzog, T, Kapp, DS, Bell, J, Young, RC; Gynecologic Oncology Group. Prognostic factors for high-risk early-stage epithelial ovarian cancer: a Gynecologic Oncology Group study. *Cancer.* 2008;112(10):2202-10.

[25] Oza, AM, Cook, AD, Pfisterer, J, Embleton, A, Ledermann, JA, Pujade-Lauraine, E, Kristensen, et al. ICON7 trial investigators. Standard chemotherapy with or without bevacizumab for women with newly diagnosed ovarian cancer (ICON7): overall survival results of a phase 3 randomised trial. *Lancet Oncol.* 2015;16(8):928-36.

[26] Moore, K, Colombo, N, Scambia, G, Kim, BG, Oaknin, A, Friedlander, M, Lisyanskaya, A, Floquet, A, Leary, A, Sonke, GS, Gourley, C, Banerjee, S, Oza, A, González-Martín, A, Aghajanian, C, Bradley, W, Mathews, C, Liu, J, Lowe, ES, Bloomfield, R., Gonzalez-Martin, A., Aghajanian, C., Bradley, W., Mathews, C., Liu, J., Lowe, E.S. and DiSilvestro, P. Maintenance Olaparib in Patients with Newly Diagnosed Advanced Ovarian Cancer. *N. Engl. J. Med.* 2018;379(26):2495-2505.

[27] Ray-Coquard, I, Pautier, P, Pignata, S, Pérol, D, González-Martín, A, Berger, R, Fujiwara, K, Vergote, I, Colombo, N, Mäenpää, J, Selle, F, Sehouli, J, Lorusso, D, Guerra Alía, EM, Reinthaller, A, Nagao, S, Lefeuvre-Plesse, C, Canzler, U, Scambia, G, Lortholary, A., Marme, F., Combe, P., de Gregorio, N., Rodrigues, M., Buderath, P., Dubot, C., Burges, A., You, B., Pujade-Lauraine, E. and Harter, P. Olaparib plus Bevacizumab as First-Line Maintenance in Ovarian Cancer. *N Engl. J. Med.* 2019;381(25):2416-2428.

[28] Soliman, AA, Elzarkaa, AA, Malik, E. Epithelial Ovarian Cancer and Cancer Stem Cells. *Adv. Exp. Med. Biol.* 2021;1330:21-32.

Chapter 16

Fertility Sparing in Ovarian Cancer Patients

Myriam Gracia, MD, PhD
Ana Peralbo, MD, PhD
and Ignacio Zapardiel*, MD, PhD
Gynecologic Oncology Unit, La Paz University Hospital, Madrid, Spain

Introduction

Ovarian cancer has an incidence of approximately 5-12 cases among 100,000 women per year [1]. Although the majority of cases are diagnosed among postmenopausal women, up to 12% of the cases are detected in women younger than 45 years, some of whom have not reached their reproductive goals at the moment of the diagnosis. Ovarian cancer has the highest mortality rate among all gynecological malignancies and less than 40% of the cases are detected in the earliest stages [1]. Most of these cases are of epithelial origin (up to 90%) whereas the rest are sex-cord or germ cell tumors.

Preserving fertility in ovarian cancer patients is more challenging than in endometrial and cervical cancer, since the affected organ is the one that we are trying to preserve. However, there are options for ovarian preservation in premenopausal women, in early stages, in borderline tumors, and in germ cell or sex cord tumors [1]. In the last decades, we have witnessed an increasing delay of the childbearing age and percentage of patients with an uncompleted gestational desire at the moment of diagnosis. This fact should be a major issue of concern for gynecological oncologists. Other main concerns are the safety of fertility sparing treatments, the uncertain efficacy of fertility options, the detrimental effects of chemotherapy to remaining reproductive organs, when to undergo fertility treatments and which candidates are the optimal for fertility sparing management [2].

About 60% of ovarian cancer are detected in advanced stages, presumably because of the default of screening tests, the absence of markers, imaging test and the unspecific symptomatology while the tumor is confined to the ovary [3]. Treatment of ovarian cancer depends on the FIGO stage at the time of diagnosis (Table 1).

Traditional treatment of advanced stage ovarian cancer unfortunately includes a primary surgical approach and adjuvant chemotherapy that leads to permanent infertility [2]. In early

* Corresponding Author's Email: ignaciozapardiel@alumni.harvard.edu.

In: Ovarian Cancer
Editors: Christos Iavazzo, Alexandros Fotiou and John Spiliotis
ISBN: 979-8-88697-633-5

stages, the standard management includes surgical staging procedures with total hysterectomy, bilateral salpingo-ooforecomy, pelvic and para-aortic lymphadenectomy (up to the left renal vein), omentectomy and peritoneal evaluation (through peritoneal washing and direct biopsies). Afterwards, adjuvant chemotherapy should be included in almost all regimes of treatment with the only exclusion of low-grade serous IA stages and IA stages-grade 1-2 of endometrioid and mucinous histology [3].

These mentioned treatments do not spare the fertility of the patient. Opposing them, conservative procedures have been developed in order to preserve fertility in patients who desire offspring. These treatments attempt to preserve the reproductive options ensuring their safety and oncological outcomes. The most important issue is to guarantee the balance between the fertility sparing and the oncological safety which requires the accurate selection of the potential candidates to these techniques, which will be discussed forwards [1].

Table 1. FIGO staging classification for cancer of the ovary, fallopian tube and peritoneum

Stage I: Tumor confined to ovaries or fallopian tube(s)
Stage IA: Tumor limited to 1 ovary (capsule intact) or fallopian tube; no tumor on ovarian or fallopian tube surface; no malignant cells in the ascites or peritoneal washings
Stage IB: Tumor limited to both ovaries (capsules intact) or fallopian tubes; no tumor on ovarian or fallopian tube surface; no malignant cells in the ascites or peritoneal washings
Stage IC: Tumor limited to 1 or both ovaries or fallopian tubes, with any of the following: • Stage IC1: Surgical spill • Stage IC2: Capsule ruptured before surgery or tumor on ovarian or fallopian tube surface • Stage IC3: Malignant cells in the ascites or peritoneal washings
Stage II: Tumor involves 1 or both ovaries or fallopian tubes with pelvic extension (below pelvic brim) or peritoneal cancer
Stage IIA: Extension and/or implants on uterus and/or fallopian tubes and/or ovaries
Stage IIB: Extension to other pelvic intraperitoneal tissues
Stage III: Tumor involves 1 or both ovaries or fallopian tubes, or peritoneal cancer, with cytologically or histologically confirmed spread to the peritoneum outside the pelvis and/or metastasis to the retroperitoneal lymph nodes
Stage IIIA1: Positive retroperitoneal lymph nodes only (cytologically or histologically proven): • IIIA1(i) Metastasis up to 10 mm in greatest dimension • IIIA1(ii) Metastasis more than 10 mm in greatest dimension Stage IIIA2: Microscopic extrapelvic (above the pelvic brim) peritoneal involvement with or without positive retroperitoneal lymph nodes
Stage IIIB: Macroscopic peritoneal metastasis beyond the pelvis up to 2 cm in greatest dimension, with or without metastasis to the retroperitoneal lymph nodes
Stage IIIC: Macroscopic peritoneal metastasis beyond the pelvis more than 2 cm in greatest dimension, with or without metastasis to the retroperitoneal lymph nodes (includes extension of tumor to capsule of liver and spleen without parenchymal involvement of either organ)
Stage IV: Distant metastasis excluding peritoneal metastases
Stage IVA: Pleural effusion with positive cytology
Stage IVB: Parenchymal metastases and metastases to extra-abdominal organs (including inguinal lymph nodes and lymph nodes outside of the abdominal cavity)

There are some options to preserve fertility, including, fertility preservation while going through potential cytotoxic treatments, assisted reproduction techniques including cryopreservation and fertility sparing surgical procedures. Nevertheless, as the majority of the diagnosis in premenopausal women are incidental (some of them during the characterization of a new diagnosed ovarian mass), the fertility sparing surgery is the most promising option for these women since there is no chance for treatments which require planification (such as cryopreservation) because the disease should be treated in a short period of time [1].

Diverse studies have shown that more than a half of patients received incomplete information about the impact of oncological treatments on their reproductive health [4]. Patients should be informed in detail about future oncological and obstetrical outcomes as well as to clearly understand that a thorough follow-up after the treatment is mandatory. Discussing these issues with patients will reduce stress, improve satisfaction with the care received, and improve long-term quality of life for these patients [2].

Indications of Fertility Sparing in Ovarian Cancer

The aim of fertility sparing treatments in ovarian cancer is to conserve the reproductive possibilities of our patients through maintaining the uterus and the other presumably healthy ovary without reducing oncological safety. There is also one more target - the preservation of the ovarian endocrine function.

Conservative management of ovarian cancer patients is limited for those cases where the disease is confined to one ovary. The best candidates for conservative management are those patients with the best prognosis [5, 6]. In order to identify those low-risk group of patients we need to evaluate parameters at the FIGO stage, the histologic subtype and grade, Ca125 serum values, the patient's age and overall performance status [2].

After determining the feasibility of a fertility sparing treatment, the patient should be informed of all possible treatments, as well as the fertility options and risks in order to achieve a consensual decision on being conservative [7]. In addition, one of the most relevant factors to consider in the initial evaluation of fertility sparing techniques are personal preferences and reproductive possibilities of the patients. Women with a desire to get pregnant, especially nulliparous women, are the main candidates for these techniques. However, it is mandatory to determine the feasibility of the fertility itself. Since fertility decreases at the decade of 40, it seems reasonable not to encourage these techniques from this age. Another reasonable approach, especially for patients among 35-40 years is to perform an ovarian reserve study, through sonography and AMH determination, in order to give a more specific recommendation [1].

In order to finally establish which are the best candidates for fertility sparing treatment, determining the histologic subtype and the FIGO stage are crucial. As mentioned before, only patients with the disease limited to one ovary are suitable, but further stages may be considered as an exception in some selected cases [8].

The oncological and fertility results of conservative treatments are still under debate in literature. Highly motivated nulliparous women with disease limited to one ovary and histological subtypes such as germ cell ovarian tumors, borderline tumors or early stages of low-grade epithelial ovarian cancer seem the best candidates for these treatments, as they have the best prognosis. Regardless, the accurate cut-off of fertility sparing treatments is still controversial [3].

According to ESMO-ESGO 2019 guidelines, fertility seems to be safe in patients with conventional low-grade stage IA *epithelial ovarian cancer (EOC)* (serous, endometrioid or mucinous expansile subtype) [8]. Clear-cell ovarian cancer has a poor prognosis and large rate of recurrences; for this reason, patients with clear-cell subtype have not traditionally been considered as candidates for fertility sparing surgery. However, the latest evidence shows that early stages IA (even IC) selected patients could be considered for this technique. As the majority of the recurrences occur within the first two years after diagnosis, the patient should be advised not to attempt pregnancy before this time, in order to avoid a recurrence during pregnancy. Nevertheless, the evidence is still limited and the recommendations remain controversial in this case [10].

Discrimination between FIGO stages IC1 to IC3 must be done using the current 2014 FIGO staging system [9]. Evidence shows safety in fertility sparing treatments in IC1 subtype (intraoperative rupture of the tumor), assuming more than 50% of recurrences in the remaining ovary but considering the possibility of a second rescue surgery. Chemotherapy could be administered, if necessary, in these cases. Recurrence risk is higher in stages IC2 -IC3 as well as high histological grade tumors, although mainly in extraovarian sites and are, therefore, not clearly correlated with the fertility-sparing approach. It is widely accepted not to recommend fertility-sparing techniques in these patients, as its safety cannot be confirmed [8, 10].

In cases of Stage II or III disease, the use of fertility sparing treatments is unconventional and not recommended, with high risk of recurrences and poor oncological outcomes reported [11].

These recommendations are valid for epithelial ovarian cancer, mostly in serous, mucinous and endometrioid tumors.

Non-epithelial ovarian tumors represent 10% of the ovarian neoplasms, and can be subclassified in two groups: Germ Cell Tumors (GCTs) and Sex Cord Stromal Tumors (SCSTs), which are diagnosed in 5% and 35% of the cases, respectively. While SCSTs are diagnosed mostly in postmenopausal women (the peak of incidence is in women between 50 and 80 years old), GCTs have the highest incidence in teenagers or young women below 30 years, the peak of incidence is around 17 years, and up to 70% of the cases are in women below 30, which, in addition to their excellent prognosis and high chemosensitivity, make these cases quite favorable for fertility sparing surgery [11, 12].

Most GCTs (60%–70%) are diagnosed at an early stage. In these cases, fertility-sparing surgery appears to be safe with excellent survival after long-term follow-up [12]. Even in higher stages, the prognosis is very favorable and current evidence supports that fertility sparing treatment should be considered up to III-IV FIGO stages, with a prior debulking surgery and adjuvant chemotherapy regime. It is not necessarily systematic biopsy of the contralateral ovary if it is macroscopically normal [13]. In dysgerminoma or immature teratoma macroscopically bilateral ovarian disease, preservation of at least a healthy part of one ovary (unilateral salpingo-oophorectomy and contralateral cystectomy) and the uterus should be encouraged [13].

SCSTs are considered for fertility sparing surgery only in stage IA due to the lack of evidence. In stage IC juvenile granulosa cell tumor (Figure 1), the safety of conservative management remains controversial, particularly in stage IC2 or IC3 disease [14].

Borderline ovarian tumors represent up to 15% of epithelial ovarian tumors. The peak of incidence is about 40 years old. The two main histological subtypes are serous and mucinous. The good prognosis, even in higher stages, requires a more conservative management. Staging surgery implies cystectomy or unilateral adnexectomy, peritoneal biopsies, omentectomy and inspection of the appendix (appendicectomy is only necessary if it looks abnormal). Fertility sparing surgery could be considered in early stages. For advanced stages or recurrences, a multidisciplinary counseling for each case should be done [14].

Finally, tumoral markers are also an important issue to consider, as high pre-surgical Ca-125 values may indicate high tumoral volume, a fertility sparing technique could be inadequate for this patient [2]. Besides, young patients must be considered for a BRCA 1-2 testing in order to evaluate the possibility of a bilateral ovarian affectation and give further advice [3].

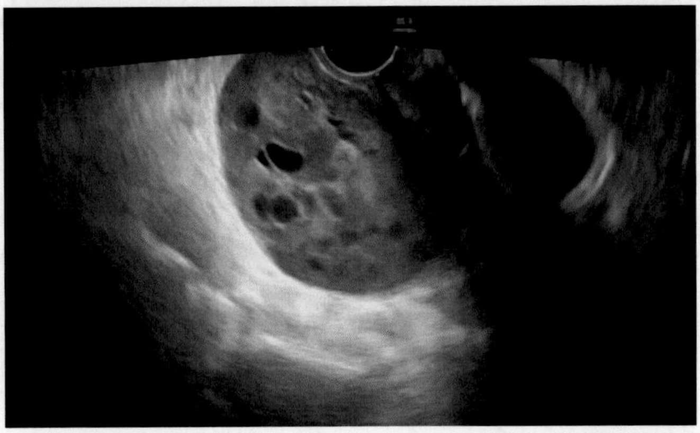

Figure 1. Granulosa cell tumor. Ultrasound image.

Fertility Sparing Procedures in Ovarian Cancer

Unfortunately, the conventional surgical treatment of ovarian cancer patients results in infertility. Conservative surgical management of ovarian cancer that allows the preservation of fertility is based on unilateral salpingo-oophorectomy and complete surgical staging. In *EOC* complete surgical staging includes pelvic and para-aortic lymphadenectomies, omentectomy and peritoneal study. Although complete lymphadenectomy can be omitted in expansile mucinous subtype [15].

There is no consensus about performing systematic lymphadenectomy in patients with GCTs. Although the omission of peritoneal staging seems to increase the recurrence rate without impacting overall survival. SCSTs present a very low incidence of retroperitoneal metastases in early-stage disease, thus, retroperitoneal staging is not mandatory [13].

In cases of non-confirmed or low risk malignancy, a cystectomy (Figure 2), could be an option, although the risk of recurrence seems to increase compared to oophorectomy in the cases of malignancy or borderline ovarian tumors. For this reason, the preferred option is oophorectomy for the majority of authors.

Additional diagnostic studies before surgical management should be considered in some histological subtypes. An endometrial curettage or biopsy could be performed in endometrioid ovarian cancer and granulosa cell tumors, as there is the possibility of a concomitant endometrial neoplasia [8]. The contralateral ovary must be examined, as well, but the recommendation is to perform a macroscopic exploration during surgery. Some authors have reported very low rates of microscopic disease (0-2.5%) in the absence of macroscopic lesions [16, 17], although the incidence of bilaterality could be as high as 33% for Stage I serious disease [2]. Besides, there is a potential risk of developing adherences in the remaining ovary, thereby affecting fertility. The biopsies should be limited to the finding of macroscopic lesions. Appendectomy as a staging procedure is not recommended even in the mucinous subtype [8]. An appendicular study could be performed with the same criteria as a contralateral ovary study, especially in mucinous subtypes, in order to rule out the possibility that the ovarian tumor could be a metastatic lesion of a primary appendicular tumor.

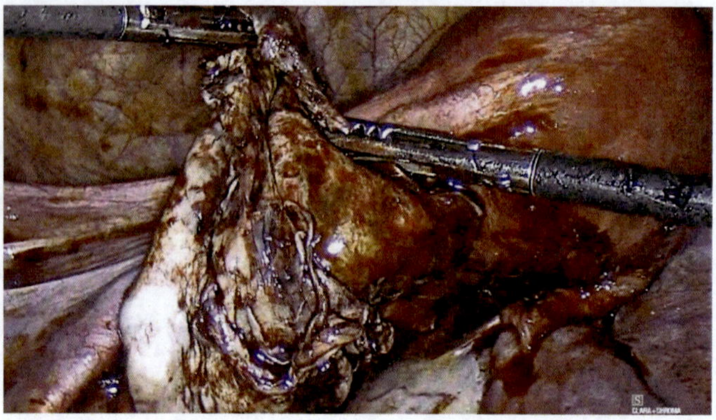

Figure 2. Laparoscopic ovarian cystectomy.

Furthermore, the approach route for surgery is as equally important to the type of surgery. Laparoscopic approach is related to higher risk of rupture of the tumor (RR=1.17), and evidence shows that women with ruptured tumors have lower overall survival rates than those with non-ruptured ones [15]. Although progression-free survival rates are lower in cases with intraoperative rupture of the cysts, some evidence shows there may be no difference between intraoperative rupture and no rupture in patients who underwent complete surgical staging operation and adjuvant platinum-based chemotherapy, if needed. It is demonstrated that the risk of recurrence increases in the event of intraoperative tumor rupture. Also, tumor volume is the main predictor of intraoperative tumor rupture [15]. Tumor rupture is also conditioned by the type of surgical procedure performed: cystectomy presents a higher risk of rupture and spillage than an adnexectomy.

Even if the risk of rupture or morcellation of the tumor during surgery is lower during a laparotomy, the potential benefits and the technical feasibility of laparoscopic approach suggests it may be a reasonable option in some cases. The precise cut-off is still uncertain, although some authors suggest the point of 10 cm, beyond which, the risk of rupture is significantly higher and the spillage of tumoral cells is unacceptable, even using protective bags [18].

The recommendation is to take all precautions to avoid rupture, including intraoperative reconversion to laparotomy and protected extraction of the specimen, especially in laparoscopic surgical treatment.

A controversial point is the need to perform a complete radical surgery after childbearing or after assuming, basing on a significant unsuccessful number of tries or the patient's age, the improbability to conceive. Considering that recurrences are reported up to 8% in IA stage and 10% in IC stage OC, performing complete radical surgery could be a reasonable option [20]. Nevertheless, in the youngest patients, the endocrine function is quite relevant, as early menopause may cause a serious detrimental in the woman's general health. Thus, the option of a close follow-up could be considered, with the counsel of a multidisciplinary committee [5].

Oncological Outcomes after Fertility Sparing Treatment in Ovarian Cancer

Fertility-sparing surgery (FSS) of *epithelial ovarian cancer* (EOC) is based on unilateral salpingo-oophorectomy and complete surgical staging. Nevertheless, many questions concerning oncological outcomes remain unclear.

EOC typically presents itself with advanced-stage disease, but premenopausal women are more likely to with exhibit early-stage disease, which is associated with a 5-year relative survival of 92.6% [19].

Literature reports that patients with early-stage EOC treated conservatively have good survival rates. Survival rates for patients with stage IA are very good (5-year survival up to 98%) and recurrence rate in the contralateral ovary is not considered high (3-5%) [2]. Regarding survival rates in early stages, two systematic reviews found recurrence rates of 11% at a median follow-up of 6 years [20, 21].

Although many studies demonstrate the safety of FSS in Stage IA, low-grade EOC, there is controversy surrounding high-risk features such as stage IC, high pathologic grade, and clear cell histology [20].

Detailing the substage of the disease, among studies that provided details about relapsing patients, 10% of recurrences occurred in stage IA and 16% in stage IC (p=0.002). Including tumor grade, recurrences were observed in 7% stage IA-grade 1, 11% stage IA-grade 2 and 29% stage IA-grade 3 (p=0-004). Likewise, data in case of stage IC were available; 11% grade 1, 11% grade 2 and 23% grade 3 (p=0.02) [22, 23]. Other authors report recurrences among stage IC subgroups; relapses occurred in 12% patients with stage IC1 and in 23% patients with stage IC2-3 (p=0.02) [12].

Focusing on histologic subtype, a systematic review found that more than a half of the tumor were mucinous subtype (53%) compared with serous (18%), endometrioid (17%) and clear cell carcinoma (9%). Recurrences occurred in 10% of mucinous tumor, 15% of serous, 13% of endometrioid and 22% of clear cell carcinoma (p=0.007) [12].

Comparing FSS with radical surgery for EOC, a recent metanalysis including 2,223 patients undergoing FSS and 5809 undergoing radical surgery, did not find statistically significant differences in overall or disease-free survival [24]. Along the same line, a recent multi-institution study adjusted for age, stage, histology, and receipt of chemotherapy, demonstrated that 5-year overall survival rates were similar between patients who underwent FSS (87.5%) and those who had conventional surgery (91.8%) [25]. In clear cell carcinoma, a retrospective study found that the number of recurrences, pattern of recurrences, and mean time to recurrence were similar between patients undergoing FSS and those undergoing conventional surgery. The number of deaths was higher in the FSS group (18% vs 8%), but this was not statistically significant, suggesting that FSS is a reasonable alternative in women with stage IA or IC clear cell carcinoma [20].

Regarding the location of the recurrent disease, a systematic review reported that 37% of recurrences involved the remanent ovary and 63% were extra-ovarian. In clear cell carcinoma, 87% of patients had extraovarian disease compared with 13% of ovarian recurrence (this rate is statistically significant compared with the rate of ovarian/extra-ovarian recurrences in the overall population; p<0.0003) [12].

The time to the first recurrence is important when a FSS is proposed. Most of the patients developed a recurrence very early, within the first 2 years after the initial treatment. Although the validity of conservative management is doubtful in clear cell carcinoma, we should not 'authorize' the patient to attempt a pregnancy before 2 years after FSS because of the potential diagnosis of a metastatic recurrence in a pregnant patient [20]. In the case of Grade 3 tumors, 95% of the recurrences were extra-ovarian (and only 22% of them were rendered disease-free) [20].

When relapse occurs in the residual ovary alone, salvage treatment may result in a cure. However, prognosis turns worse if disseminated recurrence with peritoneal carcinomatosis occurs. In some series, none of the patients with ovarian relapse died, while 11 of 14 patients (79%) who presented with distant metastases died of disease [3, 26].

In summary, FSS seems to confirm the safety of this modality, at least in patients with stage IA-IC and grade 1-2 disease. However, more research is necessary to determine the safety of FSS in women with EOC with high-risk features (IC-G3) and to determine if oncological outcomes are related to the "natural history" of the tumor rather than to the preservation of the ovary itself.

Given the fact that *non-epithelial malignant tumors* typically arise in young adolescent women, have a good prognosis even in the case of extraovarian spread and have excellent responses to adjuvant chemotherapy, fertility conservation should be always discussed in the standard practice.

Unilateral salpingo-oophorectomy with preservation of the contralateral ovary and the uterus is now considered as the standard surgical treatment for young patients with *GCTs*. Most GCTs (60%–70%) are diagnosed at an early stage. Stage I patients have an excellent prognosis with long-term disease-free status of about 90% [13].

A systematic review based on data from 29 studies and 1491 patients reported a total of 129 tumor recurrences with a cumulative relapse rate of 8.7% [27]. Other studies report a recurrence rate of 12.2% [20]. In the largest of these retrospective series, 14.6% patients undergoing FSS had a recurrence, 5 (2.9%) died of the disease, and the 5-year OS rate was 97%, which is similar to previously reported survival rates for localized GCTs [28].

Focusing on the other group of non-epithelial ovarian cancer, most *SCSTs* (60%–95%) are diagnosed at an early stage and have an excellent prognosis factor, but limited information is reported on the conservative management of these tumors. FSS preserving uterus and contralateral ovary seems to be safe in stage IA, due to the rare occurrence of bilaterality (2-8%). But in the case of juvenile granulosa cell tumors, the safety of this management approach in stage IC disease remains controversial, particularly in stage IC2 or IC3 disease. Cystectomy is not recommended for women with granulosa cell tumor who wish to maintain fertility because the risk of recurrence is higher compared to unilateral adnexectomy (16% vs 70%) [20].

Results among different retrospective studies carried out in patients treated with FSS are not homogeneous. Several retrospective studies have not found any adverse impact of FSS on tumor recurrence rates or progression free survival (PFS), but these are retrospective and with a limited number of patients [29]. One of the largest studies to date found that cancer-specific survival (CSS) was worse (11.8% vs. 4.3%; $p=0.015$) in patients with FSS but not overall survival ($P = 0.76$) compared with patients treated with complete surgery. They analyzed the risk factors associated with CSS and only tumor size was statistically associated with worse CSS. In general, SCSTs are associated with late recurrences, which highlights the need for a long-term follow up, taking into account that as many as 50% of relapses can be asymptomatic [20].

Reproductive and Obstetrics Outcomes after Fertility Sparing Treatment in Ovarian Cancer

Data regarding reproductive outcomes in patients with OC who underwent FSS should be interpreted carefully and without generalization, since rates of gestation and obstetric outcomes are not based on high-level evidence studies. In addition, many studies do not differentiate between women who decided not to try to get pregnant and those who were unable to conceive, so the resulting conception rates may be lower than they actually should be. In fact, although preserving reproductive capacity is one of the main goals of FSS, the desire to conceive postoperatively has been reported to be less than half (16%-50%) among women who undergo such techniques. Some authors have observed that the number of patients who tried to conceive, were significantly lower in high-grade than low-grade disease [3]. This could be explained by the fact that patients became more concern about recurrence risk after completing the proposed treatment and underlines the importance of adequate counseling before planning a fertility sparing treatment.

Another important consideration regarding patients who underwent FSS is the need of adjuvant treatment. It is well known that chemotherapy compromises the ovarian function, often resulting in infertility and premature menopause depending on the different drugs and dosages, although carboplatin and paclitaxel are in general less gonadotoxic compared to other cytostatic agents [3]. The main mechanism of ovarian damage includes accelerated rates of follicular apoptosis and, to a lesser extent, cortical fibrosis. Alkylating agents cause the most severe of these effects [30].

Current standards of treatment, including cisplatin, vinblastine, bleomycin and etoposide, have less effect on ovarian function. Other agents, such us cyclophosphamide present a higher rate of ovarian damage causing premature ovarian failure or persistent amenorrhea [30].

However, the need of adjuvant chemotherapy should be undertaken independently of the surgery performed and not compromising oncological outcomes [3].

It is also necessary to take into account the influence of the surgical approach. Besides lack of evidence, laparoscopic approach has been shown to be feasible and possibly associated with lower adhesion rate which could lead to higher fertility rates [3].

The successful conception rate among women with a desire to have offspring is higher than 60%, with a range from 63% to 100% depending on different studies. Also, the abortion rate has been described with acceptable percentages, around 17%. Studies that collect data about delivery rates, report that the live-birth rate ranged from 76% to 96% [20]. Otherwise, conservative treatment in ovarian cancer (surgery or surgery + chemotherapy administration) has not been associated with worse obstetric outcomes since the rate of malformations, miscarriages or preterm delivery is similar to the general population [3, 30].

All techniques of reproductive medicine in ovarian cancer patients are still under debate and are quite controversial.

Even if cryopreservation of oocytes, embryos or ovarian tissue is questionable, literature data show that ovulation induction may be a safer option after fertility sparing surgery of border line ovarian tumors. In order to induce ovulation, GnRH antagonist protocols may be a suitable option, according to their shorter stimulation period and lower risk of ovarian hyper-stimulation syndrome. In the case of estrogen-dependent tumors, protocols including aromatase inhibitors may reduce estrogen-levels, but the evidence in progression-free survival rates depending on stimulation protocol is limited. Communication between reproductive doctors and oncologists is mandatory to improve the oncological safety and fertility results [30].

Follow-up of Patients

The follow-up is quite similar to other OC patients, and it varies depending on prognostic factors and the specific treatment modality. The scheduled follow-up may include an evaluation every 3 or 4 months for the first two years, increasing the interval to 6 months between the 3rd to 5th year. Beyond the 5th year, the continuation of the follow up depends on the individual case and the centre protocol.

Imaging tests could be done periodically or conditioned to specific symptoms or Ca-125 levels. Another option for these patients that will undergo fertility sparing surgery could be to perform an ultrasonography in each visit and depending on the findings to indicate a further CT-scan if needed.

In the case of non-epithelial ovarian cancer, a tumor-specific marker should be determined in each appointment. In sex-cord stromal cells tumors, the follow-up may be maintained during the life of the patient, as late recurrences are reported [13].

Conclusion

- Fertility sparing treatments could be a suitable option to preserve fertility for conveniently informed- patients younger than 40 years old, with an early stage of ovarian cancer who want to preserve fertility.
- FIGO stage, fertility feasibility, histological subtype, image testing and tumoral markers are essential in the consideration of fertility sparing treatments.
- All fertility preserving candidates should be managed in experienced centres, where the patient will be informed of oncological risks and obstetrical outcomes.
- Fertility sparing surgery usually includes the preservation of the uterus and one ovary. Performing a complete staging surgery is mandatory, as well as close follow-up and observation. Completing radical surgery is a possibility within the evolution.

References

[1] Gorostidi M, Gil-Ibañez B, Alonso S, Gil-Moreno A, Hernandez A, Torné A, Zapardiel I. Fertility preservation treatment of gynecological cancer patients in Spain: a national survey (GOFER study). *Arch Gynecol Obstet.* 2020 Mar;301(3):793-800.

[2] Alexandros Rodolakis, Nikolaos Thomakos. Fertility preservation for gynecologic cancer patients. In: Ali Ayhan, editor. *ESGO Textbook of gynecological oncology*. p. 1051-1062.

[3] Zapardiel I, Diestro MD, Aletti G. Conservative treatment of early-stage ovarian cancer: oncological and fertility outcomes. *Eur J Surg Oncol.* 2014 Apr;40(4):387-93.

[4] Findeklee S, Radosa JC, Takacs Z, Hamza A, Sima R, Solomayer E, Sklavounos P. Fertility preservation in female cancer patients: current knowledge and future perspectives. *Minerva Ginecol.* 2019 Aug;71(4):298-305.

[5] Ditto A, Martinelli F, Lorusso D, Haeusler E, Carcangiu M, Raspagliesi F. Fertility sparing surgery in early stage epithelial ovarian cancer. *J Gynecol Oncol.* 2014 Oct;25(4):320-7.

[6] Morice P, Camatte S, El Hassan J, Pautier P, Duvillard P, Castaigne D. Clinical outcomes and fertility after conservative treatment of ovarian borderline tumors. *Fertil Steril* 2001;75(1):92–6.

[7] Fruscio R, Corso S, Ceppi L, Garavaglia D, Garbi A, Floriani I, Franchi D, Cantù MG, Bonazzi CM, Milani R, Mangioni C, Colombo N. Conservative management of early-stage epithelial ovarian cancer: results of a large retrospective series. *Ann Oncol.* 2013 Jan;24(1):138-44.

[8] Colombo N, Sessa C, du Bois A, Ledermann J, McCluggage WG, McNeish I, Morice P, Pignata S, Ray-Coquard I, Vergote I, Baert T, Belaroussi I, Dashora A, Olbrecht S, Planchamp F, Querleu D; ESMO-ESGO Ovarian Cancer Consensus Conference Working Group. ESMO-ESGO consensus conference recommendations on ovarian cancer: pathology and molecular biology, early and advanced stages, borderline tumours and recurrent disease†. *Ann Oncol.* 2019 May 1;30(5):672-705.

[9] Bentivegna E, Fruscio R, Roussin S, Ceppi L, Satoh T, Kajiyama H, Uzan C, Colombo N, Gouy S, Morice P. Long-term follow-up of patients with an isolated ovarian recurrence after conservative treatment of epithelial ovarian cancer: review of the results of an international multicenter study comprising 545 patients. *Fertil Steril.* 2015 Nov;104(5):1319-24.

[10] Thomakos N, Malakasis A, Machairiotis N, Zarogoulidis P, Rodolakis A. Fertility Sparing Management in Non-Epithelial Ovarian Cancer. Which Patients, What Procedure and What Outcome? *J Cancer.* 2018 Nov 24;9(24):4659-4664.

[11] Bentivegna E, Gouy S, Maulard A, Pautier P, Leary A, Colombo N, Morice P. Fertility-sparing surgery in epithelial ovarian cancer: a systematic review of oncological issues. *Ann Oncol.* 2016 Nov;27(11):1994-2004.

[12] Ray-Coquard I, Morice P, Lorusso D, Prat J, Oaknin A, Pautier P, Colombo N; ESMO Guidelines Committee. Non-epithelial ovarian cancer: ESMO Clinical Practice Guidelines for diagnosis, treatment and follow-up. *Ann Oncol. 2018* Oct 1;29(Suppl 4):iv1-iv18.

[13] Brown, J, Friedlander, M, Backes, FJ, Harter, P, O'Connor, DM, de la Motte Rouge, T, Lorusso, D, Maenpaa, J, Kim, JW, Tenney, ME, & Seckl, MJ. Gynecologic Cancer Intergroup (GCIG) consensus review for ovarian germ cell tumors. *Int J Gynecol Cancer* 2014; 24(9 Suppl 3): S48–S54.

[14] Bourdel N, Huchon C, Abdel Wahab C, Azaïs H, Bendifallah S, Bolze PA, Brun JL, Canlorbe G, Chauvet P, Chereau E, Courbiere B, De La Motte Rouge T, Devouassoux-Shisheboran M, Eymerit-Morin C, Fauvet R, Gauroy E, Gauthier T, Grynberg M, Koskas M, Larouzee E, Lecointre L, Levêque J, Margueritte F, D'argent Mathieu E, Nyangoh-Timoh K, Ouldamer L, Raad J, Raimond E, Ramanah R, Rolland L, Rousset P, Rousset-Jablonski C, Thomassin-Naggara I, Uzan C, Zilliox M, Daraï E. Borderline ovarian tumors: French guidelines from the CNGOF. Part 2. Surgical management, follow-up, hormone replacement therapy, fertility management and preservation. *J Gynecol Obstet Hum Reprod.* 2021 Jan;50(1):101966.

[15] Bentivegna E, Maulard A, Miailhe G, Gouy S, Morice P. Gynaecologic cancer surgery and preservation of fertility. *J Visc Surg.* 2018 Jun;155 Suppl 1: S23-S29.

[16] Benjamin I, Morgan MA, Rubin SC. Occult bilateral involvement in stage I epithelial ovarian cancer. *Gynecol Oncol.* 1999 Mar;72(3):288-91.

[17] American College of Obstetricians and Gynecologists. ACOG Practice Bulletin. Management of adnexal masses. *Obstet Gynecol.* 2007 Jul;110(1):201-14.

[18] Shiota M, Kotani Y, Umemoto M, Tobiume T, Hoshiai H. Study of the correlation between tumor size and cyst rupture in laparotomy and laparoscopy for benign ovarian tumor: is 10 cm the limit for laparoscopy? *J Obstet Gynaecol Res.* 2012 Mar;38(3):531-4.

[19] Bercow A, Nitecki R, Brady PC, Rauh-Hain JA. Outcomes after Fertility-sparing Surgery for Women with Ovarian Cancer: A Systematic Review of the Literature. *J Minim Invasive Gynecol.* 2021 Mar;28(3):527-536.e1.

[20] Nam JH, Park JY. Fertility-sparing surgery for young women with early-stage epithelial ovarian cancer. *Gynecol Obstet Invest.* 2013;76(1):14-24. doi: 10.1159/000350797.

[21] Chan JK, Tian C, Monk BJ, Herzog T, Kapp DS, Bell J, Young RC; Gynecologic Oncology Group. Prognostic factors for high-risk early-stage epithelial ovarian cancer: a Gynecologic Oncology Group study. *Cancer.* 2008 May 15;112(10):2202-10.

[22] Cheng X, Cheng B, Wan X, Lu W, Xie X. Outcomes of conservative surgery in early epithelial ovarian carcinoma. *Eur J Gynaecol Oncol.* 2012;33(1):93-5. PMID: 22439414.

[23] Kashima K, Yahata T, Fujita K, Tanaka K. Outcomes of fertility-sparing surgery for women of reproductive age with FIGO stage IC epithelial ovarian cancer. *Int J Gynaecol Obstet.* 2013 Apr;121(1):53-5.

[24] Liu D, Cai J, Gao A, Wang Z, Cai L. Fertility sparing surgery vs radical surgery for epithelial ovarian cancer: a meta-analysis of overall survival and disease-free survival. *BMC Cancer.* 2020 Apr 15;20(1):320.

[25] Kajiyama, Hiroaki & Suzuki, Shiro & Yoshikawa, Nobuhisa & Kawai, Michiyasu & Mizuno, Kimio & Yamamuro, Osamu & Shibata, Kiyosumi & Kikkawa, Fumitaka. (2019). Fertility-sparing surgery and oncologic outcome among patients with early-stage ovarian cancer ~propensity score- matched analysis. *BMC Cancer.* 19. 10.1186/s12885-019-6432-4.

[26] Fruscio R, Corso S, Ceppi L, Garavaglia D, Garbi A, Floriani I, Franchi D, Cantù MG, Bonazzi CM, Milani R, Mangioni C, Colombo N. Conservative management of early-stage epithelial ovarian cancer: results of a large retrospective series. *Ann Oncol.* 2013 Jan;24(1):138-44.

[27] Morrison A, Nasioudis D. Reproductive outcomes following fertility-sparing surgery for malignant ovarian germ cell tumors: A systematic review of the literature. *Gynecol Oncol.* 2020 Aug;158(2):476-483.

[28] Park JY, Kim DY, Suh DS, Kim JH, Kim YM, Kim YT, Nam JH. Analysis of outcomes and prognostic factors after fertility-sparing surgery in malignant ovarian germ cell tumors. *Gynecol Oncol.* 2017 Jun;145(3):513-518.

[29] Nasioudis D, Frey MK, Chapman-Davis E, Witkin, SS, Holcomb, K. Safety of Fertility-Sparing Surgery for Premenopausal Women With Sex Cord-Stromal Tumors Confined to the Ovary. *International Journal of Gynecologic Cancer* 2017;27:1826-1832.

[30] Zapardiel I, Cruz M, Diestro MD, Requena A, Garcia-Velasco JA. Assisted reproductive techniques after fertility-sparing treatments in gynaecological cancers. *Hum Reprod Update.* 2016 Apr;22(3):281-305.

Chapter 17

The Local-Regional Control of Ovarian Cancer

Paul H. Sugarbaker*, MD, FACS, FRCS

Program in Peritoneal Surface Oncology, Washington Cancer Institute, Washington, DC, USA

Introduction

As surgical treatments for advanced epithelial ovarian cancer (EOC) evolved, data emerged suggesting that a reduction in the extent of residual disease by resection correlated directly with improved survival. Griffiths presented retrospective data that showed an inverse relationship between residual tumor size and survival [1]. Hoskins et al. supported this hypothesis be defining 3 groups of patients with residual disease, microscopic, vs. <2cm vs. >2cm cancer nodules. These authors reported that survival was inversely related to the volume of residual disease [2]. In a meta-analysis, Bristow and colleagues reported that survival was directly associated with residual disease [3]. Radical debulking of the pelvic structures became an accepted strategy for the surgical treatment of advanced EOC despite the fact that gross disease may be left behind in the abdomen, especially in the subphrenic and perisplenic regions.

This data suggesting a benefit from the debulking of as much tumor as possible resulted in hysterectomy and bilateral salpingo-oophorectomyas a standard procedure for all EOC. However, the requirement for routine resection of the uterus and cervix as part of an EOC cytoreduction has never been determined. The resection of the primary malignancy requires bilateral salpingo-oophorectomy but not a hysterectomy. The lymphatic drainage of the ovaries is not through the uterus and no lymph nodes exist within the uterus [4]. The rationale for routine hysterectomy as part of the surgical management of primary EOC may be called into question. Its resection in selected patients and the requirement for technologies to protect the resection site from recurrent disease will be discussed.

Tumor Cell Entrapment (TCE)

An understanding of TCE in cancer surgery is necessary to appreciate the role of a hysterectomy in the outcome of EOC patients. TCE helps explain how cancer cells are distributed around the

* Corresponding Author's Email: Paul.Sugarbaker@outlook.com.

In: Ovarian Cancer
Editors: Christos Iavazzo, Alexandros Fotiou and John Spiliotis
ISBN: 979-8-88697-633-5

abdomen and pelvis as peritoneal metastases following surgery for EOC. This hypothesis commences with the fact that cancer cells are released prior and also from surgical trauma at the time of resection of the primary ovarian malignancy. For ovarian cancer FIGO Stage 3, both sources of cancer cells should be expected. These cancer cells free within the peritoneal space after a hysterectomy and bilateral salpingo-oophorectomy may have one of two destinies. If they remain unattached or settle on a site from which they are not nourished, they will die. However, if they attach to a surface within the abdomen and pelvis, they have the opportunity to gain vascular supply. If this occurs, they are no longer free-floating cancer but will become a cancer implant.

An important part of the TCE theory is the concept of metastatic efficiency and inefficiency developed by Weiss [5]. Some surfaces are more conducive to cancer cell adherence and progression into an implant. Although cancer cells may themselves produce enzymes that degrade barriers to implantation, there may be circumstances that are especially favorable for cancer cells to adhere at a particular anatomic site. The peritoneum is definitely a first line of body defense if the abdominal and pelvic space is challenged by bacteria or fungus. It is also the first line of defense against the adherence of cancer cells [6]. Following a surgical procedure, there are anatomic sites which are at increased risk of cancer cell adherence. An irregular (not smooth) surface will be a site for cancer cells to be sequestered. Also, if there is blood and fibrinous clot as a result of recent trauma, cancer cells will be trapped within the fibrinous matrix set up by the normal mechanism of coagulation. This accounts for the repeated observation of EOC peritoneal metastases occurring within abdominal adhesions. To use the terminology of Weiss, a traumatized peritoneal surface will be more, "Metastatically efficient" than a smooth and intact, non-inflamed peritoneal surface [5].

Not only does the surgically traumatized abdominal or pelvic peritoneal surface attract cancer cells to adhere, but it will also promote their neovascularization. Initially, the adherent cancer cell may derive its nutrition from peritoneal fluid by diffusion; however, progression to an established implant requires the cancer cell to establish its own blood supply. Inflammation and wound repair at a site of surgical trauma provides the angiogenic factors that facilitate progression from an adherent cancer cell to an implanted cell [7].

Free intraperitoneal cancer cells will develop two different configurations as a result of postoperative TCE. If single cancer cells or minute cancer nodules adhere, implant, and grow, they will develop into isolated cancer nodules at a distance from the primary site. These discrete 3-dimensional masses are not usually spherical but rather have a discoid shape upon the peritoneal surface. The implant progresses in a radial direction and then by axial invasion, penetrating into the host tissue surface. These individual hemispherical or discoid peritoneal metastases arise from widely disseminated intraperitoneal cancer cells that are disseminated at low density on the peritoneal surface [8].

The second configuration for a peritoneal implant is present at anatomic sites that have a high density of free cancer cells and are traumatized by a surgical procedure with dissection along tissue planes. This type of TCE is a layering of cancer in and around the resection site. It occurs as a result of high-density cancer cell adherence at a site of prior surgical trauma within the fibrinous matrix. It presents itself over time as a sheet of cancer of variable thickness layered out to cover specific parts of the traumatized peritoneal surface [8].

Tumor Cell Entrapment Observed with Reoperative Surgery for Ovarian Cancer

This second TCE configuration is repeatedly observed at the time of a reoperative surgery for ovarian cancer. TCE occurs post-hysterectomy but not at the time of hysterectomy for the primary disease. Consider first the condition of the ureter in a hysterectomy operation. Direct contact of ovarian cancer at discrete sites may occur. This is usually at the mid-ureter. Ureteral obstruction may be observed in advanced disease from cancerous iliac lymph nodes or from the compression (rarely invasion) of the expanding ovarian primary tumor. Now in contrast, consider the reoperative setting. A near circumferential coating of the ureter by cancer occurs. Obstruction of the distal ureter is common and complete cytoreduction may require resection of the distal ureter and its reimplantation into the dome of the bladder [9]. Alternatively, a cross ureteroureterostomy may be indicated [10]. In a great majority of ovarian cancer reoperations, the distal half of the ureters requires ureterolysis. This involvement of the ureters is usually bilateral in the reoperative setting whereas it is only unilateral with hysterectomy and on the side of the primary tumor. The layering of cancer along the distal ureter is caused by TCE.

Another example of TCE by high-density seeding is observed at the base of the bladder. A dangerous dissection in the reoperative setting is the clearance of ovarian cancer from the surface of the bladder at the prior vesicouterine space. At the time of hysterectomy, the peritoneum of the vesicouterine space is resected along with the uterus to gain access to the anterior aspect of the vagina. This portion of the bladder is, almost always, clear of all cancer at the time of a hysterectomy. In contrast, at the time of reoperation, the base of the bladder is layered by cancer. Only by sacrifice of a layer of the bladder musculature is this anatomic site, previously peritonectomized, cleared of progressive disease. TCE is responsible for cancer progression on the bladder.

TCE provides an explanation of ovarian cancer progression that is documented at reoperation at three other anatomic sites. These are the abdominal incision, laparoscopy port sites and the vaginal cuff. None of these anatomic sites are invaded by ovarian cancer prior to the hysterectomy. Unfortunately, they are involved in a large percentage of patients at reoperation. The abdominal incision may be seeded by free cancer cells present in the abdominal and pelvic spaces. As the incision is closed by sutures, these cells are fixed at this anatomic site. The same mechanism for metastases at laparoscopy port sites is postulated. For the transected vagina, no ovarian cancer is present at the completion of hysterectomy. Yet, it is usually invaded by cancer at the time of reoperation and the apex of the vagina must undergo repeat resection. The mechanism for ovarian cancer progression at these three anatomic sites is TCE.

Documentation of Tumor Cell Entrapment after Hysterectomy at the Time of Cytoreductive Surgery

A quality improvement project at the Washington Cancer Institute accumulated data on EOC patients having surgery for recurrent EOC [11]. The study was designed to enumerate and characterize the anatomic sites of recurrence/progression of high-grade serous EOC. Twenty consecutive patients had a median age of 52 with a range of 24-73 years. The interval between hysterectomy and bilateral salpingo-oophorectomy and the cytoreductive surgery for recurrence was a median of 23 months with a range of 5-77 months. The mean interval was

26.85 months. The mean time for the reoperation using peritonectomies and visceral resections was 11 hours with a range of 5-15 hours. Median was 9.53 hours. The median peritoneal cancer index (PCI) was 15 with a range of 4 to 31 [12]. The median survival from the time of reoperation until death or current status was 34 months with a range of 4 to 123 months.

In these 20 patients, there were 23 different sites with biopsy-confirmed recurrent/ progressive disease documented at the time of reoperative cytoreductive surgery. The anatomic site with the highest percentage of disease was the right subphrenic space in 14 of 20 patients (70%). Two sites had the second most frequent incidence of disease. These were the greater omentum and rectosigmoid colon both with 13 patients (65%). Anatomic sites that should be free of disease at the completion of hysterectomy but were layered by recurrence of ovarian cancer was the prior abdominal incision (11 patients, 55%), visceral surface of the bladder (10 patients, 50%), distal left ureter (10 patients, 50%), vaginal cuff (10 patients, 50%), and distal right ureter (7 patients, 35%). Three patients required resection of a distal portion of the ureter at the ureterovesical junction, one on the left and two on the right. Eight patients required a rectosigmoid colon resection with colorectal anastomosis and a single patient required an abdomino-perineal resection. Two patients underwent total abdominal colectomy with end ileostomy. Four patients had resection of disease along the iliac vessels, aorta or vena cava. Identification of this recurrence/progression as lymph node metastases in these four patients was not possible because lymphatic tissue could not be identified in these specimens.

The explanation for a high incidence of recurrence/progression of EOC at 5 of these 23 anatomic sites is TCE. The prior abdominal incision, visceral surface of the bladder, distal left ureter, vaginal cuff and distal right ureter should be dissected clean of EOC by the hysterectomy. The layering of cancer at these 5 anatomic sites must have been caused by TCE. The hysterectomy must become implicated as a component of cancer recurrence. Surgery is a part of the natural history of EOC.

Current Recommendations for Surgery in Primary Epithelial Ovarian Cancer

Hysterectomy is an essential part of the complete cytoreduction of ovarian cancer if all visible disease within the abdomen and pelvis is resected. The cytoreductive surgery requires a midline abdominal incision that extends from xiphoid to pubic bone (Figure 1). The small bowel and its mesentery are inspected to determine if complete cytoreduction is possible. The peritonectomy of the right and, if necessary, the left hemidiaphragm is usually the initial resection (Figure 2). This is followed by greater and lesser omentectomy. If these resections are complete, hysterectomy and bilateral salpingo-oophorectomy are performed. Hysterectomy usually is performed with pelvic peritonectomy (Figure 3). Often, rectosigmoid colon resection is necessary. In this group of patients with advanced EOC, hysterectomy is an essential part of the complete cytoreduction.

Rule of Least Margins and Volumes

In other patients, a hysterectomy for primary EOC may do more harm than good. The dictum of Griffin, Hoskins, Bristow is that as much ovarian tumor as possible should be debulked by a hysterectomy and that this approach improves survival needs to be reexamined [1-3]. There may be a number of reasons not to perform a hysterectomy unless, of course, its resection is required to complete the removal of all visible disease within the abdomen and pelvis. First, the essential histopathologic information will come from the ovaries, Fallopian tubes and adjacent lymph nodes. The uterine tissues are not essential for the pathologic assessment of this disease [13]. A hysterectomy creates a space within the gynecoid pelvis for the small bowel to become entrapped, causing pain and sometimes small bowel obstruction. An unnecessary hysterectomy needlessly increases operative time, blood loos and possible damage to the bladder and ureters. A hysterectomy may diminish the beneficial effects of systemic chemotherapy because cancer is trapped within poorly vascularized scar tissue. Perhaps most importantly, a hysterectomy creates a metastatically efficient site for free cancer cells within the peritoneal space to adhere. By TCE, a hysterectomy encourages cancer progression/ recurrence along the vital structures within the pelvis including bladder, apex of vagina and distal ureters.

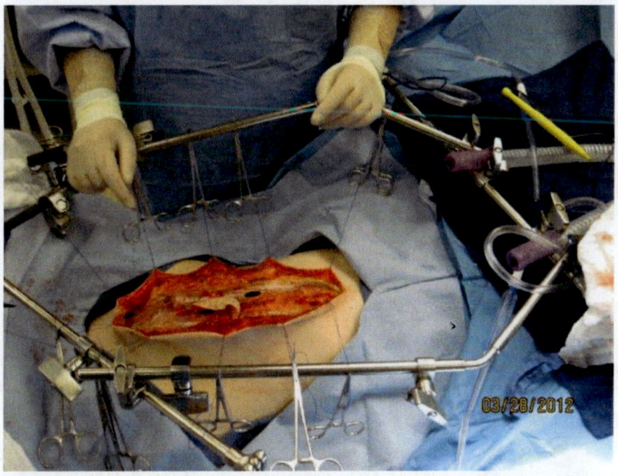

Figure 1. Midline abdominal incision for cytoreductive surgery. A long midline abdominal incision extends from the xiphoid to pubis. Skin traction sutures are used to elevate the sides of the abdominal wall. An old midline abdominal incision is removed and will be inspected by the pathologist for metastatic epithelial ovarian cancer.

The "rule of least margins and volumes" should be used to select patients with EOC for hysterectomy plus bilateral salpingo-oophorectomy versus bilateral salpingo-oophorectomy alone. By this rule, there is no rationale for a negative margin using a hysterectomy and pelvic peritonectomy in the pelvis in the presence of positive margins or gross disease on the undersurface of the diaphragms, on the spleen, or on the small bowel and its mesentery. In many patients, the decision to proceed with a complete cytoreduction will depend on the appearance of the small bowel and its mesentery. If viscera can be cleared of tumor, then by the rule of least margins and volumes, the other parts of the abdomen and pelvis should be cleared in an attempt to achieve a CC-0 score [12]. Certainly, removing all ovarian cancer from the pelvis and leaving disease behind gross disease in the abdomen does not honor the rule of least margins and volumes. In patients who have disease beneath the hemidiaphragm or on the small bowel and its mesentery that is not resected, the beneficial effects of systemic chemotherapy with paclitaxel and cisplatin are crucial to an optimal outcome. Getting started with systemic chemotherapy as soon as possible may be facilitated if a hysterectomy is not performed.

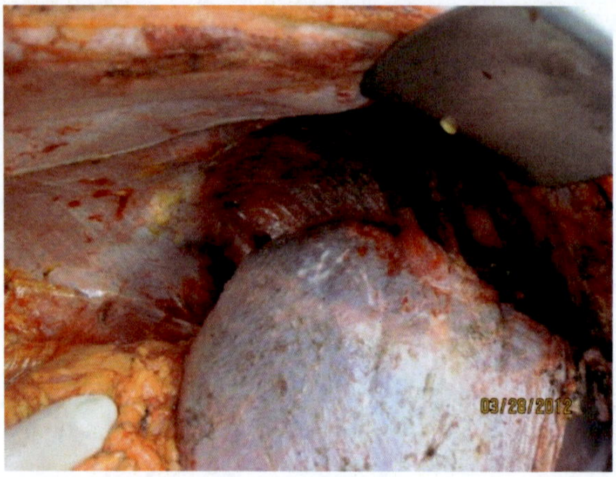

Figure 2. Right upper quadrant peritonectomy. The peritoneum from the undersurface of the right hemidiaphragm has been dissected using high-voltage electrosurgery from the diaphragm muscle. Cancer nodules that are too numerous to count can be seen layered out on the peritoneal surface of this peritonectomy specimen.

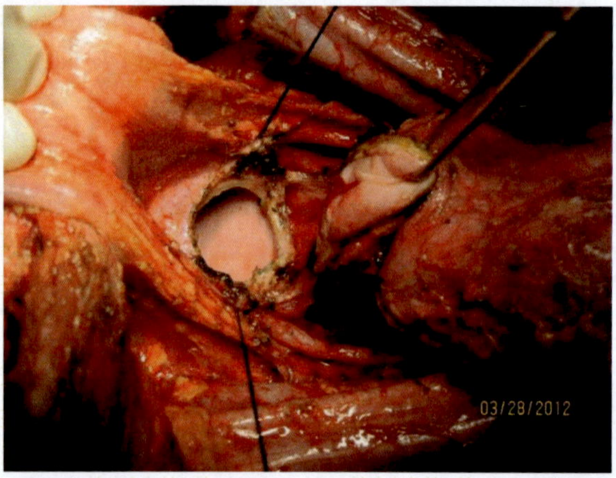

Figure 3. Total hysterectomy and pelvic peritonectomy. The uterus is removed along with a complete peritoneal stripping of the pelvis. After dividing the posterior aspect of the vagina, the peritoneum from the anterior aspect of the mid-rectum is also removed. This is a complete cul-de-sacectomy.

Perioperative Intraperitoneal Chemotherapy to Reduce Tumor Cell Entrapment

When a complete cytoreduction is performed, the number of free cancer cells to implant by TCE will be greatly reduced but not absent. To further reduce the number of free intraperitoneal cancer cells, hyperthermic intraperitoneal chemotherapy (HIPEC) is indicated (Figure 4) [14]. The benefit to the patient of having HIPEC has been demonstrated at the time of interval resection in a randomized controlled trial by Van Driel et al. and Spiliotis et al. [15, 16]. A safe and effective HIPEC regimen to use after complete cytoreductive surgery for recurrent ovarian cancer is presented in Table 1. This bidirectional (intravenous and intraperitoneal) regimen is pharmacologically designed for ovarian cancer. It has been used in over 400 patients after complete CRS and carries a low morbidity and zero mortality. It has not yet been subjected to the scrutiny of a randomized clinical trial.

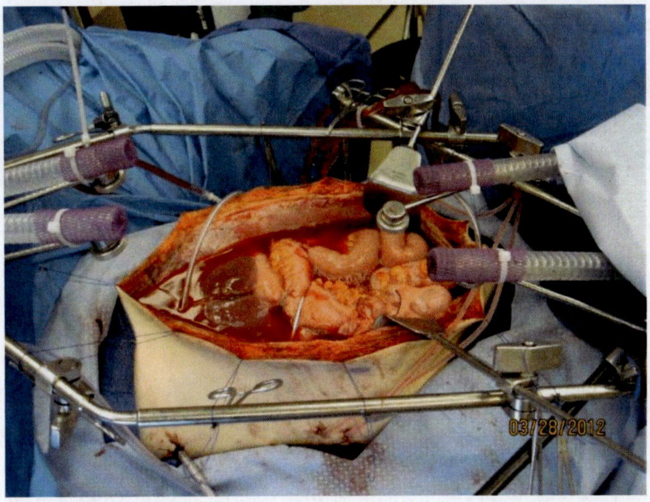

Figure 4. HIPEC is performed using the open technique. Two inflow catheters, four drainage catheters, and three temperature probes are positioned within the peritoneal space beneath the hemidiaphragms and within the pelvis. Four smoke suction tubes create a vapor barrier above the open abdomen. A standard chemotherapy regimen is used to provide a chemotherapy solution to bathe all of the structures within the abdomen and pelvis.

Perioperative Intraperitoneal Lavage Methodologies May Reduce Tumor Cell Entrapment

The number of free intraperitoneal EOC cells is at a maximum prior to the CRS. After resection of all visible disease, large volume saline can mechanically remove many of the free cancer cells. A process call extensive intraperitoneal lavage (EIPL) has been successful in gastric cancer patients [17]. Using a "limiting dilution method," one liter of physiologic saline at body temperature was instilled into the peritoneal space, extensively shaken and washed, and then completely aspirated. This lavage was repeated 10 times in a row. In a multicenter randomized trial of 88 peritoneal cytology positive gastric cancer patients, a statistically significant improvement in survival was reported ($p < 0.001$). The EIPL methodology combined with intraperitoneal cisplatin instillation for 1 hour was much more effective than intraperitoneal chemotherapy alone.

A second irrigation option to reduce the number of free cancer cells and possibly increase the cytotoxicity of HIPEC is the use of hydrogen peroxide (H_2O_2) [18]. "Oxidative stress" induced by a large volume of H_2O_2 irrigation has been associated with the disruption of cancer cells especially when combined with hyperthermia [19].

A third irrigation option to reduce the number of intraperitoneal cancer cells available to TCE is hyperthermic lavage with povidone-iodine solution. Lang-Lazdunski et al. reported positive results in a non-randomized study in patients with pleural mesothelioma [20]. They performed a brief (5 minute) lavage of the hemithoracic cavity with sterile water, and 10% povidone-iodine at 40-41°C. The lavage of the chest cavity was well tolerated, and the outcome were interpreted as favorable.

Table 1. Hyperthermic intraperitoneal chemotherapy (HIPEC) regimen pharmacologically designed to treat primary ovarian cancer following complete cytoreductive surgery (CRS)

CISPLATIN-BASED REGIMENS

Sugarbaker Regimen for Ovarian Cancer
Intraperitoneal chemotherapy
Add cisplatin to 2 L 1.5% dextrose peritoneal dialysis solution
Add doxorubicin to the same 2 L 1.5% peritoneal dialysis solution
Dose of cisplatin is 50 mg/m2 and doxorubicin is 15 mg/m2 for 90-minute HIPEC treatment
Intravenous Chemotherapy
Add ifosfamide 1300 mg/m2 to 1 L 0.9% sodium chloride. Begin continuous IV infusion over 90 minutes simultaneous with intraperitoneal chemotherapy
Add mesna disulfide 260 mg/m2 in 100 mL 0.9% sodium chloride to be given IV as a bolus 15 minutes prior to ifosfamide infusion
Add mesna disulfide 260 mg/m2 in 100 mL 0.9% sodium chloride to be given IV as a bolus 4 hours after ifosfamide infusion
Add mesna disulfide 260 mg/m2 in 100 mL 0.9% sodium chloride to be given IV as a bolus 8 hours after ifosfamide infusion

Tumor Cell Entrapment Following Hysterectomy, What Does It Cost?

When a hysterectomy is performed for the surgical treatment of FIGO 3 EOC to eliminate free tumor cells from the peritoneal space, the patient's prognosis is jeopardized. The rectosigmoid colon and rectum will be involved in a high percentage of patients. This results from the manipulation of this structure, and peritoneal trauma as a result of this manipulation, with a high concentration of cancer cells in the pelvis. Obstruction of the rectosigmoid colon from disease progression post-hysterectomy is not uncommon. Disease progression on the surface of the bladder at the site of the previous peritoneal resection to expose the vagina can result in unresectable disease associated with the base of the bladder at the time of a reoperative surgical procedure. It has created the need for total pelvic exenteration in some patients. Cancer layering as a result of TCE in and along the distal ureters is extremely dangerous for the patient's long-term survival. Manipulations and dissections required to secure the uterine artery leads to surgical trauma only millimeters away from the distal ureter. This surgical trauma causes a layering of cancer cells in and along the ureter which must be visualized in order to prevent injury at the time of the hysterectomy. Obstruction of the ureter from progressive ovarian cancer is not unusual and led to the need to resect distal ureter in 3 of our 20 patients [11]. A majority of our patients required extensive ureterolysis of scar and tumor from along the distal ureters. Finally, recurrence within the vaginal cuff is an obvious manifestation of TCE post-hysterectomy. At the time of hysterectomy, the apex of the vagina must be circumferentially excised. After this circumferential vaginal incision, the tissues are transiently free of cancer cells. However, sutures used to close the apex of the vagina can entrap tumor cells. Also, tumors cells by gravity will settle, adhere and then implant on the vaginal cuff. This led to a 50% incidence of recurrent disease on the vaginal cuff in our series of patients [11].

Data from Prior Surgical Score (PSS) Supports the Importance of Tumor Cell Entrapment (TCE)

In a previous publication, regarding reoperative surgery for EOC, our data showed that the most robust clinical factor controlling survival in the resection of recurrent EOC was the prior surgical score (PSS) [12, 21]. This phenomenon has also been described for appendiceal malignancy and colon cancer [22, 23]. The data suggests that extensive prior surgery creates surfaces that become infiltrated by cancer and make subsequent efforts, for reoperative surgery, difficult or impossible. The PSS provides survival data to demonstrate the clinical importance of TCE.

Comparisons of Initial versus Reoperative Surgery for Epithelial Ovarian Cancer

It is possible that the selection criteria for surgical interventions and the goals of these interventions may be different in the first surgery for EOC as compared to reoperative surgery. However, recent data from the DESKTOP III trial for reoperative surgery in EOC suggests that an improved outcome may be achieved with complete resection at the time of a reoperation [24]. The data seems to clearly indicate that patients who benefited from reoperative surgery were those who had a complete visible resection of their disease. This means that not only was the pelvis cleared of the malignant process but also the abdomen and the spaces beneath the hemidiaphragms were cleared of disease. Also, it has been recommended that complete resection should accompany the initial surgery in EOC patients. Certainly, TCE would be much reduced in both primary and reoperative surgery if complete visible resection of EOC occurred. Also, data to suggest that a chemotherapy washing with HIPEC which would destroy free cancer cells and eliminate TCE may be important in surgical treatment of both primary and recurrent disease [15, 16].

Conclusion

A hysterectomy is essential for the complete resection of advanced EOC. It is indicated as part of a complete abdominal and pelvic CRS because a hysterectomy is needed to complete the "modified posterior exenteration" [25]. However, from a TCE perspective, performing an ultraradical pelvic procedure but leaving gross disease within the abdomen, especially beneath the right or left hemidiaphragm, creates a "worst case scenario!" The modified posterior exenteration removes viscera and peritoneum from the pelvis. Gross disease in the abdomen and in the subphrenic spaces provides large numbers of cancer cells that move by gravity through the peritoneal space into the pelvis. The result is pelvic structures within the hysterectomy resection site layered by cancer cells. Clearing of the pelvis by modified posterior exenteration is indicated only if the remainder of the abdomen and pelvis is completely cytoreduced.

References

[1] Griffiths CT. Surgical resection of tumor bulk in the primary treatment of ovarian carcinoma. *Natl Cancer Inst Monogr,* 1975; 42:101-4.

[2] Hoskins WJ, Bundy BN, Thigpen JT, Omura GA. The influence of cytoreductive surgery on recurrence-free interval and survival in small-volume stage III epithelial ovarian cancer: A Gynecologic Oncology Group study. *Gynecol Oncol*, 1992; 47:159-66.

[3] Bristow RE, Tomacruz RS, Armstrong DK, Trimble EL, Montz FJ. Survival effect of maximal cytoreductive surgery for advanced ovarian carcinoma during the platinum era: A meta-analysis. *J Clin Oncol,* 2002; 20(5):1248-59.

[4] Eichner E, Bove ER. In vivo studies on the lymphatic drainage of the human ovary. *Obstet Gynecol,* 1954; 3(3):287-97.

[5] Weiss L. Mechanisms of metastatic patterns. (In) *Principles of Metastasis*. 1st Edition. Academic Press, 1985, pp. 200-56.

[6] Sugarbaker PH. Peritoneum as the first line of defense in carcinomatosis. *J Surg Oncol,* 2007; 95(2): 93-6.

[7] Sethna KS, Sugarbaker PH. New prospects for the control of peritoneal surface dissemination of gastric cancer using perioperative intraperitoneal chemotherapy. *Cancer Therapy,* 2004; 2:79-84.

[8] Sugarbaker PH. Update on the prevention of local recurrence and peritoneal metastases patients with colorectal cancer. *World J Gastroenterol*, 2014; 20(28):9286-91.

[9] Bristow RE, Lagasse LD. Cytoreductive surgery: Pelvis and radical oophorectomy. (In) Bristow RE, Karlan BY, Chi D (Eds). *Surgery for Ovarian Cancer*. Third Edition. CRC Press: New York, 2015, pp. 153-88.

[10] Sugarbaker PH, Gutman M, Verghese M. Transureteroureterostomy. An adjunct to the management of advanced primary and recurrent pelvic malignancy. *Int J Colorectal Dis*, 2003; 18(1):40-4.

[11] Sugarbaker PH. *Patterns of recurrence in women with ovarian cancer having hysterectomy for treatment of primary disease* (Submitted).

[12] Jacquet P, Sugarbaker PH. Current methodologies for clinical assessment of patients with peritoneal carcinomatosis. *J Exp Clin Cancer Res,* 1996; 15(1):49-58.

[13] Prat J, Olawaiye AB, Bermudez A, et al. Ovarian, Fallopian tube, and primary peritoneal carcinoma. AJCC Cancer Staging Manual, Eight Edition. In: Amin M.B., editor. *AJCC Cancer Staging Manual.* eighth ed. Springer; Switzerland: 2017. pp. 681-90.

[14] Sugarbaker PH, van der Speeten K. An overview of peritonectomy, visceral resection, and therapeutic laparoscopy for peritoneal surface malignancy. (In) Sugarbaker PH (Ed). *Cytoreductive Surgery and Perioperative Chemotherapy for Peritoneal Surface Malignancy. Textbook and Video Atlas*. 2nd Edition. Cine-Med Publishing: Woodbury, CT, 2017, pp. 17-46.

[15] Van Driel WJ, Koole SN, Sikorska K, Schagen van Leeuwen JH, Schreuder HWR, Hermans RHM, de Hingh IHJT, van der Velden J, Arts HJ, Massuger LFAG, Aalbers AGJ, Verwaal VJ, Kieffer JM, Van de Vijver KK, van Tinteren H, Aaronson NK, Sonke GS. Hyperthermic intraperitoneal chemotherapy in ovarian cancer. *N Engl J Med*, 2018; 378:230-40.

[16] Spiliotis J, Halkia E, Lianos E, Kalantzi N, Grivas A, Efstathiou E, Giassas S. Cytoreductive surgery and HIPEC in recurrent epithelial ovarian cancer: A prospective randomized phase III study. *Ann Surg Oncol*, 2015; 22(5):1570-5.

[17] Kuramoto M, Shimada S, Ikeshima S, Matsuo A, Yagi Y, Matsuda M, Yonemura Y, Baba H. Extensive intraoperative peritoneal lavage as a standard prophylactic strategy for peritoneal recurrence in patients with gastric carcinoma. *Ann Surg,* 2009; 250:242-6.

[18] Harrison LE, Tiesi G, Razavi R, Wang C-C. A phase I trial of thermal sensitization using induced oxidative stress in the context of HIPEC. *Ann Surg Oncol*, 2013; 20:1843-50.

[19] Lehmann K, Rickenbacher A, Jang J-H, Oberkofler CE, Vonlanthen R, von Boehmer L, Humar B, Graf R, Gertsch P, Clavien PA. New insight into hyperthermic intraperitoneal chemotherapy. Induction of

oxidative stress dramatically enhanced tumor killing in in vitro and in vivo models. *Ann Surg,* 2012; 256:730-8.

[20] Lang-Lazdunski L, Bille A, Belcher E, Cane P, Landau D, Steele J, Taylor H, Spicer J. Pleurectomy/ decortication hyperthermic pleural lavage with povidone-iodine followed by adjuvant chemotherapy in patients with malignant pleural mesothelioma. *J Thorac Oncol*, 2011; 6(10):1746-52.

[21] Look M, Chang D, Sugarbaker PH. Long-term results of cytoreductive surgery for advanced and recurrent epithelial ovarian cancers and papillary serous carcinoma of the peritoneum. *Int J Gynecol Cancer,* 2004; 14(1):35-41.

[22] Sugarbaker PH. Epithelial appendiceal neoplasms. *Cancer J,* 2009; 15:225-35.

[23] Paul BK, Ihemelandu C, Sugarbaker PH. Prior surgical score: An analysis of the prognostic significance of an initial nondefinitive surgical intervention in patients with peritoneal carcinomatosis of a colorectal origin undergoing cytoreductive surgery and perioperative intraperitoneal chemotherapy. *Dis Colon Rectum*, 2018; 61(3):347-54.

[24] Bommert M, Harter P, Heitz F, du Bois A. When should surgery be used for recurrent ovarian cancer? *Clin Oncol,* 2018; 30:493-7.

[25] Aletti GD, Podratz KC, Jones MB, Cliby WA. Role of rectosigmoidectomy and stripping of pelvic peritoneum in outcomes of patients with advanced ovarian cancer. *J Am Coll Surg,* 2006; 203:521-6.

Chapter 18

Surgical Management of Advanced Epithelial Ovarian Cancer

Fuat Demirkiran*, **MD, PhD**
and Ipek Betül Özçivit, MD, PhD
Department of Obstetrics and Gynecology, Division of Gynecologic Oncology,
Istanbul University-Cerrahpasa, Cerrahpasa Medical Faculty, Istanbul, Turkey

Introduction

Malignant ovarian tumors account for 3.6% of all women malignancies and 4.7% of all cancer-related deaths. More than 90% of patients with ovarian malignancies have an epithelial histology and high-grade serous ovarian carcinoma accounting for 70% of epithelial ovarian cancer. High-grade ovarian cancers are commonly seen in women of advanced age (>60 years) and have a poor prognosis with high mortality risk. A paradigm shift in the management of ovarian cancer was initiated by Joe V. Meigs in 1934, then continued by Thomas Griffiths in 1975. In the following years, cytotoxic modalities such as platinum in 1980s and taxanes in 1990s and finally targeting agents changed the treatment strategy. Currently, surgery is still an indispensable part of ovarian cancer management.

The Evolution of Debulking Surgery in Advanced Stage Ovarian Cancer

It is well known that surgery is the mainstay of ovarian cancer treatment since the 1930s. In 1934, Dr. Joe V. Meigs mentioned the importance of surgery in the management of ovarian cancer. He published a book entitled "Tumors of the Female Pelvic Organs", where he described his surgical approach to ovarian cancer. In his opinion, the fundamental treatment strategy for ovarian cancer should be operative and Dr. Meigs advocated to remove as much tumor as possible considering the condition of the patient [1, 2]. In the following years, he refined his technique by including exploration of peritoneum, diaphragm, liver, gallbladder, stomach, renal regions, spleen and intestinal tract for the detection of tumoral foci in addition

* Corresponding Author's Email: demirkiranfuat@gmail.com.

In: Ovarian Cancer
Editors: Christos Iavazzo, Alexandros Fotiou and John Spiliotis
ISBN: 979-8-88697-633-5

to hysterectomy and bilateral salpingo-oophorectomy. He suggested the resection of all tumoral masses, if possible. This approach formed the basis of debulking or cytoreductive surgery concept in ovarian cancer treatment [3].

In 1975, C. Thomas Griffiths from Boston, USA associated the primary debulking surgery with improved outcomes in ovarian cancer patients. He reported that the survival rate was inversely proportional to the size of the largest residual mass and the residual tumor size equal or less than 1.5 cm increased survival rate [4]. In his study, the effect of tumor resection on survival was studied in 102 patients with s stage II and III ovarian cancer. He reported that the histologic grade of the tumor and the postoperative size of the largest residual tumor mass were the most important factors for survival rate. In conclusion, he found that residual tumor size larger than 1.5 cm after cytoreductive surgery did not improve overall survival and it was necessary to remove all gross tumor for optimum benefit. After these studies, some authors evaluated the efficacy of debulking surgery in the management of advanced stage ovarian cancer. For example, at a GOG study published in 1992, Hoskins et al. reported that the size of residual tumor after cytoreduction is a prognostic factor besides age, grade of tumor and number of residual lesions [5]. One of the first meta-analysis addressing the role of cytoreductive surgery in ovarian cancer was published by Allen et. al in 1995. In this meta-analysis, authors evaluated the survival benefits of cytoreductive surgery in patients with 0, ≤2 cm and > 2 cm residual tumor. They reported that the cytoreduction to zero and ≤2 cm residual disease provided a clear advantage to survival compared to >2 cm residual disease [6].

Cytoreductive Surgery in Advanced Stage Ovarian Cancer

Today, it has been accepted that the standard treatment of advanced stage ovarian cancer is primary cytoreductive surgery with an abdominal open approach including a hysterectomy and bilateral salpingo-oophorectomy. In other words, the reduction of the tumor size or complete resection of the tumor is the first and the most important step in the treatment of advanced staged epithelial ovarian cancer. Briefly, the main steps of surgery in advanced stage ovarian cancer are as follows: hysterectomy, bilateral salpingo-oophorectomy, appendectomy, intragastric omentectomy and cytoreduction of all intra and retroperitoneal tumoral foci.

Every single study reported that there is a clear relationship between the residual tumor size or volume after cytoreductive surgery and the oncological outcomes in patients with advanced stage ovarian cancer. Actually, many authors consider that the biology of the tumor and the competency of the cytoreductive surgery are the two main factors affecting the treatment outcomes in ovarian cancer. The most effective residual tumor volume on oncological outcomes after cytoreductive surgery has been investigated in many study.

There are different cytoreductive surgery definitions in ovarian cancer management. While some authors use optimal and suboptimal cytoreduction (CR) terms, others use R and CC classifications in their studies. There is no consensus for the definition of optimal CR. Some authors or groups accept no gross or microscopic residual disease as optimal CR in ovarian cancer patients, while others accept ≤1 cm disease. The definition according to R calcification is as follows: R0: complete resection of all visible disease; R1: remaining ≤1 cm and R2: remaining >1 cm residual disease. At Cytoreduction score (CC score): CC-0: no residual disease after cytoreduction; CC-1: maximum residual tumor size <0.25 cm persisting after cytoreduction (but thought to be penetrable by intracavitary chemotherapy, may be accepted as complete cytoreduction); CC-2: residual tumor nodules 0,25- 2.5 cm; CC-3: residual tumor nodules >2.5 cm or a confluence of unresectable tumor at any site of abdomen or pelvis. CC-2 and CC-3 cytoreductions are accepted as suboptimal CR [7].

Cytoreduction which has an utmost positive effect on the oncological outcomes of advanced stage ovarian cancer is defined as optimal CR. Many studies evaluating the relation between residual tumor diameter and oncological outcomes following cytoreductive surgery have been published for more than 60 years. Unfortunately, the definition of optimal CR has varied over time and there is no consensus about its definition even today. Although optimal CR was accepted as ≤2 cm residual tumor size after cytoreductive surgery at first, the definition of optimal CR was altered to ≤ 1 cm residual disease a very long time ago. During the last several years, some considered the optimal CR as zero residual disease (no macroscopic residual disease) after cytoreduction and zero residual disease, which was also defined as complete or maximal CR.

One of the first studies evaluating the therapeutic efficacy of cytoreductive surgery was published in 1998 and in this prospective study, the goal was to remove all of the visible disease before platinum-based chemotherapy in patients with stage IIIC and IV epithelial ovarian cancer. Complete CR (removal all visible tumor) rate was 85.3% in 163 patients and the residual tumor diameter was 0.1- ≤1cm in 13.5% of cases. Authors reported that complete cytoreduction was associated with a median 62 months of survival and multivariate analysis showed that age, stage, histology, volume of ascites and complete cytoreduction independently influenced survival in advanced stage ovarian cancer [8]. In 1999, the survival impact of surgical cytoreduction in 84 patients with FIGO stage IV ovarian cancer was evaluated by Bristow et al. in terms of age at diagnosis, performance status, histologic subtype, tumor grade, Stage IV criteria, ascites volume, predominant peritoneal tumor pattern, surgical procedures performed, hepatic tumor residuum, extrahepatic tumor residuum and post-operative complication [9]. Optimal cytoreductive surgery was accepted as residual disease ≤1 cm in this study. Primary surgical cytoreduction was achieved optimally in 30% of the patients and the median survival time was 38.4 months in optimally cytoreduced group, compared to 10.3 months in sub-optimally cytoreduced group. The conclusion of this study was that optimal CR and performance of the patients were significant for survival in patients with stage IV ovarian cancer. In the meantime, authors reported that optimal CR achieved significant survival advantage even in patients with unresectable liver metastasis.

Optimal CR was defined as ≤2 cm residual disease in The Scottish Randomized Trial which was a prospective observational study in Ovarian Cancer (stage IIIC-IV) published in 2005. This study evaluated the relationship between progression-free survival (PFS) and residual tumor diameter, and presurgical tumor state [10]. The authors reported that the optimal debulking was associated with increased PFS mainly in patients with less extensive presurgical disease. One of the most important studies analyzing the overall survival (OS) in different residual tumor diameters was published in 2006 by Chi D.S and et al. [11]. This study which evaluated the results of 465 patients with IIIC ovarian cancer had aimed to determine the residual tumor diameter which increased OS the most. The patients were analyzed in five groups according to the residual tumor diameter following primary cytoreductive surgery. The median OS was 106, 66, 48, 33 and 34 months in patients with no macroscopic (R0), ≤ 0.5 cm, 0.6 -1 cm, 1-2 cm and >2 cm residual disease, respectively (see figure at: DOI: 10.1097/

01.OGX.0000253753.88243.F6). In this study, OS was found to be statistically significant between patients with no macroscopic residual disease, $\leq$ 1 cm residual disease and > 1cm residual disease, however not in other groups. With these findings, they concluded that removal of all visible disease (R0 CR) is associated with the longest OS time compared to other groups. Therefore, the aim in CR of advanced stage ovarian cancer should be complete CR (R0) and if it is not feasible, decreasing the residual disease below 1 cm in patients with IIIC ovarian cancer.

Another interesting study evaluating the effect of different residual tumor sizes on oncological outcomes after primary cytoreductive surgery in advanced ovarian cancer was published by du Bois A, et al. in 2009 [12]. In this trial, the authors analyzed the results of 3126 patients retrieved from 3 prospective randomized phase 3 studies (AGO-OVAR) published in 2003 and 2006. The patients with stage IIB – IV ovarian cancer were included in this study and 73% of them had serous histology. The study group was divided into 3 subgroups according to residual disease status: no visible residual disease (complete resection), 1-10 mm residual disease and >10 mm residual disease. After cytoreductive surgery, 33.5% of the patients had no residual disease, 31.2% of them had 1-10 mm residual disease and 35.3% of them had >10 mm residual disease. According to the multivariate analysis, it was found that age, ECOG score (2 vs 0-1), FIGO stage (IIIc-IV vs IIB-IIIB), grade (II-III vs I), histology (mucinous vs serous histology), residual disease (1-10 mm vs 0) (>10 mm vs 1-10 mm) and ascites (> 500 ml vs < 500 ml) affected PFS and OS. This study similar to many other studies detected a clear relationship between oncological outcomes and residual tumor size after cytoreductive surgery. The rate of recurrence was 9% in complete resection subgroup, 22% in 1-10 mm residual group and 34% in >10 mm residual group in 6 months. Surgical details were not clear at this study and median PFS and OS for the study group were 18 and 44 months in the entire group, respectively. Authors reported that the longest median survival was seen in the complete resection group. The median survival time according to the residual disease size was as follows: no residual disease (R0): 99 months, 1-10 mm residual disease: 36 months and >10mm residual disease: 29 months (see figure at: https://doi.org/10.1002/ cncr.24149). Finally, they concluded that cytoreductive surgery is the keystone for the treatment of ovarian cancer and the aim of primary cytoreductive surgery should be complete cytoreduction.

Similar results was reported in a retrospective study published in 2010 from Italy [13]. Authors evaluated the results of 259 patients who underwent an attempt of maximal primary cytoreductive surgery for advanced stage ovarian cancer. Surgery was completed with gastrointestinal resection (72% with colon resection, 5% with small bowel resection) in the 77% of patients. In this study, major complication rate was 15% and complete resection rate was 44%. This study reported that no residual disease was associated with best oncological outcomes too.

Zivanovic et al. evaluated the effect of primary CR on PFS and OS in 526 patients with ovarian cancer at FIGO stage IIIC [14]. In this study, the patients were investigated in three groups. Group 1 consisted of patients without visible or palpable upper abdominal disease (UAD) which is cephalad to greater omentum. Group 2 consisted of patients with minimal UAD (1 cm or less), and group 3 patients with bulky UAD (larger than 1 cm) at the time of exploration. The rate of no gross and 0.1- $\leq$1 cm residual disease was 49% and 34% in no UAD group, 6% and 61% in minimal UAD group and 9% and 33% in bulky UAD group, respectively. It was found that optimal CR ($\leq$ 1 cm residual disease) has significant benefit for PFS and OS in all groups. For example, optimal cytoreduction was associated with statistically significant improved median OS compared to >1 cm in patients with no UAD (80 months vs.

41 months, p = 0.001), minimal UAD (56 months vs. 26 months, p = 0.001) and bulky UAD (58 months vs. 38 months, p = 0.003), respectively. Also, authors reported that patients with upper abdominal disease who underwent optimal CR had a 28% decreased risk of relapse and 33% decreased risk of death compared to suboptimal cytoreduction. With these findings, they concluded that the appropriate management of ovarian cancer even in large volume disease should include maximal surgical effort to achieve oncological benefits.

A large-volume study published by Horowitz et al. in 2015 (GOG 182) evaluated the effects of primary surgical effort, disease burden and surgical complexity on oncological outcomes [15]. In total, 4312 ovarian cancer patients with FIGO stage III and IV were enrolled into this study and the outcomes of 2655 patients with no gross residual disease (complete surgical resection) (R0) and < 1 cm residual disease (minimal residual disease) after primary cytoreductive surgery were collected. The rate of R0 and MR disease were 23% and 68%, respectively. The cases were divided into 3 disease scores (DS) based on preoperative tumor burden (DS low, with pelvic and retroperitoneal spread; DS moderate, with additional spread to the abdomen but sparing the upper abdomen; or DS high, with the presence of upper abdominal disease affecting the diaphragm, spleen, liver or pancreas). Also, the oncological outcomes were evaluated according to a surgical complexity score (CS) calculated by a published scoring system, as follows: CS low (score 1 to 3), CS moderate (score 4 to 7), or CS high (score ≥ 8). The authors reported that the patients with MR disease had a significantly worse prognosis compared to R0 patients in terms of PFS (15 vs. 29 months) and OS (41 vs. 77 months). Also, the patients with high preoperative DS had significantly poorer survival outcomes (PFS and OS) compared to preoperative low disease burden in spite of complex surgery. For example, median OS was 86, 70 and 40 months in DS-low, DS-moderate and DS-high groups, respectively(p<0.01). Additionally, it was stated that there were statistically significant differences in PFS and OS among patients with different DS in the same residual tumor group. For example, in patients who achieved R0 disease, median OS was 83 months in DS-moderate/low group, compared to 50 months in DS-high group. There was a similar significant difference in MR disease group (median OS was 53 months DS-moderate/low group compared to 39 months in DS-high group. Another interesting result of this study was that median OS was 49, 49 and 44 months in CS low, moderate and high groups, respectively (p:191). Finally, they concluded that R0 CR was significantly associated with increased PFS and OS compared to MR disease. However, the initial disease burden remained a significant prognostic indicator despite R0 disease. Complex surgery did not seem to have an effect on survival when other confounding influences, like residual disease, were considered.

A review study involving 11,999 patients with stage III-IV ovarian cancer was published in 2016 by Chiva et al. and demonstrates the importance of cytoreductive surgery [16]. It includes more than 9,000 patients with serous histology(77%) and patients with stage IV disease (13% of whole group). The rate of zero (complete resection), 0.1-10 mm and >1 mm residual tumor size was 25%, 42% and 33% after primary debulking surgery. In the complete resection group, median DFS and OS were found as 30 and 70 months compared to 16 and 40 months in 0.1-10 mm residual disease group and 12 and 30 months in the >1 cm residual disease group. The subgroups of patients with residual disease of 0.1 to 0.5 cm reached a median survival of 53 months. With these findings, they reported that patients with 0.1-10 mm residual disease had 14 and 30 months inferior median DFS and OS compared to patients with complete resection. In the meantime, the patients with 0.1-10 mm residual disease had an advantage of

10 and 4 months in OS and DFS compared to patients with >1 cm residual disease. These differences were statistically significant.

Most of the patients analyzed in this study were in 0.1-10 mm residual disease group like in many other studies. The patients in this group had better oncological outcomes than patients in larger residual group, but worse than in complete resection group. In another study, Sorensen at al. analyzed 2092 patients with advanced stage (IIIB-IV) ovarian cancer who underwent primary cytoreductive surgery in Denmark during 2005-2017 [17]. The rates of complete cytoreduction were 47.3% and 38.4% in women with stage IIIB-IIIC and IV epithelial ovarian cancer, respectively. The longest OS time was found in complete cytoreduction group (median OS: 61 months in stage IIIB-IIIC and 43 months in stage IV) compared to those with ≤1 cm and >2 cm residual disease. Also, the patients with ≤1 cm residual disease had longer OS compared to those with > 2 cm residual disease (median OS:30 months and 20 months in stage IIIB-IIIC, respectively). Another interesting result of this study was that debulking surgery achieving complete cytoreduction had significantly increased OS compared to those with macroscopic residual disease. Additionally, it was found that the residual disease located in both upper and lower abdomen caused a significant decrease in OS compared with the residual disease located in the upper or lower abdomen only in patients with stage IIIB-IIIC disease. Finally, they concluded that complete and ≤1 cm residual tumor after cytoreduction had a positive impact on oncological results and if complete cytoreduction could be achieved, women with stage IV disease should be offered primary debulking.

All of these findings clarify the unquestionable therapeutic importance of aggressive debulking surgery in the management of advanced stage ovarian cancer (Tables 1 and 2).

Table 1. Rates of R0 and ≤1 cm residual disease in advanced stage ovarian cancer

Authors (Ref.no)	Year	n	R0 (%)	£ 1 cm (%)
Eisenkop [8]	1998	263	85.3	13.5
Bristow [9]	1999	84		30
Chi [11]	2006	465	15	15 (<0.5 cm)
				21 (0.5-1 cm)
Winter [18]	2007	1895	23	42
du Bois [12]	2009	3126	33.5	31.2
Zivanovic [14]	2010	526	18 (All patients)	42 (All patients)
			49 (No UAD)	34 (No UAD)
			6 (Minimal UAD)	61 (Minimal UAD)
			9 (Bulky UAD)	33 (Bulky UAD)
Peiretti [13]	2010	259	44	39
Rodriguez [19]	2013	2655	32.4	67.6
Horowitz [15]	2015	2655	32.4	67.6
Chiva [16]	2016	11999	25	42
Siesto [20]	2018	50	44	36
Sorensen [17]	2018	2092	47.3 (stage IIIB-IIIC)	
			38.4 (stage IV)	

UAD: Upper abdominal disease
PDS: primary debulking surgery
IDS: interval debulking surgery
NACT: neo-adjuvant chemotherapy

Debulking surgery for advanced stage ovarian cancer is an aggressive surgical attempt to obtain zero or minimal residual disease. There are a few studies demonstrating a relationship between surgical volume of center and OS [22-24]. This relationship may relate many factors such as achieving increased rate of R0 residual tumor based on high surgical competence and adequate ancillary medical support in high volume center. In a retrospective study published in 2019 by Nasioudis et al., the authors compared complete resection rate in stage III and IV ovarian cancer patients in different surgical volume centers [24]. The results of 8,894 patients which were obtained from The National Cancer Data Base were analyzed to identify the factors affecting the complete cytoreduction rate. It was found that stage, surgical complexity and hospital volume had an impact on the residual tumor volume. The rate of complete resection was concluded to be statistically significantly lower in low (<7 cases per year) and intermediate volume (7-17 cases per year) centers compared to high volume centers (>17 cases per year).

Table 2. Residual disease status and survival in advanced stage ovarian cancer

		Median Survival			
Authors (ref no.)	Year	R0	≤1 cm	≤2 cm	Bulky
Bristow [9]	1999		38.4		10.3
Chi [11]	2006	106	66 (£0.5 cm) 48 (0.6-1.0 cm)	33	34
Winter [18]	2007	71.9	42.4		35 (>1cm)
du Bois [12]	2009	99.1	36.2		29.6 (>1cm)
Zivanovic [14]	2009		80 (no UAD) 56 (minimal UAD) 58 (bulky UAD)		41 (no UAD) 26 (minimal UAD) 38 (bulky UAD)
Peiretti [13]	2010		61.3 (1-5mm) 42.4 (6-10mm)	35.3	42.6
Chi [21]	2012	78	50		36 (>1cm)
Rodriguez [19]	2013	54.6 (had UAP)	40.4 (had UAP)		
Horowitz [15]	2015	77	41		
Chiva [16]	2016	70	40		30 (>1cm)
Sorensen [17]	2018	60.8 (stage IIIB-IIIC) 43.4 (stage IV)	29.5 (stage IIIB-IIIC) 24.9 (stage IV)	27.8 (stage IIIB-IIIC) 17.2 (stage IV)	19.8 (stage IIIB-IIIC) 14.3 (stage IV)

UAD: Upper abdominal disease
UAP: Upper abdominal procedure

More than 50% of patients with advanced stage ovarian cancer present with peritoneal carcinomatosis. Paul H. Sugarbaker recommended to replace the term "Peritoneal Carcinomatosis" with the term "Peritoneal Metastasis" [25]. In his opinion, peritoneal carcinomatosis reminds one of a terminal condition, in contrast to peritoneal metastasis which may be a treatable condition. In the area of gynecologic oncology, the terminology of peritoneal carcinomatosis is used to define tumor spreading to parietal and visceral peritoneal surfaces (Figure 1).

Extra-pelvic peritoneal metastases are accepted as peritonitis carcinomatous in clinical practices, although tumoral implants in Douglas's pouch, pelvic peritoneum and sigmoid mesocolon are included in the terminology of peritonitis carcinomatous. It is not easy to assess the tumoral burden of patients at the time of diagnosis and initial perioperative evaluation (Figure 1-2). For this purpose, peritoneal cancer index (PCI) may be used to evaluate the tumoral burden of patients. In some studies, authors investigated the extent of intra-peritoneal tumor burden by using PCI in colorectal and gastric cancers [26]. In this index, peritoneal cavity was divided into 13 regions including parietal and visceral peritoneal surfaces. Also, the size of the largest tumoral mass in each region was used for calculating PCI. PCI with a maximum score of 39 may be accepted as an objective assessment method for tumoral burden.

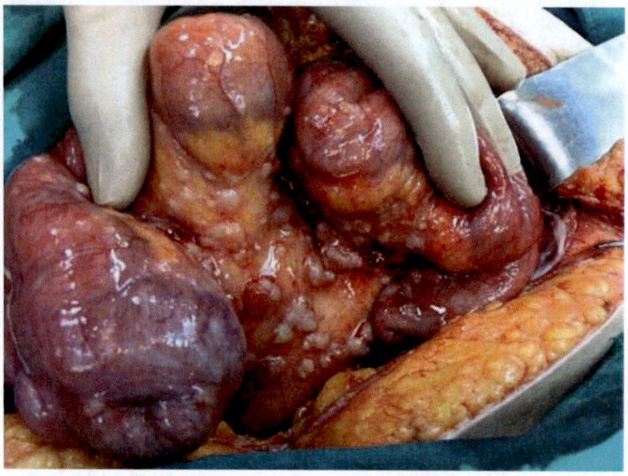

Figure 1. Peritonitis carcinomatosis, involvement small bowel mesentery.

A prospective cohort study included 96 patients with serous epithelial ovarian cancer at stage IIIB-IVA investigated the relationship between PCI and complete CR (R0) rate with using cut-off value of 13 [27]. R0 disease was achieved in 78.6% of patients with PCI score of ≤13. The median DFS of patients with PCI ≤13 was 16.4 months vs. 5.6 months of patients with PCI >13. The median OS of patients with PCI ≤13 was 22.2 months compared to 17.9 months of patients with PCI score >13 ($p<0.01$). They concluded that PCI score was a reliable tool to assess the extent of disease or tumor burden and there was a significant relationship between tumor burden and oncological outcomes. Another study published in 2019 by Uzan et al. focused on evaluating whether there is any impact of peritoneal carcinomatosis on PFS in patients with advanced stage ovarian cancer after complete cytoreductive surgery [28]. The authors found that the initial tumor burden didn't affect the PFS after complete cytoreductive surgery, but only the involvement of right mesoscopic areas was found to be associated with decreased PFS. In contrast, a GOG study reported that there was a significant relation between preoperative tumor burden and survival outcomes (PFS and OS) in patients with zero and < 1 cm residual tumor group after primary cytoreductive surgery [15]. Although it seems reasonable, the impact of tumoral burden on prognosis is still a controversial topic.

Upper Abdominal Surgery

Including GOG, lots of societies accept the optimal cytoreduction as achieving ≤ 1 cm residual disease after cytoreductive surgery. However, many studies have reported that complete CR (R0) provides nearly more than 30 months of survival advantage compared to ≤ 1 cm residual disease. Therefore, the optimal cytoreduction has recently been defined as achieving R0 disease (complete CR) after cytoreductive surgery in patients with advanced stage ovarian cancer. In other words, optimal cytoreductive surgery should be perceived as complete cytoreductive surgery according to many authors.

For this purpose, the surgery of advanced ovarian cancer should cover extragenital surgical procedures such as regional peritonectomy, gastrointestinal resection, splenectomy and hepatectomy with the goal of complete removal of macroscopic tumor (Figures 2, 3).

In other words, patients especially with upper abdominal disease need ultraradical/ extensive surgery to reach complete cytoreduction. In recent years, many surgeons have intended to increase their surgical complexity to achieve compete cytoreduction, after the demonstration of a clear and long-term survival benefit of complete resection.

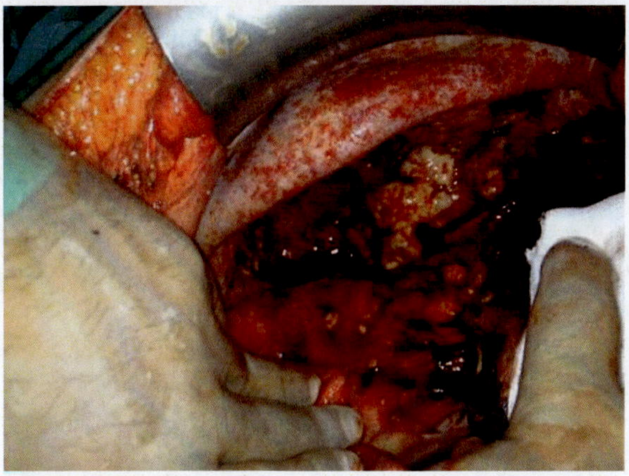

Figure 2. Metastasis to right diaphragm.

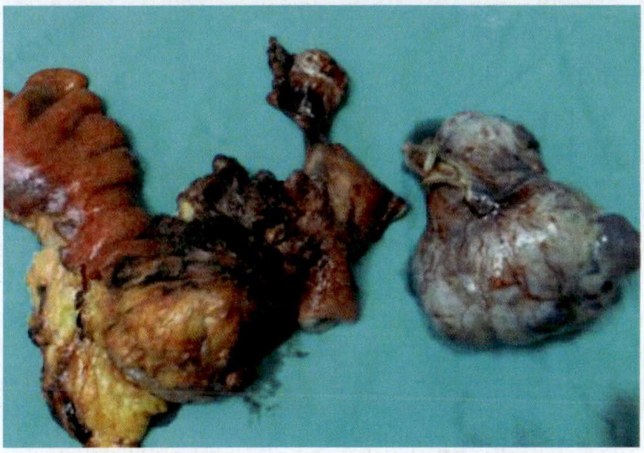

Figure 3. Recto-sigmoid resection in advanced stage ovarian cancer.

The extent of complex surgical efforts for achieving R0 disease clearly increases the rate of diaphragm stripping, gastrointestinal resection, splenectomy, partial hepatectomy and creation of ostomy. All surgical procedures are associated with an increased risk of adverse events. A study from France addressed the extent of the surgical complexity in patients who underwent maximal CR for advanced stage (IIIC-IV) ovarian cancer. In this group, small bowel, large bowel and multiple bowel resection rates were 10%, 38% and 12%, respectively. Also, 47%, 10% and 3% of patients had diaphragm stripping (right-left), splenectomy and partial hepatic resection [29].

The main problem is to predict who will benefit from ultraradical extensive surgery including the upper abdomen. It is not clear whether the patients in whom R0 disease is not achieved will benefit from this type of surgery which has increased risk of morbidity and mortality. A study published in 2016 reported that in patients with postoperative residual tumor, extensive surgery including bowel resection did not provide advantage on PFS an OS besides increasing morbidity rate [30]. Rodriguez et al. examined the upper abdominal procedures in epithelial ovarian cancer in patients enrolled in GOG 182 trial [19]. Among four hundred and eighty patients who had upper abdominal surgeries, the rate of diaphragm, liver and porta hepatis surgery were 13%, 4% and 0.2%, respectively. Also 4% and 0.5% of patients underwent splenectomy and pancreatectomy. The OS was significantly higher only when complete cytoreduction was achieved. They concluded that extensive upper abdominal procedures should only be performed for whom complete resection could be achieved. Also, some other studies have made similar suggestions [13].

The morbidity, mortality and risk-benefit ratio should be discussed in detail with the patients who are candidates for this complex surgery. The main dilemma for the surgeon is to increase the rate of adverse events while trying to increase the rate of R0 disease. Unfortunately, many studies evaluating the efficacy of extensive upper abdominal surgery had not reported sufficient data regarding the adverse events [29]. However, some centers published successful oncological outcomes with ultraradical extensive surgeries without a notable increase in morbidity [1, 19, 21]. A study published from US showed that the rate of complex surgery increased and this kind of radical surgery could be performed successfully in high volume hospitals with acceptable complication rates [1, 31].

It is known that aggressive surgery is associated with extended recovery time due to probable complications. The extent of the surgery may affect the quality-of-life parameters such as acceptance of ostomy, maintaining normal activities, continuing employment, confinement to bed, confinement to wheelchair, enjoyment of life and consuming regular diet. In a meta-analysis about the quality of life following ovarian cancer surgery, the quality of life of patients who underwent primary debulking surgery was reported similar to patients who had neoadjuvant chemotherapy except ultra-radical surgery [32]. Quality of life outcomes matters to the patients, therefore all patients with advanced ovarian cancer should be informed about the ultraradical surgery and its effect on the quality of life before the procedure.

There are many factors affecting the success of treatment in patients with advanced ovarian cancer. Only one of them is surgical quality or achieving optimal CR. Optimal CR is based on three basic factors, as follows: 1. The extent of disease, 2. The physical and medical features of the patient, 3. The skill of the surgeon and surgical equipment. Another main factor affecting the treatment success is intrinsic tumor biology and related factors such as tumor burden and sensitivity to cytotoxic therapy.

Optimization of preoperative patient selection is necessary for achieving optimal survival time. There is a group of patients having advanced stage ovarian cancer but not suitable for primary cytoreduction. Those patients are ill patients with highly advanced age and overwhelming disease burden. Therefore, it is an important matter to determine the appropriate patients for upfront debulking. Selection criteria should distinguish patients with low tumor load and high chance of complete cytoreduction. Neoadjuvant chemotherapy is an alternative treatment option for patients who are not suitable for primary cytoreduction.

Conclusion

Surgical treatment called cytoreductive surgery is the first step of ovarian management.

Standard surgical treatment of advanced stage ovarian cancer includes removing all of the tumor foci localized both intra- and retroperitoneum with hysterectomy and bilateral salpingo-oophorectomy.

The term of optimal cytoreduction has been defined as the most beneficial cytoreduction for oncological outcomes.

The accepted definition of optimal cytoreduction is achieving largest tumor diameter of 1 cm or less (≤1 cm). However, zero residual disease (R0) has more than median 25 months survival advantage compared to residual disease ≤1 cm.

It makes sense to define optimal cytoreduction as R0. The surgeon should intend to remove all of the macroscopic tumor fuci (R0 cytoreduction).

Zero residual disease (microscopic residual disease) obtained after cytoreduction increases median overall survival above 90 months.

Besides the quality of cytoreductive surgery, the initial tumor burden may affect oncological outcomes.

The balance between benefit and adverse events should be considered in patients who will have ultraradical extensive surgery. This type of surgery should be applied to the patients in whom complete cytoreduction (R0) can be achieved.

The patients with advanced stage disease who are not foreseen to be optimally cytoreduced (≤ 1 cm residual disease) should be managed with neoadjuvant chemotherapy.

References

[1] Schorge JO, Bregar AJ, Durfee J, Berkowitz RS. Meigs to modern times: the evolution of debulking surgery in advanced ovarian cancer. *Gynecologic oncology.* 2018;149(3):447-54.

[2] Meigs JV. *Tumors of the female pelvic organs: Macmillan;* 1934.

[3] MEIGS JV. The surgical treatment of cancer of the ovary. *Clinical obstetrics and gynecology.* 1961;4(3):846-54.

[4] Griffiths CT, editor Surgical Resection of Tumor Bulk in the Primary Treatment of Ovarian Carcinoma'C. Thomas Griffiths 2 METHODS SUMMARY—The effect of tumor bulk resection on survival was studied in 102 patients with stages II and III ovarian cancer. *Symposium on Ovarian Carcinoma* [held at Reston, Virginia, November 15 and 16, 1974; 1975: US Department of Health, Education, and Welfare, Public Health Service.

[5] Hoskins WJ, Bundy BN, Thigpen JT, Omura GA. The influence of cytoreductive surgery on recurrence-free interval and survival in small-volume stage III epithelial ovarian cancer: a Gynecologic Oncology Group study. *Gynecologic oncology.* 1992;47(2):159-66.

[6] Allen D, Heintz A, Touw F. A meta-analysis of residual disease and survival in stage III and IV carcinoma of the ovary. *European journal of gynaecological oncology.* 1995;16(5):349-56.

[7] Sugarbaker PH. Successful management of microscopic residual disease in large bowel cancer. *Cancer chemotherapy and pharmacology.* 1999;43(1):S15-S25.

[8] Eisenkop SM, Friedman RL, Wang H-J. Complete cytoreductive surgery is feasible and maximizes survival in patients with advanced epithelial ovarian cancer: a prospective study. *Gynecologic oncology.* 1998;69(2):103-8.

[9] Bristow RE, Montz FJ, Lagasse LD, Leuchter RS, Karlan BY. Survival impact of surgical cytoreduction in stage IV epithelial ovarian cancer. *Gynecologic oncology.* 1999;72(3):278-87.

[10] Crawford SC, Vasey PA, Paul J, Hay A, Davis JA, Kaye SB. Does aggressive surgery only benefit patients with less advanced ovarian cancer? Results from an international comparison within the SCOTROC-1 Trial. *Journal of clinical oncology.* 2005;23(34):8802-11.

[11] Chi D, Eisenhauer E, Lang J, Huh J, Haddad L, Abu-Rustum N, et al. What is the optimal goal of primary cytoreductive surgery for bulky stage IIIC epithelial ovarian carcinoma (EOC)? *Gynecologic oncology.* 2006;103(2):559-64.

[12] Du Bois A, Reuss A, Pujade-Lauraine E, Harter P, Ray-Coquard I, Pfisterer J. Role of surgical outcome as prognostic factor in advanced epithelial ovarian cancer: a combined exploratory analysis of 3

prospectively randomized phase 3 multicenter trials: by the Arbeitsgemeinschaft Gynaekologische Onkologie Studiengruppe Ovarialkarzinom (AGO-OVAR) and the Groupe d'Investigateurs Nationaux Pour les Etudes des Cancers de l'Ovaire (GINECO). *Cancer.* 2009;115(6):1234-44.

[13] Peiretti M, Zanagnolo V, Aletti GD, Bocciolone L, Colombo N, Landoni F, et al. Role of maximal primary cytoreductive surgery in patients with advanced epithelial ovarian and tubal cancer: surgical and oncological outcomes. Single institution experience. *Gynecologic oncology.* 2010;119(2):259-64.

[14] Zivanovic O, Sima CS, Iasonos A, Hoskins WJ, Pingle PR, Leitao Jr MM, et al. The effect of primary cytoreduction on outcomes of patients with FIGO stage IIIC ovarian cancer stratified by the initial tumor burden in the upper abdomen cephalad to the greater omentum. *Gynecologic oncology.* 2010;116(3):351-7.

[15] Horowitz NS, Miller A, Bunja Rungruang SDR, Rodriguez N, Bookman MA, Hamilton CA, et al. Does aggressive surgery improve outcomes? Interaction between preoperative disease burden and complex surgery in patients with advanced-stage ovarian cancer: an analysis of GOG 182. *Journal of Clinical Oncology.* 2015;33(8):937.

[16] Chiva LM, Castellanos T, Alonso S, Gonzalez-Martin A. Minimal macroscopic residual disease (0.1–1 cm). Is it still a surgical goal in advanced ovarian cancer? *International Journal of Gynecologic Cancer.* 2016;26(5).

[17] Sørensen SM, Schnack TH, Høgdall C. Impact of residual disease on overall survival in women with Federation of Gynecology and Obstetrics stage IIIB-IIIC vs stage IV epithelial ovarian cancer after primary surgery. *Acta obstetricia et gynecologica Scandinavica.* 2019;98(1):34-43.

[18] Winter III WE, Maxwell GL, Tian C, Carlson JW, Ozols RF, Rose PG, et al. Prognostic factors for stage III epithelial ovarian cancer: a Gynecologic Oncology Group Study. *Journal of Clinical Oncology.* 2007;25(24):3621-7.

[19] Rodriguez N, Miller A, Richard SD, Rungruang B, Hamilton CA, Bookman MA, et al. Upper abdominal procedures in advanced stage ovarian or primary peritoneal carcinoma patients with minimal or no gross residual disease: an analysis of Gynecologic Oncology Group (GOG) 182. *Gynecologic oncology.* 2013;130(3):487-92.

[20] Siesto GC, Raffaele; Romano, Fabrizio; Vitobello, Domenico. Primary Debulking Surgery Versus Neoadjuvant Chemotherapy in Advanced Epithelial Ovarian Cancer. *American Journal of Clinical Oncology.* 2018;41:280-5.

[21] Chi DS, Musa F, Dao F, Zivanovic O, Sonoda Y, Leitao MM, et al. An analysis of patients with bulky advanced stage ovarian, tubal, and peritoneal carcinoma treated with primary debulking surgery (PDS) during an identical time period as the randomized EORTC-NCIC trial of PDS vs neoadjuvant chemotherapy (NACT). *Gynecologic oncology.* 2012;124(1):10-4.

[22] Feng L-y, Liao S-b, Li L. Preoperative serum levels of HE4 and CA125 predict primary optimal cytoreduction in advanced epithelial ovarian cancer: a preliminary model study. *Journal of ovarian research.* 2020;13(1):1-8.

[23] Rosen B, Laframboise S, Ferguson S, Dodge J, Bernardini M, Murphy J, et al. The impacts of neoadjuvant chemotherapy and of debulking surgery on survival from advanced ovarian cancer. *Gynecologic oncology.* 2014;134(3):462-7.

[24] Nasioudis D, Kahn R, Chapman-Davis E, Frey MK, Caputo TA, Witkin SS, et al. Impact of hospital surgical volume on complete gross resection (CGR) rates following primary debulking surgery for advanced stage epithelial ovarian carcinoma. *Gynecologic oncology.* 2019;154(2):401-4.

[25] Sugarbaker PH. Pharmacology of chemotherapy treatments for peritoneal metastases: optimizing and augmenting HIPEC. *Pleura and peritoneum.* 2017;2(2):43-5.

[26] Jacquet P, Sugarbaker PH. Clinical research methodologies in diagnosis and staging of patients with peritoneal carcinomatosis. *Peritoneal carcinomatosis: principles of management.* 1996:359-74.

[27] Elzarkaa AA, Shaalan W, Elemam D, Mansour H, Melis M, Malik E, et al. Peritoneal cancer index as a predictor of survival in advanced stage serous epithelial ovarian cancer: a prospective study. *Journal of gynecologic oncology.* 2018;29(4).

[28] Uzan J, Bonsang-Kitzis H, Rossi L, Rance B, Bats A-S, Gosset M, et al. Prognostic impact of initial tumor load and intraperitoneal disease dissemination patterns in patients with advanced ovarian cancer

undergoing complete cytoreductive surgery. *European Journal of Surgical Oncology.* 2019;45(9): 1619-24.

[29] Luyckx M, Leblanc E, Filleron T, Morice P, Darai E, Classe J-M, et al. Maximal cytoreduction in patients with FIGO stage IIIC to stage IV ovarian, fallopian, and peritoneal cancer in day-to-day practice: a Retrospective French Multicentric Study. *International Journal of Gynecologic Cancer.* 2012;22(8).

[30] Oseledchyk A, Hunold LE, Mallmann MR, Domröse CM, Abramian A, Debald M, et al. Impact of extended primary surgery on suboptimally operable patients with advanced ovarian cancer. *International Journal of Gynecologic Cancer.* 2016;26(5).

[31] Fagotti A, Fanfani F, Ludovisi M, Voi RL, Bifulco G, Testa AC, et al. Role of laparoscopy to assess the chance of optimal cytoreductive surgery in advanced ovarian cancer: a pilot study. *Gynecologic oncology.* 2005;96(3):729-35.

[32] Kumar S, Long J, Kehoe S, Sundar S, Cummins C. Quality of life outcomes following surgery for advanced ovarian cancer: a systematic review and meta-analysis. *International Journal of Gynecologic Cancer.* 2019;29(8).

Chapter 19

Primary Versus Interval Debulking Surgery in Ovarian Cancer Patients

Yusuf Yildirim*, **MD, PhD**
and Volkan Karatasli, MD, PhD
OncoSurgery Private Clinic, Tepekule Congress Center, Bayrakli, Izmir, Turkey

Introduction

Treatment of advanced ovarian cancer is a combination of surgery and chemotherapy. Surgery performed with maximum effort without residual tumor in primary debulking surgery (PDS) contributes to prognosis. However, it has been reported that preoperative systemic chemotherapy (neoadjuvant chemotherapy-NACT) can provide as much survival as PDS for frail patients whose medical condition is not suitable for surgery. In recent randomized controlled trials, patients who received NACT and underwent interval debulking surgery (IDS) were compared with patients who underwent PDS, but conflicting results were obtained. Although it has been reported that NACT reduces postoperative morbidity, the information regarding its non-inferiority for survival is uncertain. Opinions differ about which patient will benefit more from PDS and which patient from NACT. The methods used in the initial clinical evaluation, the scoring systems to predict maximal cytoreduction, the regimens used in chemotherapy, the number of chemotherapy cycles, the time until IDS, management in non-serous histological types and platinum refractory disease have not been clarified. Due to the heterogeneity of the studies, generalizations could not be made to all patients with advanced ovarian cancer. The aim of this chapter was to evaluate studies involving advanced ovarian cancer patients treated with PDS and IDS in terms of morbidity, mortality, and survival.

* * *

Ovarian cancer is one of the most common gynecological malignancies leading to death [1]. Due to the lack of an effective screening test to detect it at an early stage and the occurrence of late symptoms, patients are usually in the advanced stage (Federation of International

---

* Corresponding Author's Email: dr.yusufyildirim2@yahoo.com.tr.

In: Ovarian Cancer
Editors: Christos Iavazzo, Alexandros Fotiou and John Spiliotis
ISBN: 979-8-88697-633-5

Gynaecologists and Obstetricians (FIGO) stage 3-4) at the time of diagnosis [2]. The prognosis is poor in advanced stage patients and the 5-year survival rate has been reported to be about 30% [3]. Standard treatment in advanced epithelial ovarian cancer is primary debulking surgery (PDS) followed by chemotherapy [4]. However, surgery may not always be performed in patients diagnosed at an older age due to medical comorbidities and poor performance status. The aim of surgery is to eliminate the residual tumor volume, known as complete resection, which is known as the strongest prognostic factor, by providing maximal cytoreduction [3]. A residual tumor <1 cm is defined as optimal surgery, while a residual tumor >1cm is called suboptimal surgery, and no macroscopic residue is called complete or R0 resection (Figure 1). It is known that patients undergoing suboptimal surgery have a survival disadvantage [3].

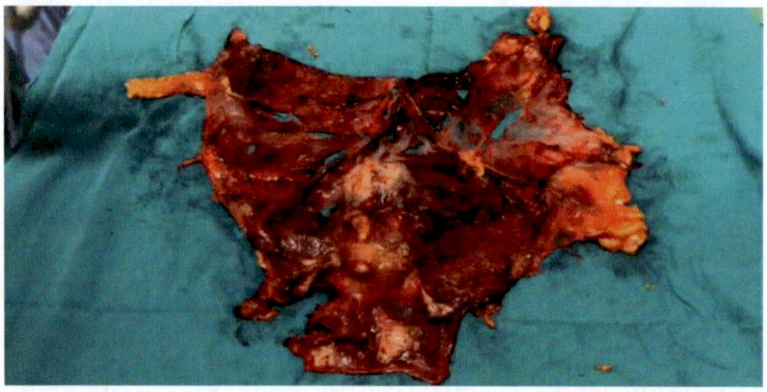

Figure 1. Macroscopic view of the specimen removed during cytoreductive surgery for advanced ovarian cancer.

Therefore, neoadjuvant chemotherapy (NACT) as chemotherapy before primary surgical treatment has been suggested as an option in frail patients with high tumor burden and in whom optimal surgery cannot be performed [5]. It is thought that interval debulking surgery (IDS) applied to patients after 3 or 4 cycles of chemotherapy may be beneficial. In 1995, van der Burg et al. found that patients who could not undergo optimal surgery and who underwent IDS after chemotherapy had better survival rates than patients who received only chemotherapy [6]. After these studies, the European Organization for Research and Treatment of Cancer (EORTC) 55971 study was initiated as the first randomized controlled trial (RCT) that NACT and IDS could provide an alternative for patients who could not undergo PDS [5]. The results in the EORTC and the second RCT (Chemotherapy or Upfront Surgery (CHORUS) study), suggested that NACT could be an alternative to PDS for advanced ovarian cancer patients, since the survival for NACT was non-inferior compared to PDS [7]. With the findings that NACT increases optimal cytoreduction rates and improves quality of life by reducing perioperative outcomes and adverse events, it has been suggested that NACT can replace PDS in advanced epithelial ovarian cancer. However, two published RCTs were criticized for their shorter survival times compared to previous studies, and it was emphasized that a generalization cannot be made to all advanced ovarian cancer patients but PDS was still the primary treatment option [8]. Although NACT has traditionally been applied to older patients with comorbidities, poor performance, and a diagnosis at an advanced stage, the fact that the survival was similar to PDS in the NACT group led to the opinion that NACT may be the primary treatment option in advanced stage ovarian cancer patients.. Therefore, other RCTs were initiated [2]. However, conflicting results were obtained in terms of survival in the Japan Clinical Oncology Group (JCOG) 0602 trial and Surgical Complications Related to Primary or Interval Debulking in

Ovarian Neoplasm (SCORPION) trial published after two RCTs [9, 10]. While NACT and PDS had similar survival in the SCORPION trial, non-inferiority could not be demonstrated for NACT in the JCOG0602 trial.

Randomized Controlled Trials

EORTC 55971 Trial

It was initiated as a multicenter non-inferiority RCT in 59 centers (Argentina, Austria, Belgium, Canada, Ireland, Italy, Netherlands, Norway, Portugal, Spain, Sweden, the United Kingdom) [5]. A total of 718 stage 3C and 4 epithelial ovarian/fallopian tube/peritoneal cancer patients were randomized into two groups, one NACT and IDS group, and the other group PDS and adjuvant chemotherapy. 48 patients from Argentina were excluded from the study due to authorization irregularities after randomization, and 670 patients were examined. As the experimental group, patients with an extra-pelvic tumor greater than 2 cm and treated with IDS after 3 cycles of platinum-based chemotherapy and at least 3 cycles of adjuvant chemotherapy were chosen. The patients who underwent PDS and received at least 6 cycles of adjuvant chemotherapy were included in the study as the control group. Patients who could not achieve optimal cytoreduction in PDS underwent IDS in the absence of progression after 3 cycles of chemotherapy, and this group was also analyzed within the PDS group. All operations were performed by gynecologist oncologists. IDS was applied to 88% of patients who received NACT. Adjuvant chemotherapy was administered in 88.4% of the PDS group. Metastatic tumor size was >5 cm in 74.5% of the patients, and >10 cm in 61.6%. Residual tumor was ≤1 cm in 41.6% of the patients in the PDS group and in 80.6% of the patients in the NACT group. Complete cytoreduction was performed in 19.4% in PDS and 51.2% in IDS. The risk of bleeding was lower in NACT. Median overall survival (OS) was 29 months in NACT and 30 months in PDS. Progression-free survival (PFS) was also similar in both groups (12 months). When subgroup analysis was performed, PDS provided better OS in the group of patients with a preoperative extra-pelvic tumor smaller than 5 cm. In addition, when FIGO stage was examined as a subgroup, it was determined that NACT provided a survival advantage in Stage 4 patients. There was no difference between the groups in terms of quality of life.

EORTC received a lot of attention as it was the first RCT, but it has also been criticized for various reasons. It was emphasized that the median OS and PFS were shorter in patients compared to previous studies [8]. In addition, it was stated that generalizations could not be made to all Stage 3C patients, since 61.6% of the patients had extra-abdominal metastases greater than 10 cm [8]. Although it was emphasized less in the study, it was stated that PDS was more beneficial in patients with metastatic tumor size less than 5 cm. It was also criticized in terms of bias because of the consideration of patients with poor prognostic factors and the remarkable differences between the participating centers (accrual range for institute was 1–125) [8]. In addition, the chemotherapy regimens used in NACT included differences. Complete cytoreduction rates have been reported to be very low in PDS and IDS [8]. Although there was an increase of 32% in the rates of complete resection after NACT, its effect was not shown in PFS and OS. OS also differed between countries [2]. It was stated that the participating centers also differed between countries and that a 'lack of qualification process' raised question marks about the demonstration of surgical effort for maximal cytoreductive surgery [8]. Although all patients who experienced mortality after diagnosis in PDS were included, perioperative mortality was calculated by including only patients who underwent IDS after chemotherapy in the NACT group. Patients who could not complete chemotherapy, who might have a high risk of mortality, and who had signs of progressive disease during chemotherapy were not included in the perioperative mortality analysis for the NACT group [8].

CHORUS Trial

It was a multicenter non-inferiority RCT that includes 87 centers in the United Kingdom and New Zealand [7]. The study was initiated by randomized 552 Stage 3 and 4 ovarian/fallopian tube/primary peritoneal cancer patients. 276 patients received surgery and 6 cycles of adjuvant chemotherapy in the PDS group, and patients with a residual tumor greater than 1 cm in PDS underwent repeat cytoreductive surgery after 3 cycles of chemotherapy. In the NACT group, 274 patients underwent IDS after 3 cycles of platinum-based chemotherapy. In NACT, 79% received IDS, and in PDS, 77% received adjuvant chemotherapy. Median OS was 24.1 months in NACT and 22.6 months in PDS, and no significant difference was detected. Median PFS was also similar (12 months for NACT, 10.7 months for PDS). The rate of complete cytoreduction was 17% in PDS and 39% in IDS. Grade 3-4 side effects and post-operative 28-day mortality were higher in PDS. There was no significant difference in terms of bleeding risk. Patients in the NACT group were more likely to be discharged within 14 days of surgery. While better quality of life was detected at 6 months in NACT, this difference was not observed at 12 months.

The CHORUS study supported the findings in the EORTC. However, it has received criticism on some issues such as EORTC [2]. In this study, optimal and complete cytoreduction rates were found to be low. In addition, it was stated that the operation times were short (median operation time was 120 minutes). There was high heterogeneity among surgical procedures performed at the 64 centers participating in the study [2]. They were also criticized for the high 28-day mortality despite the low rates of complete cytoreduction in PDS (6%). More patients (20%) in this study could not undergo IDS after NACT than in other studies (11% in EORTC, 13% in JCOG0602). They stated that the shorter survival was related to the fact that the patients were older and had poorer performance than other studies.

JCOG0602 Trial

This study was a multicenter, phase 3 non-inferiority RCT in which 301 patients with Stage 3 and 4 ovarian/fallopian tube/peritoneal cancer patients were evaluated in 34 centers in Japan [9]. In the control group, 8 courses of adjuvant chemotherapy were applied to the patients who underwent PDS. Additional surgery was performed in patients with residual tumor >1 cm in PDS and in patients whose uterus, adnexa or omentum was not removed at the initial surgery and no progression was detected. In the NACT group, 4 cycles of platinum-based chemotherapy were applied before and after the operation. Patients were evaluated for OS and adverse effects. In terms of OS, non-inferiority could not be demonstrated between NACT and PDS. Median OS was 44.3 months in the NACT group and 49 months in the PDS group. Median PFS was similar (16.4 months for NACT, 15.1 months for PDS). In NACT, the operative time was shorter and postoperative grade 3-4 side effects were less common. All macroscopic disease was resected in 12% of the PDS group and 62% of the IDS group.

This study has also been criticized from various aspects. While it had higher optimal debulking rates compared to EORTC and CHORUS, lower optimality rates were found compared to the SCORPION trial (37% for PDS, 82% for NACT). This may be due to the inclusion of all Stage 3 patients, as some of the patients initially had a lower disease burden [2]. With the application of additional debulking surgery (ADS) (PDS + 4 cycles of chemotherapy + ADS) to 33% of PDS patients (17% in EORTC), the optimal debulking rate of 37% in PDS was increased to 63%. However, it was stated that this patient group received more treatment compared to the NACT group, resulting in a high risk of bias [2].

SCORPION Trial

This RCT was initiated as a phase 3 study evaluating the superiority of NACT in 280 patients with high tumor burden at a single center in Italy [10]. Before the study groups were determined, diagnostic laparoscopy (L/S) was applied to the patients. Patients who could not undergo staging L/S were excluded from the study. Tumor burden was evaluated using the predictive index (PI) by applying L/S. Patients with PI >8 and PI <12 and no mesenteric retraction were evaluated as high tumor burden, and included in the study. Of the 225 patients who underwent L/S, only 110 were randomized to meet the study criteria. In the control group, 55 patients received 6 cycles of adjuvant chemotherapy after PDS. No additional cytoreductive surgery was performed in the PDS group. Surgery was performed in 55 patients in the NACT group who did not progress after 3 or 4 cycles of chemotherapy. Patients were compared in terms of postoperative complications, PFS, OS and quality of life. In terms of PFS, NACT (14 months) did not provide an advantage over PDS (15 months). In addition, no difference in OS was detected (43 months for NACT, 41 months for PDS). While the rate of complete cytoreduction was 47.6% in PDS, it was 67.0% in NACT. Postoperative major complications and mortality rates were higher in PDS. The NACT group had lower need for upper abdominal surgery, lower surgical complexity and less blood loss. In addition, operative time and hospital stay were shorter in NACT. Better quality of life (including emotional and cognitive functioning) was detected in patients who underwent NACT. Improvement in quality of life on 6 different scales was determined in NACT.

In the SCORPION study, the optimality rates (92.8% in PDS and 100% in IDS) were higher as a result of higher surgical effort compared to EORTC and CHORUS. In addition, according to other studies (27 months in the pooled analysis of EORTC and CHORUS), there was an increase in OS (43 months) [11]. However, this cohort was not considered to be representative of all ovarian cancer patients because only patients with a PI score of 8-12 and thought to be optimally debulking with L/S staging were included in the study [2]. In this study, compared to other RCTs, the rate of Stage 4 patients was lower and the patients were younger [2]. Therefore, it was stated in the Cochrane review that the applicability of the study is limited [2]. Patients with a PI score >12 who were considered likely to benefit more from NACT were excluded from this study. Total treatment time, that is, the time from the start of treatment to the end of treatment, was longer in PDS due to the delay in starting chemotherapy after surgery. The median duration in the CHORUS trial was 22 weeks; in the SCORPION trial, it was 38 weeks for PDS and 28 weeks for NACT.

Limitations and Criticisms of RCTs

The most criticized issue of RCTs was that although survival was reportedly higher in centers with extensive surgery experience than previous studies, their survival was much lower [3].

The median OS in the studies, especially EORTC (median OS in PDS was 29 months) and CHORUS (median OS in PDS was 22.6 months), were criticized because they were lower compared to other studies [8]. In GOG 172, median OS was 66 months in those who underwent optimal cytoreduction [12]. In the evaluations of RCTs, no difference was found between NACT and PDS in terms of survival, but high heterogeneity was reported between studies in terms of PFS and OS [2]. It was also criticized that comparisons were made between patients who had only PDS and IDS in the evaluation of postoperative complications [8]. However, among patients with low performance and high tumor burden, IDS cannot be performed on average in 15% of patients who started NACT, and this may reveal less postoperative complications in the calculation of NACT and it was thought that it may cause selection bias as well [8]. RCTs have also been criticized for their low complete cytoreduction rates [8]. However, it was stated that this conclusion was due to the extensive tumor burden of the patients included in the studies [2]. In the EORTC study, 74% had extra-pelvic metastases greater than 5 cm, while in CHORUS 1/4 of the patients and in JCOG0602 1/3 of the patients were at Stage 4 [2]. The surgical outcomes of the participating centers and countries also varied greatly [8]. It has been criticized that there was no qualification process in the selection of the centers participating in the studies and that the average number of cases was low in some centers [8]. In the Cochrane review, the heterogeneity of the tumor burden and the treatments applied in the studies was mentioned. It was also stated that chemotherapy regimens and the number of cycles differed in all studies [2].

Ongoing RCTs

Trial of Radical Upfront Surgical Therapy in Advanced Ovarian Cancer (TRUST)

This study is an ongoing multicenter international RCT to control surgical quality in advanced epithelial ovarian cancer [13]. Patients who underwent complete resection in PDS and received 6 cycles of adjuvant chemotherapy, and patients who underwent 3 cycles of NACT and IDS (complete resection) and received 3 cycles of adjuvant chemotherapy are randomized. Recruitment started in July 2016 and the results are expected in 2024. In addition, this study is important in terms of identifying various clinical and biological markers in patient selection for PDS and NACT.

Study of Upfront Surgery versus Neoadjuvant Chemotherapy in Patients with Advanced Ovarian Cancer (SUNNY)

This is a multicenter ongoing phase 3 RCT of Stage 3C and 4 ovarian cancer patients in China and Korea [14]. The study, which will evaluate OS, PFS, postoperative complications and quality of life, started in December 2015 and patient admission continues. The trial is expected to be completed in December 2022.

Systematic Reviews of Only RCTs

Vergote et al. presented their study containing long-term pooled survival data of two RCTs (EORTC and CHORUS) [11]. In the analysis of data from a total of 1220 patients, including 670 patients in the EORTC and 550 patients from the CHORUS, the patients were followed for a median of 7.6 years. There was no difference in OS between the patients who received NACT (27.6 months) and those who received PDS (26.9 months). In patients with Stage 3C and with the largest metastatic tumor size less than 5 cm, PDS provided the advantage of PFS. In Stage 4 patients, NACT increased PFS and OS.

Yang et al. presented a meta-analysis evaluating surgical outcome and quality of life, including 4 recent RCTs [15]. According to this study, the risk of grade 3-4 infections and gastrointestinal fistula were lower in the NACT group. The risk of any grade 3-4 adverse events and death within 28 days after surgery was lower in NACT, while the risk of blood transfusion was similar. In addition, the rates of achieving macroscopic and optimal debulking were higher in NACT. Residual tumor <1 cm rates were equal. In the quality of life analysis, improvement (fatigue, role functioning, emotional functioning and cognitive functioning) was higher in the NACT group at 6 months.

Machida et al. published a systematic review and meta-analysis in which the survival analysis of 4 RCTs was performed [16]. In this study, no difference was found between the NACT and PDS groups in terms of age and performance status. Tumor size was similar. In NACT, operative times were shorter, lymphadenectomy rates were higher, and intra-abdominal organ resection was less frequent. The rates of discontinuation of treatment were 17.4% in NACT and 17.3% in PDS. However, subgroup evaluations could not be made in terms of survival of patients who did not continue treatment, that is, patients who did not undergo IDS after NACT, and did not receive adjuvant chemotherapy after PDS. The most frequent discontinuation was due to disease progression and chemotherapy complications in NACT, and due to disease progression or death and postoperative complications in PDS. A meta-analysis of 4 RCTs found no significant difference in survival between groups in OS and PFS. When the complete resection rates were examined, NACT (48.2%) was more advantageous than PDS (23.2%). The optimal cytoreduction rate was also higher in NACT. In addition, the heterogeneity of the surgical procedures was emphasized. Grade 3-4 side effects, grade 3-4 venous thromboembolism and grade 3-4 infection were less common in the NACT group. Surgical mortality was lower in NACT, but in the analysis performed, patients who underwent PDS and IDS were compared, and mortality during NACT and until the operation was not included in the evaluation of the studies. In other words, a group of patients with poor medical conditions who already had advanced stage tumors were analyzed as the surgical group. However, these patients in poor conditional status in the NACT group were not included in the study. IDS could not be applied in 7% of patients who received NACT due to progressive disease. In this study, it was stated that although NACT has no advantage in terms of survival, it reduced morbidity and mortality rates and was a viable option in low-volume centers, in patients with poor performance status and unresectable tumors.

Systematic Reviews of 'RCTs and Non-randomized Studies'

Bartels et al. found that PDS and NACT group patients were similar in terms of age, performance status, FIGO stage, and Stage 4 patient ratio in their meta-analysis including 4 RCTs, 4 prospective and 9 retrospective studies [17]. Preoperative cancer antigen 125 levels were higher in the NACT group. When perioperative outcomes were evaluated, the mean operation time was 35 minutes shorter and the mean blood loss was 382 mL lower in NACT. There was no difference between blood transfusions. Hyperthermic intraperitoneal chemotherapy (HIPEC) was not used in any of the studies. While optimal cytoreduction was achieved in NACT with a rate of 71.3%, this rate was 59.8% in PDS. The rate of complete cytoreduction was 44.4% in NACT and 28.3% in PDS. The patients who underwent NACT achieved 2 times more optimal and complete cytoreduction rates. The morbidities such as moderate to severe infection, venous thromboembolism and intestinal fistula were more common in PDS. Bowel resection rate was 23.5% in PDS and 8.8% in NACT. Postoperative 30-day mortality (6.1-fold) and mean hospital stay (5 days) were higher in PDS. While 5-year survival rates were similar, mean OS was calculated as one month longer in NACT. In this meta-analysis, it was noted that the studies had low rates of complete cytoreduction and that the mean OSs were very heterogeneous (between 22.6 months and 56.4 months).

Lv et al. examined 57, 450 patients in a recent meta-analysis of 2 RCTs (EORTC and CHORUS) and 14 high-quality observational studies and evaluated surgical side effects with survival analysis [18]. According to this study, when all studies were included, OS of patients who underwent NACT was lower. PFS was examined in 11 trials and no significant differences were detected. Complete resection rates were included in 7 trials and it was stated that these rates were higher in NACT. The two groups were similar in terms of residual disease < 1 cm. While post-surgical death and major infection were lower in NACT, wound complications were similar. Contrary to the 2 RCTs, they stated that the shorter survival in patients receiving NACT was due to the worse functional status of the patients, more aggressive tumor biology and higher tumor burden, and they emphasized that these could not be adjusted in observational studies.

Qin et al. published a systematic review and meta-analysis of 2 RCTs (EORTC and CHORUS) and 22 retrospective observational studies [19]. In the analysis of 22 retrospective studies, a total of 12, 775 patients with advanced ovarian cancer were examined, and although optimal cytoreduction rates were superior in NACT, OS was higher in PDS. No differences were found in PFS in the analysis of 12 retrospective studies. In the subgroup analysis for residual tumor in retrospective studies, PDS provided better OS in all groups, regardless of the grade of the residual tumor. In the subgroup analysis for stage, OS was higher for PDS in both Stage 3 and 4.

Large Retrospective Study

Lyons et al. reviewed 36,602 patients (26,717 patients in PDS, 9,885 patients in NACT) with Stage 3 and 4 epithelial ovarian cancer, in which a large national database was retrospectively evaluated [20]. In this study, patients who received primary cytoreduction and adjuvant chemotherapy and those who received interval cytoreductive surgery and 3 or 4 cycles of chemotherapy after 3 or 4 cycles of NACT were compared in terms of surgery and survival analyses. Primary fallopian tube and primary peritoneal cancers were not included. Covariates were analyzed in terms of age, comorbidity, stage, histological type and grade. Patients with a high risk of chemo-resistance (low-grade serous and mucinous histology) and elderly/frail patients were also analyzed as high-risk patients. The group receiving NACT were older and had more comorbidities. High-grade and advanced stage patients were more common in the NACT group. The absence of gross residual disease was more common in NACT (65.4%) than in PDS (56.1%). While the 30-day and 90-day mortality rates were higher in NACT, the 90-day mortality rates were similar when high risk (advanced age, comorbidities, low-grade serous and mucinous histological type) patients were excluded. After adjusting for covariates (age, stage, histological type, grade, comorbidities, residual volume), mortality was 37% higher in NACT. Median OS in NACT was 37.6 months, while in PDS it was 50.4 months. In addition, when patients at high risk (over 75 years of age, Charlton comorbidity score >1, low-grade serous and mucinous histology) were excluded, patients with PDS had better survival. When evaluated in terms of residual disease, the median OS in patients treated with PDS-R0 (microscopic or no residual disease) resection was 62.6 months, 39.8 months in PDS-R1 (macroscopic residual disease) resection, 41.8 months in NACT-R0 resection, and 29.5 months in NACT-R1 resection. PDS-R1 had better survival compared to NACT-R0 when the analysis was done after adjusting for covariates. In this large retrospective analysis, PDS achieved better survival than NACT and lower 30-day and 90-day surgical mortality when covariates were adjusted and even high risk patients were removed. Exceptions to the PDS recommendations, regardless of tumor burden, were noted as non-removable breast, brain, liver, or bone metastases. However, in this study, patients were classified as R0 and R1 resections only, and residual tumor sizes were not presented. The authors reported that patients with advanced ovarian cancer should be treated with primary cytoreductive surgery, but patients who are not suitable for surgery should be managed with NACT.

Recent Cochrane Review

In the Cochrane review results, 1,713 Stage 3 and 4 ovarian cancer patients who underwent NACT and PDS were evaluated, including the RCTs most recently published in 2019 [2]. There was no difference between PDS and NACT in terms of OS and PFS. The need for blood transfusion, the risk of venous thromboembolism and infection were reduced in NACT. In addition, NACT reduced the risk of bowel resection and stoma formation, resulting in a decrease in postoperative mortality. It has been stated that the clinical factors of the patient, the education of the clinician and the preference of the surgeon are effective in deciding the type of surgery. While the quality of evidence was evaluated as moderate certainty in terms of survival, it was shown as low-to-moderate certainty in terms of surgical morbidity and adverse effect. It has been mentioned that further studies may change future estimates due to the risk of bias and a small number of events. It has been stated that Stage 3A and 3B patients and those with Stage 3C and PI scores below 8 who have been studied with a multidisciplinary team in a specialist center capable of performing radical procedures will benefit more from PDS. In addition, Stage 4 and stage 3C patients with tumors too large for optimal debulking as determined by imaging or L/S, elderly or morbidly obese low-performing patients who are predicted to require an extensive surgical procedure, or patients without access to an experienced ovarian cancer surgical center would benefit more from NACT. It has been reported that NACT should be offered only to those who cannot have optimal surgery performed in PDS.

Special Issues

The Number of Cycles in NACT

In all 4 RCTs, 3 or 4 cycles of chemotherapy were administered as NACT. While the median NACT cycle was 3 in EORTC and CHORUS [5, 7], it was stated that this situation caused more chemo-resistance in patients with high tumor volume, since 4 cycles were administered to patients in JCOG0602 [9]. Administration of more than 3 cycles of chemotherapy is not recommended because it does not show a survival advantage by increasing the risk of chemo-resistance [17]. Surgery is recommended after 4 cycles only if complete cytoreduction is anticipated [8].

Timing of IDS

In the EORTC study, the median time to start chemotherapy after surgery in NACT was 18 days, while it was 19 days after PDS [5]. In the SCORPION study, it was observed that this period was longer in the PDS group (40 days for PDS, 27 days for NACT) [10]. Because of this delay, the time between the start of treatment and the end of treatment was longer in PDS (38 weeks for PDS, 28 weeks for NACT) [10].

Patient Selection, Burden of Disease and Factors Determining Optimality

According to the European Society of Gynaecological Oncology (ESGO) guidelines, the tumor is considered unresectable if:: diffuse deep infiltration of the root of small bowel mesentery, diffuse carcinomatosis of the small bowel, diffuse involvement of the stomach, or duodenum, or head/middle part of the pancreas, involvement of the truncus coeliacus, hepatic arteries and left gastric artery, central or multi-segmental parenchymal liver metastases, multiple parenchymal lung metastasis, unresectable lymph node metastasis, and multiple brain metastases exist [21]. However, it is not always easy to determine this preoperatively [8]. It may be difficult to predict resectability with the use of various imaging methods [8]. Despite the fact that NACT is recommended in patients with a high tumor burden, it is not simple to predict this before abdominal exploration [20]. Although various selection methods and models have been developed to predict morbidity and mortality and optimize surgical outcomes, the usefulness of these methods is uncertain as they do not evaluate tumor biology, spread of disease and oncological outcomes and are not validated [20]. In the EORTC study, it was concluded that patients with the largest metastatic tumor size of <5 cm had a survival advantage in PDS [5]. Yıldırım et al. emphasized that PDS should be preferred because of the low response to NACT in the presence of extensive omental disease (Figure 2) [22]. NACT is also recommended in cases where extensive tumor burden is determined, such as small bowel mesentery involvement [17]. Studies were conducted to predict surgical outcome with preoperative imaging methods, but these studies could not generate predictive models that were internally validated [23].

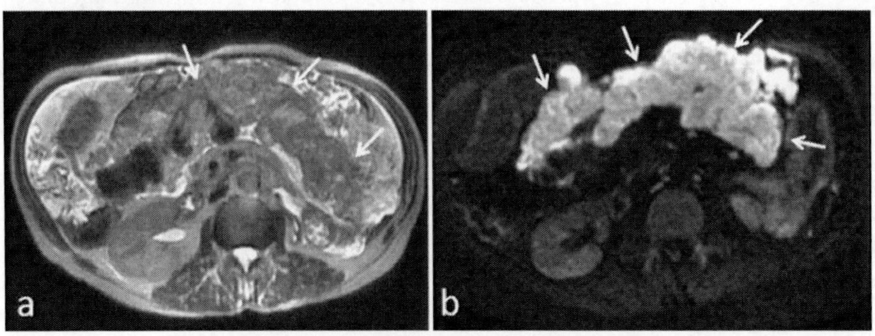

Figure 2. Omental cake with thickened heterogeneous inner structure on axial T2-weighted (a) and diffusion-weighted (b) Magnetic Resonance Imaging.

Age and Performance Status

Age is an important prognostic factor in advanced ovarian cancer [3]. The patient's operability, that is, the ability to safely tolerate surgery, is one of the primary factors in choosing PDS or NACT [8]. In the EORTC study and in the long-term pooled analysis of the two RCTs, no superiority was found between the treatments in terms of PDS and NACT when subgroup analysis was performed for age and performance status [5, 11]. In addition, in JCOG0602, NACT and PDS had similar survival among patients among patients under 60 years of age and above [9]. It was stated that NACT provided a survival advantage in case of poor performance status in JCOG0602 [9]. Morbidity in PDS can be high in the event of malnutrition and poor performance [8]. Therefore, age, medical comorbidities, nutritional status should be carefully evaluated before choosing PDS or NACT [8]. Careful evaluation before PDS is recommended because of the high risk of 30-day postoperative mortality, especially in elderly patients (over 75 years) with comorbid diseases [8]. If there is no improvement in the patient's general condition within an acceptable time, it is recommended that NACT should be started immediately in order not to delay treatment [8].

Tumor Size

In the analysis of 4 RCTs, no difference was found between NACT and PDS in terms of initial tumor size [16]. It has been stated that when the tumor size is large at the time of diagnosis, the efficacy of NACT may decrease due to the high risk of spontaneous mutation and therefore high chemo-resistance [16].

Platinum Refractory Disease

Some patients may develop progressive disease despite NACT and therefore these patients cannot be operated on [16]. In 4 RCTs, these patients account for 7% of patients receiving NACT [16]. In addition, platinum resistance is detected at a higher rate in patients who underwent NACT [17]. In the case of platinum refractory disease, the median survival is less than 1 year, and additional treatment options are still under investigation due to the poor prognosis [4]. Surgical treatment is not recommended in this patient group except in palliative conditions [4].

Other Histological Types

It is known that histological types other than high-grade serous carcinoma (low-grade serous, mucinous, clear cell carcinoma) have a higher probability of resistance to platinum-based chemotherapy and a higher risk of progressive disease [16]. Heterogeneity of histological subtypes was mentioned in the meta-analysis of RCTs and observational studies [18]. Since high-grade serous subtypes constitute the majority of the cases, it is not possible to evaluate the efficacy of NACT and PDS in the presence of other histological types [18]. In JCOG0602, patients who received NACT in the condition of chemo-resistant histology (clear and mucinous type) had a survival disadvantage [9]. However, because non-serous histological types are chemo-resistant, treatment with NACT and not performing PDS may adversely affect the prognosis [18]. It was stated that PDS should be considered as the primary option because low-grade serous types are less sensitive to chemotherapeutic agents [11]. Even if the residual tumor is more than 1 cm in low-grade serous carcinoma, the survival advantage of primary cytoreductive surgery is higher [2]. Although mucinous histology subtypes are usually detected at an early stage, the effectiveness of NACT in advanced cases is lower than high-grade serous subtypes due to platinum resistance. Due to its rarity, the efficacy of NACT in RCTs has not been clearly determined [16]. Therefore, further examination of histological subtypes other than high-grade serous carcinoma is required.

Residual Tumor

Absence of macroscopic residual tumor was determined as the most important prognostic factor [5]. In the EORTC study, median OS was calculated as 45 months in the group that underwent complete cytoreduction by applying PDS, 32 months when the residual tumor was between 1-10 mm, and 26 months in the case with a residual tumor above 1 cm [5]. Furthermore, in patients receiving NACT, median OS was 38 months for complete cytoreduction, 27 months when the residual tumor was between 1-10 mm, and 25 months when the residual tumor was over 10 mm [5]. In the SCORPION study, it was determined that NACT increased the rate of complete cytoreduction compared to PDS [10]. However, in the subgroup analysis of patients who underwent complete cytoreduction, no difference was found between NACT and PDS in terms of PFS and OS [10]. Patients with a residual tumor of 0 and <1 cm did not differ in terms of PFS in PDS (16 months and 15 months, respectively) [10]. It has been stated that this may be as a result of micro or macroscopic unrecognizable residual disease in patients undergoing complete resection with high tumor burden [10]. In a meta-analysis of retrospective studies, it was stated that PDS provided better OS compared to NACT, regardless of the grade of the residual tumor [19].

Experience and Skills of the Surgeon

It has been reported that ovarian cancer surgery performed by gynecologist oncologists increases survival and decreases morbidity [24]. In the meta-analysis that included all studies, this situation could not be evaluated because it was examined in very few studies [18]. However, as stated in the Society of Gynecologic Oncology and American Society of Clinical Oncology Clinical Practice Guidelines, it is recommended that patients with advanced ovarian cancer should be evaluated by a gynecologist oncologist before starting treatment [4]. It was determined that centers with high surgical activity had better OS in PDS and NACT than centers with low surgical activity [9]. In the JCOG0602 study, it was stated that NACT was an advantage for centers with fewer cases [9]. However, due to the lack of surgical experience, it is recommended that NACT should not be used as an alternative to PDS and that patients should be directed to centers with advanced ovarian cancer experience [8]. It has been reported that NACT is used as a compensation for poor surgical quality [20]. However, it has been suggested that patients should be managed in centers experienced in PDS to reduce complications and maximize patient benefit [20]. Experienced high-volume centers can help patients achieve complete cytoreduction and a better survival rate [17].

Upper Abdominal Surgery

The addition of upper abdominal procedures have shown to increase the optimal cytoreduction rates [4]. In the SCORPION study, all patients in PDS underwent an upper abdominal surgical procedure, while 42.3% of NACT required an upper abdominal procedure in IDS [10]. In the EORTC and CHORUS, upper abdominal surgery rates were low and optimal cytoreduction rates were lower in PDS [17].

FIGO Stage

In the EORTC study, NACT increased survival in Stage 4 patients, but in other RCTs, being in Stage 3 or 4 did not provide more benefit than NACT [2]. In the long-term analysis of the EORTC and CHORUS, patients with Stage 3C and metastatic tumor size less than 5 cm had a survival advantage in PDS, and in the case of Stage 4 disease, survival was higher in NACT compared to PDS [11]. In the meta-analysis of retrospective studies, PDS provided OS advantage in both Stage 3 and stage 4 [19]. In the SCORPION study, the survival advantage of NACT demonstrated in Stage 4 patients disappeared with increasing cytoreduction rates [10]. However, it was also reported that this situation cannot be generalized for all Stage 4 patients [10]. Presence of inguinal lymph nodes, para-cardiac nodes, focal parietal pleural involvement, isolated parenchymal lung metastases are indicated as potential extra-abdominal resectable conditions in ESGO guidelines [21]. In the last Cochrane review, the subgroup analysis could not be performed with the FIGO stage and it would be done in the future version [2].

Scoring Systems

In the initial clinical evaluation, positron emission tomography or diffusion-weighted magnetic resonance imaging is also beneficial, in addition to imaging with abdominal and chest computed tomography, in order to evaluate the extent of the tumor and the feasibility of surgery (Figures 3 and 4) [4]. Studies have been conducted on the use of L/S to predict surgical outcomes [25]. There is no clear conclusion that L/S can predict which patients will have optimal results before the first surgery. Optimal debulking can be predicted by performing L/S only in 70% of patients [25]. However, in the Cochrane review, it was stated that resectability could be determined with high specificity by the use of L/S and unnecessary laparotomy could be reduced [2]. In the SCORPION study, a PI value calculation method with staging L/S was used to evaluate the tumor burden of the patients [10]. In this defined Fagotti scoring system, PI is calculated based on seven parameters: omental cake, diffuse peritoneal or diaphragmatic surface carcinomatosis, retraction of mesentery, gastric, spleen or bowel infiltration and superficial liver metastases. If PI is greater than 8 and ≤12, it is considered as high tumor load [26]. Previously it has been reported that these patients should be managed with NACT since the optimal resectability rate of the tumor is 0% in the case of PI≥8 [26].

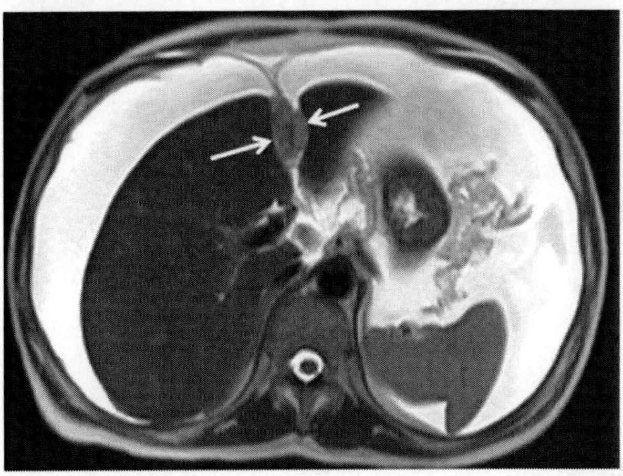

Figure 3. Implant in the falciform ligament and prominent ascites on axial T2-weighted magnetic resonance imaging.

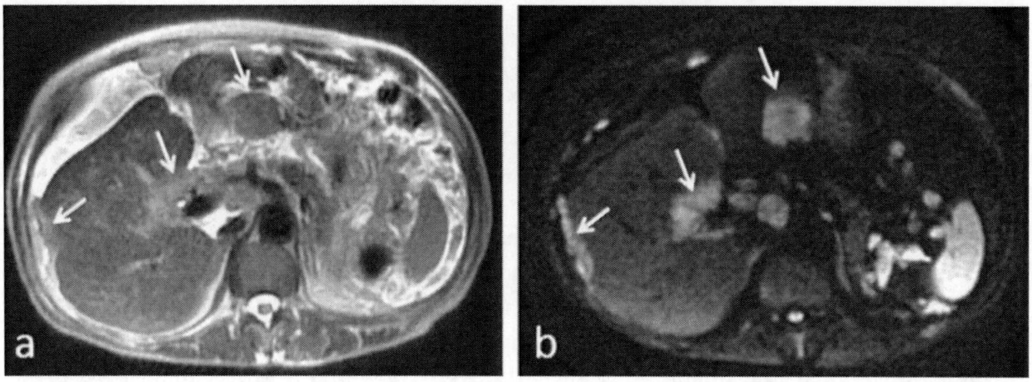

Figure 4. Extensive implants in the gastro-hepatic area, hepatic hilum, and adjacent liver right lobe capsule on T2-weighted (a) and diffusion-weighted (b) magnetic resonance imaging.

Surgical Concerns about NACT

The application of NACT may cause fibrosis and edema in the tissues, making surgery more difficult [20]. In addition, it was mentioned that tumor spread within the peritoneal cavity may be difficult to interpret, and if the perioperative evaluation is not good, incomplete resection may occur with NACT [2].

Selection Criteria

Treatment with NACT is recommended for patients with a high preoperative risk profile and who are not thought to undergo optimal cytoreductive surgery (residual tumor < 1 cm) [4]. After the EORTC study, Vergote et al. defined the Leuven selection criteria for the selection of NACT or PDS in the evaluation of patients with Stage 3C-4 ovarian cancer [27]. Accordingly, NACT and IDS are recommended in the following cases: tumors ≥ 2 cm around the superior mesenteric artery or behind the porta hepatis, intrahepatic or extra-abdominal metastases, poor performance condition, widespread serosal invasion requiring more than 1.5 meters of bowel resection, women who cannot be easily removed without residual tumor [27]. In addition, the choice of NACT and PDS depends on complex factors such as the patient's age, comorbidities, general physical condition, experience of the surgical team, preoperative imaging methods, and the decision-making process of the patient and physician [2]. Pathological and genetic studies are continuing on which patients will benefit more from NACT than PDS [8]. It is thought that the results of the studied biomarkers will benefit from the choice of treatment options in the treatment of advanced ovarian cancer [8].

Intraperitoneal Chemotherapy and HIPEC

In the previous GOG 172 study, intraperitoneal chemotherapy was found to provide a survival advantage compared to intravenous chemotherapy [12]. But there was no additional information about the use of intraperitoneal chemotherapy in RCTs [17]. In addition, no previous study specified the use of HIPEC [17].

Quality of Life

Quality of life was analyzed in 3 RCTs. While higher quality of life was found in NACT in the SCORPION, quality of life was always similar in EORTC [5, 10]. In the CHORUS study, although higher quality of life was detected in NACT at 6 months, this difference disappeared at 12 months [7]. It was reported that the results of the EORTC and SCORPION studies evaluated in the Cochrane review included inconsistent and inaccurate results [2]. In addition, the quality of life in the EORTC study was not evaluated by evaluating all participants [28]. Since the compliance was low, the centers with the best fit were analyzed in the study. Therefore, data were obtained from only 27 of the 59 centers participating in the study. Only 212 of a total of 670 patients were analyzed. However, it was stated that the patients who were not included had differences between the centers analyzed. For example, the analyzed group had longer median OS and PFS, but also had larger tumors and more optimal debulking rates. In addition, although the centers with the best compliance were selected, overall compliance was still low [2].

Cancer Genetics, Immunotherapy, Bevacizumab and New Agents

Both NACT and PDS cause immunosuppression by affecting the immune system of the patient [8]. Due to the immunological effects of NACT, its use in immunotherapies is under investigation [8]. Bevacizumab is recommended for first-line therapy in addition to adjuvant chemotherapy [4]. Although it has been reported that the use of bevacizumab as part of chemotherapy in NACT has been reported to be safe, there is no evidence of clinical benefit yet [8]. It is known that patients with BRCA gene mutations have a high response to platinum-based treatments [8]. In addition, other genetic studies trying to predict chemo-sensitivity and molecular and immunologic studies to predict complete cytoreduction are continuing [8]. Although various predictive tools are available, they were not validated due to differences in surgical techniques [8].

Cost Effectiveness

Rowland et al. evaluated the patients over the age of 65 in EORTC and found that NACT was cost-saving compared to PDS [29]. Similarly, in a cost-effectiveness analysis including 4 RCTs, a cost reduction of $7.034 per woman was reported with NACT at 7 months after treatment [30].

Conclusion

According to current evidence levels, the standard treatment of advanced ovarian cancer consists of a combination of surgery and chemotherapy. It is recommended that surgery should be performed as PDS when it is thought that optimal cytoreduction can be achieved. However, the application of NACT in patients with comorbidities, advanced age and poor performance status is as effective as the survival benefit provided by PDS. Although NACT provides higher complete and optimal cytoreduction rates, it does not provide a survival advantage over PDS. NACT reduces postoperative morbidity and mortality and provides better quality of life. NACT is a viable option in patients with advanced ovarian cancer who have high tumor burden and cannot undergo surgical cytoreduction. It is important to manage patients with advanced ovarian cancer in multidisciplinary comprehensive centers experienced in gynecological cancer surgery and to decide on the choice of PDS or NACT there.

References

[1] Bray F, Ferlay J, Soerjomataram I, Siegel RL, Torre LA, Jemal A. Global cancer statistics 2018: GLOBOCAN estimates of incidence and mortality worldwide for 36 cancers in 185 countries. *CA Cancer J Clin.* 2018;68(6):394-424.

[2] Coleridge SL, Bryant A, Lyons TJ, Goodall RJ, Kehoe S, Morrison J. Chemotherapy versus surgery for initial treatment in advanced ovarian epithelial cancer. *Cochrane Database Syst Rev.* 2019;2019(10):CD005343.

[3] du Bois A, Reuss A, Pujade-Lauraine E, Harter P, Ray-Coquard I, Pfisterer J. Role of surgical outcome as prognostic factor in advanced epithelial ovarian cancer: a combined exploratory analysis of 3 prospectively randomized phase 3 multicenter trials: by the Arbeitsgemeinschaft Gynaekologische Onkologie Studiengruppe Ovarialkarzinom (AGO-OVAR) and the Groupe d'Investigateurs Nationaux Pour les Etudes des Cancers de l'Ovaire (GINECO). *Cancer.* 2009;115(6):1234-44.

[4] Wright, Alexi A, Kari Bohlke, Deborah K Armstrong, Michael A Bookman, William A Cliby, Robert L Coleman, Don S Dizon, Joseph J Kash, Larissa A Meyer, Kathleen N Moore, Alexander B Olawaiye, Jessica Oldham, Ritu Salani, Dee Sparacio, William P Tew, Ignace Vergote, Mitchell I Edelson. Neoadjuvant chemotherapy for newly diagnosed, advanced ovarian cancer: Society of Gynecologic Oncology and American Society of Clinical Oncology Clinical Practice Guideline. *Gynecol Oncol.* 2016;143(1):3-15.

[5] Vergote, I, Tropé, CG, Amant, F, Kristensen, GB, Ehlen, T, Johnson, N, Verheijen, RHM., van der Burg, MEL, Lacave, AJ, Panici, PB, Kenter, GG, Casado, A, Mendiola, C, Coens, C, Verleye, L, Stuart, GCE, Pecorelli, S, & Reed, NS. Neoadjuvant chemotherapy or primary surgery in stage IIIC or IV ovarian cancer. *N Engl J Med.* 2010;363(10):943-53.

[6] van der Burg, MEL, van Lent, M, Buyse, M, Kobierska, A, Colombo, N, Favalli, G, Lacave, AJ, Nardi, M, Renard, J, & Pecorelli, S. The effect of debulking surgery after induction chemotherapy on the prognosis in advanced epithelial ovarian cancer. Gynecological Cancer Cooperative Group of the European Organization for Research and Treatment of Cancer. *N Engl J Med.* 1995;332(10):629-34.

[7] Kehoe, S, Hook, J, Nankivell, M, Jayson, GC, Kitchener, H, Lopes, T, Luesley, D, Perren, T, Bannoo, S, Mascarenhas, M, Dobbs, S, Essapen, S, Twigg, J, Herod, J, McCluggage, G, Parmar, M, & Swart, A-M. Primary chemotherapy versus primary surgery for newly diagnosed advanced ovarian cancer (CHORUS): an open-label, randomised, controlled, non-inferiority trial. *Lancet.* 2015;386(9990):249-57.

[8] du Bois A, Baert T, Vergote I. Role of Neoadjuvant Chemotherapy in Advanced Epithelial Ovarian Cancer. *J Clin Oncol.* 2019;37(27):2398-405.

[9] Onda, T, Satoh, T, Ogawa, G, Saito, T, Kasamatsu, T, Nakanishi, T, Mizutani, T, Takehara, K, Okamoto, A, Ushijima, K, Kobayashi, H, Kawana, K, Yokota, H, Takano, M, Kanao, H, Watanabe, Y, Yamamoto, K, Yaegashi, N, Kamura, T, & Yoshikawa, H. Comparison of survival between primary debulking surgery and neoadjuvant chemotherapy for stage III/IV ovarian, tubal and peritoneal cancers in phase III randomised trial. *Eur J Cancer.* 2020;130:114-25.

[10] Fagotti, Anna, Maria Gabriella Ferrandina, Giuseppe Vizzielli, Tina Pasciuto, Francesco Fanfani, Valerio Gallotta, Pasquale Alessandro Margariti, Vito Chiantera, Barbara Costantini, Salvatore Gueli Alletti, Francesco Cosentino, Giovanni Scambia. Randomized trial of primary debulking surgery versus neoadjuvant chemotherapy for advanced epithelial ovarian cancer (SCORPION-NCT01461850). *Int J Gynecol Cancer.* 2020;30(11):1657-64.

[11] Ignace Vergote, Corneel Coens, Matthew Nankivell, Gunnar B Kristensen, Mahesh KB Parmar, Tom Ehlen, Gordon C Jayson, Nick Johnson, Ann Marie Swart, René Verheijen, W Glenn McCluggage, Tim Perren, Pierluigi Benedetti Panici, Gemma Kenter, Antonio Casado, Cesar Mendiola, Gavin Stuart, Nick S Reed, Sean Kehoe, EORTC; MRC CHORUS study investigators. Neoadjuvant chemotherapy versus debulking surgery in advanced tubo-ovarian cancers: pooled analysis of individual patient data from the EORTC 55971 and CHORUS trials. *Lancet Oncol.* 2018;19(12):1680-7.

[12] Deborah K Armstrong, Brian Bundy, Lari Wenzel, Helen Q Huang, Rebecca Baergen, Shashikant Lele, Larry J Copeland, Joan L Walker, Robert A Burger, Gynecologic Oncology Group. Intraperitoneal cisplatin and paclitaxel in ovarian cancer. *N Engl J Med.* 2006;354(1):34-43.

[13] Alexander Reuss, Andreas du Bois, Philipp Harter, Christina Fotopoulou, Jalid Sehouli, Giovanni Aletti, Frederic Guyon, Stefano Greggi, Berit Jul Mosgaard, Alexander Reinthaller, Felix Hilpert, Carmen Schade-Brittinger, Dennis S Chi, Sven Mahner. TRUST: Trial of Radical Upfront Surgical Therapy in advanced ovarian cancer (ENGOT ov33/AGO-OVAR OP7). *Int J Gynecol Cancer.* 2019;29(8):1327-31.

[14] Jiang, R, Zhu, J, Kim, J-W, Liu, J, Kato, K, Kim, H-S, Zhang, Y, Zhang, P, Zhu, T, Aoki, D, Yu, A, Chen, X, Wang, X, Zhu, D, Zhang, W, Jia, H, Shi, T, Gao, W, Yin, S, Feng, Y, Xiang, L, Okamoto, A and Zang, R. Study of upfront surgery versus neoadjuvant chemotherapy followed by interval debulking surgery for patients with stage IIIC and IV ovarian cancer, SGOG SUNNY (SOC-2) trial concept. *J Gynecol Oncol.* 2020;31(5):e86.

[15] Yang, L, Zhang, B, Xing, G, Du, J, Yang, B, Yuan, Q, & Yang, Y. Neoadjuvant chemotherapy versus primary debulking surgery in advanced epithelial ovarian cancer: A meta-analysis of peri-operative outcome. *PloS One.* 2017;12(10):e0186725.

[16] Machida, H, Tokunaga, H, Matsuo, K, Matsumura, N, Kobayashi, Y, Tabata, T, Kaneuchi, M, Nagase, S, & Mikami, M. Survival outcome and perioperative complication related to neoadjuvant chemotherapy with carboplatin and paclitaxel for advanced ovarian cancer: A systematic review and meta-analysis. *Eur J Surg Oncol.* 2020;46(5):868-75.

[17] Bartels, HC, Rogers, AC, McSharry, V, McVey, R, Walsh, T, O'Brien, D, Boyd, WD, & Brennan, DJ. A meta-analysis of morbidity and mortality in primary cytoreductive surgery compared to neoadjuvant chemotherapy in advanced ovarian malignancy. *Gynecol Oncol.* 2019;154(3):622-30.

[18] Lv X, Cui S, Zhang X, Ren C. Efficacy and safety of neoadjuvant chemotherapy versus primary debulking surgery in patients with ovarian cancer: a meta-analysis. *J Gynecol Oncol.* 2020;31(2):e12.

[19] Qin M, Jin Y, Ma L, Zhang YY, Pan LY. The role of neoadjuvant chemotherapy followed by interval debulking surgery in advanced ovarian cancer: a systematic review and meta-analysis of randomized controlled trials and observational studies. *Oncotarget.* 2018;9(9):8614-28.

[20] Yasmin A Lyons, Henry D Reyes, Megan E McDonald, Andreea Newtson, Eric Devor, David P Bender, Michael J Goodheart, Jesus Gonzalez Bosquet. Interval debulking surgery is not worth the wait: a National Cancer Database study comparing primary cytoreductive surgery versus neoadjuvant chemotherapy. *Int J Gynecol Cancer.* 2020;30(6):845-52.

[21] Querleu, D, Planchamp, F, Chiva, L, Fotopoulou, C, Barton, D, Cibula, D, Aletti, G, Carinelli, S, Creutzberg, C, Davidson, B, Harter, P, Lundvall, L, Marth, C, Morice, P, Rafii, A, Ray-Coquard, I, Rockall, A, Sessa, C, van der Zee, A, Vergote, I and du Bois, A. European Society of Gynaecologic Oncology Quality Indicators for Advanced Ovarian Cancer Surgery. *Int J Gynecol Cancer.* 2016;26(7):1354-63.

[22] Yildirim Y, Ertas IE, Dogan A, Gultekin OE, Gultekin E. The predictors of response to neoadjuvant chemotherapy in advanced epithelial ovarian cancer. *J Surg Oncol.* 2012;105(2):200-5.

[23] Rutten, MJ, van de Vrie, R, Bruining, A, Spijkerboer, AM, Mol, BW, Kenter, GG, & Buist, MR. Predicting surgical outcome in patients with International Federation of Gynecology and Obstetrics stage III or IV ovarian cancer using computed tomography: a systematic review of prediction models. *Int J Gynecol Cancer.* 2015;25(3):407-15.

[24] Bristow RE, Chang J, Ziogas A, Randall LM, Anton-Culver H. High-volume ovarian cancer care: survival impact and disparities in access for advanced-stage disease. *Gynecol Oncol.* 2014;132(2):403-10.

[25] van de Vrie, R, Rutten, MJ, Asseler, JD, Leeflang, MM, Kenter, GG, Mol, BWJ, & Buist, M. Laparoscopy for diagnosing resectability of disease in women with advanced ovarian cancer. *Cochrane Database Syst Rev.* 2019;3(3):Cd009786.

[26] Fagotti, A, Ferrandina, G, Fanfani, F, Ercoli, A, Lorusso, D, Rossi, M, & Scambia, G. A laparoscopy-based score to predict surgical outcome in patients with advanced ovarian carcinoma: a pilot study. *Ann Surg Oncol.* 2006;13(8):1156-61.

[27] Vergote I, Amant F, Kristensen G, Ehlen T, Reed NS, Casado A. Primary surgery or neoadjuvant chemotherapy followed by interval debulking surgery in advanced ovarian cancer. *Eur J Cancer.* 2011;47 Suppl 3:S88-92.

[28] Greimel, E, Kristensen, GB, van der Burg, MEL, Coronado, P, Rustin, G, del Rio, AS, Reed, NS, Nordal, RR, Coens, C, & Vergote, I. Quality of life of advanced ovarian cancer patients in the randomized phase III study comparing primary debulking surgery versus neo-adjuvant chemotherapy. *Gynecol Oncol.* 2013;131(2):437-44.

[29] Rowland MR, Lesnock JL, Farris C, Kelley JL, Krivak TC. Cost-utility comparison of neoadjuvant chemotherapy versus primary debulking surgery for treatment of advanced-stage ovarian cancer in patients 65 years old or older. *Am J Obstet Gynecol.* 2015;212(6):763.e1-8.

[30] Arthur-Quan Tran, Daniel O Erim, Stephanie A Sullivan, Ashley L Cole, Emma L Barber, Kenneth H Kim, Paola A Gehrig, Stephanie B Wheeler. Cost effectiveness of neoadjuvant chemotherapy followed by interval cytoreductive surgery versus primary cytoreductive surgery for patients with advanced stage ovarian cancer during the initial treatment phase. *Gynecol Oncol.* 2018;148(2):329-35.

Chapter 20

Lymphadenectomy in Ovarian Cancer Surgery

Fuat Demirkiran*, MD, PhD
and Elif Akşahin, MD, PhD
Department of Obstetrics and Gynecology, Division of Gynecologic Oncology,
Istanbul University-Cerrahpasa, Cerrahpasa Medical Faculty, Istanbul, Turkey

Introduction

Lymphadenectomy (LA), like many other surgical procedures, is an important aspect of the surgical management of gynecologic malignancies. The primary controversy regarding LA is whether it is a prognostic or therapeutic procedure.

Although there is no consensus regarding this issue, LA is performed for prognostic purposes in many gynecologic malignancies. In other words, the primary goal of LA is to identify the most effective adjuvant treatment modalities.

LA or lymph node dissection (LND) is an important part of surgical management of ovarian cancer. This procedure is mainly performed for prognostic purposes and as a step of surgical staging especially in patients with early-stage ovarian cancer. LND of bulky lymph nodes has a therapeutic impact in advanced stage disease. So, LA will be discussed in early and advanced staged disease in this chapter, separately.

Lymphadenectomy in Early-Stage Ovarian Cancer

The Rate of Lymphatic Metastasis

The ovarian cancer staging systems used by FIGO and the American Joint Committee on Cancer (AJCC) are the same and Stage I-II ovarian cancer are classified as early-stage ovarian cancer (EOC) based on AJCC. In early-stage disease, cancer is limited in the ovary or ovaries or fallopian tubes without involving nearby lymph nodes. Tumors involving ovaries, tubes and other pelvic organs (rectum and bladder) without spreading pelvic nodes is also accepted in early-stage disease.

* Corresponding Author's Email: demirkiranfuat@gmail.com.

In: Ovarian Cancer
Editors: Christos Iavazzo, Alexandros Fotiou and John Spiliotis
ISBN: 979-8-88697-633-5

In EOC, the rates of nodal involvement change, based on sub-stage and histological sub-groups. A review of 14 retrospective studies including 574 cases with macroscopic Stage I-II ovarian cancer published in 2011 analyzed the relation between nodal involvement rates and sub-stage and tumor histology in patients with EOC [1]. In the whole group, lymph node metastases were found in an average of 14.3% of cases (2.9% in only a pelvic lymph node, 7.1% in only a para-aortic lymph node, and 4.3% in both pelvic and para-aortic lymph nodes) [1]. According to histological sub-groups, the highest and lowest involvement rates were detected in serous (23.3%) and mucinous (2.6%) types, respectively. In patients with unilateral tumor, the incidence of contralateral nodal metastases was 16% in pelvic and 18% in the para-aortic region. If rates of lymph node metastasis is evaluated for grade and histological sub-type in Stage I disease, it is shown that rates of nodal metastasis are 2.9%, 13.8% and 20% in Grade I, II and III tumors respectively. According to histological subtype, the rate of nodal metastasizes are 19.33% for serous and 1.9% for mucinous type. The histopathological factors affecting the rates of nodal metastases were shown in a modified table from this study.

With these findings, the authors concluded that the rate of nodal involvement was at a remarkable level and all patients with EOC cancer, except those with mucinous disease, should undergo a comprehensive pelvic and paraaortic lymphadenectomy. In fact, there are two sub-types of primary mucinous ovarian cancers, which are expansive and infiltrative. The probability of nodal involvement in infiltrative mucinous ovarian tumors is 17-30%, and pelvic-paraaortic LA should be performed in this group of mucinous tumors regardless of the stage. On the other hand, the probability of nodal involvement in expansive mucinous ovarian tumors is extremely low and LA may not be performed in patients with expansive mucinous ovarian cancer.

A study including 290 patients published in 2017 evaluated the prevalence of pelvic and para-aortic nodal involvement rate in EOC [2]. Median numbers of removed pelvic and para-aortic node were 21(1-70) and 18(2-53), respectively. 42 out of 290 (14.5%) patients had positive nodes and all patients with a positive node had a positive para-aortic node. So, the rate of positive para-aortic nod was 14.5% as well. 22 out of 290 (7.6%) cases had positive pelvic nodes. It was found that the nodal involvement rates were 18.9%, 2.7%, 13.8%, 17.4%, 7.3% and 20.8% in patients with high-grade serous, low-grade-serous, endometrioid G1, endometrioid G2&3, clear cell and undifferentiated histology when separated by histological sub-types. The rate of patients having para-aortic nodal involvement with negative pelvic node was 7% in the whole group. However, these rates were 7%, 0%, 9%, 11%, 2% and 13% in high-grade serous, low-grade-serous, endometrioid G1, endometrioid G2&3, clear cell and undifferentiated sub-groups. Also, the authors reported that high-grade serous histology and bilateral tumor are associated with increased risk of nodal involvement.

Table 1. Lymphatic metastases (LM) rates in early-stage cases (modified from [1])

Early stage OC	LM	Histologic type	LM	Grade	LM
Whole group	%14	serous	%23	I	%4
Distribution of LSs		Clear-cell	%14	II	%16
Pelvic	%20	Endometrioid	%6, 5	III	%20
Paraaortic	%50	Mucinous	%2, 6		
Pelvic-paraaortic	%30	Indifferentiated	%29		

Prognostic and Therapeutic Effects of Lymphadenectomy

There are a few randomized and large volume studies evaluating prognostic or therapeutic effects of systematic lymphadenectomy in the management of early stage EOC. While some studies include the patients who had undergone pelvic LA, other included those that underwent pelvic and paraaortic LA. There are also significant disparities in the number of lymph nodes that have been retrieved..

A randomized study (EORTC-ACTION) designed to evaluate the effect of chemotherapy on oncological outcomes in EOC was published in 2003 [3]. 448 patients (IA–IB, grade 1–3, IC, IIA and all I-IIA clear cell) were included in this study. There was no statistically significant difference found in overall survival (OS) between adjuvant chemotherapy and no adjuvant chemotherapy arm but disease-free survival (DFS) was better in the adjuvant chemotherapy group (p:0.02). In multivariant analysis, LA, grade and histological type were found to be independent prognostic factors for DFS and OS. The non-adjuvant chemotherapy group (the group that did not receive adjuvant chemotherapy) was divided into three groups: those who were not staging, those who had only peritoneal staging, and those who had peritoneal-retroperitoneal staging (full staging), the group with full staging had the best survival rates. However, it was determined that the prognostic importance of complete staging decreased in the group receiving adjuvant chemotherapy. The long-term results of the EORTC-ACTION (2003) study were published in 2010 [4]. Accordingly, it was found that chemotherapy did not affect survival in the whole groups but increased DFS. On the other hand, chemotherapy had no effect on both DFS and OS in the fully staged group, while it greatly improved DFS and OS in the un-staged group. From another perspective, it may be said that LA is not effective in patients receiving adjuvant chemotherapy in early-stage ovarian cancer.

The first and the only randomized study published in 2006 evaluated therapeutic efficacy of systematic LA by randomizing 268 cases with macroscopically EOC in two arms (systematic LA arm vs lymphatic sampling arm) [5]. The median number of removed pelvic and para-aortic was 47 in systematic LA arm and 5 in lymphatic sampling arm, and the rate positive nodes was 22% in systematic and 9% in sampling arm. At a median follow-up of 87.8 months, 5-year PFS and OS were 78% and 84% in systematic LA arm compared to 71% and 82% in the sample. These differences were not statistically significant. However, in a recent meta-analysis including 1 RCT (n: 268) 4 cohort studies (n: 14,228) Chiyoda et al. reported that lymphadenectomy improved OS(HR:0.74), but not PFS (HR:0,71) in patients having EOC [6].

The most interesting study addressing the therapeutic efficiency of LA in patients with EOC was published recently [7]. This multi-center retrospective cohort study compared women with macroscopically EOC who underwent systematic bilateral pelvic and para-aortic lymphadenectomy (defined as ≥20 lymph nodes) versus patients with no LA or node sampling. Patients with bulky nodes found in the CT scan and those without complete intra-peritoneal surgical staging were excluded and only patients who were subjected to a minimum of three cycles of platinum-based adjuvant chemotherapy were included in this study. The whole group consisted of 639 patients with stage Ia-IIIa1 disease (360 of them had comprehensive LA, 150 of them had node sampling and 129 of them no LA. At the median 63 months, 5-year DFS was 76.6% in the whole group (79.7%, 76.5% and 68.3% in those systematic LA, node sampling and no LS groups, respectively (p:0.006) (see figure at: https://ijgc.bmj.com/content/30/Suppl_3/A19). However, there were no significant differences between the systematic and sampling groups at DFS. In the meantime, authors noted no significant difference detected for 5-year OS among 3 groups (92.3% versus 94.5% versus 89.8%, respectively) (p:165).

According to the outcomes of this study, LA does not affect OS in patients with IA-IIIA ovarian cancer receiving adjuvant chemotherapy, however systematic LA and node sampling achieve DFS advantage compared to no LA.

A retrospective study published in 2021 analyzed the therapeutic effect of LA on OS and DFS in 400 patients with EOC (81 not undergone LA, 319 undergone LA) [8]. In the LA group, the median number of retrieved lymph nodes was 25 (21 pelvic and 4 paraaortic). 86% of patients in the no LA group and 91% percent of patients in the LA group were subjected to adjuvant chemotherapy. The 5-year PFS and OS were 83% and 93% in the no LA group compared to 82% and 91% in LA group, respectively ($p > 0.05$). According to these results, LA has no benefit on PFS and OS in EOC and an increased risk of adverse events. A low volume study analyzed the effectiveness of LA on oncological results in three groups. These groups consisted of patients who underwent no LA or lymph node sampling (less than 10 pelvic nodes), those who underwent pelvic LA (more than 10 pelvic nodes) and those who underwent systematic LA (more than 10 pelvic and 5 para-aortic) [9]. In conclusion, the authors reported that systematic LA might be omitted in patients with apparent early-stage low-grade mucinous and endometrioid ovarian cancer since it did not significantly improve prognosis and increased surgical risk.

Some studies evaluated the impact of the number of retrieved lymph nodes in the oncological outcome. For example, a study published in 2018 reported that to remove more than 12 nodes from the pelvis had a more positive oncological outcome compared to less than 12 nodes [10]. Another study published in 2021investigated the same interaction in 184 EOC cases [11]. In this study, the median removed node count was 29 and 9 in pelvic and para-aortic region. Authors found that para- aortic node number (<10 vs ≥ 10) was independently and significantly associated with PFS and OS in multivariate analyses.

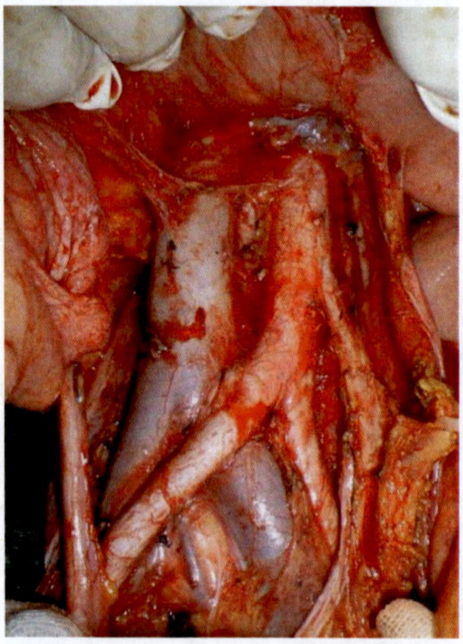

Figure 1. Paraaortic lymphadenectomy in patients with early-stage ovarian cancer.

No doubt, LA is one of the important parts of surgical staging of EOC. Societies and organizations such as ESGO and GOG recommend that "bilateral pelvic and para-aortic node dissection up to the level of the left renal vein (with the exception of stage I expansible-type mucinous adenocarcinomas) should be performed in all patients with macroscopically EOC (grade B) [12]. According to the National Comprehensive Cancer Network (NCCN) Guidelines "Para-aortic lymph node dissection should be performed by stripping the nodal tissue from the vena cava and the aorta bilaterally to at least the level of the inferior mesenteric artery and preferably to the level of the renal vessels" [13]. The therapeutic effect of LA on DFS and OS is open to discussion. Some studies have reported that there is a survival benefit of systematic LA in patients especially receiving adjuvant therapy. A few retrospective studies demonstrated the benefit of LA in oncological outcomes in patients with an increased number of removed lymph nodes. The general acceptance including our opinion, is that LA is a prognostic procedure which determines the necessity of adjuvant treatment and that it is an important part of surgical staging of EOC. In conclusion, systematic pelvic and para-aortic LA should be performed in all the patients with macroscopic EOC with the exception of stage I expansible-type mucinous cancer (Figure 1).

Lymphadenectomy in Advanced Staged Ovarian Cancer

Nearly 75-80% of women with ovarian cancer are in advanced stages of the disease. In contrast to early stage disease, Lymphadenectomy (LA) may not be a part of surgical staging in patients with advanced stage ovarian cancer. Dissection of bulky lymph node is a therapeutic procedure in this group of patients. It is well-known that primary cytoreductive surgery with optimal cytoreduction is the most effective treatment of advance staged ovarian cancer. Therefore, a bulky lymph node dissection is necessary to achieve optimal cytoreduction in some patients. The prognostic role of LA is highly discussible in advanced stage disease.

In this chapter, the prognostic and therapeutic role of LA will be discussed in primary cytoreductive surgery.

The Rate of Lymphatic Metastasis

The rate of pelvic, paraaortic and pelvic-para-aortic nodal involvement is high in patients with advanced stage ovarian cancer. In some studies, lymph node metastasis has been reported between 43% and 55.7% during systematic lymphadenectomy performed in patients [14, 15, 25]. Some other studies reported that when lymphadenectomy was performed in advanced stage ovarian cancer, the likelihood of the detection of metastatic lymph node was around 60% in literature [16, 17].

The Role of Prognostic and Therapeutic Effect in Primary Cytoreduction

Since it was discovered that the size of the postoperative residual tumor is a significant prognostic factor, primary cytoreductive surgery (removal of as much of the tumor as possible during the initial operation, as well as resection of the bulky lymph nodes) has become an important part of the treatment of advanced stage ovarian cancer. However, whether systematic lymphadenectomy should be included in maximal cytoreductive surgery is still debatable. In advanced ovarian cancer, removal bulky nodes to achieve complete CR is a standard procedure, but unlike in early ovarian cancer, staging for clinically negative nodes is highly discussible because the histologic lymph node status has no bearing on the systemic treatment options (Figure 2, 3).

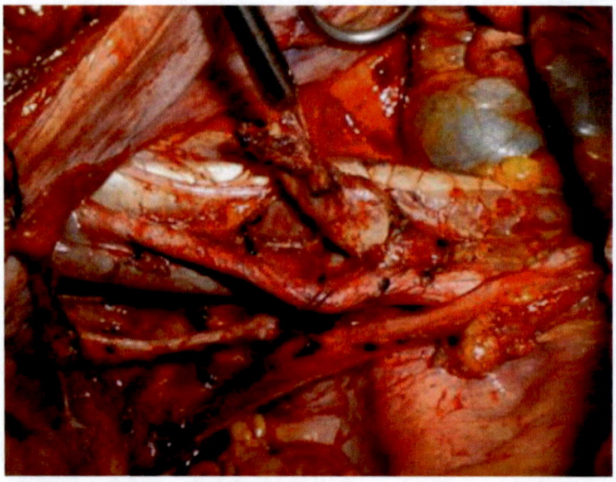

Figure 2. Bulky lymph nodes at aortic bifurcation.

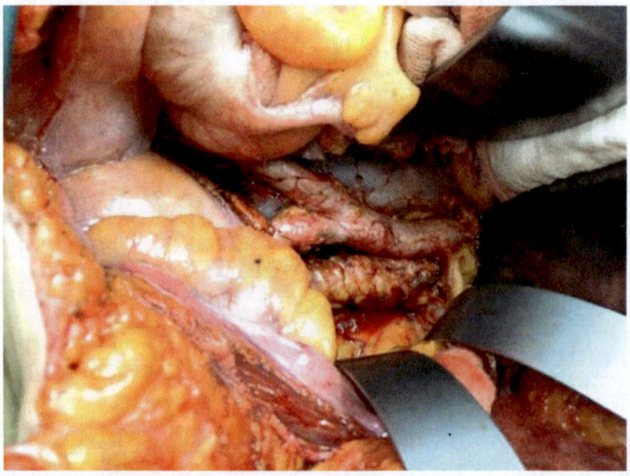

Figure 3. Bulky lymph node along the lateral side of the aorta.

One of the first studies published in 1995 reported that in patients with advanced ovarian cancer, up to 41% had macroscopic lymph node involvement during primary surgical exploration, so that lymph node resection should be a part of primary surgery to achieve optimal cytoreduction [18]. Additionally, some retrospective studies determined that LA has a positive effect on survival in advanced staged ovarian cancer, and the increase in survival becomes more pronounced as the number of lymph nodes are removed [19, 20].

The first prospective randomized study examining the effectiveness of systematic pelvic and para-aortic LA on PFS an OS in patients with advanced stage ovarian cancer (IIIB-IV) was published by Panici et al. in 2005 [21]. In this trial, oncological outcomes of patients (n:216) undergoing systematic LA compared with patients(n:211) resected only bulky nodes. Complete cytoreduction rate was nearly equal (37% vs 37.4) in two arms and the rates of $\leq$1 cm residual disease were 62.2% in LA group and 55.9% in no systematic LA group. Optimal cytoreduction rate was 96% in the entire group. The median number of removed pelvic, aortic and pelvic-aortic lymph node was 28, 23, 51 in study arm and 1,1 and 4 in the control arm. The complication rate was much greater in the LA arm due to lymphocytes and lymphedema. With a median survival of 68 months, it was reported in this study that systematic LA significantly increased PFS (29 months vs 22 months) in the group with a residue $\leq$1 cm but did not affect the OS. The authors concluded that systematic pelvic and paraaortic LA did not affect OS in patients with optimal cytoreduction (<1 cm residual disease). The main problem related to this study was that there was no subgroup analysis for the complete(R0) cytoreduction group. Another randomized study addressing the role of systematic LA on oncological outcome was published by du Bois in 2010 [22]. Data analyzed in this study was obtained from the three prospectively randomized phase III trials in advanced epithelial ovarian cancer coordinated and performed by the Arbeitsgemeinschaft Gynaekologische Onkologie Stu-diengruppe Ovarialkarzinom. The study included a total of 1,942 patients with advanced stage ovarian cancer (IIB-IV), including 966 patients with no residual disease and 946 patients with 1-10 mm residual disease. The patients were classified into three groups according to LA status. These were no LA group, incomplete LA group (pelvic or para-aortic) and systematic pelvic and paraaortic group. Systematic pelvic and paraaortic LA was performed in 39% of patients in R0 residual group and 24% of patients in 1-10 mm residual group. The median OS is 103 and 39 months in R0 and 1-10 mm residual disease groups, in median observation period of 56 months, respectively. In the R0 group, the 5-year survival was found to be 59% in those who did not undergo LA, and 67% in those who did systematic any LA (p:0.016). A comparison of incomplete LA with systematic pelvic and paraaortic LA revealed no statistically significant difference (68% vs 67%). Same ratios were 29% and 32% in patients with 1-10 mm residual group for no LA and any LA (p:0.06). Also there were no significant differences in patients with 1-10 mm residual group between any LA and systematic pelvic and paraaortic LA for 5-year survival (32% vs 32%). In the same study, it was observed that LA significantly affected survival in the R0 residual group in patients without pre-intraoperative suspicious lymph nodes (p:0.0081). On the other hand, it was found that LA did not increase survival in patients with 1-10 mm residuals without suspicious nodes, but increased survival in patients with suspicious nodes. With these findings, the researchers concluded that lymphadenectomy had a survival advantage in patients with complete cytoreduction and should be performed in advanced stage ovarian cancers (IIB-IV), especially in this group of patients.

A meta-analysis including 14 relevant studies with 3,488 patients was published by Jingwei G et al. in 2015 [23]. In this meta-analysis, the therapeutic effect of lymphadenectomy was compared between those of systematic LA and no LA groups in patients with advanced staged ovarian cancer, A subgroup analysis of this study showed that systematic LA significantly increased the OS compared to no systematic LA in patients with advanced stage (III-IV) ovarian cancer, but not in early-stage ovarian cancer.

Zhou et al. investigated the effect of lymphadenectomy on the survival outcomes of patients with advanced (IIIC-IV) epithelial ovarian cancer and all data was collected from the Surveillance, Epidemiology, and End Results (SEER) database records according to residual disease status [24]. They analyzed the outcomes of 3048 patients and divided them into four groups based on their LA status as no lymphadenectomy group (0 LN), 1–10 LNs removed group, 11–20 LNs removed group, and >20 LNs removed group. A total of 1904/3048 (62.5%) patients underwent lymphadenectomy and 1355 (71%) them had nodal metastasis. According to residual disease size, the patients were divided into the following three classifications: no residual tumor; residual tumor ≤1 cm; and residual tumor >1 cm. More than a half of patients had 1-10 retrieved lymph nodes, and there was no significant relation between rate of nodal metastasis and residual tumor size in the LA group. In the whole group, LA had a survival advantage compared to those of no LA. However, in the subgroup analysis, authors reported that patients with 1–10 LNs removed had similar survival rates compared to patients with non-LA group and the patients with >10 lymph nodes removed had better survival rates compared with non-lymphadenectomy and 1–10 lymph nodes removed groups. In this study, there was only a significant association between LA and survival in patients with no gross residual tumor. In contrast, there was no survival benefit of the extent of lymphadenectomy in the residual tumor ≤1 cm or >1 cm. In summary, their results indicated that the survival benefit of LA was related to residual tumor size.

Until this time, the most important study evaluating the effectiveness of systematic pelvic and paraaortic LA in advanced stage ovarian cancer was called the LION study and it was published in 2019 [25]. This well-designed prospective randomized 647 patients with stage IIB-IV in two groups compared to those of systematic LA (323 patients) and those of (234) no LA. All patients included in this study had undergone macroscopically complete resection and had normal lymph nodes both before and during surgery. The median number of resected lymph nodes was 57 (35 pelvic and 22 paraaortic nodes) and the rate of nodal metastasis was 55.7% in the lymphadenectomy group. Nearly half of patients had undergone gastrointestinal tract resection in both groups. In the meantime, the rate of splenectomy, partial hepatic-pancreatic resection and stoma placement were 19%, 11% and 10% in LA group, respectively. Same ratios were 17%, 11% and 7% in no LA group. The edition of LA to the cytoreductive surgery had significantly affected the median duration of surgery, median blood loss, the percentage of patients with postoperative admission to an intermediate or intensive care unit, the percentage of relaparotomy for complications and percentage of death. Also, lymphedema and lymphocyte formation were seen in 11% of the LA group. In the whole group, the median progression-free and overall survival rates were 25.5 months and 67.2 months, respectively. The median PFS was 25 months in both groups, and the median overall survival was 65.5 months in the LA group and 69.2 months in the no LA group (P:0.65). The authors concluded that systematic pelvic and paraaortic lymphadenectomy was not associated with better outcomes than no lymphadenectomy for PFS and OS in patients with macroscopically complete resection of advanced ovarian cancer and clinically negative lymph nodes. Also, they concluded that LA increased significantly some complications rate. With the results of this randomized study, it could be said that there was no beneficial role of systematic LA in patients achieving complete resection in advanced ovarian cancer. Only bulky lymph nodes detected intraoperatively and postoperatively should be removed..

There were two meta-analyses published after the LION trial in 2020. One of them evaluated the effect of LA on oncologic outcomes in 2425 patients (IIB-IV ovarian cancer) achieving <1cm residual disease. In this study, it was determined that systematic LA did not affect PFS in the <1 cm residual disease group, but it had a statistically significant positive effect on survival [26]. However, a subgroup analysis showed that systematic LA did not affect PFS and survival in the complete(R0) cytoreduction group. Another study published in the same year analyzed the effectiveness of systematic lymphadenectomy in patients treated with optimal cytoreduction for ovarian cancer [27]. A total of 1607 patients with ovarian cancer (stage I-IV) were included in the meta-analysis. Authors reported that systematic LA had no benefit on PFS and OS compared to unsystematic LA in patients with achieving optimal cytoreduction.

It is quite clear that the removal of bulky lymph nodes should be a part of an attempt to achieve maximum cytoreduction. In addition, according to NCCN Guidelines "Suspicious and/or enlarged nodes should be respected in patients with advanced stage ovarian cancer. It can be said that since the LION trial, there was a paradigm shift from systematic lymphadenectomy to removing bulky lymph nodes. The main dilemma is what was the definition of suspicious lymph nodes. Unfortunately, generally, it is a subjective decision. In conclusion, further studies and molecular innovations are still needed for this subject to be more certain.

References

[1] Kleppe M, Wang T, Van Gorp T, Slangen BF, Kruse AJ, Kruitwagen RF. Lymph node metastasis in stages I and II ovarian cancer: a review. *Gynecol Oncol.* 2011 Dec;123(3):610-4.

[2] Bogani G, Tagliabue E, Ditto A, Signorelli M, Martinelli F, Casarin J, Chiappa V, Dondi G, Leone Roberti Maggiore U, Scaffa C, Borghi C, Montanelli L, Lorusso D, Raspagliesi F. Assessing the risk of pelvic and para-aortic nodal involvement in apparent early-stage ovarian cancer: A predictors- and nomogram-based analyses. *Gynecol Oncol*. 2017 Oct;147(1):61-65.

[3] Trimbos JB, Vergote I, Bolis G, Vermorken JB, Mangioni C, Madronal C, Franchi M, Tateo S, Zanetta G, Scarfone G, Giurgea L, Timmers P, Coens C, Pecorelli S; EORTC-ACTION collaborators. European Organisation for Research and Treatment of Cancer-Adjuvant ChemoTherapy in Ovarian Neoplasm. Impact of adjuvant chemotherapy and surgical staging in early-stage ovarian carcinoma: European Organisation for Research and Treatment of Cancer-Adjuvant ChemoTherapy in Ovarian Neoplasm trial. *J Natl Cancer Inst*. 2003 Jan 15;95(2):113-25.

[4] Trimbos B, Timmers P, Pecorelli S, Coens C, Ven K, van der Burg M, Casado A. Surgical staging and treatment of early ovarian cancer: long-term analysis from a randomized trial. *J Natl Cancer Inst*. 2010 Jul 7;102(13):982-7.

[5] Maggioni A, Benedetti Panici P, Dell'Anna T, Landoni F, Lissoni A, Pellegrino A, Rossi RS, Chiari S, Campagnutta E, Greggi S, Angioli R, Manci N, Calcagno M, Scambia G, Fossati R, Floriani I, Torri V, Grassi R, Mangioni C. Randomised study of systematic lymphadenectomy in patients with epithelial ovarian cancer macroscopically confined to the pelvis. *Br J Cancer*. 2006 Sep 18;95(6):699-704.

[6] Chiyoda T, Sakurai M, Satoh T, Nagase S, Mikami M, Katabuchi H, Aoki D. Lymphadenectomy for primary ovarian cancer: a systematic review and meta-analysis. *J Gynecol Oncol*. 2020 Sep;31(5):e67.

[7] Bizzarri N, du Bois A, Fruscio R, De Felice F, De Iaco P, Casarin J, Vizza E, Chiantera V, Corrado G, Cianci S, Magni S, Ferrari D, Giuliani D, Harter P, Ataseven B, Bommert M, Perrone AM, Scambia G, Fagotti A. Is there any therapeutic role of pelvic and para-aortic lymphadenectomy in apparent early stage epithelial ovarian cancer? *Gynecol Oncol*. 2021 Jan;160(1):56-63.

[8] Deng T, Huang Q, Wan T, Luo X, Feng Y, Huang H, Liu J. The impact of lymph node dissection on survival in patients with clinical early-stage ovarian cancer. *J Gynecol Oncol*. 2021 May;32(3):e40.

[9] Chen J, Yin J, Li Y, Gu Y, Wang W, Shan Y, Wang YX, Qin M, Cai Y, Jin Y, Pan L. Systematic Lymph Node Dissection May Be Abolished in Patients With Apparent Early-Stage Low-Grade Mucinous and Endometrioid Epithelial Ovarian Cancer. *Front Oncol*. 2021 Sep 6;11:705720.

[10] Matsuo K, Machida H, Mariani A, Mandelbaum RS, Glaser GE, Gostout BS, Roman LD, Wright JD. Adequate pelvic lymphadenectomy and survival of women with early-stage epithelial ovarian cancer. *J Gynecol Oncol*. 2018 Sep;29(5):e69.

[11] Günakan E, Akıllı H, Kara AT, Altundağ Ö, Haberal AN, Meydanlı MM, Ayhan A. Survival impact of number of removed para-aortic lymph nodes in stage I epithelial ovarian cancer. *Arch Gynecol* Obstet. 2021 Aug 19.

[12] Ledermann JA, Raja FA, Fotopoulou C, Gonzalez-Martin A, Colombo N, Sessa C; ESMO Guidelines Working Group. Newly diagnosed and relapsed epithelial ovarian carcinoma: ESMO Clinical Practice Guidelines for diagnosis, treatment and follow-up. *Ann Oncol.* 2013 Oct;24 Suppl 6:vi24-32.

[13] Armstrong DK, Alvarez RD, Bakkum-Gamez JN, Barroilhet L, Behbakht K, Berchuck A, Chen LM, Cristea M, DeRosa M, Eisenhauer EL, Gershenson DM, Gray HJ, Grisham R, Hakam A, Jain A, Karam A, Konecny GE, Leath CA, Liu J, Mahdi H, Martin L, Matei D, McHale M, McLean K, Miller DS, O'Malley DM, Percac-Lima S, Ratner E, Remmenga SW, Vargas R, Werner TL, Zsiros E, Burns JL, Engh AM. Ovarian Cancer, Version 2. 2020, NCCN Clinical Practice Guidelines in Oncology. *J Natl Compr Canc Netw*. 2021 Feb 2;19(2):191-226.

[14] Harter P, Gnauert K, Hils R, et al. Pattern and clinical predictors of lymph node metastases in epithelial ovarian cancer. *Int J Gynecol Cancer* 2007;17:1238-44.

[15] Morice P, Joulie F, Cammatte S, et al. Lymph node Involvement in epithelial ovarian cancer: Analysis of 276 pelvic and paraaortic lymphadenectomies and surgical implications. *J Am Coll Surg* 2003;197:198-205.

[16] Zhou J, Zhang WW, Zhang QH, et al. The effect of lymphadenec- tomy in advanced ovarian cancer according to residual tumor status: A population-based study. *Int J Surg*. 2018; 52: 11–15.

[17] Eoh KJ, Lee JY, Yoon JW, et al. Role of systematic lymphadenectomy as part of primary debulking surgery for optimally cytoreduced advanced ovarian cancer: Reappraisal in the era of radical surgery. *Oncotarget*. 2017; 8(23): 37807–37816.

[18] Spirtos N, Gross G, Freddo J, et al. Cytoreductive surgery in advanced epithelial cancer of the ovary: the impact of aortic and pelvic lymphadenectomy. *Gynecol Oncol* 1995;56:345-52.

[19] di Re F, Baiocchi G, Fontanelli R, et al. Systematic pelvic and paraaortic lymph- adenectomy for advanced ovarian cancer: prognostic significance of node metasta- ses. *Gynecol Oncol* 1996;62:360-5.

[20] Scarabelli C, Gallo A, Visentin MC, Canzonieri V, Carbone A, Zarrelli A. Sys- tematic pelvic and para-aortic lymphade- nectomy in advanced ovarian cancer pa- tients with no residual intraperitoneal disease. *Int J Gynecol Cancer* 1997;7:18- 26.

[21] Panici PB, Maggioni A, Hacker N, Landoni F, Ackermann S, Campagnutta E, Tamussino K, Winter R, Pellegrino A, Greggi S, Angioli R, Manci N, Scambia G, Dell'Anna T, Fossati R, Floriani I, Rossi RS, Grassi R, Favalli G, Raspagliesi F, Giannarelli D, Martella L, Mangioni C. Systematic aortic and pelvic lymphadenectomy versus resection of bulky nodes only in optimally debulked advanced ovarian cancer: a randomized clinical trial. *J Natl Cancer Inst*. 2005 Apr 20;97(8):560-6.

[22] du Bois A, Reuss A, Harter P, Pujade-Lauraine E, Ray-Coquard I, Pfisterer J; Arbeitsgemeinschaft Gynaekologische Onkologie Studiengruppe Ovarialkarzinom; Groupe d'Investigateurs Nationaux pour l'Etude des Cancers Ovariens. Potential role of lymphadenectomy in advanced ovarian cancer: a combined exploratory analysis of three prospectively randomized phase III multicenter trials. *J Clin Oncol*. 2010 Apr 1;28(10):1733-9.

[23] Gao J, Yang X, Zhang Y. Systematic lymphadenectomy in the treatment of epithelial ovarian cancer: a meta-analysis of multiple epidemiology studies. *Jpn J Clin Oncol*. 2015 Jan;45(1):49-60.

[24] Zhou J, Zhang WW, Zhang QH, He ZY, Sun JY, Chen QH, Wu SG. The effect of lymphadenectomy in advanced ovarian cancer according to residual tumor status: A population-based study. *Int J Surg*. 2018 Apr;52:11-15.

[25] Harter P, Sehouli J, Lorusso D, Reuss A, Vergote I, Marth C, Kim JW, Raspagliesi F, Lampe B, Aletti G, Meier W, Cibula D, Mustea A, Mahner S, Runnebaum IB, Schmalfeldt B, Burges A, Kimmig R, Scambia G, Greggi S, Hilpert F, Hasenburg A, Hillemanns P, Giorda G, von Leffern I, Schade-Brittinger C, Wagner U, du Bois A. A Randomized Trial of Lymphadenectomy in Patients with Advanced Ovarian Neoplasms. *N Engl J Med*. 2019 Feb 28;380(9):822-832.

[26] Wang Y, Ren F, Song Z, Wang X, Zhang C, Ouyang L. Prognostic Significance of Systematic Lymphadenectomy in Patients With Optimally Debulked Advanced Ovarian Cancer: A Meta-Analysis. *Front Oncol*. 2020 Feb 11;10:86.

[27] Lin Q, Liu W, Xu S, Li J, Tong J. The value of systematic lymphadenectomy during debulking surgery in the treatment of ovarian cancer: a meta-analysis of randomized controlled trials. *J Ovarian Res*. 2020 May 8;13(1):56.

Chapter 21

Serous Papillary Primary Peritoneal Carcinoma

Marcello Deraco[1,*], MD
Navinakathiresu Muthukumarasamy[2], MD
Dario Baratti[1], MD, Marcello Guaglio[1], MD
and Shigeki Kusamura[1], MD, PhD
[1]Peritoneal Surface Malignacies Unit, Fondazione IRCCS Istituto Nazionale dei Tumori, Milan, Italy
[2]ESPSO Fellow from Hospital Selayang, Lebuhraya Selayang-Kepong, Batu Caves,
Selangor Malaysia Hospital, Selayang, Selagor, Malaysia

Introduction

Previously identified as Cancer of Unknown Primary (CUP), Serous Papillary Primary Peritoneal Carcinoma (SPPC) has been distinguished from patients with unknown primaries with multiple visceral metastases from the histological, molecular, therapeutic, and prognostic standpoints [1]. SPPC is a rare malignancy arising from the peritoneal epithelium, and it was first reported by Swerdlow in 1959 [2]. SPPC rarely involves the ovaries. When this happens, it usually affects the surface. Serous carcinomas are the most common epithelial ovarian cancer subtype with a predilection for peritoneal spread. Hence serous carcinoma is a common pathological diagnosis in patients with peritoneal metastases [3]. There is a clinicopathological similarity between ovarian, tubal, and peritoneal serous carcinomas, however these different cancers should be distinguished as separate entities because of their differing management and prognostic implications [4-6].

Incidence: the estimated incidence of SSPC is unclear but is reported to be 10-18% in a series of epithelial ovarian carcinoma [7]. It has also been reported that the incidence is 6.78 cases per 1,000,000 individuals in the United States [8]. The peak incidence of epithelial ovarian carcinoma (EOC) has been reported at age 50-75, with a median age of 63 years [9]. The incidence of patients with fallopian tube cancer is in the range of 60–74 years [10]. The age-specific peak incidence of SPPC is 75–79 years. Therefore SPPC is most commonly seen in older women than tubal-ovarian carcinoma [11].

* Corresponding Author's Email: info@marcelloderaco.com.

In: Ovarian Cancer
Editors: Christos Iavazzo, Alexandros Fotiou and John Spiliotis
ISBN: 979-8-88697-633-5

Risk factors: female gender, obesity, elderly patients, and post-menopausal women have been commonly identified in patients with SPPC [12]. However, there have rarely been any reported cases in males [13].

BRCA1/2 germline mutations have been reported in 15.8–40.9% and are commonly associated with a higher prevalence of a multifocal tumor. For patients with germline BRCA mutations, the lifetime risk of SPPC is 1.3%. Prophylactic bilateral salpingo-oophorectomy does not seem to reduce the risk of SPPC, which may occur at intervals reaching 12–84 months. Moreover, it is not associated with BRCA mutation in men in the cases reported [14]. Inactivation of Mismatch Repair genes (MMR) leads to the accumulation of mutations, leading to microsatellite instability. MSI was reported to be in 3.8–7% of cases with SPPC, which is higher than in ovarian cancer [15].

Pathogenesis: SPPC pathogenesis can be explained by the theory of mesothelial cells retaining their 'differentiating potential'. The same embryonal mesoderm forms the germinal epithelium of ovaries and mesothelial cells of the peritoneum, which explains the resemblance between the two tumors.

There are several theories to explain the development of SPPC. Malignant transformation of embryonic germ cells derived from Mullerian ducts that remain along the gonadal embryonic pathway is one of the pathways that lead to SPPC. Another theory is that carcinogenesis takes place in the coelomic epithelium which lines the abdominal cavity [16].

The oncogenic stimulus occurs when there is the loss of heterozygosity at p53 or BRCA1, chromosome X inactivation and HER2/neu overexpression seen in extraovarian Mullerian adenocarcinoma [17].

The pathogenesis of extraovarian SPPC is also explained by the multifocal origin of the tumor. However, different patterns of inactivation result in tumors that have independent sites of development. Gu et al. did a study regarding the clonality of peritoneal and ovarian cancer. 54% of patients showed non-random inactivation, and most had different patterns [18].

In the last decade, there was some evidence that suggests that most extrauterine high-grade serous carcinomas originate from the fimbriated end of the fallopian tubes. Serous tubal intraepithelial carcinoma (STIC) is a precursor lesion of the fallopian tubes that have been found in many cases of both primary ovarian and SPPC. Therefore STIC is considered to be the source of a significant proportion of SPPC which is in approximately 45%-56% of cases. These tumor cells migrate to the peritoneum via tumor cell sheddings which then disseminate in the peritoneal cavity or through hematogenous spread with affinity to implant on the omentum [19].

There are some fundamental differences in the tumorigenesis and pathogenetic presentation between SPPC and EOC. Firstly, SPPC tends to show a more diffuse micronodular pattern of spread in the omentum and peritoneal surfaces suggesting that SPPC is a more aggressive malignancy and is more likely to have widespread disease at the same stages of ovarian cancer. Different genetic events take place at different peritoneal sites in the same patient, explaining the multifocality of SPPC. This means that the tumor cells present at multiple peritoneal sites within the same patient may have a different genetic make-up and clonality and may have the ability to give rise to an independent primary tumor at multiple anatomic sites, unlike ovarian cancer which is unifocal. This inherent multifocality and polyclonality of SPPC, therefore, necessitate a more extensive surgery. In order to improve the rates of optimal cytoreduction, neoadjuvant chemotherapy (NACT) has been recommended for SPPC and EOC. Another feature identified showed that SPPC has significantly lower expression of estrogen and progesterone receptor positivity and increased ki-67 expression than ovarian carcinomas [20-24].

Clinical Features

SPPC is commonly diagnosed following incidental symptoms due to massive ascites in advanced stages. As a result, non-specific symptoms like abdominal discomfort with bloating, distension, breathlessness, nausea, indigestion, anorexia, weight loss, lethargy, constipation, and abdominal or back pain can occur. Upon clinical examination, there may be a palpable abdominal mass and ascites [26, 29]. Occasionally, mesothelium involvement in the absence of primary is seen as an incidental finding in laparotomy or for a post mortem to identify the cause of death.

Peritoneal carcinomatosis usually presents symptoms from the primary tumor and non-specific symptoms in patients with a primary from the peritoneum itself. The secondary metastatic deposits may range from microscopic involvement to nodules to large, infiltrating disease. More extensive involvement and location of involvement determine the severity of the symptoms. Progression of both primary and secondary tumors can exert pressure effects, leading to mechanical obstruction to the intestine or urinary tract.

Diagnosis

SPPC shares a similar clinical presentation with EOC with elevated levels of CA125 and radiological findings such as diffuse peritoneal disease, omental nodules or cake, and ascites. The absence of a pelvic mass may suggest the diagnosis of SPPC. The two tumors are indistinguishable during a pathological examination. A morphological analysis of SPPC shows a papillary growth pattern of the tumor with a poorly differentiated structure, atypical cells with large nuclei and prominent nucleoli, and the presence of calcifications called psammoma bodies [25]. The immunohistochemistry expression of SPPC includes CK7(+), S-100(+), CA125 (+), CK20(-), ER/PR (+/-) and CEA (-) [26]. PAX-8 and Claudin-4 are reactive in SPPC and distinguish SPPC from epithelioid peritoneal mesothelioma, especially in the tubule-papillary variant [27]. To distinguish SPPC from papillary serous adenocarcinoma of the ovary, the Gynecology Oncology Group (GOG) developed specific criteria to diagnose SPPC when [28]:

1. Ovaries are absent, normal-sized, or enlarged due to a benign mass;
2. Extraovarian involvement is more significant than involvement of ovarian surface;
3. Ovarian involvement is either limited to the surface or measures less than 5×5 mm within the cortex; and
4. Serous histopathological/cytological characteristics.

Therefore, intraoperative assessment, either laparoscopically or through an exploratory laparotomy, and mainly histological examination, will lead to a reliable diagnosis of SPPC.

Investigation

Tumor Markers: CA-125 was slightly higher in patients with advanced EOC; however, on analysis, this finding was found not to be significant compared to the levels in patients with SPPC. Yedema et al. reported that CA125/CEA ratio >25 will be able to differentiate EOC and SPPC from primary colorectal carcinoma spreading to the peritoneum [28]. Regarding the significance of tumor marker measurement in ascites, different studies have reported varying results using different cut-off levels of tumor markers. Hence, due to their low sensitivity, serum tumor markers have been used as a prognostic indicator and as a monitoring tool [29].

Guaglio et al. reported that in a series of rare peritoneal surface malignancies (PSM) who did not have a complete pre-operative tumor marker evaluation, patients received an improper treatment tailored for EOC, with consequences on outcomes, underlining the need for full pre-operative workup with a comprehensive assessment with serum tumor markers that could help in the differential diagnosis [30].

CT Scan: is the modality of choice for patients with abdominal pain and distension symptoms. An ultrasound is readily available in almost all centers and almost routinely done; however, it is unable to accurately diagnose lesions less than 2 cm in size. In peritoneal carcinomatosis, ultrasonographic features include ascites which are hypo- or anechoic and hyperechogenic nodules representing tumor deposits in the peritoneum [7].

CT scans are able to demonstrate calcified peritoneal-based soft tissue masses, especially involving the omentum, and this finding is highly suggestive of high-grade serous carcinoma. It is even more evocative of SPPC in a post-menopausal female. The diagnosis of SPPC over ovarian cancer can be explored when the adnexal or pelvic tumor is minimally involved. Without calcification, diagnosing SPPC is challenging as it will appear similar to peritoneal carcinomatosis from secondaries [31].

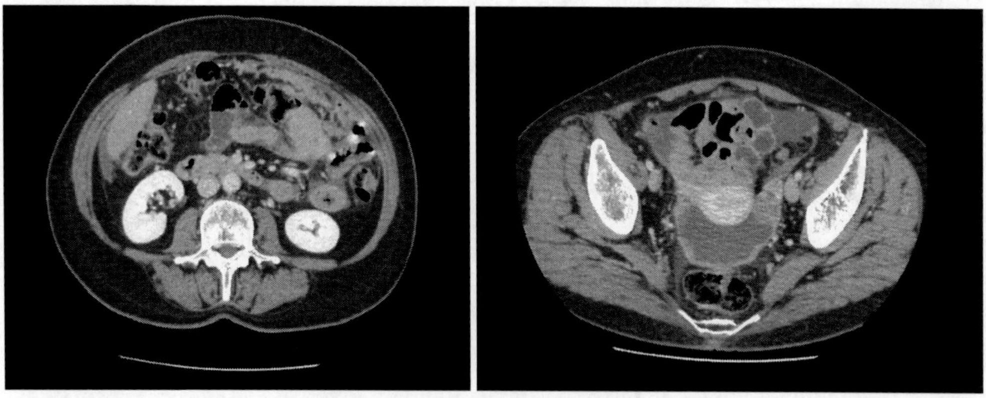

(a) (b)

Figure 1. CT scan and SPPC. (a) Upper abdomen with ascites and omental cake; (b) pelvis with ascites, parietal peritoneum thickened, no pelvic mass.

On CT scan, clumping and compartmentalization of bowel loops, omental cake, and lymphadenopathy can be seen. CT scans can detect lesions as small as 5mm. In peritoneal carcinomatosis, it has a sensitivity of 70% if the lesion is 2 cm, which is further reduced to 28% in the case of a tumor size of 5 mm. Moreover, CT scan findings are non-specific and similar in both neoplastic and benign conditions at such a small dimension. Ascites is a common finding together with contrast-enhanced diffuse or nodular thickening of the peritoneum. With a contrast-enhanced CT scan, omental cakes can also be appreciated as an increased density of large cell mass between the bowel and anterior abdominal wall (Figure 1).

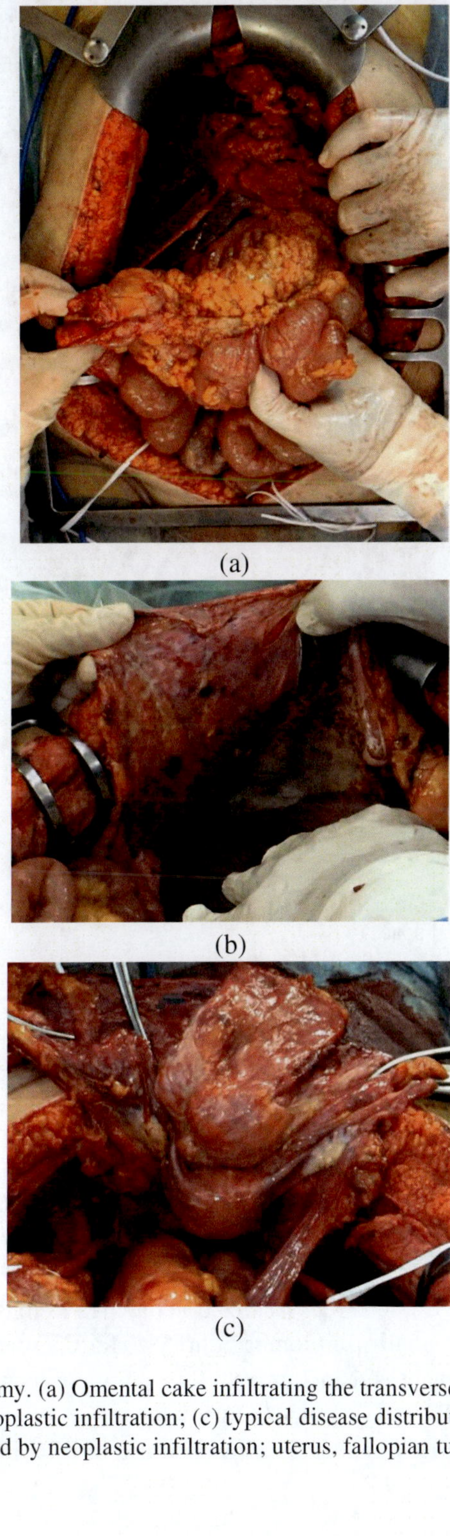

Figure 2. SPPC at Laparotomy. (a) Omental cake infiltrating the transverse colon; (b) diafragmatic peritoneum thickened by neoplastic infiltration; (c) typical disease distribution in the pelvis with parietal peritoneum thickened by neoplastic infiltration; uterus, fallopian tubes and ovaries with small and superficial lesions.

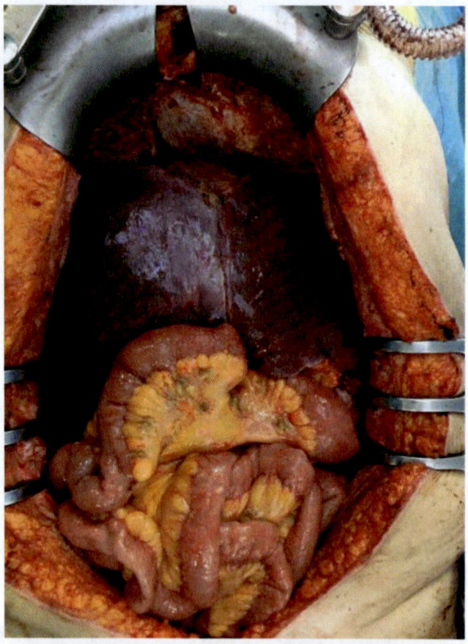

(a)

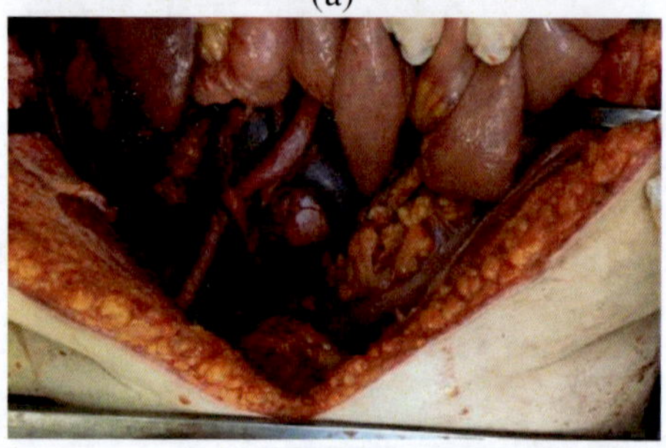

(b)

Figure 3. SPPC after CRS with retroperitoneal and pelvic lymphadenectomy. (a) abdomen; (b) pelvis with retroperitoneal space.

The CT scan findings in SPPC are similar to those in EOC, except for ovaries of normal appearance. Chiou et al. reported common CT scan findings in primary peritoneal carcinomas: ascites (82%), peritoneal nodules (73%), omental caking (64%), and pelvic mass (36%) [32, 33]. In comparison to malignant peritoneal mesothelioma, the CT scan will be able to identify a solid, heterogeneous mass with irregular margins and ascites are present in about 60-100% of cases.

Hence, the CT scan is the primary diagnostic modality and helps the interventional radiologists conduct guided biopsies and guide surgeons to perform optimal cytoreductive surgeries.

An MRI is better than the CT scan for visualization of small lesions as the detection sensitivity of MRI is 84% for tumors of all sizes compared to 54% for CT scans. The sensitivity increases for tumors with dimensions less than 1 cm (85-90%). For peritoneal tumors, T1 images show an intermediate signal, T2 images appear hypointense for solid lesions, and contrast with Gadolinium will enhance lesions seen in MRI. The use of MRI in peritoneal malignancy has increased over time, and it is commonly used for diagnosing and staging subcentimeter lesions due to its higher contrast resolution [35].

PET Scan: The mainstay of imaging modalities for peritoneal tumors is CT scans and MRIs. However, smaller peritoneal implants are not visible by these modalities. In such cases, FDG PET-CT scan (Fluorine -18- deoxyglucose positron emission tomography) has the potential to improve detection. It identifies malignant cells due to their increased glucose metabolism. This radionuclide imaging helps early detection, staging, monitoring treatment response, and long-term follow-up. The sensitivity of fused PET-CT scan (unenhanced) and PET-MDCT scan (multidetector) ranges between 58% to 100% [34].

Invasive Procedures for Diagnosis

A histological diagnosis is always required to plan an appropriate treatment strategy for the patient. This can be reached by obtaining ascitic fluid for cytology or histopathological examination of a specimen resected by laparoscopy.

Abdominal percutaneous paracentesis: In peritoneal carcinomatosis, ascites is exudative with high protein content (2.5 mg/dl), elevated LDH, and low glucose. Frank blood ascitic fluid is seen in peritoneal carcinomatosis in only 10% of cases, and blood-tinged (RBC >10,000 mm) ascites are seen in 8.3% of cases [35].

The sensitivity for detecting malignant cells was reported to be 53.3% in EOC and an incidence of 55.1% of free cancer cells in patients with colorectal peritoneal metastasis [36, 37].

Laparoscopy: A minimally invasive procedure that allows a reliable obtention of tissue specimens to diagnose and accurately evaluate disease extension. The diagnostic sensitivity is 100%. Laparoscopy is useful to calculate the peritoneal cancer index (PCI) [38].

Treatments

Traditional Treatment

Traditionally, SPPC was managed similarly to Figo Stage III-IV-4 EOC with systemic chemotherapy (sCT) either as neoadjuvant (NACT) or adjuvant (ADCT) and debulking surgery (DBK). Results of the traditional approach are summarized in Table 1 [21, 24, 39-42]. According to the retrospective series; the median Overall Survival is not exciting ranging from 17-42 months, with a progression-free survival ranging from 7-17 months. Most of the studies were conducted to compare the outcome of patients with SPPS vs. EOC treated with the association of sCT and DBK and evaluate the response to NACT and the rate of platinum resistance. Iavazzo et al. concluded, in their limited series of patients, that SPPC mimics EOC regarding the clinical and laboratory characteristics, but it has a worse prognosis [43]. Eisenhauer et al. [21] argues that SPPC was associated with a similar initial response but a higher rate of platinum resistance and shorter PFS and OS. Consideration of these results may be useful for patient counseling, trial stratification, and molecular comparisons. On the other hand, in the Bloss study, patients with SPPC and EOC exhibit a similar probability of response to cisplatin and cyclophosphamide and a similar overall survival [44].

Table 1. Summary of SPPC study outcomes following debulking surgery and chemotherapy

Authors	No. of Cases	Year	Stage	Debulking surgery + mmChemotherapy	Progression free survival (months)	Median Overall survival (months)
Bloss JD et al. [44]	36	2003	III/IV	NACT +DBK	11	22
Iavazzo C et al. [43]	9	2008	III/IV	DBK + ADCT	7	30
Roh SH et al. [42]	22	2007	IIIc/IV	NACT +DBK	9,9	23,1
Eisenhauer et al. [21]	43	2008	IIIc/IV	NACT +DBK	17	42
Eltabbakh et al. [46]	75	1998	IIc/III/IV	DBK+ ADCT	N/A	23.5
Halperin et al. [39]	28	2001	IIb/III/IV	DBK + ADCT	N/A	17
Dubenard et al. [24]	37	2004	IIIc/IV	DBK + ADCT	3- yr DFS 29%	Not reached
Qi Liu et al. [41]	22	2011	IIIc/IV	NACT + DBK + ADCT	N/A	22
Blontzos et al. [40]	19	2019	IIIc/IV	DBK + ADCT		13-46(29)

NACT: Neo Adjuvant Chemotherapy, DBK: Debulking Surgery, ADCT: Adjuvant Chemotherapy.

Innovative Treatment

A growing body of evidence suggests that CRS with HIPEC is recommended for peritoneal surface malignancies such as peritoneal metastasis from colorectal cancers, pseudomyxoma peritonei, and primary peritoneal tumors, such as peritoneal mesothelioma. Promising oncological results have also been reported in treating the peritoneal dissemination from gastric and ovarian cancers [45, 46]. There is a strong rationale for patients receiving HIPEC following cytoreductive surgery after neoadjuvant chemotherapy in advanced stage IIIc/IV ovarian cancer. Yet, a definite conclusion on optimal management is still under investigation. SPPC is usually confined within the intraperitoneal cavity, and therefore it fits for a locoregional treatment as CRS+HIPEC [47].

Management of SPPC requires vast resources and specialized surgical methods. Therefore the current practice to manage SPPC is to seek opinion from a referral center with expertise in peritoneal surface malignancy that will be able to manage SPPC based on platinum/taxane-based neoadjuvant systemic chemotherapy (NACT) followed by extensive cytoreductive surgery (CRS) and hyperthermic intraperitoneal chemotherapy (HIPEC). Recent evidence has shown this to have a beneficial effect on survival, described below.

Omitting neoadjuvant chemotherapy in patients with SPPC resulted in suboptimal debulking with a poorer prognosis. Therefore, neoadjuvant chemotherapy has also been advocated before a CRS and HIPEC [48, 49].

Cytoreductive surgery (CRS): The reasons to treat SPPC with CRS through extensive peritonectomy procedures are twofold: extensive disease usually involving all the parietal peritoneal at the outset and the multifocality. This complex surgery is conducted via a laparotomy. At the abdominal exploration, the disease extension is assessed with the PCI [38] (Figure 2).

CRS was first described by Sugarbaker and is composed of five different procedures allowing for the removal of all the parietal peritoneum, greater and lesser omentum. According to the disease involvement, multiorgan resection is also performed, including resection of the gallbladder, spleen, left/correct or total colon, uterus, fallopian tubes, and ovaries en bloc with a pelvic peritonectomy [50]. In cases of mesentery involvement, removing the mesenteric peritoneum is required, according to the technique proposed by Deraco et al. [51]. Depending on the center, systematic pelvic and retroperitoneal lymph node dissection is also recommended. Following an extensive cytoreductive surgery and HIPEC, lymph node dissection would be challenging to perform if there is a recurrence in the future due to postoperative adhesions. Therefore, for this reason, systematic lymph node dissection has been advocated, although the prognostic implications of positive nodal status in both histology are still under investigation [52]. A covering ileostomy is not routinely performed unless the anastomosis is below the sacral promontory (Figure 3). At the end of CRS, the residual disease is quantified according to the completeness of cytoreduction score (CC-Score) [47, 53].

Hyperthermic Intraperitoneal Chemotherapy (HIPEC): A prerequisite for effective HIPEC is optimal cytoreduction. No residual disease or minimal lesions are left behind because the penetration depth of intraperitoneally delivered drugs is limited.

HIPEC is done after completing the CRS, with the technique described elsewhere [48]. Briefly, four silicone catheters are placed in the right subphrenic space, deep pelvic cavity, left subphrenic space, and the last one in the superficial pelvic space. Thermal probes are inserted in the abdominal cavity to monitor peritoneal temperature during intraperitoneal hyperthermic chemotherapy continuously. At our center, HIPEC is conducted with the closed-abdomen technique; therefore, the skin is closed with a running suture to ensure no fluid leakage. The catheters are then connected through an extracorporeal circuit to a roller pump coupled with a heat exchanger. Chemotherapy regimens used Cisplastin (43 mg/L of perfusate) and doxorubicin (15.25 mg/L of perfusate) accordingly to the Phase One study dose-finding reported in the past [54]. Patients aged >70 years received a 30% dose reduction of both drugs. Different approaches have been performed with similar outcomes, such as the open, coliseum technique whereby the abdomen is left open, and the intraperitoneal cavity is irrigated with chemotherapeutic agents, and this is performed in other centers. Various extracorporeal perfusion equipment with CE (European) and some with FDA approved has been used as well [55, 56].

This procedure has some challenges, such as high cost, high morbidity, and technically demanding with a steep learning curve. Few studies have addressed the learning curve of CRS and HIPEC, whereby literature data have demonstrated trends toward better surgical outcomes (morbidity rates, operating time, etc.) as the surgeon gained experience and improved proficiency by performing more cases.. Kusamura et al. quoted a case breakpoint of 86 to overcome the learning curve. Incomplete cytoreduction, procedure-related mortality, severe morbidity, and early oncologic failure were indicators used as a learning curve [57]. As CRS and HIPEC is not regularly performed surgery, centralization of cases is the key to increasing case numbers and hence proficiency of the procedure. It is imperative to establish study protocols, a multidisciplinary team, and troubleshooting to improve patient selection criteria to improve outcomes [57].

Results with CRS HIPEC

Intraperitoneal chemotherapy has recently demonstrated a survival benefit in patients with Stage IIIc/IV advanced ovarian cancer compared to those treated with surgery alone or surgery combined with systemic chemotherapy. Recently, Ceresoli et al. performed a retrospective case-control propensity score-matched analysis, which pointed out that HIPEC can affect the relapse pattern with lesser peritoneal recurrence and better overall survival [58]. Similarly, Van Driel et al. showed improved survival of patients with advanced ovarian cancer who underwent HIPEC in addition to interval debulking surgery (IDS) vs. IDS alone. All patients received preoperative neoadjuvant chemotherapy (NACT) with cisplatin/ carboplatin and paclitaxel. All patients received six cycles of NACT before cytoreductive surgery. Following chemotherapy, patients were evaluated with thoracic and abdominal contrast-enhanced tomography and serum tumor marker measurements. Patients with stable disease or partial response were subjected to CRS and HIPEC. The median overall survival was 33.9 months in the surgery group and 45.7 months in surgery with HIPEC group [59].

Table 2 illustrates the results of the management of SPPC with CRS HIPEC in addition to sCT [1, 52, 60, 61].The median survival ranged from 31-68 months, and in two studies, it was not reached [49, 56]. Bakrin et al. reported the results of a multi-institutional study comprising nine institutions over ten years with 36 patients of SPPC treated by CRS with HIPEC. All patients underwent neoadjuvant platinum-based chemotherapy, most of the patients underwent HIPEC for 90 minutes, and only seven patients received adjuvant chemotherapy following surgery. This study reported a 5-year OS of 57.4%, a median DFS of 16.7 months, and a 5-year DFS of 24%. Their study found PCI as the only prognostic factor affecting survival on univariate analysis [56].

Table 2. Summary of SPPC study outcomes following CRS + HIPEC

Authors	No. of Cases	Year	Stage	Complete Cytoreduction + HIPEC	Progression free survival (months)	Median Overall survival (months)
Bakrin et al. [60]	36	2013	N/A	NACT + CRS + HIPEC	DFS 16.7	Not reached
Sun JH et al. [61]	22	2016	N/A	CRS +HIPEC	N/A	31
Sardi et al. [62]	30	2017	II/III/IV	CRS + HIPEC	PFS at 1/3/5 years (%) 80/75/59	68
Deraco et al. [52]	22	2019	III/IV	CRS + HIPEC	32.9 months	Not reached 5y = 65%

NACT: Neoadjuvant Chemotherapy.

As for the Milan study published in 2019, with an initial 22 patients, the 5-year overall survival (OS) was 64.9%, the median progression-free survival was 32.9 months, and progression-free survival at 5-years was 33.2%. More than 50% of the patients were alive at the analysis time, and median OS was not reached. In this study, survival analyses were performed from the date of surgery and not from initial diagnosis and so may well underestimate survival. However, there were no significant prognostic factors influencing survival in univariate and multivariate analyses. Importantly, this study demonstrated a better OS and PFS in patients with SPPC when treated with CRS & HIPEC after NACT compared to patients treated with traditional treatment. In this study, in 60% of the resected parietal peritoneal specimens, a microscopic residual disease was present despite grossly normal-appearing peritoneum at surgical exploration, further strengthening the case for a total peritonectomy. At the time of cytoreductive surgery, the median PCI was 10.5 (range 1-31), which indicates a moderate extent of peritoneal carcinomatosis, if not greater. The study demonstrated a high rate of lymph node involvement whereby 46% of patients had lymph node metastasis in both retroperitoneal and pelvic lymph nodes. Systematic lymph node dissection in SPPC has been proposed to limit lymph node recurrence. After total parietal peritonectomy, eventual lymph node recurrence would be hard to treat surgically due to postoperative adhesions and scar formation. One of the reasons clinicians are skeptical about adopting CRS & HIPEC routinely is the concerns of morbidity and mortality related to the combined procedure. Overall surgical morbidity rate reported in the Milan study was 18%, which is in the lower range of the reported morbidity rates elsewhere following a complete CRS & HIPEC, and there was no mortality amongst the 22 patients [52].

Conclusion

SPPC is a distinct disease entity, and treating this disease as EOC should be avoided. There should be awareness of the existence of SPPC when abdominal distension, gross ascites, and a raised level of CA125 are present in women without ovarian enlargement. Despite similarities in histology and an overlap with biological characteristics, SPPC is associated with widespread peritoneal dissemination, which is more aggressive, has a higher recurrence, and has a poorer outcome than EOC. Patients with SPPC, when treated with DBK and sCT, have poor outcomes. According to cohort studies, the prognosis of SPPC has improved with the advances in NACT, CRS & HIPEC. Therefore, SPPC necessitates a thorough peritonectomy of all quadrants and requires radical surgical approaches to obtain the best results from experts trained in treating peritoneal surface malignancies. The efficacy of this complex treatment has been proven but needs to be confirmed through further prospective studies.

References

[1] Pentheroudakis, G. and Pavlidis, N., 2010. Serous papillary peritoneal carcinoma: unknown primary tumour, ovarian cancer counterpart or a distinct entity? A systematic review. *Critical reviews in oncology/hematology*, 75(1), pp.27-42.

[2] Swerdlow M. Mesothelioma of the pelvic peritoneum resembling papillary cystadenocarcinoma of the ovary; case report. *Am J Obstet Gynecol* 1959 Jan;77(1):197-200.

[3] Ledermann, J.A., Raja, F.A., Fotopoulou, C., Gonzalez-Martin, A., Colombo, N. and Sessa, C., 2013. Newly diagnosed and relapsed epithelial ovarian carcinoma: ESMO Clinical Practice Guidelines for diagnosis, treatment and follow-up. *Annals of oncology*, 24, pp.vi24-vi32.

[4] Ben-Baruch, G., Sivan, E., Moran, O., Rizel, S., Menczer, J. and Seidman, D.S., 1996. Primary peritoneal serous papillary carcinoma: A study of 25 cases and comparison with stage III–IV ovarian papillary serous carcinoma. *Gynecologic oncology*, 60(3), pp.393-396.

[5] Hou, T., Liang, D., He, J., Chen, X. and Zhang, Y., 2012. Primary peritoneal serous carcinoma: a clinicopathological and immunohistochemical study of six cases. *International journal of clinical and experimental pathology*, 5(8), p.762.

[6] Komiyama, S., Nishijima, Y., Kondo, H., Nomura, H., Yamaguchi, S., Futagami, M., Arai, H., Yokoyama, Y., Suzuki, N., Mikami, M. and Kubushiro, K., 2018. Multicenter Clinicopathological study of high-grade serous carcinoma presenting as primary peritoneal carcinoma. *International Journal of Gynecologic Cancer*, 28(4).

[7] Dalrymple, J.C., Bannatyne, P., Russell, P., Solomon, H.J., Tattersall, M.H.N., Atkinson, K., Carter, J., Duval, P., Elliott, P., Friedlander, M. and Murray, J., 1989. Extraovarian peritoneal serous papillary carcinoma. A clinicopathologic study of 31 cases. *Cancer*, 64(1), pp.110-115.

[8] Goodman, M.T., Shvetsov, Y.B. Incidence of Ovarian, Peritoneal, and Fallopian Tube Carcinomas in the United States, 1995-2004. *Cancer Epidemiol Biomarkers Prev* 2009;18:132-9.

[9] Edmondson, R.J. and Monaghan, J.M., 2001. The epidemiology of ovarian cancer. *International journal of gynecological cancer*, *11*(6), pp.423-429.

[10] Stewart, S.L., Wike, J.M., Foster, S.L. and Michaud, F., 2007. The incidence of primary fallopian tube cancer in the United States. *Gynecologic Oncology*, *107*(3), pp.392-397.

[11] Hattori, S., Kajiyama, H., Fuji, U., Furui, Y., Ishibashi, Y., Hattori, Y., et al. Clinical characteristics of primary peritoneal carcinoma patients: a single-institution experience involving 8 patients. *Nagoya J Med Sci* 2016 Dec;78(4):407-14.

[12] Jordan, S.J., Green, A.C., Whiteman, D.C., Moore, S.P., Bain, C.J., Gertig, D.M., Webb, P.M. and Australian Cancer Study Group (ovarian cancer) and the Australian Ovarian Cancer Study Group, 2008. Serous ovarian, fallopian tube and primary peritoneal cancers: a comparative epidemiological analysis. *International journal of cancer*, 122(7), pp.1598-1603.

[13] Neuhausen, S.L., Shani, H., Boker, L.K., et al. Primary peritoneal serous carcinoma in men: a rare and non-BRCA-associated entity. *Anticancer Res* 2017; 37(6): 3069–3072.

[14] Pentheroudakis, G. and Pavlidis, N., 2010. Serous papillary peritoneal carcinoma: unknown primary tumor, ovarian cancer counterpart or a distinct entity? A systematic review. *Critical reviews in oncology/hematology*, 75(1), pp.27-42.

[15] Huang, L.W., Garrett, A.P., Muto, M.G., et al. Identification of a novel 9cM deletion unit on chromosome 6q23-24 in papillary serous carcinoma of the peritoneum. *Hum Pathol* 2000;31:367–73.

[16] Kusamura, S., Baratti, D., Zaffaroni, N., Villa, R., Laterza, B., Balestra, M.R. and Deraco, M., 2010. Pathophysiology and biology of peritoneal carcinomatosis. *World journal of gastrointestinal oncology*, 2(1), p.12.

[17] Kowalski, L.D., Kanbour, A.I., Price, F.V., et al. A case-matched molecular comparison of extraovarian versus primary ovarian adenocarcinoma. *Cancer* 1997;79:1587-94.

[18] Gu, J., Roth, L.M., Younger, C., Michael, H., Abdul-Karim, F.W., Zhang, S., Ulbright, T.M., Eble, J.N. and Cheng, L., 2001. Molecular evidence for the independent origin of extra-ovarian papillary serous tumors of low malignant potential. *Journal of the National Cancer Institute*, 93(15), pp.1147-1152.

[19] Horn, L.C., Kafkova, S., Leonhardt, K., Kellner, C. and Einenkel, J., 2013. Serous tubal in situ carcinoma (STIC) in primary peritoneal serous carcinomas. *International Journal of Gynecological Pathology*, 32(4), pp.339-344.

[20] Huang LW, Garrett AP, Schorge JO, Michael G, BellAD, Welch RW, et al. Distinct allelic loss patterns in papillary serous carcinoma of the peritoneum. *Am J Clin Pathol* 2000;114:93-9.

[21] Eisenhauer EL, Sonoda Y, Levine DA, Abu-Rustum NR, Gemignani ML, Sabbatini PJ, et al. Platinum resistance and impaired survival in patients with advanced primary peritoneal carcinoma: matched-case comparison with patients with epithelial ovarian carcinoma. *Am J Obstet Gynecol* 2008 Feb;198(2). 213.e1-7.

[22] Kawaguchi, R., Tanase, Y., Haruta, S., Nagai, A., Yoshida, S., Furukawa, N., et al. Paclitaxel plus carboplatin chemotherapy for primary peritoneal carcinoma: a study of 22 cases and comparison with stage IIIeIV ovarian serous carcinoma. *Case Rep Oncol* 2012 Apr 13;5(1):173e80.

[23] Luyckx, M., Leblanc, E., Filleron, T., Morice, P., Darai, E., Classe, J.-M., et al. Maximal cytoreduction in patients with FIGO stage IIIC to stage IV ovarian, fallopian, and peritoneal cancer in day-to-day practice: a Retrospective French Multi- centric Study. *Int J Gynecol Cancer Off J Int Gynecol Cancer Soc* 2012 Oct;22(8):1337-43.

[24] Dubernard, G., Morice, P., Rey, A., Camatte, S., Fourchotte, V., Thoury, A., et al. Prognosis of stage III or IV primary peritoneal serous papillary carcinoma. *Eur J Surg Oncol J Eur Soc Surg Oncol Br Assoc Surg Oncol* 2004 Nov;30(9): 97-e8.

[25] Levy, A.D., Arnáiz, J., Shaw, J.C. and Sobin, L.H., 2008. Primary peritoneal tumors: imaging features with pathologic correlation. *Radiographics*, *28*(2), pp.583-607.

[26] Bollinger, D.J., Wick, M.R., Dehner, L.P., Mills, S.E., Swanson, P.E. and Clarke, R.E., 1989. Peritoneal malignant mesothelioma versus serous papillary adenocarcinoma. A histochemical and immunohistochemical comparison. *The American journal of surgical pathology*, *13*(8), pp.659-670.
[27] Ordóñez, N.G., 2013. Value of PAX8, PAX2, claudin-4, and h-caldesmon immunostaining in distinguishing peritoneal epithelioid mesotheliomas from serous carcinomas. *Modern Pathology*, *26*(4), pp.553-562.
[28] Yedema, C.A., Kenemans, P., Wobbes, T., Thomas, C.M.G., Bon, G.G., Mulder, C., Voorhorst, F.J., Verstraeten, A.A., Van Kamp, G.J. and Hilgers, J., 1992. Use of serum tumor markers in the differential diagnosis between ovarian and colorectal adenocarcinomas. *Tumor biology*, *13*(1-2), pp.18-26.
[29] Pentheroudakis, G.E.O.R.G.E. and Pavlidis, N.I.C.H.O.L.A.S., 2008. Serum tumor markers. *Metastatic carcinomas of unknown origin. New York, NY: Demos Medical Publishing*, pp.165-75.
[30] Guaglio, M., Baratti, D., Kusamura, S., Reis, A.C., Montenovo, M., Bartolini, V., Battaglia, L. and Deraco, M., 2021. Impact of Previous Gynecologic Surgical Procedures on Outcomes of Non-Gynecologic Peritoneal Malignancies Mimicking Ovarian Cancer: Less Is More*?*. *Annals of Surgical Oncology*, 28(5), pp.2899-2908.
[31] Voultsinos, V., Semelka, R.C., Elias Jr, J., Altun, E., Huertas, C., Woosley, J.T. and Balci, N.C., 2008. Primary peritoneal carcinoma: computed tomography and magnetic resonance findings. *Journal of computer assisted tomography*, 32(4), pp.541-547.
[32] Chiou, S.Y., Sheu, M.H., Wang, J.H. and Chang, C.Y., 2003. Peritoneal serous papillary carcinoma: a reappraisal of CT imaging features and literature review. *Abdominal imaging*, 28(6), pp.815-819.
[33] Pickhardt, P.J., Perez, A.A., Elmohr, M.M. and Elsayes, K.M., 2021. CT imaging review of uncommon peritoneal-based neoplasms: beyond carcinomatosis. *The British journal of radiology*, 94(1119), p.20201288.
[34] Rakheja, R., Makis, W. and Hickeson, M., 2012. Extraovarian primary peritoneal carcinoma: staging with 18F-FDG PET/CT. *Abdominal imaging*, 37(2), pp.304-308.
[35] Milingos, S., Protopapas, A., Papadimitriou, C., Rodolakis, A., Kallipolitis, G., Skartados, N., Markaki, S., Dimopoulos, M.A. and Antsaklis, A., 2007. Laparoscopy in evaluating women with unexplained ascites: an invaluable diagnostic tool. *Journal of Minimally Invasive Gynecology*, 14(1), pp.43-48.
[36] Ayhan, A., Gultekin, M., Taskiran, C., Dursun, P., Firat, P., Bozdag, G., Celik, N.Y. and Yuce, K.U.N.T.E.R., 2007. Ascites and epithelial ovarian cancers: a reappraisal with respect to different aspects. *International Journal of Gynecological Cancer*, *17*(1), pp.68-75.
[37] Sugarbaker, P.H., Deng, T. and Chang, D., 2021. Peritoneal cytology as an indicator of peritoneal metastases in colorectal cancer. *Journal of Surgical Oncology*, *124*(3), pp.361-366.
[38] Jacquet, P. and Sugarbaker, P.H., 1996. Clinical research methodologies in diagnosis and staging of patients with peritoneal carcinomatosis. *Peritoneal carcinomatosis: principles of management*, pp.359-374.
[39] Halperin, R., Zehavi, S., Langer, R., Hadas, E., Bukovsky, I. and Schneider, D., 2001. Primary peritoneal serous papillary carcinoma: a new epidemiologic trend? A matched-case comparison with ovarian serous papillary cancer. *International Journal of Gynecologic Cancer*, *11*(5).
[40] Blontzos, N., Vafias, E., Vorgias, G., Kalinoglou, N. and Iavazzo, C., 2019. Primary peritoneal serous papillary carcinoma: a case series. *Archives of Gynecology and Obstetrics*, 300(4), pp.1023-1028.
[41] Liu, Q., Lin, J.X., Shi, Q.L., Wu, B., Ma, H.H. and Sun, G.Q., 2011. Primary peritoneal serous papillary carcinoma: a clinical and pathological study. *Pathology & Oncology Research*, *17*(3), pp.713-719.
[42] Roh, S.Y., Hong, S.H., Ko, Y.H., Kim, T.H., Lee, M.A., Shim, B.Y., Byun, J.H., Woo, I.S., Kang, J.H., Hong, Y.S., Lee, K.S. Clinical characteristics of primary peritoneal carcinoma. *Cancer Res Treat.* 2007;39:65–8.
[43] Iavazzo, C., Vorgias, G., Katsoulis, M., Kalinoglou, N., Dertimas, V., Akrivos, T. Primary peritoneal serous papillary carcinoma: clinical and laboratory characteristics. *Arch Gynecol Obstet.* 2008;278:53–6.
[44] Bloss, J.D., Brady, M.F., Liao, S.Y., Rocereto, T., Partridge, E.E., Clarke-Pearson, D.L. Extraovarian peritoneal serous papillary carcinoma: a phase II trial of cisplatin and cyclophosphamide with comparison to a cohort with papillary serous ovarian carcinoma-a Gynecologic Oncology Group Study. *Gynecol Oncol.* 2003;89:148–54.

[45] Ben-Baruch, G., Sivan, E., Moran, O., Rizel, S., Menczer, J. and Seidman, D.S., 1996. Primary peritoneal serous papillary carcinoma: a study of 25 cases and comparison with stage III–IV ovarian papillary serous carcinoma. *Gynecologic oncology*, 60(3), pp.393-396.

[46] Eltabbakh, G.H., Werness, B.A., Piver, S. and Blumenson, L.E., 1998. Prognostic factors in extraovarian primary peritoneal carcinoma. *Gynecologic oncology*, 71(2), pp.230-239.

[47] Deraco, M., Baratti, D. and Kusamura, S., 2007. Morbidity and quality of life following cytoreduction and HIPEC. *Peritoneal Carcinomatosis*, pp.403-418.

[48] Jacquet, P., Sugarbaker, P.H. Clinical research methodologies in diagnosis and staging of patients with peritoneal carcinomatosis. *Cancer Treat Res* 1996;82:359–374.

[49] Yang, F., Wang, J., Li, H. and Tong, X., 2012. Prognosis of primary peritoneal carcinoma: effect of cytoreductive surgery combined with neoadjuvant chemotherapy after laparoscopic diagnosis and evaluation: a multi-center trial. *Eur. J. Gynaec. Oncol.-ISSN*, *33*(1), p.2012.

[50] Sugarbaker, P.H. and Chang, D., 1999. Results of treatment of 385 patients with peritoneal surface spread of appendiceal malignancy. *Annals of surgical oncology*, 6(8), pp.727-731.

[51] Deraco, M., Baratti, D., Kusamura, S., Laterza, B. and Balestra, M.R., 2009. Surgical technique of parietal and visceral peritonectomy for peritoneal surface malignancies. *Journal of surgical oncology*, *100*(4), pp.321-328.

[52] Deraco, M., Sinukumar, S., Salcedo-Hernández, R.A., Rajendra, V.J., Baratti, D., Guaglio, M., Nizri, E. and Kusamura, S., 2019. Clinico-pathological outcomes after total parietal peritonectomy, cytoreductive surgery and hyperthermic intraperitoneal chemotherapy in advanced serous papillary peritoneal carcinoma submitted to neoadjuvant systemic chemotherapy-largest single institute experience. *European Journal of Surgical Oncology*, *45*(11), pp.2103-2108.

[53] González-Moreno, Santiago, Kusamura, Shigeki, Baratti, Dario, Deraco, Marcello. Postoperative residual disease evaluation in the locoregional treatment of peritoneal surface malignancy *J Surg Oncol* 2008, Volume 98, Issue 4 p. 237-241 https://doi.org/10.1002/jso.21072.

[54] Rossi, C.R., Foletto, M., Mocellin, S., Pilati, P., De, S.M., Deraco, M., Cavaliere, F., Palatini, P., Guasti, F., Scalerta, R., Lise, M. Hyperthermic intraoperative intraperitoneal chemotherapy with cisplatin and doxorubicin in patients who undergo cytoreductive surgery for peritoneal carcinomatosis and sarcomatosis: phase I study. *Cancer.* 2002 Jan 15;94(2):492-9. PubMed PMID: 11900234.

[55] Halkia, E., Tsochrinis, A., Vassiliadou, D.T., Pavlakou, A., Vaxevanidou, A., Datsis, A., Efstathiou, E. and Spiliotis, J., 2015. Peritoneal carcinomatosis: intraoperative parameters in open (coliseum) versus closed abdomen HIPEC. *International Journal of Surgical Oncology*, 2015.

[56] Glehen, O., Cotte, E., Kusamura, S., Deraco, M., Baratti, D., Passot, G., Beaujard, A.C. and Noel, G.F., 2008. Hyperthermic intraperitoneal chemotherapy: nomenclature and modalities of perfusion. *Journal of surgical oncology*, *98*(4), pp.242-246.

[57] Kusamura, S., González-Moreno, S., Nizri, E., Baratti, D., Guadagni, S., Guaglio, M., Battaglia, L. and Deraco, M., 2018. Learning curve, training program, and monitorization of surgical performance of peritoneal surface malignancies centers. *Surgical Oncology Clinics*, 27(3), pp.507-517.

[58] Ceresoli, M., Verrengia, A., Montori, G., Busci, L., Coccolini, F., Ansaloni, L. and Frigerio, L., 2018. Effect of cytoreductive surgery and hyperthermic intraperitoneal chemotherapy on relapse pattern in primary epithelial ovarian cancer: a propensity score based case-control study. *Journal of Gynecologic Oncology*, 29(3).

[59] Van Driel, W.J., Koole, S.N., Sikorska, K., Schagen van Leeuwen, J.H., Schreuder, H.W., Hermans, R.H., De Hingh, I.H., Van Der Velden, J., Arts, H.J., Massuger, L.F. and Aalbers, A.G., 2018. Hyperthermic intraperitoneal chemotherapy in ovarian cancer. *New England Journal of Medicine*, 378(3), pp.230-240.

[60] Bakrin, N., Gilly, F.N., Baratti, D., Bereder, J.M., Quenet, F., Lorimier, G., Mohamed, F., Elias, D., Glehen, O. and Association Française de Chirurgie, 2013. Primary peritoneal serous carcinoma treated by cytoreductive surgery combined with hyperthermic intraperitoneal chemotherapy. A multi-institutional study of 36 patients. *European Journal of Surgical Oncology* (EJSO), 39(7), pp.742-747.

[61] Sun, J.H., Ji, Z.H., Peng, K.W., Wu, H.T., Zhang, Q., Yonemura, Y. and Li, Y., 2016. Cytoreductive surgery combined with hyperthermic intraperitoneal chemotherapy for the treatment of primary

peritoneal serous carcinoma: Results of a Chinese retrospective study. *International Journal of Hyperthermia,* 32(3), pp.289-297.

[62] Sardi, A., Sipok, A., Díaz-Montes, T.P., Sittig, M., Nieroda, C., Studeman, K. and Gushchin, V., 2017. Outcomes of cytoreductive surgery and hyperthermic intraperitoneal chemotherapy in the treatment of primary peritoneal carcinoma. *Journal of Peritoneum* (and other serosal surfaces), 2(2).

Chapter 22

Ovarian Carcinosarcoma

Ilker Kahramanoglu[1,*], MD, PhD
and Olcay Ilhan[2], MD, PhD
[1]Emsey Hospital, Department of Gynecologic Oncology, Istanbul, Turkey
[2]Diyarbakir Gazi Yasargil Training and Research Hospital, Department of Gynecologic Oncology, Diyarbakir, Turkey

Introduction

This chapter is aimed at clarifying the epidemiology, pathology, diagnosis, prognostic factors, surgical and medical treatment options of ovarian carcinosarcoma.

Carcinosarcomas of the female genital tract are mostly identified in the uterus [1, 2]. Carcinosarcomas comprise 1-4% of ovarian cancers [3, 4]. These tumors differ from epithelial ovarian cancers as they contain sarcomatous tissue that arise from the connective tissue, in addition to carcinomatous tissue that arise from the epithelial tissue [5]. Similar to uterine carcinosarcoma, the carcinomatous component is similar to conventional epithelial carcinoma (serous, endometrioid, undifferentiated adenocarcinoma, squamous cell carcinoma, or clear cell adenocarcinoma) [2]. The sarcomatous component may arise from the ovary itself (homologous, such as endometrial stromal sarcoma, fibrosarcoma, and leiomyosarcoma) or may be different from the mesencyhmal tissue of the ovary (heterologous, such as rhabdomyosarcoma, chondrosarcoma, osteosarcoma, liposarcoma, or angiosarcoma) [3, 6, 7]. A similar etiopathogenic pathway for both uterine and ovarian carcinosarcomas was proposed [1, 8, 9]. According to this, tumorogenesis is initiated by the epithelial component and the sarcomatous component represents a metaplastic phenomenon. However, the sarcomatous component becomes a driving component in metastatic lesions. The lesions are biologically aggressive, and their presentation is similar to that of most epithelial ovarian malignancies. At diagnosis, more than 80% of patients have extra-ovarian intraabdominal spread [5].

Ovarian carcinosarcoma is not expected to be involved in inherited cancer syndromes. However, Carnevali et al., [10] presented two cases of ovarian carcinosarcoma which occurred in patients with hereditary cancer syndromes. One of the cases had a BRCA 1 mutation, and

* Corresponding Author's Email: ilkerkahramanoglu@gmail.com.

In: Ovarian Cancer
Editors: Christos Iavazzo, Alexandros Fotiou and John Spiliotis
ISBN: 979-8-88697-633-5

the other had Lynch Syndrome. Thus, when carcinosarcoma of the ovary is diagnosed at a young age, a hereditary cancer susceptibility syndrome should be suspected.

Comparing to serous and other epithelial ovarian cancers, ovarian carcinosarcomas are diagnosed at an older age. It is usually seen in postmenopausal women with the average age of 65 years old [3, 11]. Similar to high-grade serous ovarian tumors, a majority of patients are diagnosed at an advanced stage. Ovarian carcinosarcoma has a significantly worse prognosis than serous carcinoma. In a large study of the Surveillance, Epidemiology, and End Results (SEER) Program, the 5-year disease free survival was found to be 28.2% and 38.4% ($p < 0.001$) in patients with ovarian carcinosarcoma and those with high-grade serous ovarian carcinoma, respectively [12]. Survival difference remained against carcinosarcoma in each FIGO stage [12]. In another SEER study, involving 1,763 women with ovarian carcinosarcoma and 25,974 women with serous carcinoma, the outcomes between the two were compared [4]. After adjusting for other prognostic factors, patients with ovarian carcinosarcoma were found to be 72% more likely to die of cancer (HR = 1.72; 95CI, 1.52-1.96). The five year survival for Stage I was 65.2% (95% CI, 58.0-71.4%) for ovarian carcinosarcoma and 80.6% (95% CI, 78.9-82.2%) for serous carcinomas. For Stage IIIC patients, the 5-year survival was reported to be 18.2% (95% CI, 14.5-22.4%) for ovarian carcinosarcoma compared to 33.3% (95% CI, 32.1-34.5%) for serous carcinomas.

Similar to those of high-grade serous ovarian carcinoma, patients with ovarian carcinosarcoma present with non-specific symptoms were related to abdominal distension and weight loss [3]. The most common ultrasound appearance is a large solid tumor with irregular margins and heterogenous echogeneity of the solid tissue. The most second common appearance is multilocular-solid tissue with heterogenous echogeneity of the solid tissue [13]. The stained-glass appearance, hemorrhage and necrosis are frequently seen in Magnetic Resonance Imaging [14]. Compared to serous ovarian carcinoma, patients' performance status is usually poorer at the time of diagnosis, after adjusting for stage [15].

On initial investigation, more than 90% of cases are found to have distant spread. Nearly all patients express CA 125 with a value more than 75 U/ml [16]. A recent review on carcinosarcoma of the ovary demonstrated that 12 of 13 patients had elevated CA 125 with the lowest level of 80 U/mL and the highest of 4872 U/mL [3]. One third of cases had bilateral ovarian involvement [15, 17]. Pelvic and paraaortic nodal metastasis was present in half of patients [15].

Traditionally, the primary treatment of ovarian carcinosarcoma has been cytoreductive surgery followed by chemotherapy [5]. Cytoreductive surgery is aimed to remove all macroscopic tumor or as much of the tumor as possible. As ovarian carcinosarcoma is a rare histology, no randomized prospective study has been conducted. Patients with early-stage tumors should undergo staging surgery, including total hysterectomy, bilateral salpingooophorectomny, pelvic and paraaortic lymphadenectomy to the left renal vein, omentectomy, peritoneal biopsies and washing [18]. However, due to rarity of this tumor, the effect of lymphadenectomy on prognosis has not been clarified. A SEER database study including 363 patients with early stage ovarian carcinosarcoma (186 patients underwent lymphadenectomy vs 177 did not) demonstrated a significantly higher survival in lymphadenectomy group in American Joint Committee on Cancer (AJCC) T2 tumor ($p = 0.002$ for overall survival) [19]. Nevertheless, no significant difference was found in AJCC T1 disease.

Several retrospective studies showed significantly improved survival with maximal and optimal cytoreduction [20-24]. The principal goal of cytoreductive surgery should be the removal of the primary cancer and all metastatic disease. Patients whose disease has been completely resected have the best prognosis. If complete rection is feasible, then the surgical aim should be reducing the tumor burden to optimal status, where the largest tumor size is smaller than 1 cm. Silasi et al., [1] showed that the median survival was 46 months for 18 optimally debulked patients and 27 months for four suboptimally debulked patients. Another data series of 40 patients over 10 years demonstrated a 40% 1-year survival rate and a 7.5% 5-year survival rate [25]. In this series, bulk residual disease was associated with a worse survival.

In their multicenter study, Yalcin et al., showed similar disease-free survival and overall survival between ovarian carcinosarcoma and high-grade serous ovarian carcinoma when optimal cytoreduction is achieved [26].

As there is yet no randomized trial on chemotherapy regimen for ovarian carcinosarcoma, the decision has been made based on data from epithelial ovarian cancer and other sarcoma subtypes. All available treatment guidelines are extropolated from the epithelial ovarian tumor. In addition, ifosfamide has been incorporated into the treatment of ovarian carcinosarcoma based on the efficacy of ifosfamide in uterine carcinosarcoma [27]. Ifosfamide and cisplatin either as single agents or in combination were shown to have response rates between 18-100% [17, 21, 28]. Outcomes of patients who received ifosfamide-based regimens and those who received carboplatinum-paclitaxel combination have been compared in several studies, however, the results remained controversial [12, 17, 21, 23, 24, 26, 29, 30].

A Gynecologic Oncology Groups study by Thigpen et al., [31] presented the results of 136 patients with ovarian carcinosarcoma who were given cisplatin 50 mg/m2 every 3 weeks. Cisplatin was found to be active as initial therapy for these tumors. The median overall survival was 11.7 months.

A case control study including 50 women with ovarian carcinosarcoma and 100 women with serous ovarian carcinoma treated who received platinum and taxane-based chemotherapy demonstrated a 62% and 83% response rate, respectively ($p = 0.03$). Median progression-free survival was 11 months versus 16 months ($p = 0.02$) and median overall survival was 24 months versus 41 months ($p = 0.002$) [20].

A single institution, retrospective study compared first-line chemotherapy regimens in ovarian carcinosarcoma [30]. Fifteen patients received carboplatin and paclitaxel, 7 received ifosfamide and paclitaxel, and six received a different regimen. The stage of disease and residual tumor status after surgery were similar between groups. A significant longer progression-free survival was found in patients treated with carboplatin and paclitaxel comparing to those who received ifosfamide and paclitaxel (17.8 vs 8.0 months, $p = 0.02$). Overall survival was similar between groups.

Signorelli et al., [32] reported 41 patients with ovarian carcinosarcoma over 11 years. All women underwent cytoreductive surgery and received platinum-based chemotherapy. Complete response was achieved in 46% of the patients. The median overall survival and progression-free survival was 20 and 12 months, respectively.

A study at Memorial Sloan Kettering Cancer Center used platinum and paclitaxel in 30 women with ovarian carcinosarcoma [33]. Twelve patients (40%) had complete response, seven (23%) partial response, two (7%) stable disease, and nine (30%) progression of disease. The median overall survival was 43 months. The 3- and 5-year survival rates were 53% and 30%, respectively.

A retrospective study including 29 women with ovarian carcinosarcoma found a longer two-year overall survival in patients who received ifosfamide and cisplatin compared to carboplatin and paclitaxel (81% and 55%, respectively, p = 0.003) [21].

A Cochrane review was performed to see the effectiveness of therapy options in ovarian carcinosarcoma [5]. No study was found to include for qualitative analysis. Only two prospective studies and 15 retrospective studies were discussed. Finally, authors found no evidence to support any adjuvant therapy regimens.

The results of two prospective studies are awaited. First, GOG-261 is a randomized phase III study of paclitaxel and carboplatin versus ifosfamide, mesna, and paclitaxel in newly diagnosed Stage I-IV, persistent or recurrent carcinosarcoma of the fallopian tube, peritoneum or ovary (NCT00954174). Recently, the primary results of GOG 261 was published [34]. This study demonstrated that carboplatin and paclitaxel were not inferior to paclitaxel plus ifosfamide with regards to overall survival. A longer progression-free survival was achieved with carboplatin and paclitaxel. Secondly, the expected study is a MITO 26 study which is a phase II multicenter study investigating the efficacy and toxicity of trabectedin in advanced or recurrent ovarian carcinosarcoma (NCT02993705). Recruitment has been completed and we are awaiting the results.

Data on second line treatment options for recurrent or progressing ovarian carcinosarcoma is limited. Currently, a multicentric, randomized phase II/III study evaluating dostarlimab plus niraparib versus niraparib alone compared to chemotherapy in the treatment of endometrial/ovarian carcinosarcoma is ongoing (NCT03651206).

Highlights

- Ovarian carcinosarcomas are rare and a highly aggressive tumor of the ovary.
- Presentation of the patients is similar to those with epithelial ovarian cancer.
- Optimal debulking surgery is an important prognostic factor.
- Platinum and paclitaxel is the most common regimen used for ovarian carcinosarcoma.
- Prognosis is worse than high-grade serous ovarian cancer.

References

[1] Silasi D A, Illuzzi J L, Kelly M G, Rutherford T J, Mor G, Azodi M, Schwartz P E. Carcinosarcoma of the ovary. *Int. J. Gynecol. Cancer.* 2008;18(1):22-9.

[2] Kahramanoglu I, Demirkiran F, Turan H, Bese T, Cebi S, Ilvan S, Arvas M. Adjuvant Treatment Modalities, Prognostic Factors, and Outcome of the Uterine Carcinosarcoma. *J. Obstet. Gynaecol. Can.* 2021 Jan;43(1):34-42. doi: 10.1016/j.jogc.2020.06.021. Epub 2020 Jul 18. PMID: 33041218.

[3] Kozłowski M, Nowak K, Kordek A, Cymbaluk-Płoska A. Therapeutic Management of Rare Primary Ovarian Neoplasms: Carcinosarcoma, Leiomyosarcoma, Melanoma and Carcinoid. *Int. J. Environ. Res. Public Health* 2021;18,7819. doi: 10.3390/ijerph18157819. PMID: 34360112; PMCID: PMC8345663.

[4] George E M, Herzog T J, Neugut A I, Lu YS, Burke WM, Lewin SN, Hershman DL, Wright JD. Carcinosarcoma of the ovary: Natural history, patterns of treatment, and outcome. *Gynecol. Oncol.* 2013;131:42–45. doi: 10.1016/j.ygyno.2013.06.034. Epub 2013 Jul 6. PMID: 23838036; PMCID: PMC4230696.

[5] Shylasree T, Bryant A, Athavale R. Chemotherapy and/or radiotherapy in combination with surgery for ovarian carcinosarcoma. *Cochrane Database Syst. Rev.* 2013 Feb 28;2013(2):CD006246.

[6] Dasgupta S, Bose D, Bhattacharyya N, Biswas PK. Carcinosarcoma of ovary with its various immunohistochemical expression: Report of a rare case. *J. Cancer Res. Ther.* 2015;11:1022. doi: 10.4103/0973-1482.147390. PMID: 26881579.

[7] Jain V, Pundir S, Sekhon R, Mishra A, Nayyar N, Vishwakarma G, Kamboj M, Rawal S. Carcinosarcoma of the Ovary: A Single-Institute Experience with Surgical Cytoreduction and Platinum-Based Chemotherapy. *J. Gynecol. Surg.* 2019;35:224–231.

[8] Kounelis S, Jones M W, Papadaki H, Bakker A, Swalsky P, Finkelstein S D. Carcinosarcomas (malignant mixed mullerian tumors) of the female genital tract: comparative molecular analysis of epithelial and mesenchymal components. *Hum. Pathol.* 1998;29:82–7. doi: 10.1016/s0046-8177(98) 90394-x. PMID: 9445138.

[9] Amant F, Vloeberghs V, Woestenborghs H, Moerman P, Vergote I. Transition of epithelial toward mesenchymal differentiation during ovarian carcinosarcoma tumorigenesis. *Gynecol. Oncol.* 2003;90:372–7. doi: 10.1016/s0090-8258(03)00326-3. PMID: 12893202.

[10] Carnevali I W, Cimetti L, Sahnane N, Libera L, Cavallero A, Formenti G, Riva C, Tibiletti M G. Two Cases of Carcinosarcomas of the Ovary Involved in Hereditary Cancer Syndromes. *Int. J. Gynecol. Pathol.* 2017;36:64–70. doi: 10.1097/PGP.0000000000000290. PMID: 27167672.

[11] Chandra S, Gaur D S, Saini S, Pathak V P. Malignant mixed Müllerian tumour of the ovary with probable prognostic factors. *J. Obstet. Gynaecol.* 2011;31:457–458. doi: 10.3109/01443615. 2011.573106. PMID: 21627442.

[12] Rauh-Hain J A, Diver E J, Clemmer J T, Bradford L S, Clark R M, Growdon W B, Goodman A K, Boruta D M 2nd, Schorge J O, del Carmen M G. Carcinosarcoma of the ovary compared to papillary serous ovarian carcinoma: a SEER analysis. *Gynecol. Oncol.* 2013;131:46–51. doi: 10.1016/j.ygyno. 2013.07.097. Epub 2013 Jul 29. PMID: 23906658.

[13] Ciccarone F, Biscione A, Moro F, Fischerova D, Savelli L, Munaretto M, Jokubkiene L, Sladkevicius P, Chiappa V, Fruscio R, Franchi D, Epstein E, Timmerman D, Froyman W, Valentin L, Scambia G, Testa A C. Imaging in gynecological disease: clinical and ultrasound characteristics of ovarian carcinosarcomas. *Ultrasound Obstet. Gynecol.* 2021 Jul 5. doi: 10.1002/ uog.23733.

[14] Saida T, Mori K, Tanaka Y O, Sakai M, Amano T, Kikuchi S, Masuoka S, Yoshida M, Masumoto T, Satoh T, Minami M. Carcinosarcoma of the ovary: MR and clinical findings compared with high-grade serous carcinoma. *Jpn. J. Radiol.* 2021 Apr;39(4):357-366. doi: 10.1007/s11604-020-01072-7. Epub 2020 Nov 20. PMID: 33216290.

[15] Brown E, Stewart M, Rye T, Al-Nafussi A, Williams A R, Bradburn M, Smyth J, Gabra H. Carcinosarcoma of the ovary: 19 years of prospective data from a single center. *Cancer* 2004;100:2148–2153. doi: 10.1002/cncr.20256. PMID: 15139057.

[16] Sood A K, Sorosky J I, Gelder M S, Buller R E, Anderson B, Wilkinson E J, Benda J A, Morgan L S. Primary ovarian sarcoma: analysis of prognostic variables and the role of surgical cytoreduction. *Cancer* 1998;82:1731–1737. PMID: 9576296.

[17] Boussios S, Karathanasi A, Zakynthinakis-Kyrikaou N, Tsiouris A K, Chatziantoniou A A, Kanellos F S, Tatsi K. Ovarian carcinosarcoma: Current developments and future perspectives. *Critical Reviews in Oncology* 2019;134:46-55. doi: 10.1016/j.critrevonc.2018.12.006. Epub 2018 Dec 24. PMID: 30771873.

[18] Berton-Rigaud D, Devouassoux-Shisheboran M, Ledermann J A, Leitao MM, Powell MA, Poveda A, Beale P, Glasspool RM, Creutzberg CL, Harter P, Kim JW, Reed NS, Ray-Coquard I. Gynecologic Cancer InterGroup (GCIG) consensus review for uterine and ovarian carcinosarcoma. *Int. J. Gynecol. Cancer.* 2014 Nov;24(9 Suppl 3):S55-60. doi: 10.1097/IGC.0000000000000228. PMID: 25341582.

[19] Wang W P, Li N, Zhang Y Y, Gao Y T, Sun Y C, Ge L, Wu L Y. Prognostic significance of lymph node metastasis and lymphadenectomy in early-stage ovarian carcinosarcoma. *Cancer Manag. Res.* 2018;10:1959-1968. doi: 10.2147/CMAR.S166524. PMID: 30022854; PMCID: PMC6044428.

[20] Rauh-Hain J A, Growdon W B, Rodriguez N, Goodman A K, Boruta D M 2nd, Schorge J O, Horowitz N S, del Carmen M G. Carcinosarcoma of the ovary: a case-control study. *Gynecol. Oncol.* 2011;121:477–481. doi: 10.1016/j.ygyno.2011.02.023. Epub 2011 Mar 21. PMID: 21420726.

[21] Rutledge T L, Gold M A, McMeekin D S, Huh W K, Powell M A, Lewin S N, Mutch D G, Johnson G A, Walker J L, Mannel R S. Carcinosarcoma of the ovary-a case series. *Gynecol. Oncol.* 2006;100:128–132. doi: 10.1016/j.ygyno.2005.07.119. Epub 2005 Oct 5. PMID: 16213011.

[22] Doo D W, Erickson B K, Arend R C, Conner MG, Huh WK, Leath CA 3rd. Radical surgical cytoreduction in the treatment of ovarian carcinosarcoma. *Gynecol. Oncol.* 2014;133:234–237. doi: 10.1016/j.ygyno.2014.03.002. Epub 2014 Mar 11. PMID: 24631447; PMCID: PMC7307700.

[23] Cicin I, Ozatlı T., Turkmen E, Özturk T, Özçelik M, Çabuk D, Gökdurnalı A, Balvan Ö, Yıldız Y, Şeker M, Özdemir N, Yapar B, Tanrıverdi Ö, Günaydin Y, Menekşe S, Öksüzoğlu B, Aksoy A, Erdogan B, Bekir Hacıoglu M, Arpaci E, Sevinç A. Predictive and prognostic factors in ovarian and uterine carcinosarcomas. *Balkan Med. J.* 2016;33:517–524. doi: 10.5152/balkanmedj.2016.151268. Epub 2016 Sep 1. PMID: 27761279; PMCID: PMC5056654.

[24] Lu C H, Chen I H, Chen Y J, Wang K L, Qiu J T, Lin H, Lin W C, Liou W S, Huang Y F, Lin Y S, Tee Y T, Hung Y C. Primary treatment and prognostic factors of carcinosarcoma of the ovary, fallopian tube, and peritoneum: a Taiwanese Gynecologic Oncology Group Study. *Int. J. Gynecol. Cancer* 2014;24:506–512. doi: 10.1097/IGC.0000000000000083. PMID: 24557435.

[25] Harris M A, Delap L M, Sengupta P S, Wilkinson P M, Welch R S, Swindell R, Shanks JH, Wilson G, Slade R J, Reynolds K, Jayson G C. Carcinosarcoma of the ovary. *Br. J. Cancer.* 2003 Mar 10;88(5):654-7. doi: 10.1038/sj.bjc.6600770. PMID: 12618869; PMCID: PMC2376340.

[26] Yalcin I, Meydanli M M, Turan A T, Taskin S, Sari ME, Gungor T, Akbayir O, Ayhan A. Carcinosarcoma of the ovary compared to ovarian high-grade serous carcinoma:impact of optimal cytoreduction and standard adjuvant treatment. *Int. J. Clin. Oncol.* 2018;23(2):329–337. doi: 10.1007/s10147-017-1215-x. Epub 2017 Nov 16. PMID: 29143144.

[27] Sutton G P, Blessing J A, Homesley H D, Malfetano J H. A phase II trial of ifosfamide and mesna in patients with advanced or recurrent mixed mesodermal tumors of the ovary previously treated with platinum-based chemotherapy: a Gynecologic Oncology Group study. *Gynecol. Oncol.* 1994 Apr;53(1):24-6. doi: 10.1006/gyno.1994.1081. PMID: 8175017.

[28] Crotzer D R, Wolf J K, Gano J B, Gershenson D M, Levenback C. A pilot study of cisplatin, ifosfamide and mesna in the treatment of malignant mixed mesodermal tumors of the ovary. *Gynecol. Oncol.* 2007;105:399–403. doi: 10.1016/j.ygyno.2006.12.023. Epub 2007 Feb 9. PMID: 17292457.

[29] Inthasorn P, Beale P, Dalrymple C, Carter J. Malignant mixed mullerian tumour of the ovary: prognostic factor and response of adjuvant platinum-based chemotherapy. *Aust. N. Z. J. Obstet. Gynaecol.* 2003;43:61–64. doi: 10.1046/j.0004-8666.2003.00003.x. PMID: 12755351.

[30] Brackmann M, Stasenko M, Uppal S, Erba J, Reynolds R K, McLean K. Comparison of first-line chemotherapy regimens for ovarian carcinosarcoma: a single institution case series and review of the literature. *BMC Cancer* 2018;18:172. doi: 10.1186/s12885-018-4082-6. PMID: 29426293; PMCID: PMC5810191.

[31] Thigpen J, Blessing J A, DeGeest K, Look K Y, Homesley H D; Gynecologic Oncology Group. Cisplatin as initial chemotherapy in ovarian carcinosarcomas: a Gynecologic Oncology Group study. *Gynecol. Oncol.* 2004;93:336–9. doi: 10.1016/j.ygyno.2004.01.007. PMID: 15099942.

[32] Signorelli M, Chiappa V, Minig L, Fruscio R, Perego P, Caspani G, Battistello M, Colombo N. Platinum, anthracycline, and alkylating agent-basedchemotherapy for ovarian carcinosarcoma. *Int. J. Gynecol. Cnacer* 2009;19(6):1142-6. doi: 10.1111/IGC.0b013e3181a8ef22. PMID: 19820383.

[33] Leiser A L, Chi D S, Ishill N M, Tew W P. Carcinosarcoma of the ovary treated with platinum and taxane: the memorial Sloan-Kettering Cancer Center experience. *Gynecol. Oncol.* 2007 Jun;105(3):657-61. Epub 2007 Mar 28. PMID: 17395252.

[34] Powell M A, Filiaci V L, Hensley M L, Huang H Q, Moore K N, Tewari K S, Copeland L J, Secord A A, Mutch D G, Santin A, Warshal D P, Spirtos N M, DiSilvestro P A, Ioffe O B, Miller D S. A randomized phase 3 trial of paclitaxel (P) plus carboplatin (C) versus paclitaxel plus ifosfamide (I) in chemotherapy-naïve patients with stage I-IV, persistent or recurrent carcinosarcoma of the uterus or ovary: an NRG oncology trial. *J. Clin. Oncol.* 2019;37:5500. doi: 10.1200/JCO.21.02050. Epub 2022 Jan 10. PMID: 35007153; PMCID: PMC8937015.

Chapter 23

Krukenberg Tumors

Federico Coccolini[1,*], MD
Riccardo Guelfi[1], MD
Enrico Cicuttin[1], MD
Camilla Cremonini[1], MD
Dario Tartaglia[1], MD
Marta Carretto[2], MD
Tommaso Simoncini[2], MD
and Massimo Chiarugi[1], MD
[1]General, Emergency and Trauma Surgery Department, Pisa University Hospital, Pisa, Italy
[2]Gynecology Department, Pisa University Hospital, Pisa, Italy

Introduction

In 1896 a German gynecologist and pathologist, Friedrich Ernst Krukenberg (1871-1946), described for the first time a supposedly new type of primary ovarian cancer and he called it "fibrosarcoma ovarii mucocellulare, carcinomatodes" [1]. Five years later, Kraus revealed the metastatic nature of this tumor, taking origin from the primary gastrointestinal [9]. Kraus was probably the first who proposed the eponym "Krukenberg tumor" [22].

Krukenberg tumors (KTs) make up about 1% to 2% of all ovarian tumors and they are histopathologically defined as carcinomas that have a significant component (arbitrarily defined as >10% of the tumor) of mucin-filled signet-ring cells [1]. The correct diagnosis of secondary ovarian tumors may be challenging: KTs are frequently diagnosed incorrectly as primary ovarian cancer, particularly in the case of mucinous adenocarcinomas. Even though KT are probably the best-known secondary tumors of the ovary (STOs), they represent only about 30–40% of all STOs [24]. They are often bilateral (over 80%), given their metastatic nature. The most common primary tumors that give origin to ovarian metastases are colorectal carcinoma (32%) [23], breast carcinoma (15.4%), endometrial carcinoma (12.9%), gastric carcinoma (9.2%) [20] appendiceal carcinoma (6.7%), uterine cervix carcinoma (2.4%),

* Corresponding Author's Email: Federico.coccolini@gmail.com.

In: Ovarian Cancer
Editors: Christos Iavazzo, Alexandros Fotiou and John Spiliotis
ISBN: 979-8-88697-633-5

pancreatic carcinoma (2.2%), small intestine carcinoma (1.6%), and carcinoma of the gallbladder and biliary tract (1.5%) [16]. Other tumors such as lung carcinoma, skin tumors, kidney cancer, and esophageal carcinoma each accounted for less than 1% [9-26]. The primary source of the metastatic tumors could be unknown in about 12.2% [25]. It is not rare that the detection of STOs precedes the diagnosis of the primary tumor, which may be small and asymptomatic: it's a great challenge, for both clinicians and pathologists, making the correct diagnosis and choosing the adequate treatment. Although the prognosis of STOs is generally poor, there are differences across various primary tumors [1]. The distinction from the latter is essential, as it requires different treatment. Immunohistochemistry plays an important role in distinguishing primary ovarian tumors from extra-ovarian metastases and may suggest the primary tumor site. Furthermore, metastasectomy may improve the prognosis in select cases [1]. Several intriguing questions are encountered in daily practice, including diagnostic algorithm, the role of cytoreductive surgery (CRS) and of consequent adjuvant therapies.

Epidemiology

The age at diagnosis of secondary ovarian tumors seems to be associated with the origin of the primary tumor and women affected by STOs are generally younger than those with primary epithelial ovarian cancer (EOC). If the primary tumors have origin from the gastrointestinal (GI) tract, patients are generally older than those with a primary tumor located outside the GI tract. Conversely, patients with breast cancer metastasizing to ovaries are significantly younger than those with primary tumors originated elsewhere than the breast [27]. Patients with KTs represent the youngest subgroup with an average age of 45 years at the time of diagnosis [28]. Probably, a greater ovary vascularization in young women facilitates hematogenous spread. Meer et al. showed that approximately one in twenty young female colorectal cancer patients will present with or develop ovarian metastases [1]. The incidence is higher in countries like Korea, Japan, and China where the tumor makes up about 20% of all ovarian cancers [9] and gastric cancer accounts for 23.4 and 30.4% of STOs in Japan and Korea, respectively. Asian countries have been consistently reporting higher rates of secondary ovarian tumors compared to European Countries. In Europe and the USA, breast cancer and colorectal cancer are the most common primary tumors spread to the ovaries [1].

Pathogenesis

All tumors spread through different mechanisms:

- the lymphatic system
- the hematogenous system
- the transcoelomic pathway.

The first two pathways involve the spreading of tumor cells via lymphatic and blood vessels, respectively, whereas transcoelomic dissemination means the direct spreading of the tumor cells through the abdominal route to adjacent organs across the peritoneal cavity [32].

The *lymphatic route* is believed to be the most likely route of cancer spread with several supporting evidence: microscopically, the hilum and cortex have demonstrated lymphatic permeation. Many cases have been reported where the primary tumor is confined to mucosa and submucosa and given the rich lymphatic network in the GI mucosa and submucosa, the only logical explanation is that the tumor spread through this pathway. The risk of metastasis is higher with an increased number of positive metastatic lymph nodes [20]. Furthermore, it seems that different tumors metastasize through different pathways; for example, a hematogenous spread seems to be the most frequent pathway in colon cancer [1]. This observation is further supported by immunohistochemical analyses revealing a higher rate of vascular invasion and a lower rate of lymphangio-invasion in ovarian metastases from colorectal cancer compared to gastric cancer. Conversely, a retrograde lymphogenous spread seems to be involved in gastric cancer metastases [33]. There are several possible explanations. First, a rich mucosal and submucosal lymphatic plexus in the stomach enables lymphogenous metastases even at an early stage of the disease. The anatomy and evolution of the lymphatic system provides another explanation [1]. The urogenital lymph vessel tract gives rise to the receptaculum chyli via the lumbar trunks. The receptaculum chyli joins intestinal trunks, which connect via celiac lymph nodes to the gastric, hepatic, pancreaticolienal, and mesenteric (superior mesenteric and mesocolic) nodes. The short distance from the receptaculum chyli to the gastric nodes enables the gastric cancer cells to metastasize easily via the receptaculum chyli to the urogenital lymph vessel trunks, which supply the ovaries [1]. Moreover, tumor infiltration of retroperitoneal lymphatic nodes by GI cancers may lead to lymphatic vessel obstruction and subsequently countercurrent of the lymph flow into the ovaries [1]. Transcoelomic dissemination, which is the main pathway of metastasis in primary ovarian cancer [34], does not seem to play a major role in secondary ovarian tumors development. A study proposes a hypothesis of transcoelomic spread and ruptured ovary during ovulation, providing a seeding site for metastasizing tumor cells as the possible route of metastasis in KTs' cases [18].

Metastatic Organotropism

Several mechanisms explain the propensity of tumors to metastasize to specific secondary, including the attraction of tumor cells to specific organs, adhesion of cells to the endothelium in a specific organ, survival in the metastatic site, angiogenesis at the metastatic site, the pre-metastatic niche, and the ability of tumor cells to extravasate into a specific organ [35]. Generally, the principle of organotropism can be described as a cross-talk between intrinsic molecular properties of the primary tumor cells and the specific features of the metastatic site microenvironment [36]. However, no specific markers associated with ovarian metastatic progression have yet been identified. A retrospective study including 38 cases of ovarian metastases from colorectal cancer used next-generation somatic mutation profiling to assess 341 cancer-associated genes [30], finding an increased number of mutations in the KRAS, SMAD4, and NTRK1 genes in ovarian metastases, compared to a cohort of 543 cases with no metastases of the ovaries. However, whether the presence of these mutations is responsible for ovarian organotropism remains unclear. Another study compared somatic mutation profiles in 26 primary colorectal cancer and matched ovarian metastases [37], and while the known driver genes were mostly concordant, the primary colorectal showed a considerably higher number of passenger mutations than corresponding ovarian metastases. They could speculate that many sub-clones are present within the primary tumor, out of which only certain sub-clones possess the ability of homing into ovaries [37]. Mutated KRAS is a universal driver of the metastatic disease in women with KRAS-mutated colorectal cancer with ovarian metastases. Future studies may investigate the efficacy of KRAS inhibitors in the treatment of these patients [7]. Recent evidence demonstrated that most high-grade serous ovarian cancers (HGSOC) have their origin from the fimbria of the fallopian tube and subsequently metastasize into the ovaries [38]: could HGSOC and STOs share some molecular patterns related to ovarian organotropism? Further studies are needed to identify specific molecular patterns associated with preferential ovarian metastatic spread: if these patterns are found within the primary tumor, they might aid in treatment decision-making.

Clinical Signs

Generally, there are no clear differences between the symptoms arising from primary and secondary ovarian malignancies [40]. Both of them can be asymptomatic or may manifest with non-specific GI signs and symptoms like abdominal or pelvic pain (42%), bloating, dyspareunia, weight loss (6%), and an increase of abdominal circumference (15%) [9, 31]. Sometimes, these tumors could cause vaginal bleeding (18%) or menstrual cycle irregularities: vaginal bleeding and change in menstrual cycles can be attributed to luteinization of the ovarian stroma and consequent hormonal production [39]. These changes are induced by STOs and sometimes may lead to hirsutism and virilization. Ascites is present in 39% of cases at diagnosis, which is less common than in primary ovarian cancer [1]. Patients with STOs that originate from the appendix may be present with pseudomyxoma peritonei [26]. Compared to KTs from colorectal cancer, KTs from gastric cancer cause higher incidence of ascites, higher proportion of solid ovarian masses and a trend of higher incidence of synchronous KTs [15]. Like primary ovarian cancer, STOs remain asymptomatic until the tumor grows into a certain size. This is the reason why most patients attend the clinic with advanced disease.

Diagnosis

The detection of KTs precedes diagnosis of the primary tumor in up to 40% of cases, especially in patients with colorectal or stomach cancer [40]. The method to distinguish STOs from primary ovarian tumors comes through histopathological examination, preferably performing immunohistochemistry (IHC). Unfortunately, despite thorough diagnostic evaluation, the primary tumor remains unknown in about 12.2% of cases [41]. The diagnostic criteria of KT diagnose were proposed by Novak and Gray and consist of ovarian neoplasm, signet- ring cells producing mucin, and sarcomatoid proliferation of the ovarian stroma [42].

Imaging Methods

The role of imaging methods is to provide information on the extent of the disease and to identify a potential primary site of the tumor. On ultrasound examination, Krukenberg metastases can appear solid (if stomach or breast are the primary tumor), mixed solid and cystic (when colon, rectum, appendix, or biliary tract are the primary tumor), or less commonly, predominantly cystic masses (when colon or appendix are primary tumor) with clear well-defined margins [20]. A computed tomography (CT) scan of the chest, abdomen, and pelvis, with the use of intravenous contrast material, should be performed as a baseline evaluation, as this is considered a standard in cancer of an unknown primary site [43]. None of the routinely used imaging methods, including CT, ultrasonographic (US), and magnetic resonance (MR) imaging has proved reliable in distinguishing primary ovarian cancer from STOs, although primary ovarian tumors tend to be multilocular more frequently than STOs on US and MR images [44]. On MRI, the solid components appear to be T1 and T2 hypointense because of dense stromal reaction, and they show corresponding diffusion restriction and enhancement on contrast-enhanced sequences. T2 hyperintensity is seen in the cystic areas, representing mucin that does not enhance. Hypointense T2 solid components in an ovarian mass are characteristic of KT, particularly if the tumors are bilateral with uniform cystic locules, have sharp margins, and have an oval configuration [20]. Also, 2-[fluorine-18]-fluoro-2-deoxy-d-glucose positron emission tomography integrated with computed tomography (18F-FDG PET/CT) is unable to distinguish STOs from primary ovarian tumors. Despite the superior sensitivity of PET/CT over CT, there are several limitations, including the inability to detect smaller lesions (<1.0 cm) and tumors with low or no FDG uptake (e.g., renal cell carcinoma, breast carcinoma, and some GI cancers). PET/CT might be useful in select patients [45]: the potential efficacy of this functional imaging for KT is still in the exploratory phase, but its applications in diagnosis, disease prognostication, therapeutic response monitoring, and follow-up recurrence detection are superior to other imaging modalities [6].

The Role of CA 125

More than 80% of women with primary EOC have an elevated CA 125 and the same marker increases in 70% of patients affected by STOs [27, 46]. However, the pre-operative level of serum CA 125 does not differ between primary and STOs, the sensitivity of CA 125 in detecting STOs is significantly lower than in detecting primary ovarian cancer. CA 125 does not seem to be a useful biomarker for the diagnosis of STOs. The CA 125/CEA ratio might be useful for a differential diagnosis between primary ovarian tumors and colorectal carcinoma (CRC) metastases [1]. Additionally, serum CA 125 level could have a high positive predictive value (95.7%) for primary ovarian cancer when it's above 170 U/mL in combination with a complex ovarian mass with papillary projections presenting on the US [40]. Pre-operative level for serum CA-125 can be decreased after tumor resection. Checking postoperative levels of serum CA-125 can be useful for:

- Follow-up of patients after surgery to document complete resection as levels will decline;

- Follow-up of patients to diagnose metastatic spread to ovaries in patients with a history of other cancers (e.g., gastrointestinal, breast);
- To predict the prognosis of patients with KT [9]. One study showed that levels greater than 75 U/ml were associated with decreased 5-year survival than patients with lower levels [10].

Endoscopic Methods

Endoscopic investigation is a reasonable approach because the majority of STOs take their origin from GI and it also provides a non-invasive method to obtain a histopathological specimen. In countries with a high incidence of gastric and colorectal cancer, the endoscopic evaluation (esophagogastroduodenoscopy and/or colonoscopy) should always be considered as a frontline for anatomic localization and diagnostic tool in STOs of an unknown primary site [1]. Endoscopically, the tumor can appear as a friable, ulcerated mass or a nodular appearing mucosa. The mucosal architecture can appear expanded or elongated as if it has been "stretched". Signet ring cell carcinoma of the stomach often tend to infiltrate the sub-mucosa and muscularis propria extensively, and there may be minimal mucosal findings on standard white light endoscopy. An important clue to the presence of these tumors could be the poor distensibility of the stomach: use of defoaming and mucolytic agents may help improve visibility, and adequate air insufflation can help assess distensibility. Identifying subtle irregularities in mucosal glands and microvasculature could be possible using magnification endoscopy. Advanced imaging technologies, such as narrow-band imaging (NBI) and chromoendoscopy, may be useful. During an endoscopic evaluation, every suspicious-appearing area in the stomach should be biopsied, even if sometimes superficial mucosal biopsies may be falsely negative. Larger biopsies with jumbo forceps can be employed when this is suspected. When endoscopic biopsies are non-diagnostic, endoscopic ultrasound (EUS) may be helpful to confirm the hypothesis of a suspicious gastric cancer. EUS guided fine-needle aspiration (FNA) of the gastric wall may help confirm the diagnosis. Use of Elastography to help guide FNA can improve the diagnostic yield [47].

Histopathological Diagnosis

Macroscopic Description

The ovaries are asymmetrically enlarged with an irregular external capsule. They are usually solid, but they can occasionally be cystic. The capsular surface is mostly free of any tumor infiltrates, adhesions, implants, or deposits which can be deceptive and appear as a primary ovarian tumor. The diagnostic criteria of WHO are:

- presence of stromal involvement,
- ovarian stromal sarcomatoid proliferation,
- presence of mucin-producing signet-ring cells [9].

Metastases to ovaries are generally smaller than primary ovarian carcinomas and usually contain cysts. Most secondary ovarian tumors have a diameter smaller than 10 cm. Notably, metastases from breast cancer are usually smaller, while metastases from the GI tract (especially from colon cancer) are bigger and may resemble primary ovarian tumors [27, 29]. Bilateralism is more frequent than in primary ovarian cancer: the tendency toward metastasizing into both ovaries is even more obvious in KTs, which are bilateral in more than 80% of cases [23]. While tumor metastases from breast, stomach, and appendix carcinomas are mostly bilateral, the metastases from colorectal carcinoma tend to be unilateral [42] [48]. Both primary and metastatic mucinous ovarian tumors are characterized by several macroscopic and microscopic features, which may be helpful in their differential diagnosis (Fig. 1). Most primary ovarian mucinous carcinomas are large, unilateral tumors that are cystic, multilocular, with intact smooth surface, with no discrete nodularities. Cystic and solid areas in these tumors are evenly distributed throughout the tumor. The predominant type of invasion is usually expansile, with the infiltrative type of invasion being absent or only focal in most cases. On the contrary, metastatic tumors are often smaller, bilateral, and involve the ovarian surface or superficial cortex [16].

The nodularity is usually visible macroscopically, however, even cases without macroscopically distinct nodules usually show at a microscopic level, where they are characterized by aggregates (groups, nodules) of tumor cells surrounded by normal ovarian stroma, especially in the superficial cortex. Metastatic tumors often have a predominantly infiltrative pattern of development. There is no specific features which would allow for a clear distinction between a primary and a metastatic tumor [16].

Histology

The histology of STOs usually corresponds to the primary tumor and mucinous adenocarcinoma is the most common histological finding. A poorly cohesive/signet-ring cell morphology can be observed in most metastases from gastric cancer [28]. The predominant histological type of breast cancer metastasizing to ovaries is invasive ductal carcinoma, followed by invasive lobular carcinoma, with the latter not uncommonly manifesting as KT [27, 49]. Metastatic endometrial malignancies are mainly adenocarcinomas, while squamous cell carcinomas are the most common histological type of cervical metastases [49]. Other rarer histological types include metastatic sarcoma, melanoma, and lung cancer [27]. Metastatic adenocarcinomas with mucinous features represent a diagnostic issue, as they might be misdiagnosed as primary ovarian neoplasms [50]. Tubular KT with luteinization of the ovarian stroma (i.e., cells arranged in tubules) must be distinguished from ovarian tumors with an annular or tubular pattern including Sertoli-Leydig cell tumor (lack of signet-ring cells, stain positive for inhibin and negative to cytokeratin), endometrioid carcinoma, and tumor of Wolffian origin [9, 39]. Classic KT (i.e., tumors with signet ring cells that lack tubular formation) must be distinguished from ovarian tumors that contain signet ring cells with mucinous or non-mucinous material. Ovarian tumors with mucin stain like KT, but they also stain positive for chromogranin and synaptophysin, which can differentiate them from KT. Ovarian tumor with signet ring cell without mucin is divided into:

- a signet-ring stromal tumor (benign, unilateral, devoid of epithelial differentiation, stain positive for vimentin, and negative for cytokeratin)
- sclerosing stromal cell tumor (contain lipid with no reactivity to periodic acid-Schiff stain and stain positive for inhibin stain)
- clear cell adenocarcinoma of the ovary (contains glycogen that stains with periodic acid-Schiff, papillary and tubulocystic pattern with hobnail cells)

Previous history of malignancy may raise suspicion of STOs, but the metastatic nature of any ovarian mass always must be considered as it may be the first finding in previously undiagnosed extra-ovarian cancer. An intra-operative frozen section biopsy is used to tailor the surgical effort, even if systematic pelvic and para-aortic lymphadenectomy (with staging purpose) is generally not considered in primary ovarian cancers with peritoneal spread.

The Role of Immunohistochemistry

Cytokeratin 7 and 20 (CK7 and CK20) are the most determined antigens in ovarian tumors. Primary ovarian carcinomas are almost always CK7 positive (90–100%), whereas the immunoreactivity to CK20 is generally negative [28]. A cytokeratin 7 (CK7)–positive and cytokeratin 20 (CK20)–negative immunophenotype favors a primary ovarian carcinoma, whereas a CK7-negative and CK20-positive immunophenotype or a CK7-positive and CK20-positive immunophenotype (note that both feature CK20 positivity) in commonly reported in metastatic gastrointestinal carcinoma. Other frequently used markers include WT1 and CA 125, which are associated with primary ovarian carcinoma. However, their expression varies in different histologic subtypes: they are positive in most primary ovarian serous adenocarcinomas (both high-grade and low-grade) but are negative in the majority of ovarian clear cell and mucinous carcinomas [51]. In addition, a carcinoembryonic antigen–positive and cancer antigen 125–negative profile favors metastatic origin [20]. The expression of both progesterone receptors (PRs) and estrogen receptors (ERs) in primary ovarian carcinomas is highly variable, depending on the tumor type. In general, ERs are more commonly expressed than PRs and the expression of ERs and PRs is detected only in about 10% of mucinous and clear cell carcinomas. ERs positivity may be observed in more than 80% of serous and endometrioid carcinomas and the expression of PRs in 30–70% of these tumor types [48].

Moreover, ovarian mucinous adenocarcinomas are negative for β-catenin and positive for MUC5AC, whereas mucinous colorectal cancer exhibits a reverse pattern [1,51]. CDX2 is a sensitive marker for mucinous colorectal cancer, but it is non-specific and can also be expressed in ovarian mucinous carcinoma. A novel marker, dipeptidase 1 (DPEP1), was found to be clinically useful in distinguishing primary mucinous ovarian cancer from ovarian metastasis of GI cancers [68]; if combined with other IHC markers (CDX2 and CK7), together with a single clinical factor (tumor size), DPEP1 can provide an accuracy of 93%. A very potent biomarker for differentiating metastasis of breast and gastric cancer is hepatocyte nuclear factor 4A (HNF4A): it is positive in gastric carcinoma and negative in breast carcinoma [52].

When IHC is inconclusive, molecular profiling may aid differential diagnosis between primary ovarian tumors and secondary ovarian tumors: performing comprehensive genomic analysis (a single nucleotide polymorphism [SNP] assay) and transcriptomic analysis could help to discriminate primary ovarian tumors from cancer metastases in accordance with pathological diagnosis [53].

Staging

The KT are metastatic disease from the gastrointestine or other sites, so they are classified as Stage IV disease [9].

Management

There are no international standard guidelines for the treatment of KTs: they represent an extremely heterogeneous group of tumors with distinct biological characteristics and prognosis. Moreover, the rarity of KTs makes any prospective randomized clinical trials practically unfeasible. The management of STOs should be based on a diagnostic process to assess the primary tumor site, their biological features, and the diffusion of disease. If the primary tumor is detected, it should be treated according to its histological type [54].

The Role of CRS for STOs

Recently, evidence demonstrated that primary surgical cytoreduction in primary ovarian cancer benefits survival, but there are no prospective trials regarding the role of cytoreductive surgery for STOs. A multidisciplinary consensus is essential for appropriate selection of asymptomatic patients who may benefit from prophylactic surgery [21]. Bilateral oophorectomy should be performed during the surgery for ovarian metastasis, even in the case of a tumor confined to a single ovary, as the contralateral ovary can be a site for metachronous metastases, thus preventing the patient from undergoing additional tumor resection [1]. Most retrospective studies agreed that cytoreductive surgery may provide a survival benefit in a select sub-groups of patients. A retrospective analysis showed that patients who underwent palliative surgeries including unilateral or bilateral salpingo-oophorectomy alone, or a total combined with bilateral salpingo-oophorectomy, had a median overall survival of 17 months [11]. The primary tumor site is the most relevant factor in choosing the management. Patients with ovarian metastases from colorectal cancer appear to be the best candidates because the survival benefit from cytoreductive surgery has been confirmed in most studies [1, 55]. Patients with disease confined to the pelvis have better prognosis than those with extra-pelvic metastases [56]. Literature confirms that an optimal surgical cytoreduction in patients with colorectal cancer confined to ovaries may result in a higher 5-year survival rate than in those with optimally resected isolated pulmonary or liver metastases [57]. Moreover, STOs of gastric origin have poorer prognosis, compared with other primary tumors, and they are usually associated with lower performance status (PS), anemia, coagulation dysfunction, and cachexia, often preventing the patient from undergoing surgery [55]. There is a difference between synchronous and metachronous STOs of gastric origin in terms of higher feasibility of R0 resection and better survival following resection in metachronous fashion. Taking this into consideration, it seems reasonable to perform a cytoreductive surgery in metachronous STOs of gastric origin confined to ovaries in patients with good performance status. In the case of synchronous metastases, the benefit of this approach is less clear, although when combined with hyperthermic intraperitoneal chemotherapy (HIPEC), it might provide a survival benefit with acceptable morbidity and mortality rates [58]. Therefore, the decision to perform cytoreductive surgery must be tailored to the patients. Ayhan et al. observed that cytoreductive surgery in breast cancer metastasizing into ovaries did not provide any survival benefit [59]. There was a trend toward better survival in patients with no visible residual disease after metastasectomy for abdominal/pelvic masses originating from breast cancer compared with those left with gross disease; however, it did not reach any statistical significance [1]. At present, there is not enough evidence supporting the routine use of metastasectomy in STOs of breast origin. Similar to primary ovarian cancer, the extent of cytoreductive surgery is an important prognostic factor, as it was found that 5-year survival in patients with residual disease less than 2 cm in diameter is significantly higher than in those with residual disease greater than 2 cm in diameter, especially in patients with primary colorectal cancer [8]. An aggressive debulking surgery seems to be beneficial and a maximal surgical effort should be made in patients with secondary ovarian tumors [60]. In conclusion, there is a subgroup of patients (good PS, metastases limited to ovaries, primary tumor of colorectal origin, a feasibility of no or minimal residual disease) who may benefit from cytoreductive surgery. The data supporting cytoreductive surgery in patients with STOs of gastric origin is less clear, and this approach should be evaluated for every single patient [22].

Palliative surgery for patients with KTs can be performed safely in an experienced unit with acceptable complication rates. The decision to proceed with metastasectomy is influenced by several factors including the presence of symptoms, synchronous disease, and tumor response to chemotherapy, and should be made as part of a multidisciplinary team consensus. Proper selection is essential for asymptomatic patients who may benefit from prophylactic surgery. Further studies can be done to determine if symptom-free survival can be prolonged, or quality of life improved with palliative surgery [14].

Adjuvant Chemotherapy Following CRS

There are not promising results about the effectiveness of adjuvant chemotherapy, and it couldn't replace surgery in a satisfactory way [19]. Platinum-based chemotherapy regimens seem to provide a survival benefit in gastric cancer [61]. Cheong et al. found no difference regarding OS when comparing intravenous and intraperitoneal adjuvant chemotherapy in patients with resected STOs of gastric origin [1]. Instead, Rosa et al. described a significantly longer median OS in patients who received a combination of HIPEC and systemic chemotherapy compared with those who received only systemic chemotherapy (33 vs. 20 months, $P = 0.0005$) [58].

Hyperthermic Intraperitoneal Chemotherapy (HIPEC)

In literature, only a few studies have analyzed HIPEC for KTs. Rosa et al. assessed the association of HIPEC with CRS and adjuvant chemotherapy. They showed that this association significantly increased OS compared with CRS and adjuvant chemotherapy protocol or chemotherapy alone, supporting the independent prognostic value of HIPEC. Wu et al. evaluated the effectiveness of HIPEC in combination with surgery, showing that this association increased the OS about three times on average compared to CRS alone. Finally, Cheong et al. investigated the difference in OS between the CRS with HIPEC Protocol and CRS with chemotherapy protocol. They did not find any significant difference between the two protocols, concluding that chemotherapy and HIPEC might have the same effectiveness when associated with CRS. Despite the low number of studies, HIPEC seems to be effective both alone and in combination with CRS. Therefore, also given the less severe adverse effects compared to chemotherapy, HIPEC seems to be a preferable adjuvant approach for KT. CRS with no residual disease improves OS in KT patients, but results about chemotherapy are conflicting. The association of CRS with HIPEC seems to be the most effective and safe therapeutic protocol for KT patients, but further studies are needed [19].

Prognosis

Patients will usually die within 2 years. Literature reports a median survival of 14 months. The median overall survival (OS) of patients with KTs is reportedly 11, 21.5, 31, and 19.5 months for gastric, colorectal, breast, and other origins respectively [12]. The survival of patients with secondary ovarian tumors is significantly worse than those with primary ovarian cancer (5-year survival rate of 18.5 vs. 40.0%) [1], although there are differences in prognosis according with the primary tumor [1]. The prognosis of advanced gastric cancer is worse compared with that of advanced colorectal cancer; and patients with KTs of gastric origin usually have a lower performance status score and severe anemia [15]. If the secondary ovarian tumors originate from the genital tract, the prognosis is significantly better than of those originating outside the genital tract (median overall is 48 vs. 12 months) [29]. The poorest prognosis seems to be associated with STOs originating from pancreatic and small intestine cancer [25]. Several prognostic factors have been identified: pre-operative carbohydrate antigen 125 (CA 125) level in serum, age at diagnosis of secondary ovarian tumor, pre-operative secondary ovarian tumor size, primary tumor origin, presence of peritoneal dissemination, extent of CRS, and unilaterality versus bilaterality [1]. Obviously, the median OS was also shorter for patients younger than 50 years old, patients with a pre-operative American Society of Anaesthesiologists (ASA) score of 3 vs 2, larger tumors $\geq$ 12 cm, those with peritoneal metastases and those with Hepatic metastases [31]. Recently, evidence suggested the role of molecular profiling: mutations of the SMAD family member 4 (SMAD4) and lysine methyltransferase 2D (KMT2D) genes are associated with a reduced median overall in ovarian metastases from colorectal cancer [30], indicating that somatic mutation profiling may provide additional prognostic information.

Conclusion

The metastasis to ovaries from various primary tumor sites is not a common event. Several metastatic pathways (lymphogenous, hematogenous, and transcoelomic spread) have been suggested, highlighting that different primary tumor probably use different preferential metastatic routes. STOs may be confused with primary ovarian cancer, especially in the case of suspicious mucinous adenocarcinomas. Therefore, the potential metastatic nature of all newly diagnosed adnexal masses should always be considered. Furthermore, immunohistochemistry plays a major role in distinguishing primary from metastatic ovarian tumors and may suggest the potential primary tumor site. Though the role of adjuvant chemotherapy following resection of metastases is not clear, it seemingly provides a survival benefit in the case of gastric and colorectal cancer [1]. The diagnosis and management of the KTs are complex and should involve a multidisciplinary team that includes oncologists, oncologic surgeons, hospice, palliative care nurses, pain specialists, dedicated pathologists, and radiologists. Peritoneal involvement, ascites, synchronous presentation, and increased serum CEA levels appear as significant unfavorable prognostic factors. The assessment of such factors may be considered in a prognostic algorithm for the risk stratification in KTs, to achieve a more tailored management of patients. On the other hand, age, menopausal status, KTs' size, bilateral ovarian involvement, non-peritoneal extaovarian metastases, signet ring cell morphology and levels of CA125 does not show significant association with the OS [17]. The prognosis is generally poor, although there are differences according to histological subtypes, most patients will die within 12-24 months [13]. In most cases, patients are frail and debilitated, aggressive surgery is not recommended as it does not extend life span. Most patients may benefit from hospice care and pain control.

References

[1] Kubeček O, Laco J, Špaček J, Petera J, Kopecký J, Kubečková A, Filip S. The pathogenesis, diagnosis, and management of metastatic tumors to the ovary: a comprehensive review. *Clin Exp Metastasis*. 2017 Jun;34(5):295-307. doi: 10.1007/s10585-017-9856-8. Epub 2017 Jul 20. PMID: 28730323; PMCID: PMC5561159.

[2] Sakio R, Ito H, Ota G, Tahara M, Yano T, Koinuma K, Horie H, Lefor AK, Yamamoto H, Sata N. Metachronous Krukenberg tumor from adenocarcinoma in a Meckel's diverticulum: a case report. *J Surg Case Rep*. 2021 Aug 31;2021(8):rjab374. doi: 10.1093/jscr/rjab374. PMID: 34476080; PMCID: PMC8407034.

[3] Goidescu IG, Nemeti G, Preda A, Kovacs T, Surcel M, Eniu DT, Cruciat G, Mureșan D. Krukenberg tumor in pregnancy: a rare case and review of the literature. *J Matern Fetal Neonatal Med*. 2021 Sep 1:1-6. doi: 10.1080/14767058.2021.1946788. Epub ahead of print. PMID: 34470118.

[4] van der Meer R, Bakkers C, Rostamkhan E, de Hingh I, Roumen R. Ovarian metastases from colorectal cancer in young women: a systematic review of the literature. *Int J Colorectal Dis*. 2021 Aug 25. doi: 10.1007/s00384-021-04012-7. Epub ahead of print. PMID: 34432125.

[5] Creffier C, Broome K, Palmer D. Ovarian metastasis from a urachal adenocarcinoma primary in a young female. *Urol Case Rep*. 2021 Aug 2;39:101797. doi: 10.1016/j.eucr.2021.101797. PMID: 34401351; PMCID: PMC8353346.

[6] Kumar N, Lata K, Tripathy S, Shamim SA, Ray MD. Renal Cell Carcinoma Mimicking with Peritoneal Carcinomatosis and Krukenberg Tumor: Diagnosis Seen on Fluorodeoxyglucose Positron Emission Tomography-Computed Tomography. *Indian J Nucl Med*. 2021 Apr-Jun;36(2):207-209. doi: 10.4103/ijnm.IJNM_197_20. Epub 2021 Jun 21. PMID: 34385798; PMCID: PMC8320827.

[7] Kemps PG, Bol M, Steller EJA, de Pont LMH, Holterhues C, van Gerven L, Kolkman W. Colon carcinoma presenting as ovarian metastasis. *Radiol Case Rep*. 2021 Jul 23;16(9):2799-2803. doi: 10.1016/j.radcr.2021.06.072. PMID: 34367398; PMCID: PMC8326593.

[8] Kim C, Hu YH, Lee K, Lee HA, Lee DH, Ouh YT. Metastatic gallbladder cancer to the ovary presenting as primary ovarian cancer: a case report. *J Med Case Rep.* 2021 Aug 5;15(1):413. Doi: 10.1186/s13256-021-03001-2. PMID: 34348771; PMCID: PMC8340448.

[9] Aziz M, Kasi A. *Krukenberg Tumor.* 2021 Jul 25. In: StatPearls [Internet]. *Treasure Island* (FL): StatPearls Publishing; 2021 Jan–. PMID: 29489206.

[10] Al-Agha OM, Nicastri AD. An in-depth look at Krukenberg tumor: an overview. *Arch Pathol Lab Med.* 2006 Nov;130(11):1725-30.

[11] Seow-En I, Hwarng G, Tan GHC, Ho LML, Teo MCC. Palliative surgery for Krukenberg tumors - 12-year experience and review of the literature. *World J Clin Oncol.* 2018 Feb 10;9(1):13-19.

[12] Wu F, Zhao X, Mi B, Feng LU, Yuan NA, Lei F, Li M, Zhao X. Clinical characteristics and prognostic analysis of Krukenberg tumor. *Mol Clin Oncol.* 2015 Nov;3(6):1323-1328.

[13] Seow-En I, Hwarng G, Tan GHC, Ho LML, Teo MCC. Palliative surgery for Krukenberg tumors - 12-year experience and review of the literature. *World J Clin Oncol.* 2018 Feb 10;9(1):13-19.

[14] Seow-En I, Hwarng G, Tan GHC, Ho LML, Teo MCC. Palliative surgery for Krukenberg tumors – 12-year experience and review of the literature. *World J Clin Oncol.* 2018 Feb 10;9(1):13-19. Doi: 10.5306/wjco.v9.i1.13. PMID: 29468133; PMCID: PMC5807888.

[15] Xie H, Erickson BJ, Sheedy SP, Yin J, Hubbard JM. The diagnosis and outcome of Krukenberg tumors. *J Gastrointest Oncol.* 2021 Apr;12(2):226-236. doi: 10.21037/jgo-20-364. PMID: 34012621; PMCID: PMC8107606.

[16] Dundr P, Singh N, Nožičková B, Němejcová K, Bártů M, Stružinská I. Primary mucinous ovarian tumors vs. ovarian metastases from gastrointestinal tract, pancreas and biliary tree: a review of current problematics. *Diagn Pathol.* 2021 Mar 11;16(1):20. doi: 10.1186/s13000-021-01079-2. PMID: 33706757; PMCID: PMC7953678.

[17] Lionetti R, De Luca M, Travaglino A, Raffone A, Saccone G, Di Cicco A, Insabato L, Mascolo M, D'Armiento M, Zullo F, Corcione F. Prognostic factors in Krukenberg tumor. *Arch Gynecol Obstet.* 2019 Nov;300(5):1155-1165. doi: 10.1007/s00404-019-05301-x. Epub 2019 Sep 21. PMID: 31542818.

[18] Shah B, Tang WH, Karn S. Transcoelomic spread and ovarian seeding during ovulation: A possible pathogenesis of Krukenberg tumor. *J Cancer Res Ther.* 2017 Jan-Mar;13(1):152-153. Doi: 10.4103/0973-1482.206234. PMID: 28508852.

[19] Lionetti R, De Luca M, Travaglino A, Raffone A, Insabato L, Saccone G, Mascolo M, D'armiento M, Zullo F, Corcione F. Treatments and overall survival in patients with Krukenberg tumor. *Arch Gynecol Obstet.* 2019 Jul;300(1):15-23. Doi: 10.1007/s00404-019-05167-z. Epub 2019 May 1. PMID: 31044302.

[20] Zulfiqar M, Koen J, Nougaret S, Bolan C, VanBuren W, McGettigan M, Menias C. Krukenberg Tumors: Update on Imaging and Clinical Features. *AJR Am J Roentgenol.* 2020 Oct;215(4):1020-1029. doi: 10.2214/AJR.19.22184. Epub 2020 Jul 13. PMID: 32755184.

[21] Seow-En I, Hwarng G, Tan GHC, Ho LML, Teo MCC. Palliative surgery for Krukenberg tumors – 12-year experience and review of the literature. *World J Clin Oncol.* 2018 Feb 10;9(1):13-19. Doi: 10.5306/wjco.v9.i1.13. PMID: 29468133; PMCID: PMC5807888.

[22] Kraus E (1901) Über das zustandekommen der krebsmetastasen im ovarium bei primärem kerbs eines anderen bauchorgans. *Monatsschr Geburtsh Gynakol* 14:1–30.

[23] Al-Agha OM, Nicastri AD (2006) An in-depth look at Krukenberg tumor: an overview. *Arch Pathol Lab Med* 130(11):1725–1730. doi:10.1043/1543-2165(2006)130[1725:ailakt]2.0.co;2.

[24] Fujiwara K, Ohishi Y, Koike H, Sawada S, Moriya T, Kohno I (1995) Clinical implications of metastases to the ovary. *Gynecol Oncol* 59(1):124–128. doi:10.1006/gyno.1995.1278.

[25] de Waal YR, Thomas CM, Oei AL, Sweep FC, Massuger LF (2009) Secondary ovarian malignancies: frequency, origin, and characteristics. *Int J Gynecol Cancer* 19(7):1160–1165. doi:10.1111/IGC.0b013e3181b33cce.

[26] Moore RG, Chung M, Granai CO, Gajewski W, Steinhoff MM (2004) Incidence of metastasis to the ovaries from nongenital tract primary tumors. *Gynecol Oncol* 93(1):87–91. doi:10.1016/j.ygyno.2003.12.039.

[27] de Waal YR, Thomas CM, Oei AL, Sweep FC, Massuger LF (2009) Secondary ovarian malignancies: frequency, origin, and characteristics. *Int J Gynecol Cancer* 19(7):1160–1165. doi:10.1111/IGC.0b013e3181b33cce.

[28] Al-Agha OM, Nicastri AD (2006) An in-depth look at Krukenberg tumor: an overview. *Arch Pathol Lab Med* 130(11):1725–1730. doi:10.1043/1543-2165(2006)130[1725:ailakt]2.0.co.

[29] Kondi-Pafiti A, Kairi-Vasilatou E, Iavazzo C, Dastamani C, Bakalianou K, Liapis A, Hassiakos D, Fotiou S (2011) Metastatic neoplasms of the ovaries: a clinicopathological study of 97 cases. *Arch Gynecol Obstet* 284(5):1283–1288. doi:10.1007/s00404-011-1847-4.

[30] Ganesh K, Shah RH (2017) Clinical and genetic determinants of ovarian metastases from colorectal cancer. *Cancer* 123(7):1134–1143. doi:10.1002/cncr.30424.

[31] T Kikkawa F, Shibata K, Ino K, Nomura S, Kajiyama H, Suzuki T, Kawai M, Mizutani S (2002) Preoperative findings in non-gynecologic carcinomas metastasizing to the ovaries. *Gynecol Obstet Invest* 54(4):221–227. doi:10.1159/000068388.

[32] Tan DS, Agarwal R, Kaye SB (2006) Mechanisms of transcoelomic metastasis in ovarian cancer. *Lancet Oncol* 7(11):925–934. doi:10.1016/s1470-2045(06)70939-1.

[33] Yamanishi Y, Koshiyama M, Ohnaka M, Ueda M, Ukita S, Hishikawa K, Nagura M, Kim T, Hirose M, Ozasa H, Shirase T (2011) Pathways of metastases from primary organs to the ovaries. *Obstet Gynecol Int* 2011:612817. doi:10.1155/2011/612817.

[34] Tan DS, Agarwal R, Kaye SB (2006) Mechanisms of transcoelomic metastasis in ovarian cancer. *Lancet Oncol* 7(11):925–934. doi:10.1016/s1470-2045(06)70939-1.

[35] Kall SL, Koblinski JE (2013) Metastatic cancer: clinical and biological perspectives. Genes that mediate metastasis organotropism. *Landes Bioscience*, Austin.

[36] Lorusso G, Ruegg C (2012) New insights into the mechanisms of organ-specific breast cancer metastasis. *Semin Cancer Biol* 22(3):226–233. doi:10.1016/j.semcancer.2012.03.007.

[37] Crobach S, Ruano D, van Eijk R, Schrumpf M, Fleuren G, van Wezel T, Morreau H (2016) Somatic mutation profiles in primary colorectal cancers and matching ovarian metastases: identification of driver and passenger mutations. *J Pathol Clin Res* 2(3):166–174. doi:10.1002/cjp2.45.

[38] Carlson JW, Miron A, Jarboe EA, Parast MM, Hirsch MS, Lee Y, Muto MG, Kindelberger D, Crum CP (2008) Serous tubal intraepithelial carcinoma: its potential role in primary peritoneal serous carcinoma and serous cancer prevention. *J Clin Oncol* 26(25):4160–4165. doi:10.1200/jco.2008.16.4814.

[39] Kiyokawa T, Young RH, Scully RE (2006) Krukenberg tumors of the ovary: a clinicopathologic analysis of 120 cases with emphasis on their variable pathologic manifestations. *Am J Surg Pathol* 30(3):277–299. doi:10.1097/01.pas.0000190787.85024.cb.

[40] Bruchim I, Ben-Harim Z, Piura E, Tepper R, Fishman A (2013) Preoperative clinical and radiological features of metastatic ovarian tumors. *Arch Gynecol Obstet* 288(3):615–619. doi:10.1007/s00404-013-2776-1.

[41] Antila R, Jalkanen J, Heikinheimo O (2006) Comparison of Secondary and primary ovarian malignancies reveals differEnces in their pre- and perioperative characteristics. *Gynecol Oncol* 101(1):97–101. doi:10.1016/j.ygyno.2005.09.046.

[42] Bruls J, Simons M, Overbeek LI, Bulten J, Massuger LF, Nagtegaal ID (2015) A national population-based study provides Insight in the origin of malignancies metastatic to the ovary. *VirChows Arch* 467(1):79–86. doi:10.1007/s00428-015-1771-2.

[43] National Comprehensive Cancer Network (2016) *Occult primary* (cancer of unknown primary [CUP]) (version 2.2016). https://www.nccn.org/professionals/physician_gls/pdf/occult.pdf. Accessed 1 August 2016.

[44] Willmott F, Allouni KA, Rockall A (2012) Radiological manifestations of metastasis to the ovary. *J Clin Pathol* 65(7):585590. doi:10.1136/jclinpath-2011-200390.

[45] Park HL, Yoo Ie R, O JH, Han EJ, Kim SH (2015) F-18 FDG PET/CT findings of metastatic ovarian tumors from gastrointestinal tract origin. *J Cancer Res Clin Oncol* 141(10):18711878. doi:10.1007/s00432-015-1978-2.

[46] Pepin K, del Carmen M, Brown A, Dizon DS (2014) CA 125 And epithelial ovarian cancer: role in screening, diagnosis, and Surveillance. *Am J Hematol Oncol* 10(6):22–29.

[47] Ramrakhiani H, Thaker AK, Pisani A, Sangoi A, Triadafilopoulos G. Magnifying Power: New Endoscopic Tools for the Diagnosis of Krukenberg Tumor. *Dig Dis Sci.* 2021 Oct;66(10):3296-3299. doi: 10.1007/s10620-020-06799-x. Epub 2021 Jan 12. PMID: 33433803.

[48] Kurman RJ, International Agency for Research on Cancer, World Health Organization. (2014) WHO classification of Tumours of female reproductive organs. *World Health OrganiZation classification of tumours*, 4th edn. International Agency For Research on Cancer, Lyon.

[49] Kondi-Pafiti A, Kairi-Vasilatou E, Iavazzo C, Dastamani C, Bakalianou K, Liapis A, Hassiakos D, Fotiou S (2011) MetaStatic neoplasms of the ovaries: a clinicopathological study of 97 cases. *Arch Gynecol Obstet* 284(5):1283–1288. doi:10.1007/S00404-011-1847-4.

[50] McCluggage WG (2006) The value of immunohistochemistry as a diagnostic aid in ovarian neoplasia: a review. *AJSP* 11(1):31–37.

[51] Mittal K, Soslow R, McCluggage WG (2008) AppliCation of immunohistochemistry to gynecologic Pathology. *Arch Pathol Lab Med* 132(3):402–423. doi:10.1043/1543-2165(2008)132[402:aoitgp]2.0.co;2.

[52] van der Post RS, Bult P, Vogelaar IP, Ligtenberg MJ, Hoogerbrugge N, van Krieken JH (2014) HNF4A immunohistochemistry facilitates distinction between primary and metastatic breast and gastric carcinoma. *Virchows Arch* 464(6):673–679. doi:10.1007/s00428-014-1574-x.

[53] Meyniel JP, Cottu PH, Decraene C, Stern MH, Couturier J, Lebigot I, Nicolas A, Weber N, Fourchotte V, Alran S, Rapinat A, Gentien D, Roman-Roman S, Mignot L, Sastre-Garau X (2010) A genomic and transcriptomic approach for a differential diagnosis between primary and secondary ovarian carcinomas in patients with a previous history of breast cancer. *BMC Cancer* 10:222. doi:10.1186/1471-2407-10-222.

[54] Pavlidis N, Pentheroudakis G (2012) Cancer of unknown priMary site. *The Lancet* 379(9824):1428–1435. doi:10.1016/S0140-6736(11)61178-1.

[55] Jiang R, Tang J, Cheng X, Zang RY (2009) Surgical treatment For patients with different origins of Krukenberg tumors: outComes and prognostic factors. *Eur J Surg Oncol* 35(1):92–97. doi:10.1016/j.ejso.2008.05.006.

[56] Rayson D, Bouttell E, Whiston F, Stitt L (2000) Outcome after ovarian/adnexal metastectomy in metastatic colorectal carcinoma. *J Surg Oncol* 75(3):186–192.

[57] McCormick CC, Giuntoli RL 2nd, Gardner GJ, Schulick RD, Judson K, Ronnett BM, Vang R, Bristow RE (2007) The Role of cytoreductive surgery for colon cancer metastatic to The ovary. *Gynecol Oncol* 105(3):791–795. doi:10.1016/j.Ygyno.2007.02.025.

[58] Rosa F, Marrelli D, Morgagni P, Cipollari C, Vittimberga G, Fra-Marini M, Cozzaglio L, Pedrazzani C, Berardi S, Baiocchi GL, Roviello F, Portolani N, de Manzoni G, Costamagna G, Doglietto GB, Pacelli F (2016) Krukenberg tumors of gastric origin: the Rationale of surgical resection and perioperative treatments in a multicenter western experience. *World J Surg* 40(4):921–928. doi:10.1007/s00268-015-3326-8.

[59] Ayhan A, Guvenal T, Salman MC, Ozyuncu O, Sakinci M, BasaRan M (2005) The role of cytoreductive surgery in nongenital Cancers metastatic to the ovaries. *Gynecol Oncol* 98(2):235–241. doi:10.1016/j.ygyno.2005.05.028.

[60] Sal V, Demirkiran F, Topuz S, Kahramanoglu I, Yalcin I, Bese T, Sozen H, Tokgozoglu N, Salihoglu Y, Turan H, Iyiboz-Kurt C, Kolomuc T, Sofiyeva N, Berkman S, Arvas M (2016) Surgical treatment of metastatic ovarian tumors from extraGenital primary sites. *Int J Gynecol Cancer* 26(4):688–696. doi:10.1097/igc.0000000000000673.

[61] Lu LC, Shao YY, Hsu CH, Hsu C, Cheng WF, Lin YL, Cheng AL, Yeh KH (2012) Metastasectomy of Krukenberg tumors may be associated with survival benefits in patients with metastatic gastric cancer. *Anticancer Res* 32(8):3397–3401.

Chapter 24

Pseudomyxoma Peritonei

John Spiliotis[1,*], MD, PhD
Alexandros Fotiou[2], MD
and Christos Iavazzo[2], MD, PhD
[1]Department of Surgical Oncology and HIPEC, European Interbalkan Medical Center, Thessaloniki, Greece
[2]Department of Gynecologic Oncology, Metaxa Memorial Cancer Hospital, Piraeus, Greece

Introduction

Pseudomyxoma peritonei (PMP) is a rare malignant clinical syndrome with an incidence of 2-4 per million people [1, 2]. The main feature of PMP is the extensive dissemination of copious mucus-containing tumor cells in the abdominal cavity. Mucus accumulation causes progressive abdominal distention, intestinal obstruction, malnutrition, cachexia, and ultimately death. As a rare disease, an early and accurate diagnosis of PMP is difficult, which often leads to the clinically advanced stage at the time of optimal clinical treatment.

Currently, CRS + HIPEC are the recommended treatment for PMP, vastly enhancing the prognosis of patients.

There are still many controversies regarding the treatment of PMP, such as the HIPEC regimen, efficacy of systemic chemotherapy, and early postoperative intraperitoneal chemotherapy (EPIC).

Since the first consensus statement by the PSOGI was published in 2008, sequential HIPEC treatment after CRS has gradually become the standard treatment of PMP in many countries or regions. Currently, there are five up-to-date consensuses in different regions, coming from PSOGI/EURACAN, CCWG (U. S. A.) [3], CACA (Chine) [4], LARPD (Latin America) [5], and BSSO (Brazil) [6].

The greatest differences among the five consensuses are the exclusion criteria, HIPEC regimen, and systemic chemotherapy, which still exist in the PSOGI/EUROCAN 2020 Guideline. Consensuses had a significant impact on consensus making around the world, which implies the important leading role of the PSOGI in PMP management.

---

* Corresponding Author's Email: jspil@hotmail.gr.

In: Ovarian Cancer
Editors: Christos Iavazzo, Alexandros Fotiou and John Spiliotis
ISBN: 979-8-88697-633-5

Consensus on Preoperative Evaluation

A consensus on preoperative evaluation for PMP was reached in the 2008 PSOGI Consensus, which greatly facilitated patient diagnosis and selection, mainly including 4 aspects [4]. (1) Serum tumor markers, which mainly combined testing of carcinoembryonic antigen (CEA), carbohydrate antigen 125 (CA125), and carbohydrate antigen 199 (CA199). CEA, CA125, and CA199 are helpful indicators for evaluating the degree of tumor invasion, ascites production and tumor burden, and the proliferation of cancer cells, respectively. (2) A computed tomography (CT) examination +3D reconstruction is the optimal choice for routine preoperative examination. Typically, a CT scan of PMP revealed a right lower abdominal cystic or cystic-solid mass frequently with calcification; copious mucinous ascites in the abdominal cavity; extensive organ invasion or compression; Laparoscopic exploration and exfoliative cytology are both optional.

Intraoperative Evaluation

The peritoneal cancer index (PCI) score is a standard parameter used to evaluate tumor burden during comprehensive abdominal exploration. The PCI scoring system helps to evaluate tumor load in the abdominal cavity and has important significance for confirming regions in the peritoneum that need to be removed or stripped or whether an optimal CRS can be performed. A high PCI score is an independent factor for poor PFS [8].

The completeness of cytoreduction (CC) score is the main prognostic factor for PC patients. It is suitable for PMP, colon cancer peritoneal metastasis, peritoneal sarcomatosis, and peritoneal malignant mesothelioma. The specific evaluation is as follows: CC-0, no residual tumor nodule after cytoreduction; CC-1: residual tumor diameter <2.5 mm; CC-2: residual tumor diameter 2.5 mm-2.5 cm; and CC-3: residual tumor diameter >2.5 cm or the residual tumor cannot be removed or palliatively removed.

Operating Procedures of CRS + HIPEC

The implementation of standardized CRS and complete resection of all visible malignant tumors is the basis for long-term survival. Sugarbaker elaborated on the PMP peritonectomy procedure as early as 1995 [9]. Complete CRS may require a 6-step peritonectomy to completely remove all tumors implanted on the peritoneum. These six procedures include greater omental excision + splenectomy; left upper peritoneal resection; right upper peritoneal resection; lesser omental excision + cholecystectomy + omental bursa peritonectomy; pelvic peritonectomy + sleeve resection of the sigmoid colon; and antrectomy. In 2003, Sugarbaker further improved the surgical principles and technical specifications for peritoneal resection in the pelvic peritoneum, left upper peritoneum, right upper peritoneum, greater omentum + spleen, and lesser omentum + gallbladder [10]. After four decades of clinical practice, the surgical procedures and details have been refined and standardized, which are accepted by PC centers all over the world.

Perioperative Management

When PMP patients receive CRS + HIPEC, perioperative safety management is of paramount importance. The main high-risk factors for PMP patients include heavy tumor burden, multiple previous operations and chemotherapies, long anesthesia and operation time, extensive resections, high-volume bleeding and blood infusion, and central venous catheter. The main adverse events include perioperative venous thrombosis, anastomotic leakage, bleeding, infection, and postoperative hypermyoglobinemia. Therefore, the clinical consensus on the perioperative management of CRS + HIPEC has also become important for preventing complications. The most important aspect of perioperative period of perioperative management is the graded evaluation system of adverse events.

Controversies on HIPEC Regimens

Among the frequently applied HIPEC regimens, most are based on oxaliplatin and mitonycin C. A consensus is almost impossible to reach due to the lack of high-level evidence from well-designed randomized controlled trials. Similarly, the dosage and intraperitoneal concentration of mitomycin C are also under heated debate [11, 12].

The date, HIPEC regimen-related studies have been mostly single or multicenter large-simple analyses [7, 8, 13-27]. In 2018, Levine et al. published the first multicenter randomized controlled trial on appendix-derived PMP. The study compared the safety, quality of life (QOL), 3-year disease-free survival (DFS), and 3-year overall survival (OS) after HIPEC (oxaliplatin 200 mg/m^2 *vs.* mitomycin C 40 mg) [28].

No significant differences were found regarding the 3-year DFS and OS rates between the two groups.

The Role of Systemic Chemotherapy

Systemic chemotherapy in PMP includes neoadjuvant systemic chemotherapy, adjuvant systemic chemotherapy, and palliative systemic chemotherapy. The expert panel of the PSOGI/EUROCAN 2020 Guideline reached a consensus on the application of palliative systemic chemotherapy in patients with unrespectable tumors or who are not suitable for surgery. In addition, its combination with bevacizumab might contribute to prolonged PFS. With respect to neoadjuvant [8, 30-38] and adjuvant [31, 39-41] chemotherapy, no definite survival benefits were proven in low-grade PMP, high-grade PMP, or high-grade PMP with signet ring cells, which is quite controversial. Neoadjuvant or adjuvant chemotherapy should not be totally abandoned in low-grade PMP (92.7% and 74.5%, respectively) and can be considered in patients with high-grade PMP with signet ring cells (76.4% and 85.5%, respectively). If neoadjuvant or adjuvant systemic chemotherapy is needed, a combination of fluoropyrimidine and an alkylating agent (e.g., oxaliplatin) is recommended (87.3% for both).

Controversies on HIPEC Methods

There is a consensus that the efficacy evaluation of different HIPEC regimens relies largely on randomized clinical trials. However, an unified HIPEC method, duration, and temperature are required to guarantee the accuracy and reliability of both multicenter clinical trials and retrospective analyses of large samples. The randomized trial conducted by Levine et al. provided valuable experience for HIPEC regimen-related clinical trials. With the strengthening cooperation among PC centers worldwide and the promotion of standardized CRS + HIPEC technology, a larger randomized clinical trial of higher quality might promote a HIPEC regimen with better efficacy and less toxicity.

Controversies on EPIC

EPIC is usually performed from postoperative days 1 to 4/5 without heating and is easier to perform than HIPEC. At present, one multicenter, prospective randomized clinical trial is being conducted at Memorial Sloan Kettering Cancer Center to evaluate the efficacy and toxicity between CRS + HIPEC and CRS + EPIC [29], the results of which might provide strong evidence for the efficacy and toxicity of EPIC.

Conclusion

In conclusion, the up-to-date reached consensus in PMP clinical management includes. (a) pathological classification; (b) terminology; (c) preoperative evaluation and eligibility for surgical treatment; (d) intraoperative evaluation; (e) standard CRS procedures and intraoperative criteria for non-respectability; and (f) SAE classification system.

This is also the root cause for controversies regarding the HIPEC regimen, systemic chemotherapy, and EPIC. In the near future, consensuses or guidelines are still indispensable for the development in the management and research of PMP.

References

[1] Smeenk RM, van Velthuysen ML, Verwaal VJ, Zoetmulder FA. Appendiceal neoplasms and pseudomyxoma peritonei: a population based study. *Eur. J. Surg. Oncol.* 2008;34:196-201.

[2] Mittal R, Chandramohan A, Moran B. Pseudomyxoma peritonei: natural history and treatment. *Int. J. Hyperthermia*. 2017;33:511-9.

[3] Chicago Consensus Working Group. The Chicago consensus on peritoneal surface malignancies: management of appendiceal neoplasms. *Cancer*. 2020;126;2525-33.

[4] Li Y, Xu HB, Peng Z, Cui SZ, Wu W. Chinese expert consensus on cytoreductive surgery and hyper thermic intraperitoneal chemotherapy for pseudomyxoma peritonei. *Natl. Med. J. China*. 2019;99:1527-35.

[5] Latin American Registry of Peritoneal Diseases. Current practice of Latin American centers in the treatment of peritoneal diseases with cytoreductive surgery with HIPEC. *Eur. J. Surg. Oncol.* 2018;44:1800-4.

[6] Batista TP, Sarmento BJQ, Loureiro JF, Petruzziello A, Lopes A, Santos CC, et al. A proposal of Brazilian Society of Surgical Oncology (BSSO/SBCO) for standardizing cytoreductive surgery (CRS) plus hyper thermic intraperitoneal chemotherapy (HIPEC) procedures in Brazil: pseudomixoma peritonei, appendiceal tumors and malignant peritoneal mesothelioma. *Revista do Colegio Brasileiro de Cirurgioes* [Magazine of the Brazilian College of Surgery]. 2017;44:530-44.

[7] Baratti D, Kusamura S, Milione M, Bruno F, Guaglio M, deraco M. Validation of the recent PSOGI pathological classification of pseudomyxoma peritonei in a single-center series of 265 patients treated by cytoreductive surgery and hyper thermic intraperitoneal chemotherapy. *Ann. Surg. Oncol.* 2018;25:404-13.

[8] Chua TC, Moran BJ, Sugarbaker PH, Levine EA, Glehen O, Gilly FN, et al. Early-and long-term outcome data of patients with pseudomyxoma peritonei from appendiceal origin treated by a strategy of cytoredictive surgery and hyper thermic intraperitoneal chemotherapy. *J. Clin. Oncol.* 2012;30:2449-56.

[9] Sugarbaker PH. Peritonectomy procedures. *Ann. Surg*. 1995;221:29-42.

[10] Sugarbaker PH. Peritonectomy procedures. *Surg. Oncol. Clin. N. Am.* 2003;12:703-27.

[11] Mohamed F, Cecil T, Moran B, Sugarbaker P. A new standard of care for the management of peritoneal surface malignancy. *Curr. Oncol*. 2011;18:e84-96.

[12] Levine EA, Stewart JH, Shen P, Russell GB, Loggie BL, Votanopoulos Kl. Interperitoneal chemotherapy for peritoneal surface malignancy: experience with 1.000 patients. *J. Am. Coll Surg.* 2014;218:573-85.

[13] Chua TC, Yan TD, Smigielski ME, Zhu KJ, Ng KM, Zhao J, et al. Long-term survival in patients with pseudomyxoma peritoneal treated with cytoreductive surgery and perioperative intraperitoneal chemotherapy: 10 years of experience from a single institution. *Ann. Surg. Oncol.* 2009;16:1903-11.

[14] Elias D, Gilly F, Quenet F, Bereder JM, Sidéris L, Mansvelt B, Lorimier G, & Glehen O. Pseudomyxoma peritonei: a French multicentric study of 301 patients treated with cytoreductive surgery and intraperitoneal chemotherapy. *Eur. J. Surg. Oncol*. 2010;36:456-62.

[15] Saxena A, Yan TD, Chua TC, Morris DL. Critical assessment of risk factors for complications after cytoreductive surgery and perioperative intraperitoneal chemotherapy for pseudomyxoma peritonei. *Ann. Surg. Oncol*. 2010;17:1291-301.

[16] Chua TC, Liauw W, Zhao J, Morris DL. Upfront compared to delayed cytoreductive surgery and perioperative intraperitoneal chemotherapy for pseudomyxoma peritonei is associated with considerably lower perioperative morbidity and recurrence rate. *Ann. Surg*. 2011;253:769-73.

[17] Youssef H, Newman C, Chandrakumaran K, Mohamed F, Cecil TD, Moran BJ. Operative findings, early complications, and long-term survival in 456 patients with psuedomyxoma peritonei syndrome of appendiceal origin. *Dis. Colon. Rectum.* 2011;54:293-9.

[18] Dayal S, Taflampas P, Riss S, Chandrakumaran K, Cecil TD, Mohamed F, & Moran BJ. Complete cytoreduction for pseudomyxoma peritonei is optimal but maximal tumor debulking may be beneficial in patients in whom complete tumor removal cannot be achieved. *Dis. Colon Rectum.* 2013;56:1366-72.

[19] Ro Robella M, Vaira M, Mellano A, Cinquegrana A, Marsanic P, & De Simone M. Treatment of pseudomyxoma peritonei with cytoreductive surgery and hyperthermic intraperitoneal chemotherapy (HIPEC): a single center experience. *Minerva Chir*. 2013;68:569-77.

[20] Sparks DS, Morris B, Xu W, Fulton J, Atkinson V, Meade B, & Lutton N. Cytoreductive surgery and heated intraperitoneal chemotherapy for peritoneal carcinomatosis secondary to mucinous adenocarcinoma of the appendix. *Int. Surg*. 2015;100:21-8.

[21] Ansari N, Chandrakumaran K, Dayal S, Mohamed F, Cecil TD, Moran BJ. Cytoreductive surgery and hyperthermic intraperitoneal chemother- apy in 1000 patients with perforated appendiceal epithelial tumours. *Eur. J. Surg. Oncol*. 2016;42:1035-41.

[22] Azzam AZ, Alyahya ZA, Wusaibie AAA, Amin TM. Cytoreductive surgery and hyperthermic intraperitoneal chemotherapy in the management of pseudomyxoma peritonei: a single-center experience. *Indian J. Gastroenterol*. 2017;36:452-8.

[23] Grotz TE, Royal RE, Mansfield PF, Overman MJ, Mann GN, Robinson KA, Beaty KA, Rafeeq S, Matamoros A, Taggart MW, & Fournier KF. Stratification of outcomes for mucinous appendiceal

adeno-carcinoma with peritoneal metastasis by histological grade. *World J. Gastrointest. Oncol.* 2017;9:354-62.

[24] Choudry HA, Pai RK, Shuai Y, Ramalingam L, Jones HL, Pingpank JF, Ahrendt SS, Holtzman MP, Zureikat AH, Zeh HJ, & Bartlett DL. Impact of cellularity on oncologic outcomes following cytoreductive surgery and hyperthermic intraperitoneal chemoperfusion for pseudomyxoma peritonei. *Ann. Surg. Oncol.* 2018;25:76-82.

[25] Delhorme JB, Severac F, Averous G, Glehen O, Passot G, Bakrin N, Marchal F, Pocard M, Lo Dico R, Eveno C, Carrere S, Sgarbura O, Quenet F, Ferron G, Goéré D, Brigand C, Abba J, Abboud K, Alyami M, Arvieux, C, Averous, G, Bakrin, N, Balagué, G, Barrau, V, Rejeb, HB, Bereder, J-M, Berton-Rigaud, I, Bibeau, F, Bonnefoy, I, Bouzard, D, Bricault, I, Brigand, C, Carrère, S, de Chaisemartin, C, Chassang, M, Chevallier, A, Courvoisier, T, Dartigues, P, Dohan, A, Dubreuil, J, Dumont, F, Eveno, C, Faruch-Bilfeld, M, Ferron, G, Fontaine, J, Fournier, L, Gagniere, J, Geffroy, D, Ghouti, L, Gilly, F-N, Gladieff, L, Glehen, O, Goéré, D, Guibal, A, Guilloit, J-M, Guyon, F, Heyd, B, Hoeffel,C, Hordonneau, C, Isaac, S, Jourdan-Enfer, P, Kaci, R, Kianmanesh, R, Labbé-Devilliers, C, Lacroix, J, Lelong, B, Leroux-Broussier, A, Lherm, Y, Lo Dico, R, Lorimier, G, Malhaire, C, Marchal, F, Mariani, P, Mathiotte, E, Meeus, P, Mery, E, Msika, S, Nadeau, C, Ortega-Deballon, P, Passot, G, Pellet, O., Peyrat, P, Pezet, D, Pirro, N, Pocard, M, Poizat, F, Porcheron, J, Poulet, A, Quenet, F, Rat, P, Rousselot, P, Rousset, P, Senellart, H, Serrano, M, Servois, V, Sgabura, O, Skanjeti, A, Svrcek, M, Tetreau, R, Thibaudeau, E, Touchefeu, Y, Tuech, J-J, Valmary-Degano, S, Vaudoyer, D, Velasco, S, Verriele-Beurrier, V, Villeneuve, L, Wernert, R and Zinzindohoue, F. Cytoreductive surgery and hyperthermic intraperitoneal chemotherapy for pseudomyxoma peritonei of appendicular and extra-appendicular origin. *Br. J. Surg.* 2018;105:668-76.

[26] Lansom J, Alzahrani N, Liauw W, Morris DL. Cytoreductive surgery and hyperthermic intraperitoneal chemotherapy for pseudomyxoma peritonei and appendix tumours. *Indian J. Surg. Oncol.* 2016;7:166-76.

[27] Vaira M, Cioppa T, Marco GD, Bing C, D'Amico S, D'Alessandro M, et al. Management of pseudomyxoma peritonei by cytoreduction HIPEC (hyper thermic intraperitoneal chemotherapy): results analysis of a twelve-year experience. *Vivo.* 2009;23:639-44.

[28] Levine EA, Votanopoulos KI, Shen P, Russell G, Fenstermaker J, Mansfield P, et al. A multicenter randomized trial to evaluate hematologic toxicities after hyper thermic intraperitoneal chemotherapy with oxaliplatin or mitomycin in patients with appendiceal tumors. *J. Am. Coll. Surg.* 2018;226:434-43.

[29] *ICARuS Post-operative Intraperitoneal Chemotherapy (EPIC) and Hyper-thermic Intraperitoneal Chemotherapy (HIPEC) After Optimal Cytoreductive Surgery (CRS) for Neoplasms of the Appendix, Colon or Rectum With Isolated Peritoneal Metastasis (ICARuS).* https://www.clinicaltrials.gov/ct2/show/NCT01815359.

[30] Baratti D, Kusamura S, Nonaka D, Cabras AD, Laterza B, Deraco M. Pseudomyxoma peritonei: biological features are the dominant prognostic determinants after complete cytoreduction and hyperthermic intraperitoneal chemotherapy. *Ann. Surg.* 2009;249:243-9.

[31] Blackham AU, Swett K, Eng C, Sirintrapun J, Bergman S, Geisinger KR, Votanopoulos K, Stewart JH, Shen P, & Levine EA. Perioperative systemic chemotherapy for appendiceal mucinous carcinoma peritonei treated with cytoreductive surgery and hyperthermic intraperitoneal chemotherapy. *J. Surg. Oncol.* 2014;109:740-5.

[32] Bijelic L, Kumar AS, Stuart OA, Sugarbaker PH. Systemic chemotherapy prior to cytoreductive surgery and HIPEC for carcinomatosis from appendix cancer: impact on perioperative outcomes and short-term survival. *Gastroenterol. Res. Pract.* 2012;2012:163284.

[33] Lieu CH, Lambert LA, Wolff RA, Eng C, Zhang N, Wen S, Rafeeq S, Taggart M, Fournier K, Royal R, Mansfield P, & Overman MJ. Systemic chemotherapy and surgical cytoreduction for poorly differentiated and signet ring cell adenocarcinomas of the appendix. *Ann. Oncol.* 2012;23:652-8.

[34] Van Sweringen HL, Hanseman DJ, Ahmad SA, Edwards MJ, Sussman JJ. Predictors of survival in patients with high-grade peritoneal metastases undergoing cytoreductive surgery and hyperthermic intraperitoneal chemotherapy. *Surgery.* 2012;152:617-24 (discussion 24-5).

[35] Raghav KPS, Shetty AV, Kazmi SMA, Zhang N, Morris J, Taggart M, Fournier K, Royal R, Mansfield P, Eng C, Wolff RA, & Overman MJ. Impact of molecular alterations and targeted therapy in appendiceal adenocarcinomas. *Oncologist*. 2013;18:1270-7.

[36] Turner KM, Hanna NN, Zhu Y, Jain A, Kesmodel SB, Switzer RA, et al. Assessment of neoadjuvant chemotherapy on operative parameters and outcome in patients with peritoneal dissemination from high-grade appendiceal cancer. *Ann. Surg. Oncol*. 2013;20:1068-73.

[37] Milovanov V, Sardi A, Ledakis P, Aydin N, Nieroda C, Sittig M, et al. Systemic chemotherapy (SC) before cytoreductive surgery and hyperthermic intraperitoneal chemotherapy (CRS/HIPEC) in patients with peritoneal mucinous carcinomatosis of appendiceal origin (PMCA). *Eur. J. Surg. Oncol*. 2015;41: 707-12.

[38] Spiliotis J, Kopanakis N, Efstathiou E, Vassiliadou D, Argiriou O, Rogdakis A, et al. Perioperative systemic chemotherapy for peritoneal mucinous appendiceal carcinomas treated with cytoreductive surgery & HIPEC. *J BUON*. 2017;22:783-9.

[39] Asare EA, Compton CC, Hanna NN, Kosinski LA, Washington MK, Kakar S, et al. The impact of stage, grade, and mucinous histology on the efficacy of systemic chemotherapy in adenocarcinomas of the appendix: analysis of the National Cancer Data Base. *Cancer*. 2016;122:213-21.

[40] Schomas DA, Miller RC, Donohue JH, Gill S, Thurmes PJ, Haddock MG, Quevedo JF, & Gunderson LL. Intraperitoneal treatment for peritoneal mucinous carcinomatosis of appendiceal origin after operative management: long-term follow-up of the Mayo Clinic experience. *Ann. Surg*. 2009;249:588-95.

[41] Cummins KA, Russell GB, Votanopoulos KI, Shen P, Stewart JH, Levine EA. Peritoneal dissemination from high-grade appendiceal cancer treated with cytoreductive surgery (CRS) and hyperthermic intraperitoneal chemotherapy (HIPEC). *J. Gastrointest. Oncol*. 2016;7:3-9.

Chapter 25

Ovarian Malignancies during Pregnancy

Miriam Turiel Miranda, MD
Ignacio Cristobal, MD
Elena Martin-Boado, MD
and Ignacio Zapardiel*, MD, PhD
Gynecologic Oncology Unit, La Paz University Hospital, Madrid, Spain

Introduction

Fortunately, cancer and pregnancy are two conditions that rarely coexist with an incidence rate of approximately 1 in 1,000 pregnancies [1]. However, although rare, it is not uncommon and can lead to complex situations where the diagnosis and management during pregnancy may not be well understood for several reasons. Firstly, there is a lack of prospective studies; secondly, the type, stage, diagnosis, treatment and prognosis vary widely; last, the diagnosis of cancer during pregnancy is not easy because the symptoms and signs may mimic the physiologic changes or common complaints reported during pregnancy leading to delayed diagnosis and eventual progression to an advanced stage.

The aim of this chapter is to describe the clinical characteristics, diagnostic process, treatment and prognosis of ovarian malignancies detected during pregnancy.

Epidemiology

As the routine use of ultrasonography in prenatal care has spread, the finding of an incidental adnexal mass in pregnancy has become more common. 1-4% of pregnant women are diagnosed with an adnexal mass in the first trisemester. The majority of these masses are corpus luteum or other functional cysts that usually resolve before 20 weeks of gestation. However, some of them may persist and approximately 1-6% of these are malignant [2].

In a population-based hospital registry with a series of malignancies identified during pregnancy using birth records linked to hospital discharge data, ovarian cancer was the 5th most

* Corresponding Author's Email: ignaciozapardiel@hotmail.com.

In: Ovarian Cancer
Editors: Christos Iavazzo, Alexandros Fotiou and John Spiliotis
ISBN: 979-8-88697-633-5

common cancer diagnosed during pregnancy after breast, thyroid, cervical cancer, and Hodgkin's Lymphoma [3]. There was also a high proportion of tumors of low malignant potential (n = 115) reported separately, with the majority caught in its early stages and associated with favorable maternal and neonatal outcomes.

Patient Presentation

Most pregnant women with an adnexal mass have asymptomatic masses. The incidental detection of adnexal masses is most common in the first and second trimester of pregnancy. Detection at delivery by cesarean section and in the postnatal period is much less common [4].

On the other hand, there are symptoms and signs that may lead to the diagnosis of adnexal masses. They include:

- Nonspecific symptoms such as abdominal or back pain, constipation, abdominal swelling, and urinary symptoms. In any case, their presence is unlikely to trigger a diagnostic evaluation since these symptoms are present in normal pregnancies.
- Palpable mass may be identified during a physical examination and later evaluated by an ultrasound.
- Acute abdominal pain may be due to bleeding or torsion of the adnexal mass. Torsion is an important concern of pregnancy-associated adnexal masses which has a much higher incidence (13.8%) than malignancy. In one review, two main risk factors were identified. 1) Size: adnexal masses between 6 and 8 cm in diameter had a significantly higher rate of torsion than either smaller or larger masses [5]. 2) Gestational Age: 60% of the torsions occurred between the 10th and 17th week of gestation when the adnexal tumor had been carried out of the pelvis and had a larger surrounding environment.
- Alteration of analytical parameters – Elevated concentrations of oncofetal proteins such as alpha-fetoprotein (AFP), human chorionic gonadotropin (hCG), CA125 and CE 19.9 during pregnancy can be due to their involvement in biological functions. Thus, these antigens cannot be used as reliable markers of cancer in pregnant patients [6]. However, an unexplained elevation in maternal serum analytes, obtained while screening for neural tube defects or Down syndrome, may be the first alarm sign of these tumors.

Types of Adnexal Masses in Pregnancy: Sonographic Evaluation

After the identification of the mass, the following step is its characterization via an ultrasound. Similar to the evaluation of an adnexal mass in a non-pregnant woman, the principal goals during its evaluation are to determine whether the mass is "almost certainly benign," has a "reasonable chance of being malignant" and whether there is an urgent condition that requires prompt treatment. Any adnexal mass should be described and measured. Follow-up recommendations must be based on its characteristics [2].

In the following paragraphs, we present a brief differential diagnosis of benign adnexal masses during pregnancy. They are characterized by their ultrasonographic appearance and, in some cases, associated clinical findings.

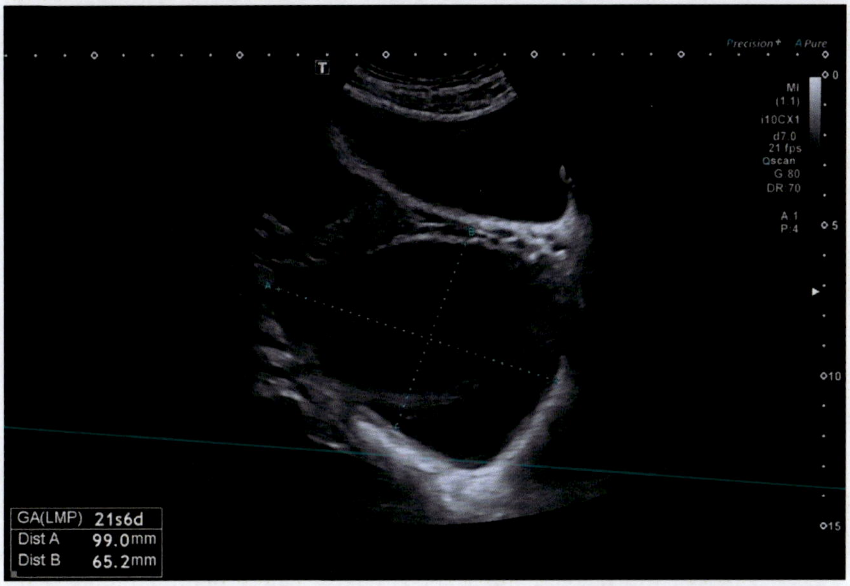

Figure 1. Patient with 21 weeks of gestational age, with a cystic formation of 99 x 65 x 96 mm with thin walls without septa or papillae inside that corresponds to a cyst in the left ovary.

Cysts

- Clear cysts: Functional ovarian cysts that occur as part of the normal physiological function are seen as an echoic fluid sonolucent area with clear margins within the ovarian parenchyma. Usually, they are accompanied by an enhanced posterior wall and posterior echo. Color doppler shows mild blood flow into de capsule. Approximately 70% of all adnexal cystic masses detected in the first trimester spontaneously resolve by the early part of the second trimester [7]. Rarely, they can continue to increase in size beyond this date.
- Hemorrhagic cysts: Most hemorrhagic cysts are corpus luteum cysts that have developed bleeding. Depending on the timing, their appearance may change. While an acute hemorrhage can be present as echogenic masses, with time, the cysts become anechoic. During this process, it can present itself with debris-filled fluid, organized clots or fibrin stranding.

Pregnancy Associated Masses

- Theca lutein cysts: Theca lutein cysts are anechoic, irregular, bilateral, multiseptated cysts that are form as a result of overstimulation from high hCG levels or hypersensitivity to hCG. They are related to conditions with high levels of these hormone such as gestational trophoblastic disease, multiple gestation or a pregnancy complicated by fetal hydrops.

- Luteomas: Luteoma is an uncommon solid benign lesion specific to pregnancy that can simulate a neoplasm as they are hypoechoic, well demarcated and thick walled. They tend to be heterogeneous with irregular internal borders and can be very vascular. The diagnosis should be suspected when a solid adnexal mass is associated with maternal hirsutism or virilization as these tumors tend to produce androgens. They regress spontaneously after delivery.

Masses

- Leiomyomas: Fibroids are the most common solid tumor identified in the pelvis and are detected in 1.4% of pregnancies. On a sonography, they are typically well demarcated, round and hypoechoic, found in or extending from the uterus, demonstrating a feeding vessel and diffuse vascular flow. However, it is not uncommon that they vary their appearance dramatically as the pregnancy progresses. Imbalances in vascular perfusion may result in degeneration that is clinically referred to as pain. During this process, it may acquire a concerning aspect. In these circumstances, the magnetic resonance imaging can be helpful to make the differential diagnosis with an ovarian malignancy.
- Ovarian torsion: As it has already been said, ovarian torsion is usually associated with 6-8 cm ovarian mass or cysts and occurs in the late first trimester. Classic ultrasound findings include ovarian enlargement, dense edematous stroma, peripheral follicles, lack of vascular flow on color doppler and free fluid in pelvis. It is almost exclusively unilateral, with the right ovary affected in two thirds of cases.

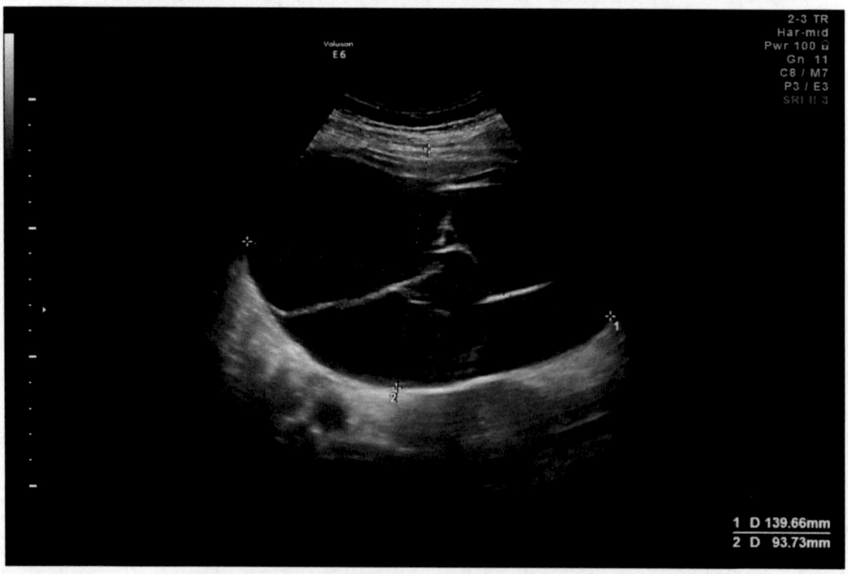

Figure 2. Patient with 19 + 6 weeks of gestational age present with a giant multiloculated cyst of 140 x 94 x 90. Patient underwent ovarian torsion. Urgent left anexectomy was performed. (Hospital Universitario La Paz).

Complex Masses

- Mature teratomas: The majority of persistent adnexal masses 5 cm or greater in diameter are mature teratomas. Most of the time they are heterogeneous, well-circumscribed cystic masses that can present a wide range of sonographic characteristics. It may contain echogenic material that may show "layering," calcifications or punctate, linear echogenic foci. Equally, strong posterior acoustic shadowing or loss of posterior attenuation due to dense lipid material may be demonstrated.
- Endometriomas: The typical aspect of an endometrioma is not always recognized during pregnancy. Exposure to progesterone causes decidualization resulting in glandular mucous production and accumulation and stromal vascularity. These changes can create intraluminal papillary projections with increased vascular flow mimicking ovarian malignancies.
- Serous and mucinous cystadenomas: Cystadenomas tend to be either simple cysts or multiseptated cysts with thin septations. Serous cysts are anechoic, whereas mucinous cysts tend to have low level echoes. Cystadenomas usually increase in size during pregnancy but malignant transformation is rare. Nevertheless, serial examinations must be performed if conservative management is being considered.

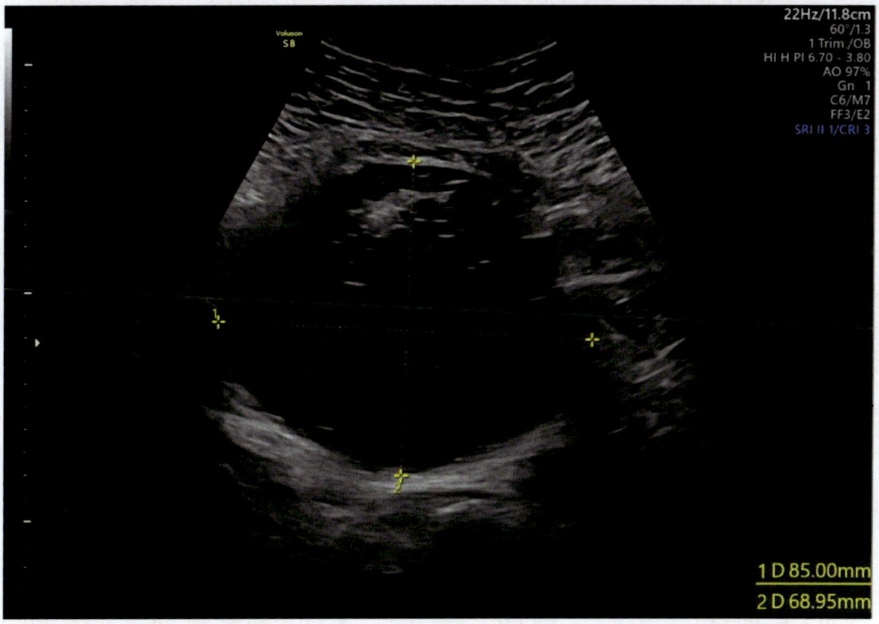

Figure 3. Patient with 9 weeks of gestational age present with an extrapelvic cystic image, compatible with a 85 x 69 x 82 mm mesogastrial teratoma (Hospital Universitario La Paz).

Malignant Neoplasms

As it has already been said, although rare, up to 6% of persistent adnexal masses on prenatal ultrasound are malignant. Various sonographic characteristics of adnexal masses have been associated with an increased risk of malignancy. They are shown in Table 1.

Table 1. Sonographic characteristics of malignant adnexal masses in pregnant patients

Size > 7 cm
Solid components or complex appearance
Excrescences or papillary structures
Internal septations (especially if they are thick or vascular)
Irregular borders
Increased vascularity
Low-resistance blood flow
Ascites
Persistence or progression on follow-up imaging

Efforts have been made to establish a sonographic scoring system in order to optimize the ultrasound examination as a diagnostic test for ovarian malignancies, but none of them have demonstrated sufficient accuracy to become the standard approach. In general, sonographic characteristics have a strong negative predictive value, but often suboptimal positive predictive value. In other words, sonographic evaluation suggestive of benign adnexal masses by highly trained sonologist can be of considerable use in reassuring pregnant women that her risk of malignancy is low and that the expectant management is appropriate [8].

Anatomopathological Diagnosis

In any case, without the intention of discrediting the role of an ultrasound, definitive diagnosis can only be made through microscope analysis performed by an experienced pathologist. Pregnancy-related changes in the histologic appearance of tumors of low malignant potential such as nuclear enlargement, anisocytosis and multifocal microinvasion can result in atypical characteristics suggestive of invasive cancer [9]. It is very important that the pathologist is informed of the ongoing pregnancy.

Focusing on the tumor line, solid ovarian tumors can be divided in primary ovarian malignancies or, more rarely, metastatic cancer. Epithelial ovarian tumors are comprised of approximately one-half of all ovarian malignancies in pregnant patients, germ cell ovarian malignancies make up approximately one-third, and stromal tumors and a variety of other tumor types account for the remainder [2].

- Epithelial ovarian tumors: Approximately 50% are of low malignant potential (formerly called "borderline") and the other 50% are invasive.
- Germ cell tumors: Approximately three-fourths of malignant ovarian germ cell tumors in pregnancy are dysgerminomas. Endodermal sinus tumors, immature teratomas, and mixed germ cell tumors comprise the remainder [10]. Most germ cell tumors are grossly limited to one adnexa, but lymphatic spread to pelvic or para-aortic nodes occurs, most commonly in dysgerminoma. Dysgerminomas are bilateral in 10-15% of cases; other germ cell tumors are almost always unilateral.
- Sex cord-stromal tumors: Approximately half of all pregnancy-associated stromal tumors are granulosa cell tumors, one-third are Sertoli-Leydig cell tumors, and the remainder are unclassified stromal tumors [11]. Most of these tumors are limited to one ovary at the time of diagnosis. Prior to the routine use of prenatal ultrasound,

approximately 20% of these lesions presented with intraperitoneal hemorrhage and/or hemorrhagic shock, but this has become less common with an earlier diagnosis. Between 10-15% of stromal tumors secrete androgens and produce virilization. Although estrogen secretion also occurs, symptoms of a hyperestrogenic state are masked by the already high estrogen concentration associated with pregnancy. Pregnancy-related histologic changes in these tumors include a disorderly arrangement of cells, edema and unusually large number of lutein or Leydig cells.

- Metastatic tumors: Their most common etiology is the gastrointestinal tract, such as the colon or Krükenberg tumors. Further evaluation of the GI tract is recommended if metastatic disease is suspected.

Patient Evaluation for Treatment

Patient Selection for Surgery

Adnexal masses that do not have concerning features can be managed expectantly and often resolve during pregnancy, avoiding unnecessary surgery. For any ovarian mass, if the diagnosis is uncertain, further evaluation is required. The general consensus regarding management of adnexal masses in pregnancy is to surgically resect asymptomatic masses that are present after the first trimester, especially if they have developed suspicious features (solid, contain solid and cystic areas, papillary areas, or septum). These findings increase the likelihood of malignancy, and it is desirable to diagnose malignancy, if present, at an early stage. In addition, the resection of large adnexal masses (>10 cm) reduces the risk of complications such as adnexal torsion, rupture, or obstruction of labor. Asymptomatic masses detected in the second trimester can be dealt with in a similar manner. Asymptomatic masses detected in the third trimester with no features of malignancy are best left undisturbed until its evaluation during caesarean or six weeks postpartum [12].

Timing

In pregnancy, besides an optimal surgical outcome, the main objectives to consider are also the maternal and fetal safety [13]. Surgery can be performed throughout pregnancy, if specific measures are taken. However, the optimal time for semi-elective surgery during pregnancy is after the first trimester for a number of reasons:

1. The most likely is that functional cysts would have disappeared by this time.
2. Organogenesis is mainly completed, so it would reduce the risk of teratogenesis.
3. The placenta has replaced the corpus luteum in his hormonal function, so reduction in progesterone secretion from oophorectomy or cystectomy does not result in loss of the pregnancy if not replaced.
4. Spontaneous miscarriages are likely to have already happened and will not be incorrectly attributed to the surgery.

Emergency surgery during pregnancy for management of a twisted or ruptured adnexal mass is uncommon and can lead to preterm delivery. That is the reason why, if intervention is needed before fetal pulmonary maturity, steroid treatment should be considered.

Preoperative Assessment

Secondary Imaging

In most cases, an ultrasound provides enough data to guide a decision for an exploratory surgery against an expectant management with ultrasound checks, and occasionally, other radiologic assessments.

Magnetic Resonance Image (MRI) has excellent resolution for soft tissue pathology and does not produce ionizing radiation, being safe for both mother and fetus. Consequently, a MRI is particularly useful in typifying leiomyomas, endometriomas, and ovarian edema and differentiating these from ovarian cancer [14]. Although, commonly gadolinium-based contrast should be avoided in pregnancy as fetal safety is yet unclear.

Computed tomography (CT) has to be avoided in these patients if other techniques can provide the desired data. A single pelvis CT produces 0.035 Gy of ionizing radiation dose for the fetus. However, an increased risk of abortion, congenital anomalies, growth restriction, or perinatal mortality have not been observed with less than 0.05 Gy of fetal radiation, though there are concerns considering a potential risk of developing childhood cancer. Furthermore, the use of iodinated contrast could cause fetal thyroid suppression and should be avoided.

Tumor Markers in Ovarian Malignancy

As it has already been explained, it is not suggested during pregnancy to draw serum tumor markers routinely preoperatively as several of them are difficult to interpret during pregnancy because oncofetal antigens are involved in the fetal development. The levels are usually high during pregnancy and vary with gestational age, or they can be elevated due to abnormal placentation or fetal abnormalities (for example, preeclampsia, Down syndrome) [6]. Contrarywise, HE4 serum marker is unaffected, and therefore may be helpful in the assessment of pelvic masses during pregnancy [15].

Surgery

Previously, pregnancy was thought to be a contraindication for laparoscopy of benign adnexal masses, although currently there are numerous publications showing acceptable maternal and fetal outcomes. In a meta-analysis with a total of 240 patients evaluating laparoscopic versus open surgery for management of adnexal masses in the second trimester, it was concluded that laparoscopy was associated with better surgical outcomes but longer operative times [16].

A laparoscopic approach is recommended to be scheduled between 16 and 20 weeks, to optimize the visualization of the mass and to decrease the ratio of preterm labor. The location of the first trocar should be at least 3-4 cm above the uterine fundus. Experts recommended a maximal laparoscopic procedure time of 90-120 minutes, a pneumoperitoneum with a maximal intra-abdominal pressure of 10-13 mmHg, Hasson technique and an experienced surgeon. It has to be taken into account that laparoscopic surgery can cause hypercapnia, perforation of the uterus, and reduced blood flow due to increased abdominal pressure [17]. Careful preparation and adequate monitoring of the maternal condition is mandatory since cardiotocography monitoring during surgery is impossible. Postoperative Kleihauer test should be performed. Routinely, Rh negative patients must receive 300 μg of Rh immune globulin (RhIg). Patients with a positive Kleihauer test should receive more RhIg, with an additional 300 μg for every 15 ml of fetal red blood cells in maternal blood [18].

The most common findings at surgery are persistent functional cysts, benign dermoid cysts, and serous/mucinous cystadenomas. If the preoperative imaging and intraoperative gross findings are consistent with a benign diagnosis, it is reasonable to attempt only a cystectomy.

If the mass has features suggesting malignancy, then ipsilateral salpingo-oophorectomy is suitable. If it is possible, the mass should be sent to the pathologist, and if confirmed to be of a malignant nature, the surgeon should be prepared to complete an adequate surgical staging procedure. Obviously, a hysterectomy is not performed if preservation of the pregnancy is desired, and it is necessary to weigh the pros and cons of staging versus potential risks. In certain malignant germ cell tumors of the ovary (for example endodermal sinus tumors), lymph node dissection may be omitted, as the patient will require chemotherapy based on histopathology alone [19].

If a malignant mass is suspected from the start, a laparotomy should be performed, with a midline laparotomy being optimal for correct exposure [13]. However, minimal uterine manipulations should be performed as significant more preterm contractions are evident in these patients than women undergoing laparoscopy.

Staging procedures during pregnancy may include infracolic omentectomy, peritoneal washings, appendectomy, pelvic-peritoneal biopsies, and lymph nodes dissection. Even contralateral ovarian biopsy can be performed if the ovary appears to be affected, but routine biopsy of a normal-appearing contralateral ovary is unnecessary. A general recommendation is that, if the pelvic peritoneum cannot be properly examined, restaging surgery should be planned postpartum. In patients who are motivated for pregnancy preservation, an adnexectomy should be performed, followed by platinum-based chemotherapy. In these cases, cytoreductive surgery commonly is planned after delivery, if possible, as surgery to define residual disease cannot be carried out during pregnancy [17].

Satisfactory surgical staging is really important for Stage I cancers, as many are satisfactorily treated with surgery alone. Surgical staging is less critical in advanced disease (for example, Stage IIIB/C disease), as these tumors will require chemotherapy.

If a metastatic ovarian cancer is discovered, cytoreduction should be attempted, personalizing each case. It is unusual that the removal of the gravid uterus is necessary for optimal cytoreductive surgery at the first surgery, as it is possible to return for secondary cytoreduction following chemotherapy and after pregnancy. This surgery can be performed following vaginal delivery or in conjunction with cesarean delivery [20]. This strategy is not thought to negatively influence survival rates, it has a poor outcome for advanced stage disease. Despite the importance of initial surgical debulking, it should be noted the sensitivity to platinum-based chemotherapy, with approximately 70% responding, even if they have residual disease remaining after cytoreductive surgery [21].

Any adnexal mass that appears suspicious for malignancy incidentally detected at a C section should be completely removed and sent for intraoperative analysis. In these cases, if the analysis indicates malignancy, the patient habitually will not have a suitable incision for surgical staging. Salpingo-oophorectomy must be performed and postpartum the patient should be referred to a gynecologist oncologist for advice and full surgical staging if necessary within 1-2 weeks [17].

Chemotherapy

Chemotherapy during pregnancy arise concerns as it kills rapidly proliferating cells, and the fetus is a rapidly proliferating cell mass. All chemotherapy agents used in the treatment of ovarian cancers are category D of the FDA. However, the decision of chemotherapy should consider the individual circumstances and preferences of the mother, highlighting the role of patient autonomy and the concept of beneficence and nonmaleficence for both the mother and fetus.

Although previous data suggested that the administration of chemotherapy increased malformations, most data currently suggest this is not the case. Nowadays, it is observed that the effects depend on when treatment is administered:

- During the first four weeks of gestation, fetal exposure to cytotoxic agents results in a "all or none" phenomena [22].
- The administration of cytotoxic drugs, particularly antimetabolites and alkylating agents, during the period of organogenesis (weeks 5 to 10 of gestation) carries an increased risk of malformations. The majority of stillborn infants and infants with congenital anomalies occur when it was administered during the first trimester [23].
- When chemotherapy is delivered to the mother during the second and third trimesters of pregnancy, the risk of fetal malformation is lower. Administration of chemotherapy within three weeks of anticipated delivery or beyond 35 weeks of gestation may induce neonatal myelosuppression producing low bone marrow reserves. Additionally, neonatal toxicity may be higher if chemotherapy is administered peripartum because hepatic and renal drug clearance is lower in the neonate [24].

Though we must consider all the above general premises, each histologic type requires specific medical treatment. Specifically for epithelial ovarian cancer, the use of a platinum drug plus taxane is recommended as this results in the best survival outcomes. During pregnancy, carboplatin is preferred as is better tolerated and reduces the risk of renal and neurotoxicity. Paclitaxel is also preferred as it is less myelotoxic than other taxanes. Targeted therapy and angiogenesis inhibitors have demonstrated potential embryotoxicity, intrauterine growth restriction, skeletal malformation and a risk of adverse fetal outcomes in animal models [17, 25]. Therefore, these latter agents should not be used during pregnancy.

Regarding germ cell tumors, chemotherapy is recommended in those with a complete resected germ cell tumor except those with Stage IA dysgerminoma or Stage I grade one immature teratoma. A consensus report proposed paclitaxel-carboplatin or cisplatin-vinblastine-bleomycin as alternatives to BEP (bleomycin, etoposide and platinum) in pregnancy [26].

According to sex cord-stromal tumors, most of them are limited to one ovary and have low malignant potential. It is suggested that oophorectomy alone could be enough. Most of the times, the decision for chemotherapy, if necessary, is postponed after delivery [27].

Prognosis: Obstetrical Outcomes after Ovarian Cancer in Pregnancy

Pregnancies complicated by maternal cancer are considered as high-risk pregnancies and should be followed in a multidisciplinary high-risk obstetric unit. Recently, a systematic review of the literature has been performed on the feto-maternal outcome of pregnancy complicated by ovarian epithelial, sex-cord stromal and malignant germ cell tumors [28].

Approximately half of ovarian cancers are detected in the first trimester, pushing the obstetrician and the patient to make decisions regarding the continuation of the pregnancy and the treatment that must be followed. Comparing the obstetrical outcome of patients diagnosed with cancer in pregnancy to the outcome of normal pregnancies, three complications occur more commonly: prematurity, fetal growth restriction and fetal loss.

In reference to fetal loss, elective abortion is the most common reason for non-viable pregnancies. However, pregnancy preservation has been increasingly accepted resulting in overall favorable outcomes for both mother and fetus. In relation to maternal survival, there is no evidence of a worse prognosis of ovarian cancer during pregnancy compared with nonpregnant patients matched for histology, stage, and grade [29]. Early-stage disease represents approximately 75% of invasive ovarian malignancies in pregnant patients. Therefore, the five-year survival rate is between 72% and 90%. Nevertheless, the presence of ascites implies advanced disease and poor prognosis. An early termination of pregnancy during the first trimester does not improve the outcome of ovarian cancer, and it should be individualized and made by a fully informed patient. Some factors that should be considered in these patients:

- If she is willing to assume a potential risk of fetal toxicity or adverse consequences from the treatment.
- The prognosis and ability to care for the newborn.
- The effect of treatment on future fertility.

To sum up, pregnancy itself does not appear to alter the survival outcomes for patients with ovarian cancer while treatment delay based on the presence of a pregnancy could negatively impact a patient’s outcome.

As with any pregnancy complicated by malignancy, the timing of delivery must be balanced to account for both fetal maturity and maternal well-being. Although the rate of preterm delivery is approximately 5% in the general population, almost half of pregnancies that coincide with a malignancy will deliver preterm. It is particularly common in pregnancies undergoing chemotherapy. However, the rate of preterm delivery due to spontaneous preterm labor however was far less than that of iatrogenic preterm delivery (12% versus □50%, respectively). This is particularly important, as the majority of neonatal intensive care unit admissions in pregnancy associated with cancer are due to prematurity. As evidence is accumulating that preterm and even early-term births are associated with increased neonatal morbidity and mortality, it is preferable to initiate treatment during gestation and delaying delivery until full-term instead of scheduling early delivery for the purpose of avoiding fetal chemotherapy exposure [30].

Initiating chemotherapy while the pregnancy is ongoing is one possible strategy to improve both maternal outcomes and delay delivery, however, as it has already been explained that chemotherapy carries risks for the fetus. Restriction of intrauterine growth is one of the main concerns associated with chemotherapy administration in the second and third trimesters. In the mentioned review, the small for gestational age (SGA) rate in our study was 26%, which is significantly higher than the rate of 4-8% seen in the general population. These differences are attributed to the chemotherapy cytotoxic effect as the rate of SGA in pregnancies complicated by malignancy that do not receive treatment in-utero is similar to that seen in the general population. Apart from the prevention of prematurity, in patients receiving chemotherapy in pregnancy, a 3-week interval between the last cycle of chemotherapy and delivery should be maintained in order to avoid problems associated with hematopoietic suppression (bleeding, infection, anaemia) in the patient and neonate, and to avoid drug accumulation in the fetus. There is an additional concern regarding the impact of chemotherapy on the developing fetal brain however data on neuro-behavioral outcomes is too sparse to allow for definitive associations at this time.

Conclusion

Persistent adnexal masses diagnosed during pregnancy are malignant in about 5%. Surgery should be considered in every tumor with a diameter > 5 cm, persisting until the 16th week with sonographic signs of possible malingnancy. In some situations, MRI scans can provide additional information. Optimal timing for planned surgery is the second trimester. If ovarian cancer is diagnosed, it is mostly at an early stage. As in non-pregnant women, optimal outcome depends on early diagnosis, resection of unbroken ovarian lesion, adequate staging and resection of any visible mass in cases of advanced disease. In any case, information of ovarian cancer management in treatment is limited and decisions must be tailored to each patient.

References

[1] Pavlidis N. A. Coexistence of pregnancy and malignancy. *Oncologist.* 2002;7(4):279–87.

[2] Webb K. E., Sakhel K., Chauhan S. P., Abuhamad A. Z. Adnexal mass during pregnancy: a review. *Am J Perinatol.* 2015 Sep;32(11):1010–6.

[3] Shim M. H., Mok C. W., Chang K. H. J., Sung J. H., Choi S. J., Oh S., Soo-young Oh, Cheong-Rae Roh, and Jong-Hwa Kim. Clinical characteristics and outcome of cancer diagnosed during pregnancy. *Obstet Gynecol Sci*. 2016;59(1):1.

[4] Palmer J., Vatish M., Tidy J. Epithelial ovarian cancer in pregnancy: a review of the literature. *BJOG.* 2009 Mar;116(4):480–91.

[5] Yen C. F., Lin S. L., Murk W., Wang C. J., Lee C. L., Soong Y. K., Aydin Arici. Risk analysis of torsion and malignancy for adnexal masses during pregnancy. *Fertil Steril* [Internet]. 2009;91(5):1895–902. Available from: http://dx.doi.org/10.1016/j.fertnstert.2008.02.014.

[6] Sarandakou A., Protonotariou E., Rizos D. Tumor markers in biological fluids associated with pregnancy. *Crit Rev Clin Lab Sci.* 2007;44(2):151–78.

[7] Giuntoli R. L. 2nd, Vang R. S., Bristow R. E. Evaluation and management of adnexal masses during pregnancy. *Clin Obstet Gynecol.* 2006 Sep;49(3):492–505.

[8] Bromley B., Benacerraf B. Adnexal masses during pregnancy: accuracy of sonographic diagnosis and outcome. *J ultrasound Med Off J Am Inst Ultrasound Med.* 1997 Jul;16(7):444–7.

[9] Mooney J., Silva E., Tornos C., Gershenson D. Unusual features of serous neoplasms of low malignant potential during pregnancy. *Gynecol Oncol.* 1997 Apr;65(1):30–5.

[10] Bakri Y. N., Ezzat A., Akhtar, Dohami, Zahrani. Malignant germ cell tumors of the ovary. Pregnancy considerations. *Eur J Obstet Gynecol Reprod Biol.* 2000 May;90(1):87–91.

[11] Young R. H., Dudley A. G., Scully R. E. Granulosa cell, Sertoli-Leydig cell, and unclassified sex cord-stromal tumors associated with pregnancy: a clinicopathological analysis of thirty-six cases. *Gynecol Oncol.* 1984 Jun;18(2):181–205.

[12] Aggarwal P., Kehoe S. Ovarian tumours in pregnancy: a literature review. *Eur J Obstet Gynecol Reprod Biol.* 2011 Apr;155(2):119–24.

[13] Fruscio R., de Haan J., Van Calsteren K., Verheecke M., Mhallem M., Amant F. Ovarian cancer in pregnancy. *Best Pract Res Clin Obstet Gynaecol.* 2017 May;41:108–17.

[14] Telischak N. A., Yeh B. M., Joe B. N., Westphalen A. C., Poder L., Coakley F. V. MRI of adnexal masses in pregnancy. *Am J Roentgenol.* 2008;191(2):364–70.

[15] Gucer F., Kiran G., Canaz E., Kilinc M., Ekerbicer H. C., Avci F., H. Kiran, A. Coskun, D. C. Arikan. Serum human epididymis protein 4 can be a useful tumor marker in the differential diagnosis of adnexal masses during pregnancy: a pilot study. *Eur J Gynaecol Oncol.* 2015;36(4):406–9.

[16] Liu Y. X., Zhang Y., Huang J. F., Wang L. Meta-analysis comparing the safety of laparoscopic and open surgical approaches for suspected adnexal mass during the second trimester. *Int J Gynaecol Obstet Off organ Int Fed Gynaecol Obstet.* 2017 Mar;136(3):272–9.

[17] Amant F., Berveiller P., Boere I. A., Cardonick E., Fruscio R., Fumagalli M., M. J. Halaska, A. Hasenburg, A. L. V. Johansson, M. Lambertini, C. A. R. Lok, C. Maggen, P. Morice, F Peccatori, P. Poortmans, K. Van Calsteren, T. Vandenbroucke, M. van Gerwen, M. van den Heuvel-Eibrink, F. Zagouri, I. Zapardiel. Gynecologic cancers in pregnancy: guidelines based on a third international consensus meeting. *Ann Oncol Off J Eur Soc Med Oncol.* 2019 Oct;30(10):1601–12.

[18] Katiyar R., Kriplani A., Agarwal N., Bhatla N., Kabra M. Detection of fetomaternal hemorrhage following chorionic villus sampling by Kleihauer Betke test and rise in maternal serum alpha feto protein. *Prenat Diagn.* 2007 Feb;27(2):139–42.

[19] Perry M. F., Jackson A. L., Herzog T. J., Billingsley C. C. Early diagnosis and treatment challenges of endodermal sinus tumors: A case report. Vol. 27, *Case reports in women's health. 2020*. p. e00198.

[20] Méndez L. E., Mueller A., Salom E., González-Quintero V. H. Paclitaxel and carboplatin chemotherapy administered during pregnancy for advanced epithelial ovarian cancer. *Obstet Gynecol.* 2003 Nov;102(5 Pt 2):1200–2.

[21] Runowicz C. D., Brewer M. Adnexal mass in pregnancy. *UpToDate.* 2021.

[22] Leslie K. K., Koil C., Rayburn W. F. Chemotherapeutic drugs in pregnancy. *Obstet Gynecol Clin North Am.* 2005 Dec;32(4):627–40.

[23] Selig B. P., Furr J. R., Huey R. W., Moran C., Alluri V. N., Medders G. R., Christina D. Mumm, H. Gene Hallford, John J. Mulvihill. Cancer chemotherapeutic agents as human teratogens. *Birth Defects Res A Clin Mol Teratol.* 2012 Aug;94(8):626–50.

[24] Boulay R., Podczaski E. Ovarian cancer complicating pregnancy. *Obstet Gynecol Clin North Am.* 1998 Jun;25(2):385–99.

[25] Zagouri F., Sergentanis T. N., Chrysikos D., Filipits M., Bartsch R. Taxanes for ovarian cancer during pregnancy: a systematic review. *Oncology.* 2012;83(4):234–8.

[26] Amant F., Halaska M. J., Fumagalli M., Dahl Steffensen K., Lok C., Van Calsteren K., Sileny N. Han, Olivier Mir, Robert Fruscio, Cathérine Uzan, Cynthia Maxwell, Jana Dekrem, Goedele Strauven, Mina Mhallem Gziri, Vesna Kesic, Paul Berveiller, Frank van den Heuvel, Petronella B. Ottevanger, Ignace Vergote, Michael Lishner, Philippe Morice, Irena Nulman, ESGO task force 'Cancer in Pregnancy.' Gynecologic cancers in pregnancy: guidelines of a second international consensus meeting. *Int J Gynecol Cancer.* 2014;24(3):394–403.

[27] Carolyn D. Runowicz M. B. Chemotherapy of ovarian cancer. *UpToDate.* 2021.

[28] Blake E. A., Kodama M., Yunokawa M., Ross M. S., Ueda Y., Grubbs B. H., Koji Matsuo. Feto-maternal outcomes of pregnancy complicated by epithelial ovarian cancer: A systematic review of literature. *Eur J Obstet Gynecol Reprod Biol* [Internet]. 2015;186(2015):97–105. Available from: http://dx.doi.org/10.1016/j.ejogrb.2015.01.010.
[29] Grimm D., Woelber L., Trillsch F., Keller-v Amsberg G., Mahner S. Clinical management of epithelial ovarian cancer during pregnancy. *Eur J Cancer*. 2014 Mar;50(5):963–71.
[30] Reddy U. M., Ko C. W., Raju T. N. K., Willinger M. Delivery indications at late-preterm gestations and infant mortality rates in the United States. *Pediatrics*. 2009 Jul;124(1):234–40.

Index

N

O

P

R

S

Editors' Contact Information

Christos Iavazzo
Metaxa Memorial Cancer Hospital
Piraeus, Greece
Email: christosiavazzo@hotmail.com.

Alexandros Fotiou
Metaxa Memorial Cancer Hospital
Alexandrosfotiou92@gmail.com.

John Spiliotis
Department of Surgical Oncology and HIPEC,
Athens Medical Centre, Athens, Greece
Department of Surgical Oncology and HIPEC,
European Interbalkan Medical Centre, Thessaloniki, Greece
Email: jspil@hotmail.gr.